ATLAS OF
PEDIATRIC
ORTHOPEDIC
SURGERY

ATLAS OF
PEDIATRIC
ORTHOPEDIC
SURGERY

Volume I

MIHRAN O. TACHDJIAN, M.D.
Professor of Orthopedic Surgery
Northwestern University Medical School
Attending Orthopedic Surgeon
The Children's Memorial Hospital
Chicago, Illinois

W.B. SAUNDERS COMPANY
A Division of Harcourt Brace & Company
Philadelphia   London   Montreal   Toronto   Sydney   Tokyo

W.B. SAUNDERS COMPANY
A Division of
Harcourt Brace & Company

The Curtis Center
Independence Square West
Philadelphia, Pennsylvania 19106

Library of Congress Cataloging-in-Publication Data

Tachdjian, Mihran O.
Atlas of pediatric orthopedic surgery/Mihran O. Tachdjian.—1st ed.

p. cm.

ISBN 0–7216–3733–7

1. Pediatric orthopedics—Atlases.   I. Title.
[DNLM: 1. Orthopedics—in infancy & childhood—atlases.
WS 17 T117a 1994]

RD732.3.C48T328 1994

617.3'0083—dc20

DNLM/DLC   93–31640

ATLAS OF PEDIATRIC ORTHOPEDIC SURGERY

Volume One   ISBN 0–7216–5448–7
Volume Two   ISBN 0–7216–5449–5
Two Volume Set   ISBN 0–7216–3733–7

Last digit is the print number: 9   8   7   6   5   4   3   2   1

Dedicated to Dr. Paul P. Griffin

. . . my close friend,
who has devoted his life to teaching
and the care of the disabled child
and who is a master of the art of
the practice of pediatric orthopedic surgery.

Preface

This atlas describes and illustrates the standard and attested operative procedures performed in pediatric orthopedics. Of the surgical techniques described, 124 are taken from the second edition of *Pediatric Orthopedics;* these have been revised. One hundred thirty-two new surgical procedures have been added.

The resident and fellow in training will learn details of surgical technique by first observing, next assisting, and then operating under the supervision of an experienced surgeon and teacher. This atlas is intended to serve as a guide; modifications can be made, depending on the individual deformity, findings at surgery, and complexity of the problem. Each operative case is different. One should follow the principles that are based on biologic facts and past experience of successful surgery. It is vital to pay meticulous attention to detail—preoperatively, at surgery, and postoperatively.

On the page opposite each plate, indications, requisites, and requirements for blood for transfusion, image intensifier radiographic control, or special instrumentation are listed for each procedure. Preoperative planning is crucial!

In the beginning of the atlas I have given an overview of the total care of the child and some practical points of basic surgical technique. The practice of orthopedic surgery is an art. The operative procedure is only a portion of what is involved in the management of the whole child.

Preparation of this atlas has been a challenging task. I have tried to describe and illustrate my preferred methods of operative procedures learned from personal experience for the past four decades. I hope that the reader will find it useful as a guide to the surgical care of children with neuromusculoskeletal disorders.

MIHRAN O. TACHDJIAN

Acknowledgments

I wish to thank the three new illustrators of this atlas, Ms. Marguerite Aitken, Ms. Cynthia Eller, and Ms. Janice Ruvido, with whom I have greatly enjoyed working. I am also greatly indebted to the late Mr. Ernie Beck, whose superb artistry has been a landmark for medical illustrators.

I also thank the staff at W. B. Saunders for their efforts.

Special thanks to Dr. Robert Winter for his assistance in preparing the chapter on the spine.

Finally, I would like to express my deep gratitude to Mrs. Lynn Ridings, without whose editorial assistance and collaboration this difficult task would not have come to fruition.

Principles of the Practice of Pediatric Orthopedic Surgery

The practice of surgery is an art as well as a science. The following practical points and general principles of surgery are presented for the sake of thoroughness in provision of total care to the child.

INDICATIONS AND OBJECTIVES OF SURGERY

Objectives and indications for surgery should be clearly defined, discussed with the parents and patient, and recorded. Explain clearly what you propose to do, the reasons for performing the operation, and the results to be expected. Be realistic in your goals. Alternate methods of management should be discussed and reasons given why you propose to perform the operative procedure for that particular problem. Often the parents and patient want to know the natural history of the deformity if left untreated. Is open surgery absolutely necessary? Can the deformity be corrected by intensive physical therapy, casts, or orthotic devices? Prolonged immobilization in cast causes muscle atrophy and joint contracture, whereas early open surgery will rapidly correct deformity and restore function. The effectiveness and safety of surgery and its advantages and disadvantages should be compared with that of nonoperative methods of management. The philosophy and practice among most physicians is that nonsurgical methods of treatment should always be tried initially and only after they fail should operative procedures be employed. In certain deformities, however, such as rigid intrinsic talipes equinovarus, surgery is more conservative and simpler than nonoperative methods of management.

Parents often like to know the worst outcome that can occur following surgery. *Non nocere*—Do no harm!—is one of the basic requisites of surgery. The problems, complications, and dangers of the operation should be clearly explained to the parents and to the adolescent patient.

TIMING OF THE OPERATION

Timing is important. What is the best age? Should a clubfoot be corrected surgically at three months, six months, or one year of age? Should a congenital high scapula be transferred distally at one year or at three years of age? What are the risks of early surgery versus the drawbacks of postponing it to a later date? For example, a septic hip should be drained immediately because it is an emergency procedure; a heel cord lengthening to correct equinus deformity in spastic cerebral palsy should be delayed until the child is three to four years of age, when adequate postoperative care can be provided.

SEQUENCE OF OPERATIVE PROCEDURES

When involvement is bilateral, should you operate on both sides during the same procedure or should you stage them? What should be the interval between the two operations? A child may need two, three, or more surgical procedures for treatment of a complex problem. For example, with a high dislocation of a hip (antenatal or teratologic), open reduction with femoral shortening and possibly innominate osteotomy are needed; should you operate on both hips on the same day or stagger them two or three weeks apart? Most surgeons prefer to stage such extensive operative procedures, whereas a patient with spastic cerebral palsy can readily tolerate multilevel surgery, such as bilateral hip adductor myotomy, iliopsoas tenotomy and hamstring and heel cord lengthening. Some surgeons prefer to operate on both feet for correction of talipes equinovarus at the same sitting; others prefer to stage the procedures because of the potential for excessive blood loss and the necessity for blood transfusion with its inherent risks.

BLOOD LOSS

Blood loss may be significant during a major orthopedic operation. An estimate of the probable amount of blood loss should be forecast and arrangements made for obtaining adequate blood and cross-matching. In the modern era of autoimmune deficiency (human immunodeficiency virus, or HIV) syndrome and hepatitis B, the family should be given the option to donate blood by a designated donor or, in the older patient, to have autologous blood available. As a general policy, a patient who is donating autologous blood should weigh at least 110 pounds and be 17 years of age. He may be younger with parental consent. A red blood cell saver may be used, especially in spine surgery. Arrangements should be made in advance for the blood saver and its possible problems, and complications should be discussed with the family and patient. Certain religious groups, such as Jehovah's Witnesses, will refuse blood transfusion. This can create special problems, which should be handled individually.

PREOPERATIVE LABORATORY STUDIES

Preoperative studies should consist of a complete blood count and urinalysis.

Sickle Cell Disease

For African American children, a sickle cell preparation should be arranged when scheduling the operation. Order it far ahead of the day of surgery. If findings are positive, a hemoglobin electrophoresis should be done to determine the exact hemoglobinopathy. It behooves the surgeon to remember that a sickle cell test may be negative in an infant under four months of age but can subsequently change to positive; therefore, a negative sickle cell preparation in a young infant needs to be performed again when he or she is older.

Pregnancy Test

A pregnancy test in teenagers who have reached menarche is appropriate, provided that first a recent menstrual history is taken and the patient and parents are informed. A routine chest radiogram should not be made unless there is cardiopulmonary pathology. HIV and hepatitis B screenings are still a controversial issue.

Contagious Diseases

It is vital to inquire whether the child has been recently exposed to a contagious disease, such as chickenpox or measles. A child would be extremely uncomfortable in a cast with the skin lesions caused by these diseases.

Allergies and Medications

The surgeon should know whether the child has any allergies, whether he or she has been or is presently taking medication, and whether there have been any adverse reactions to the drugs. Most importantly, ask whether there has been any unusual bruising or bleeding; it is best to detect a bleeding disorder *before* surgery. Ask about previous surgical procedures and how they were tolerated. A family history of difficulty with surgery or anesthesia should be investigated.

Latex gloves and other products, such as Penrose drains, should not be used for patients with myelomeningocele during surgery because of the great probability of allergy and anaphylactic shock. It is best to use non-latex gloves, such as those made of neoprene. Other patients who may have similar allergies to latex products include those who have experienced multiple catheterizations and latex exposure.

Chronic Illness

Chronically ill patients who have been taking long-term medication require special preoperative assessment and laboratory studies. For patients with cerebral palsy and other central nervous system disorders who are taking seizure medications, a recent neurologic assessment and blood level determinations of anticonvulsant medications are indicated. After neurologic clearance—and if the blood levels of the medications are within normal, not toxic ranges—the child should take seizure medication on the morning of surgery with a small sip of water. It is my policy that children who are receiving anti-seizure medication see the anesthesiologist preoperatively because many of these medications can affect cardiopulmonary, liver, and kidney function and blood coagulation. The anesthesiologist should be familiar with the patient's history long before the day of surgery. Children with shunts should be provided with appropriate neurosurgical consultation.

Asthma

Asthmatic children require special preoperative assessment by an allergist to determine whether their medications are adequate. In the past, it was a common practice to start an aminophylline infusion; however, this rarely is needed now because beta$_2$ agonists, like nebulized albuterol, are very effective and less cardiotoxic. Nebulized albuterol is often provided just before surgery.

Occasionally, children with asthma may require prednisone treatment several days prior to surgery. Patients who have received steroid therapy treatment for rheumatoid arthritis, asthma, or organ transplantation during the past year require administration of steroids perioperatively.

Diabetes

The diabetic patient who is insulin-dependent will require glucose infusion and insulin injection in divided doses administered the day before surgery, during surgery, and postoperatively. The primary physician in charge of medication management should be the endocrinologist or pediatrician, who, in conjunction with the anesthesiologist, will plan the perioperative management.

Patients who have received *salicylates* or *nonsteroidal anti-inflammatory agents,* such as tolmetin sodium (tolectin), naprosyn, or ibuprofen, may experience bleeding problems on the operating table. It is best to stop such medications three to four weeks before surgery.

Prematurity

Premature infants up to six months of age are at high risk for apnea spells during recovery and postoperatively. They should be admitted and observed with an apnea monitor for at least 12 hours. Do not schedule the premature baby for outpatient surgery; however, a morning admission on the day of surgery can be arranged.

Upper Respiratory Disease

The most common problem associated with an anesthetic concerns patients with upper respiratory infection, including coughing, rhinorrhea, and pulmonary congestion. These children are at high risk for airway obstruction, laryngospasm, and a stormy anesthetic course. They should not be anesthetized until after the symptoms have disappeared unless it is an emergency.

Malignant Hyperthermia

Because malignant hyperthermia is a very serious complication of some anesthetics, it is crucial to interrogate the family about any temperature control problems, any difficulties with previous operations or anesthesia, or symptoms compatible with the syndrome in the patient, the parents, and immediate family. The surgeon must remember that patients with malignant hyperthermia syndrome show a greater incidence of kyphoscoliosis, clubfoot, winged scapula, hyperlaxity of joints, and repeated dislocations than do healthy children. As a rule, I recommend that children with myopathies, arthrogryposis, and central core disease also be managed as if they are in the high-risk group.

Atlantoaxial Instability

Atlantoaxial instability can be a serious problem, such as in Down syndrome, skeletal dysplasias (such as Morquio's disease), and rheumatoid arthritis. It is vital to assess stability of the cervical spine by flexion-extension views and magnetic resonance imaging (MRI) studies.

Physical Health

When elective surgical procedures are to be performed, it is prudent to have the patient in the best physical condition possible. If in doubt, obtain preoperative pediatric and anesthesia consultations. The anesthesiologist should discuss risks of anesthesia with the family.

PREOPERATIVE ORTHOPEDIC CONSULTATION

When a surgical procedure is being discussed with the family and patient, the approximate site and length of incisions should be mentioned. Often an adolescent is more concerned with the cosmesis of the scar than the surgery itself. The possibility of a drain and the type and extent of cast immobilization—below-knee, above-knee, or hip spica—should be discussed: I also give my patients a choice of color of cast. Other details of interest are whether the child will be able to bear full weight or whether crutches with partial or non-weight bearing will be used. Instructing the child in how to walk with crutches before surgery is much simpler than teaching the patient who is in discomfort in the cast after surgery. The expected total length of time in the cast should be estimated and the physical therapy program after cast removal outlined. If internal fixation devices are to be used, explain when removal will be necessary, what is involved, whether a general or local anesthetic with sedation will be used, and whether or not another cast will be applied. Mention the possibility that you may not be able to remove the fixation device or that it may break.

When special physical or occupational therapy is required, especially after surgery for neuromuscular disorders such as cerebral palsy or myelomeningocele, it is best that the postoperative therapy program be outlined and discussed by the physical therapist and occupational therapist and the appropriate arrangements made. A patient-therapist and surgeon-therapist rapport should be established to ensure optimal results.

Discuss the length of the hospital stay, and indicate whether the parents can stay with the child. The child should be allowed to bring an object of comfort, such as a favorite teddy bear or blanket. Address the transport of the child from the hospital to the home and any special equipment required in the home, such as a sitting or reclining wheelchair or hospital bed with a trapeze, or whether the child will be in home traction. The discharge nurse from the hospital should be involved preoperatively to assist in solving difficult problems of home management.

Because the nursing staff interacts with the patients and families more than any other members of the health care team, they are in the best position to provide the physician with information regarding obvious or subtle changes in a patient's condition or response to treatment. It is therefore essential that the nurses and physicians maintain an environment that is conducive to collaboration in an effort to best meet the physical as well as psychosocial needs of the patients and their families.

PAIN CONTROL

A great concern for children and their families is postoperative pain. Assure these patients that they will be made as comfortable as possible but that a slight degree of discomfort is desirable to prevent total inactivity, atelectasis, and pulmonary complications. At present, patient-controlled analgesia in the older child and adolescent is used. The anesthesiologist may perform one caudal anesthetic injection at the end of surgery to provide significant analgesia for lower extremity procedures that lasts for several hours postoperatively. Epidural anesthesia has its drawbacks, especially because there is a potential for compartment syndrome following procedures such as osteotomy of the tibia. It is best that the anesthesiologist be involved in the discussion of postoperative pain control with the family, patient, and surgeon.

If possible, arrangements should be made for the parents to bring the child to the operating room and recovery area preoperatively so that the child is familiarized with the area.

PSYCHOLOGIC STATE OF THE PATIENT

The patient's psychologic state is not always easy to assess, but it is important, particularly when the child's cooperation is required after surgery. The adequacy of postoperative care often dictates the difference between success or failure of a surgical procedure, especially one affecting the muscular system.

HOME AND FAMILY SITUATION

The family should be well informed and prepared for provision of an intensive postoperative care and therapy training program. These questions should be addressed: Who will take care of the child after discharge? Are both parents working, or is there a single parent? How interested are they in the child?

OUTPATIENT PROCEDURES

Outpatient surgery has become very popular because of the demands of insurance companies to curtail health care costs. There are advantages and disadvantages. It minimizes the disturbances of life for the patient and family. However, there is increased risk of postoperative complications from early discharge. *The surgeon should demand and dictate what is best for the child.*

The prerequisites for outpatient surgery are as follows:

1. The child should be in good general health, with only a minimal possibility of surgical and anesthesia problems and complications arising.

2. The procedure should not be very painful; only minimal medication for pain control, such as simple acetaminophen (Tylenol) or Tylenol with codeine, is anticipated.

3. The patient should not be sent home with a drain.

Before discharge, it is vital that the patient be fully awake and responsive, is not vomiting, and can tolerate oral fluids. Neurovascular function should be normal. If in doubt, the cast must be bivalved. Clear instructions should be given, preferably in writing as to cast or wound care and when to return for follow-up. The patient and family should understand the potential complications that can develop and they should be reported.

PATIENT TRANSFER

During transfer of the patient from the waiting-holding area to the operating room, it is reassuring and comforting to the patient and the parents if the surgeon accompanies and assists in this move. The surgeon should again confirm with the parents and patient that the correct limb is being operated on. The surgeon should reiterate the expected length of time during which the patient will be in the operating room and that the parents will be able to speak with the surgeon after the procedure. A few words of assurance, such as, "I'll take good care of Billy—don't worry," will relax the nervous parents and patient.

THE OPERATING ROOM

When the child is wheeled to the operating room, there should be a professional demeanor, an atmosphere of tranquility, and a minimum level of noise. Demand that the assisting staff turn off loud music. Assist in transferring the patient to the operating table. Provide for the privacy of the patient by appropriate cover by sheets or clothing. If radiograms are to be made during surgery, be sure that the table is radiolucent. The radiopaque strips of the heating pad will obscure the operative site; pull them out of the field proximally—this is a problem, particularly with hip surgery.

Before anesthetizing the patient, be sure the image intensifier machine is functioning and a competent x-ray technician is available. When scheduling, specify image intensifier radiographic control. If only one or two machines are available, the orchestration of cases is important.

Do not anesthetize the child unless recent radiograms are on the x-ray viewing box and you personally verify and check the correct limb and site of surgery. Bring the pertinent office or outpatient preoperative notes to the operating room. It is the personal responsibility of the surgeon to see that the correct limb is operated on. Do not depend on the operating room schedule, the nursing staff, or resident staff.

After the proper level of anesthesia is achieved, if tourniquet ischemia is to be used, the surgeon should personally supervise or apply the tourniquet and the level of tourniquet pressure.

PATIENT POSITION

The surgeon directs the proper positioning of the patient on the operating table. Secure the proper posture by sandbags or adhesive strapping. Bony prominences are adequately padded to prevent pressure sores. Nerves, such as the ulnar nerve at the elbow or the common peroneal nerve at the fibular head-neck, must be relieved of all pressure. When the patient is placed on a fracture table, the greater sciatic notch and perineum should be well padded. Discuss any special positions, such as prone or lateral, with the anesthesiologist before the anesthetic is administered.

SPECIAL INSTRUMENTATION

When an operative procedure is expected to take more than two hours, insert a Foley catheter into the bladder for urine drainage. Catheterization is carried out under sterile conditions.

The surgeon should consult with the operating room nurse well in advance of the surgery time so that the proper instruments can be obtained and sterilized. This is particularly true when special instruments are required for a particular operation. Such planning ahead will prevent unnecessary delay during surgery.

THE INCISION

In planning the site and extent of the incision, the surgeon should obtain adequate exposure but should not ignore cosmesis. The appearance of the scar should be pleasing, not unsightly. Draw the proposed incision with a sterile pencil. As a rule, straight incisions look less conspicuous than S-shaped or curved ones. When making an ilioinguinal approach to the hip, use Salter's "bikini" incision, not that described for a Smith-Peterson approach. Also, a transverse adductor incision is preferable to that of a longitudinal one in adductor myotomy of the hip. When performing a procedure around the upper arm, employ an axillary medial incision if possible. For wound closure, use the subcuticular technique; an absorbable suture may be used in the fearful child. I prefer 00 subcuticular nylon; it is very easy to remove, causes little pain, and avoids problems of foreign body reaction, allergy, and rejection and discharge of absorbable suture material.

OPERATIVE TECHNIQUE

Gentle handling of tissues is vital. Rough and forceful retraction of skin and muscles causes tissue necrosis and increases the chance of infection. Atraumatic technique is the hallmark of a good surgeon. The growth plate and articular cartilage are sacred; they should not be injured.

Repeat irrigation of the wound during surgery removes all debris and dead tissue. Blood vessels should be clamped and coagulated before division; such a technique controls bleeding and conserves blood. Venous drainage of the limb should be preserved as much as possible. Do not divide sensory nerves. After completion of the operation prior to wound closure, the wound is thoroughly irrigated and Ace bandage compression is applied and the tourniquet released. The wound should be completely dry before closure. Insert closed suction drainage in all cases, particularly when bone work has been performed. Blood oozing from the divided surfaces of cancellous bone will cause hematoma and infection.

A fast surgeon who is fighting the clock is not necessarily technically superb. Manual dexterity and eye-hand coordination are important. Plan and think ahead. A surgeon and the assistants should know the steps of the procedure. The competent surgeon knows what to do and how to do it. The scrub nurse should anticipate the needs of the surgeon and should be prepared to hand over the next instrument before being asked for it. Such teamwork can decrease the actual operating time.

IMMOBILIZATION IN A CAST

Operations on bones and joints often necessitate immobilization in a cast. Children ordinarily do not respect Ace or other bandages; they take them off. Therefore, the surgeon may prefer to use a cast as a method of postoperative dressing and support. The trauma of repeated dressing care and bandage changes is more disturbing to a child than cast care. Frequently I recommend the use of a posterior cast mold and Ace bandage support if postoperative swelling is anticipated; this is particularly important when there is a possibility of compartment syndrome, such as following osteotomy of the tibia or both bones of the forearm. The splint is applied in the operating room, and before the child goes home, a plaster of Paris or plastic cast is applied. All bony prominences and nerves should be adequately padded, and the cast should be well molded.

The parents and patients are indoctrinated on cast care; written instructions are provided. I insist that parents sign a statement that written instructions on cast care and details of postoperative care, such as when to be seen again, have been provided. There should be no diversity of opinion between the surgeon, resident, nurse, or therapist. Instructions given should be uniform.

THE OPERATIVE RECORD

The operation should be dictated in detail. The operative record includes the following: (1) name of the patient, (2) medical record number, (3) name of attending physician, (4) name of assisting physician, (5) preoperative diagnosis, (6) postoperative diagnosis, (7) indications for surgery, (8) surgical procedures performed, (9) alternate methods of management, (10) possible problems and complications, (11) type of anesthesia, (12) position of the patient, (13) technique of preparing the operative site, (14) surgical exposure, (15) findings at surgery, (16) operative procedure, (17) total tourniquet time and pressure, (18) blood loss, (19) wound closure, (20) sponge count, (21) cast application and dressings, (22) return visit or readmission, and (23) weight-bearing status.

PHYSIOTHERAPY AND OCCUPATIONAL THERAPY

The therapist is a vital member of the team who provides care of the patient's neuromusculoskeletal system. It is beyond the scope of this volume to cover details of therapy. The therapist should be involved preoperatively and should develop a working relationship and communication between the child and parent. It is unfortunate that most orthopedic residents have a limited knowledge of the usefulness of physiotherapy and occupational therapy; such modalities of therapy in the child are different from those of the adult.

The surgeon and therapist should work together. For neuromuscular disorders and complex problems of the upper and lower limbs, I strongly recommend that the therapist assess the child preoperatively and be involved in the decision-making process. In certain cases, I invite the therapist to come to the operating room and observe surgery. Such a professional working relationship between the therapist and surgeon should improve the overall care of the child.

When making a request for physical or occupational therapy, include the following: diagnosis, aim of treatment, previous treatment (especially surgery), and special precautions. Attach a copy of the office notes and operative report for the therapist's information.

Always remember to show warmth, gentleness, and consideration of the child as a whole person. An orthopedic surgeon must remember that there is a fourth dimension to pediatric orthopedic surgery—growth. Treatment is not concluded until the child becomes an adult.

Contents

Volume II

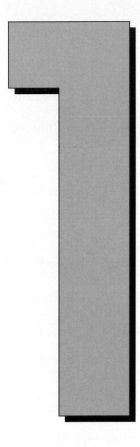

1

Neck-Shoulder

PLATE 1   Operative Treatment for Congenital Muscular Torticollis

Indications. Fixed contracture of sternocleidomastoid muscle not responding to conservative nonsurgical measures in a child one year of age or older.

Preoperative Assessment

1. Neurologic examination to rule out other causes of torticollis. Eye examination to detect visual disturbances.

2. Anteroposterior and lateral radiograms of the cervical spine. Rule out congenital deformities of the vertebrae, widening of the spinal canal.

Blood for Transfusion. Yes.

Presurgical Measures. Arrange preoperatively with orthotist for a torticollis brace.

Patient Position. The patient is placed in supine position, and the head and neck are prepared and draped so that they can be manipulated to check correction of the contractural deformity during the operation. Ensure that the opposite clavicle is draped free and that the sternal notch is readily palpable. With a sterile indelible pencil, mark the outline of the clavicles and sternal notch with the neck in some flexion. *Caution!* When the neck is hyperextended, the skin incision may be distal to the clavicle.

Operative Technique

A. A transverse incision 4 to 5 cm. long is made in line with the skin creases and centered over the lower part of the sternocleidomastoid muscle. It should be one fingerbreadth proximal to the clavicle. The skin incision should not be made inferior to the clavicle, as the resulting healed scar will spread and be cosmetically objectionable.

B. and **C.** Next, the subcutaneous tissue and superficial fascia are divided in line with the skin incision and the wound flaps are retracted by traction with skin hooks. Then, the platysma muscle is divided with electrocautery. Avoid injury to the anterior and external jugular veins, the carotid vessels, and other deep structures.

D. and **E.** By dull dissection, the clavicular and sternal parts of the distal attachments of the sternocleidomastoid muscle are exposed.

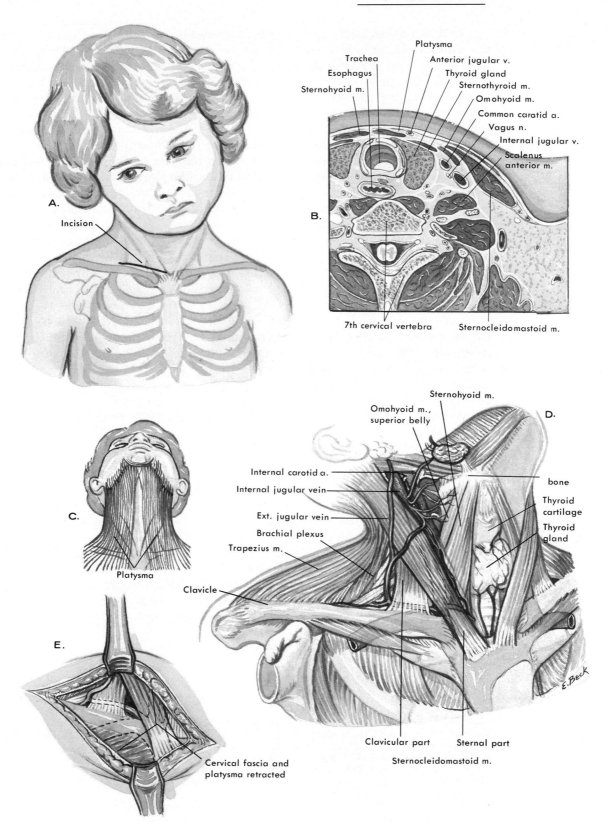

A.

Incision

B.

Trachea
Esophagus
Sternohyoid m.

Platysma
Anterior jugular v.
Thyroid gland
Sternothyroid m.
Omohyoid m.
Common caratid a.
Vagus n.
Internal jugular v.
Scalenus anterior m.

7th cervical vertebra

Sternocleidomastoid m.

C.

Platysma

E.

Cervical fascia and
platysma retracted

D.

Omohyoid m.,
superior belly

Sternohyoid m.

Internal carotid a.
Internal jugular vein
Ext. jugular vein
Brachial plexus
Trapezius m.
Clavicle

bone
Thyroid cartilage
Thyroid gland

Clavicular part
Sternal part
Sternocleidomastoid m.

E.Beck

Plate 1. A.–I., Operative treatment for congenital muscular torticollis.

F. A staphylorrhaphy probe is gently passed posterior to the clavicular part of the sternocleidomastoid muscle to protect the deep structures. Then a large hemostat is used to clamp the clavicular part of the attachment of the sternocleidomastoid muscle, and with electrocautery, 2 cm. of its distal part is cautiously excised. Next, the sternal part is released by clamping and division with electrocautery following the same technique as the clavicular part. The degree of correction obtained is checked by manipulating the head and neck—rotating the chin toward the affected side and flexing the head laterally so that the opposite ear touches the contralateral shoulder. Often one has to divide contracted bands of deep fascia. The shortened deep structures are explored digitally and sectioned under direct vision. After complete hemostasis is obtained, the wound is closed.

G. and H. If it is desirable to preserve the V contour of the neck, especially in girls, the clavicular attachment of the sternocleidomastoid muscle is divided transversely; however, the sternal head is lengthened by an oblique cut and the muscle ends are sutured. The technique that I prefer is a Z-lengthening of the tendinous segment of the sternal part. Elevate the muscle fibers proximally, and expose the tendinous segment, which is usually 3 cm. in length, and perform a Z-lengthening.

I. Sometimes, when the deformity is not severe, the sternocleidomastoid muscle can be released at its origin. The resultant scar will be hidden behind the ear. A small transverse incision is made immediately inferior to the mastoid process. The subcutaneous tissue is divided in line with the skin incision, and the muscle is gently divided and elevated near the bone. *Caution!* Do not damage the spinal accessory nerve. A bipolar release, i.e., by detaching the sternocleidomastoid muscle at its origin from the mastoid and its distal insertions, is indicated in severe, neglected cases.

Postoperative Care. In the child younger than two years of age, a postoperative orthosis or cast is not necessary. As soon as the child is comfortable, passive exercises are performed to maintain range of motion.

In the older patient with moderate deformity, a torticollis orthosis is worn as soon as the patient is comfortable. In the older patient, when the deformity is quite severe, a Minerva cast is applied on the second or third postoperative day. The cast maintains the head in the overcorrected position. There should be distal traction on the shoulder of the operated side with a strap on the clavicle.

In four weeks the cast is removed, and the patient wears a night orthosis to maintain the head in the corrected position. The brace is worn *only* at night, and passive and active exercises are performed to restore normal alignment of the head and neck.

REFERENCES

Canale, S. T., Griffin, D. W., and Hubbard, C. N.: Congenital muscular torticollis. J. Bone Joint Surg., 64–A:810, 1982.
Chandler, F. A.: Muscular torticollis, J. Bone Joint Surg., 30-A:566, 1948.
Coventry, M. B., and Harris, L.: Congenital muscular torticollis in infancy. Some observations regarding treatment. J. Bone Joint Surg., 41-A:815, 1959.
Ferkel, R. D., Westin, G. W., Dawson, E. G., and Oppenheim, W. L.: Muscular torticollis. A modified surgical approach. J. Bone Joint Surg., 65–A:894, 1983.
Ling, C. M.: The influence of age on the results of open sternomastoid tenotomy in muscular torticollis. Clin. Orthop., 116:142, 1976.
Ling, C. M., and Low, Y. S.: Sternomastoid tumor and muscular torticollis of infancy: familial occurrence. Am. J. Dis. Child., 132:422, 1978.
Staheli, L. T.: Muscular torticollis: Late results of operative treatment. Surgery, 69:469, 1971.
Tillaux, P. J., and Lange, C.: Quoted in Lange, C.: Zur Behandlung der Schiefhalses. Wochenschr. Orthop. Chir. (Stuttg.), 27:440, 1910.

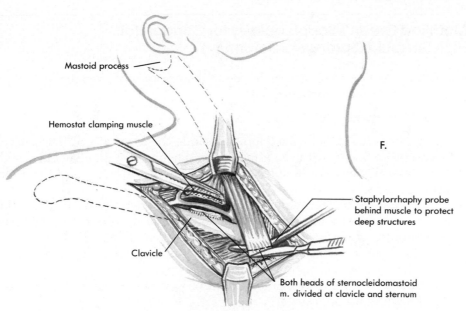

Mastoid process

Hemostat clamping muscle

F.

Staphylorrhaphy probe behind muscle to protect deep structures

Clavicle

Both heads of sternocleidomastoid m. divided at clavicle and sternum

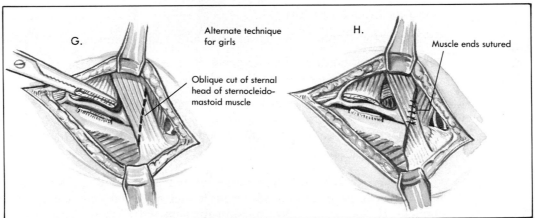

G.

Alternate technique for girls

H.

Muscle ends sutured

Oblique cut of sternal head of sternocleido-mastoid muscle

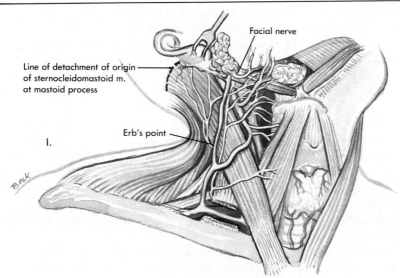

Facial nerve

Line of detachment of origin of sternocleidomastoid m. at mastoid process

Erb's point

I.

Beck

Plate 1. (Continued)

PLATE 2

Modified Green's Scapuloplasty for Congenital High Scapula (Sprengel's Deformity)

Indications. Moderate or severe degree of deformity with impairment of shoulder function and cosmetic disfiguration.

Preoperative Assessment

1. Radiograms of both shoulders to include the cervical and thoracic spine: (a) anteroposterior views, with the arms at the side and maximal shoulder abduction, and (b) lateral views. Rule out congenital scoliosis, Klippel-Feil syndrome, and omovertebral bar.

2. Computed tomography (CT) or magnetic resonance imaging (MRI) as necessary to delineate omovertebral bar and site of its cervical attachment. Rule out spina bifida occulta and intraspinal lesions such as lipoma.

3. Rule out associated visceral abnormalities, especially anomalies of the kidneys, i.e., ultrasonography and intravenous pyelogram.

4. Muscle testing to determine extent of muscle weakness and fibrosis.

5. Photographs of patient.

Blood for Transfusion. Yes.

Radiographic Control. The patient lies on a radiolucent operating table.

Special Instrumentation. Rib stripper.

First, an osteotomy of the clavicle is performed.

Patient Position. The patient is placed in supine position, and the upper half of the chest and the entire neck are fully prepared and draped. It is vital that the level of the contralateral normal scapula be visible during surgery.

Operative Technique

A. A supraclavicular transverse incision is made 2 cm. above the clavicle in line with the skin creases of the neck and centered over the midportion of the clavicle. It is best to make the skin incision with the neck in slight flexion (not hyperextension). The subcutaneous tissue is divided in line with the skin incision, and the wound is pulled down directly over the clavicle.

B. The deep fascia is incised; any superficial veins are clamped and coagulated. The periosteum of the clavicle is divided longitudinally on its anterosuperior aspect and, with a periosteal elevator, is gently elevated circumferentially around the clavicle. Two small Chandler elevators are placed deep to the clavicle, protecting the subclavian vessels and the brachial plexus.

C. With a bone cutter or an oscillating electric saw, the clavicle is sectioned at its middle third. If the clavicle is tilted too cephalad, it is sectioned at two sites, which should be 3 cm. apart. Leave the posteroinferior cortex intact. Then, by gentle force, a greenstick fracture of the clavicle is produced. The periosteum is closed. A small Hemovac suction tube is used for drainage. Skin closure is with subcuticular running sutures. Morcellation of the clavicle is not recommended because it will cause marked shortening of the clavicle and forward drooping of the shoulder.

In the older patient, the incision may be extended laterally so that the tip of the coracoid process and the origins of the short head of the biceps brachii and the coracobrachialis muscle are exposed. The cartilaginous tip of the coracoid process is sectioned, and the wound is closed as already described. The purpose of this step in the child older than ten years of age is to prevent compression of the neurovascular bundle against the rib. Sterile dressings are applied.

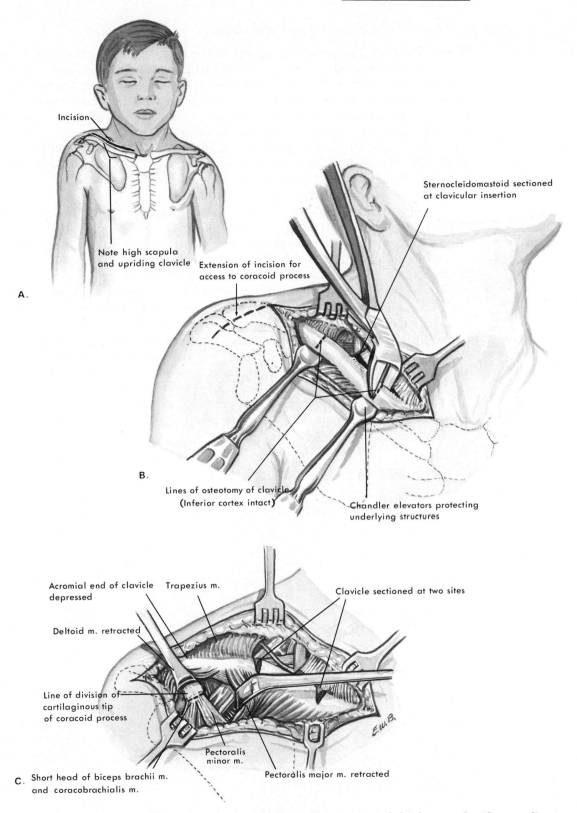

A.

Incision

Note high scapula
and upriding clavicle

Extension of incision for
access to coracoid process

Sternocleidomastoid sectioned
at clavicular insertion

B.

Lines of osteotomy of clavicle
(Inferior cortex intact)

Chandler elevators protecting
underlying structures

Acromial end of clavicle
depressed

Trapezius m.

Clavicle sectioned at two sites

Deltoid m. retracted

Line of division of
cartilaginous tip
of coracoid process

Pectoralis
minor m.

Pectoralis major m. retracted

C. Short head of biceps brachii m.
and coracobrachialis m.

E.W.B.

Plate 2. A.–T., Modified Green's scapuloplasty for congenital high scapula (Sprengel's deformity).

Next, the scapula is transferred distally.

Patient Position. The patient is turned to the prone position very gently, with the head and neck extending beyond the operating table and supported on a headrest. The chin piece of the headrest should be well padded. During the procedure, the anesthesiologist should frequently check the chin for pressure areas. Anchoring the patient's buttocks to the operating table with 2- or 3-inch-wide adhesive tape will prevent the patient from slipping caudally. Care should be taken to guard the sterility of the operating field. First, the vertebral border, the level of the inferior angle and the spine of the elevated scapula, and those of the opposite normal scapula are palpated and marked with indelible ink.

D. A midline skin incision is made that begins at the spinous process of the fourth cervical vertebra and extends distally to terminate at the spinous process of the tenth thoracic vertebra (C-4 to T-10).

E. The skin and the subcutaneous tissue are divided in line with the skin incision, and a plane between the subcutaneous tissue and fascia underlying the trapezius muscle is developed. Dissection is extended laterally to expose the spine of the scapula. Next, the inferior margin of the trapezius muscle, which runs obliquely upward and laterally to the scapular spine, is isolated. Its free lateral border is mobilized and retracted proximally and medially. The insertion of the entire trapezius muscle (superior, middle, and inferior parts) on the scapular spine is sectioned, elevated extraperiosteally, and marked with 0 Tycron sutures. Inferiorly, the lower fibers of the trapezius muscle are separated from the subjacent latissimus dorsi muscle with Metzenbaum scissors.

F. The detached trapezius muscle is reflected medially, exposing underlying muscles and the scapula. The spinal accessory nerve, which is the motor nerve of the trapezius, should not be injured.

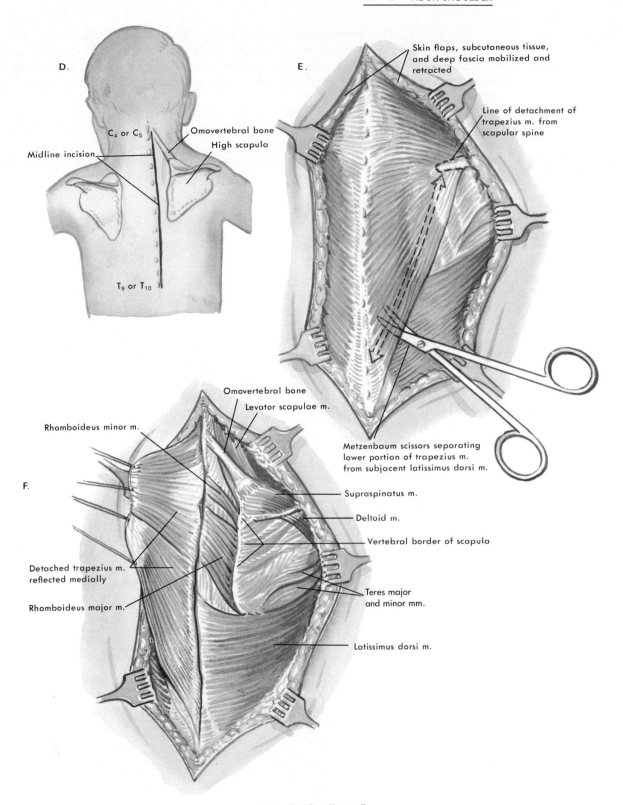

D.

C₄ or C₅

Midline incision

Omovertebral bone

High scapula

T₉ or T₁₀

E.

Skin flaps, subcutaneous tissue, and deep fascia mobilized and retracted

Line of detachment of trapezius m. from scapular spine

Metzenbaum scissors separating lower portion of trapezius m. from subjacent latissimus dorsi m.

Omovertebral bone

Levator scapulae m.

Rhomboideus minor m.

F.

Supraspinatus m.

Deltoid m.

Vertebral border of scapula

Detached trapezius m. reflected medially

Rhomboideus major m.

Teres major and minor mm.

Latissimus dorsi m.

Plate 2. (Continued)

G. and **H.** The supraspinatus muscle is then detached from the scapula extraperiosteally to the greater scapular notch. The transverse scapular artery and suprascapular vessels and nerve must be identified and protected in the lateral portion of the wound as they enter the infraspinatus fossa, passing through the greater scapular notch.

I. The omovertebral bar (bony, cartilaginous, or fibrous) is excised by first sectioning it at the scapular end with a bone cutter and then gently detaching its attachment to the cervical vertebra. At the cervical level it may be attached to the spinous process, lamina, or transverse process of one of the lower cervical vertebra (fourth to seventh).

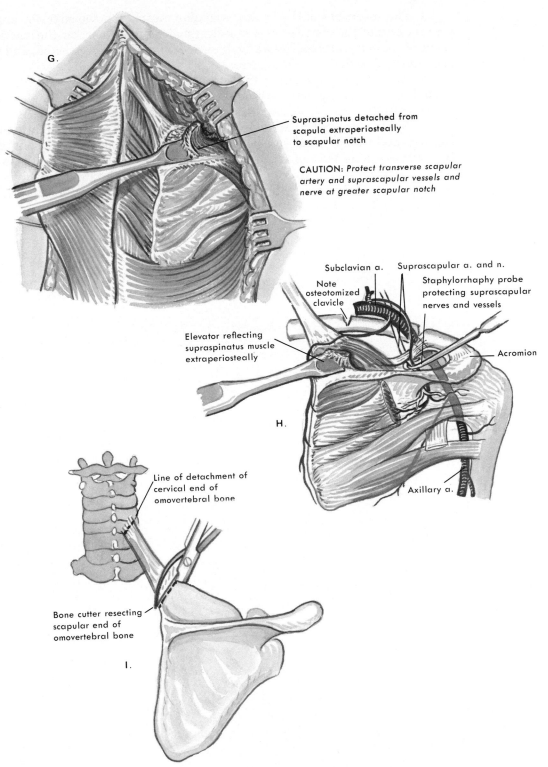

G.

Supraspinatus detached from scapula extraperiosteally to scapular notch

CAUTION: *Protect transverse scapular artery and suprascapular vessels and nerve at greater scapular notch*

Subclavian a.   Suprascapular a. and n.

Note osteotomized clavicle   Staphylorrhaphy probe protecting suprascapular nerves and vessels

Elevator reflecting supraspinatus muscle extraperiosteally

Acromion

H.

Axillary a.

Line of detachment of cervical end of omovertebral bone

Bone cutter resecting scapular end of omovertebral bone

I.

Plate 2. (Continued)

J. The insertions of the levator scapulae muscles on the superior angle of the scapula and of the rhomboideus muscles, major and minor, on the medial border of the scapula are extraperiosteally dissected, divided, and retracted, and their free ends marked with 0 Tycron sutures.

K. The superior margin of the scapula is then retracted posteriorly; starting medially, the supraspinous portion of the subscapularis muscle is elevated extraperiosteally from the anterior surface of the scapula.

L. Next, a staphylorrhaphy probe is placed in the scapular notch to protect the suprascapular nerves and vessels, and with bone-cutting forceps or an osteotome, the supraspinous part of the scapula along with its periosteum is excised. (I preserve the normal anatomy of the scapula because often its supraspinous portion is tilted anteriorly toward the rib cage, in which case a greenstick fracture is produced and the tilted portion is elevated.)

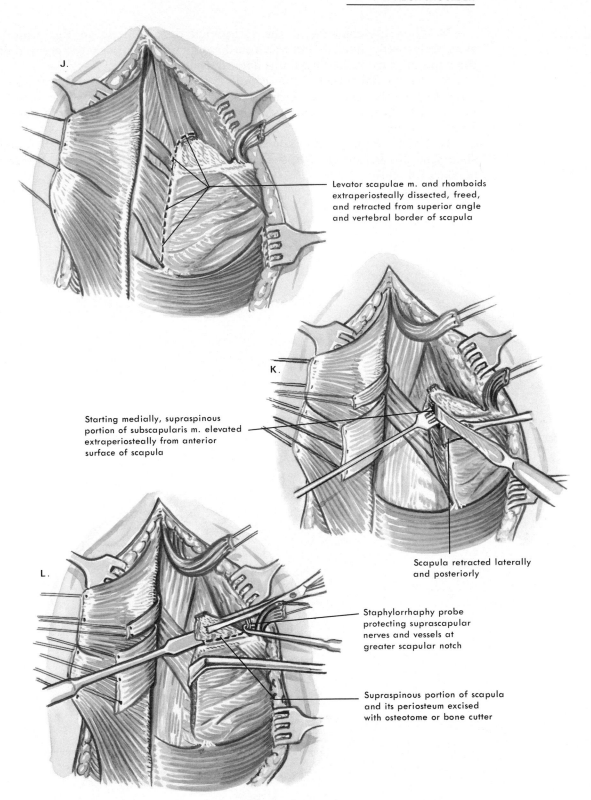

J.

Levator scapulae m. and rhomboids extraperiosteally dissected, freed, and retracted from superior angle and vertebral border of scapula

K.

Starting medially, supraspinous portion of subscapularis m. elevated extraperiosteally from anterior surface of scapula

Scapula retracted laterally and posteriorly

L.

Staphylorrhaphy probe protecting suprascapular nerves and vessels at greater scapular notch

Supraspinous portion of scapula and its periosteum excised with osteotome or bone cutter

Plate 2. (Continued)

M. Then attachments of the latissimus dorsi muscle to the scapula are extraperiosteally divided, and by blunt dissection a large pocket is created deep to the superior part of the latissimus dorsi muscle.

N. The medial border of the scapula is everted by retracting it posteriorly and laterally, and the insertions of the serratus anterior muscle to the vertebral margin and to the angle of the scapula are freed extraperiosteally and marked with 0 Tycron sutures.

O. Thick fibrous bands may connect the scapula to the chest wall. The bands should be divided to mobilize the scapula so that the scapula can be adequately displaced distally.

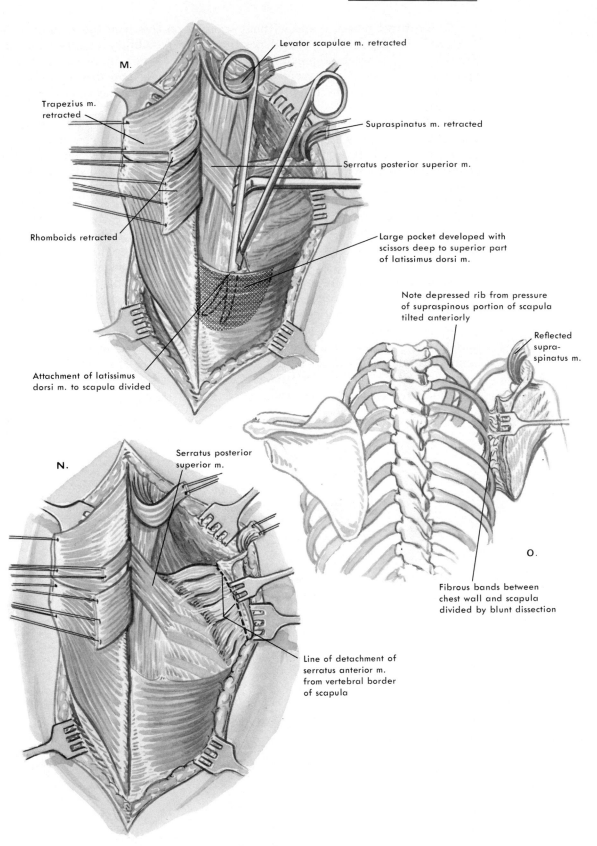

M.

Levator scapulae m. retracted

Trapezius m. retracted

Supraspinatus m. retracted

Serratus posterior superior m.

Rhomboids retracted

Large pocket developed with scissors deep to superior part of latissimus dorsi m.

Note depressed rib from pressure of supraspinous portion of scapula tilted anteriorly

Reflected supra-spinatus m.

Attachment of latissimus dorsi m. to scapula divided

N.

Serratus posterior superior m.

O.

Fibrous bands between chest wall and scapula divided by blunt dissection

Line of detachment of serratus anterior m. from vertebral border of scapula

Plate 2. (Continued)

P. By direct pressure and without traction on the arm, the scapula is gently displaced distally to the desired position. The possibility of stretching of and damage to the brachial plexus must always be kept in mind, and vigorous manipulations should be avoided. The inferior angle and distal quarter of the scapula should be in the large pocket deep to the superior part of the latissimus dorsi muscle.

Q. To prevent superior migration and winging of the scapula, the inferior pole and distal one fourth of the vertebral border of the scapula are attached to the adjacent rib with two or three large absorbable sutures (such as Vicryl). If the rhomboid muscles and other scapulocostal muscles are hypoplastic or fibrotic and there is marked winging of the scapula, this author recommends fixing the scapula on the rib cage in a lowered and more laterally rotated position with nonabsorbable sutures, such as Mersilene strips. The winging will be corrected, and the laterally rotated fixed position of the scapula will enable the patient to abduct the shoulder fully at the glenohumeral joint. (See Plate 12.) A posteroanterior radiogram is made to double-check that the scapula has been lowered adequately.

Note: The scapula in Sprengel's deformity is hypoplastic, and symmetry of the level of the superior border is the important determination. The inferior border may be higher as compared with the normal side because of its small size.

R. Next, while the assistant holds the scapula in its lowered position, the divided and marked muscles are reattached in the following order: (1) The supraspinatus to the base of the scapular spine. (2) The subscapularis to the vertebral border. (3) The serratus anterior to the vertebral border at a level more proximal than its original position.

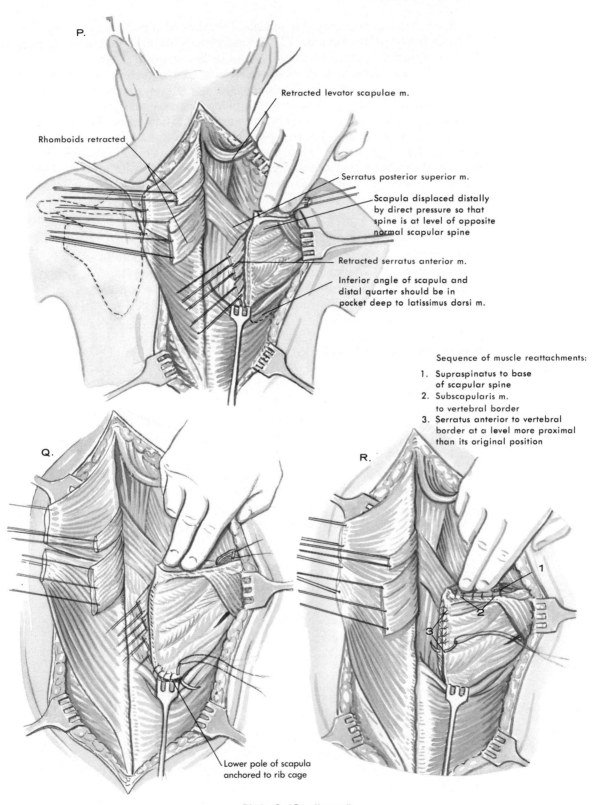

P.

Rhomboids retracted

Retracted levator scapulae m.

Serratus posterior superior m.

Scapula displaced distally
by direct pressure so that
spine is at level of opposite
normal scapular spine

Retracted serratus anterior m.

Inferior angle of scapula and
distal quarter should be in
pocket deep to latissimus dorsi m.

Sequence of muscle reattachments:

1. Supraspinatus to base
   of scapular spine
2. Subscapularis m.
   to vertebral border
3. Serratus anterior to vertebral
   border at a level more proximal
   than its original position

Q.

R.

Lower pole of scapula
anchored to rib cage

Plate 2. (Continued)

S. (4) The levator scapulae muscle, lengthened if necessary, is attached to the superior border of the scapula. (5) The rhomboids are attached to the medial border of the scapula at a more proximal site than the original position.

T. (6) The superior part of the trapezius is reattached to the scapular spine about 3 to 4 cm. medial to its original position. (7) The inferior part of the trapezius is attached to the spine of the scapula more laterally and proximally than before. (8) The superior edge of the latissimus dorsi is attached to the inferolateral edge of the laterally advanced lower part of the trapezius. In the distal part of the incision, the origin of the lower part of the trapezius is followed, the excess tissue is excised, and the free muscle edges are overlapped and sutured. The increased tension in this part of the muscle will serve as an added measure to hold the scapula in its lowered position.

The wound is closed in layers. Closure of the skin should be subcuticular. If there is an associated pterygium colli, a Z-plasty repair may be performed.

Postoperative Care. The shoulder is immobilized in a Velpeau cast. Make sure that the elbow is not elevated. The patient is discharged from the hospital in three or four days. Periodic radiograms are made to be sure that the clavicular osteotomy is healing appropriately. About four to six weeks postoperatively, the cast is removed and active shoulder abduction and scapular depression exercises are performed to increase muscle strength. Passive exercises of the glenohumeral and scapulocostal joints are carried out to increase range of joint motion.

REFERENCES

Chung, S. M. K., and Farahvar, H.: Surgery of the clavicle in Sprengel's deformity. Clin. Orthop., 116:138, 1976.

DeBastiani, G., Boscaro, C., and Coletti, N.: Green's operation in treatment of elevated scapula. Chir. Organi Mov., 64:1, 1978.

Green, W. T.: The surgical correction of congenital elevation of the scapula (Sprengel's deformity). Proceedings of the American Orthopedic Association. J. Bone Joint Surg., 39-A:1439, 1957.

Klisic, P., Filipovic, M., Uzelac, O., and Milinkovic, Z.: Relocation of congenitally elevated scapula. J. Pediatr. Orthop., 1:43, 1981.

Robinson, A. R., Braun, R. M., Mack, P., and Zadek, R.: The surgical importance of the clavicular component of Sprengel's deformity. J. Bone Joint Surg., 49-A:1481, 1967.

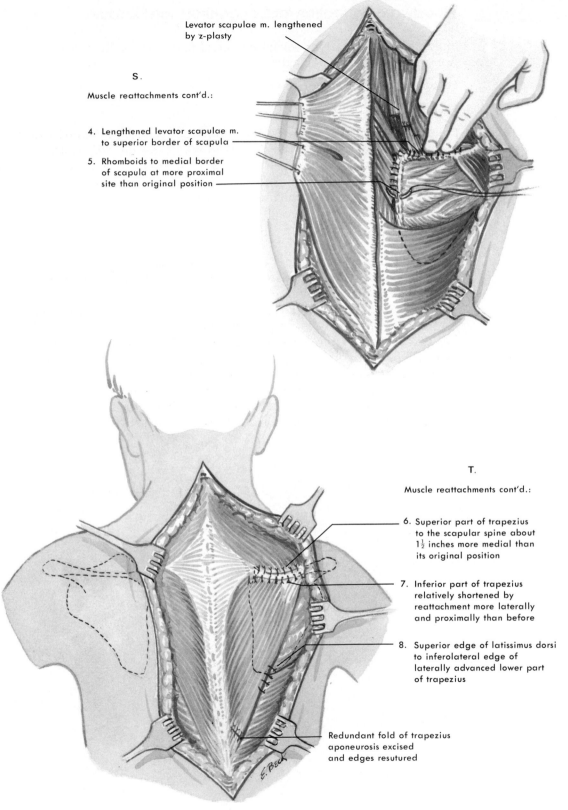

Levator scapulae m. lengthened
by z-plasty

S.

Muscle reattachments cont'd.:

4. Lengthened levator scapulae m.
   to superior border of scapula

5. Rhomboids to medial border
   of scapula at more proximal
   site than original position

T.

Muscle reattachments cont'd.:

6. Superior part of trapezius
   to the scapular spine about
   1½ inches more medial than
   its original position

7. Inferior part of trapezius
   relatively shortened by
   reattachment more laterally
   and proximally than before

8. Superior edge of latissimus dorsi
   to inferolateral edge of
   laterally advanced lower part
   of trapezius

Redundant fold of trapezius
aponeurosis excised
and edges resutured

E. Beck

Plate 2. (Continued)

PLATE 3   Woodward Operation for Congenital High Scapula

Indications. Moderate or severe degree of deformity with impairment of shoulder function and cosmetic disfiguration.

Preoperative Assessment. Same as for Plate 2.

Blood for Transfusion. Yes.

Patient Position. The patient is in prone position. The head is supported on a craniotomy headrest, and the neck is in slight flexion. The sides and back of the neck, both shoulders, the trunk down to the iliac crests, and the upper limb on the involved side are prepared and draped. One should be able to manipulate the shoulder girdle and arms during the operation without contaminating the surgical field.

Operative Technique

A. A midline longitudinal incision is made, extending from the spinous process of the first cervical vertebra to that of the ninth thoracic vertebra.

B. The subcutaneous tissue is divided in line with the skin incision. The wound margins are undermined laterally to the medial border of the scapula. The muscle arrangement should be clearly visualized.

C. Next, the lateral border of the trapezius muscle is identified at the distal part of the wound. By blunt dissection, the lower portion of the trapezius is separated from the subjacent latissimus dorsi muscle.

D. With a sharp scalpel, the tough and tendinous origin of the trapezius muscle is detached from the spinous process. Numerous sutures are passed at the entire origin of the muscle for marking it and for use at later reattachment.

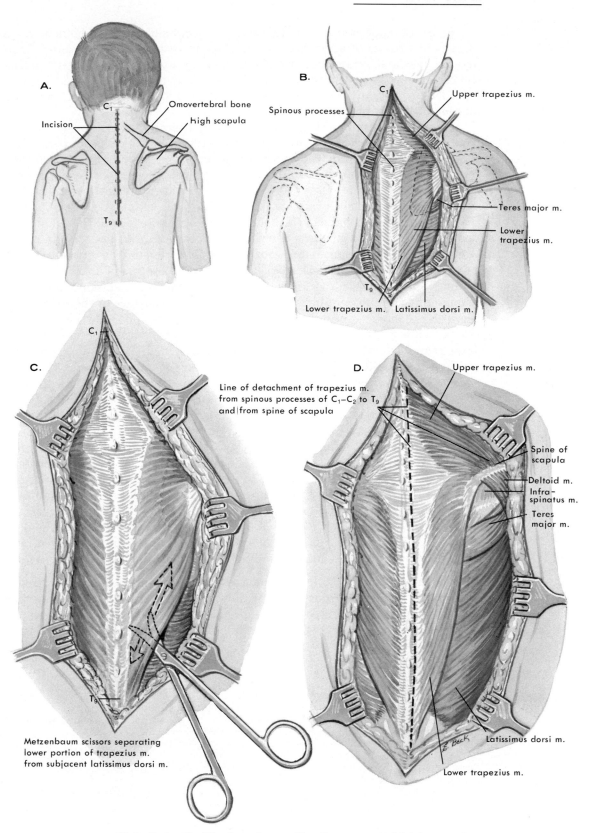

A.

Incision

C₁

Omovertebral bone

high scapula

T₉

B.

Spinous processes

C₁

Upper trapezius m.

Teres major m.

Lower trapezius m.

T₉

Lower trapezius m.   Latissimus dorsi m.

C.

C₁

T₉

Metzenbaum scissors separating
lower portion of trapezius m.
from subjacent latissimus dorsi m.

D.

Line of detachment of trapezius m.
from spinous processes of C₁–C₂ to T₉
and from spine of scapula

Upper trapezius m.

Spine of
scapula

Deltoid m.

Infra-
spinatus m.

Teres
major m.

Latissimus dorsi m.

Lower trapezius m.

Plate 3. A.–G., Woodward operation for congenital high scapula.

E. In the upper part of the incision, the origins of the rhomboideus major and minor muscles are sharply divided and tagged with sutures. A well-defined deep layer of fascia separates the rhomboids and the upper part of the trapezius from the serratus posterior superior and erector spinae muscles. It is vital to maintain a proper tissue plane. Preserve the aponeurosis and muscle sheet intact for secure fixation of the scapula at its lowered level.

Next, the entire muscle sheet is retracted laterally, exposing the omovertebral bone or fibrous band, if present. The omovertebral bar is excised *extraperiosteally;* it usually extends from the superior angle of the scapula to one of the lower cervical vertebrae. It is best to use a bone cutter for resection. Avoid injury to the spinal accessory nerve, the nerves to the rhomboids, and the descending scapular artery. The contracted levator scapulae muscle is sectioned at its attachment to the scapula. Fibrous bands attached to the anterior surface of the scapula usually restrict its downward displacement; if present, they are sectioned. Next, the scapula is everted and the serratus anterior muscle is detached from its insertion on the vertebral border of the scapula. A periosteal elevator is used to elevate the supraspinatus muscle extraperiosteally from the supraspinous portion of the scapula and the subscapularis muscle from the deep surface of the scapula midway between the superior and inferior angles. The supraspinous portion of the scapula is resected with its periosteum. Suprascapular vessels and nerves and the transverse scapular artery should be protected from injury. These steps are illustrated in Plate 2, Steps **K** and **L** of the modified Green's scapuloplasty.

F. Next, the scapula is lowered to its normal level and held in the corrected position by an assistant. The subscapularis muscle is reattached to the vertebral border of the scapula, and the supraspinatus muscle is resutured to the scapular spine. The serratus anterior muscle is reattached to the vertebral border of the scapula at a more proximal level. The latissimus dorsi muscle is reattached to the scapula. Proceeding cephalocaudally, the surgeon sutures the thick aponeurosis of the trapezius and rhomboid muscles to the spinous processes at a more distal level. It is essential that an assistant maintain the corrected level of the scapula.

G. Since the origin of the trapezius muscle distal to the ninth thoracic vertebra is not disturbed, a redundant fold of aponeurotic tissue is created in the distal end of the trapezius muscle. This fold of soft tissue is excised and resutured.

The wound is closed in the usual fashion. The skin closure is subcuticular.

Postoperative Care. A Velpeau bandage is applied and is worn for three to four weeks. The patient is allowed to be up and around the day after the operation. After removal of the Velpeau bandage, postoperative exercises similar to those described for the modified Green's scapuloplasty are carried out.

REFERENCES

Carson, W. G., Lovell, W. W., and Whitesides, T. E., Jr.: Congenital elevation of the scapula. Surgical correction by the Woodward procedure. J. Bone Joint Surg., 63-A:1199, 1981.

Grogan, D. P., Stanley, E. A., and Bobechko, W. P.: The congenital undescended scapula. Surgical correction by the Woodward procedure. J. Bone Joint Surg., 65–B:598, 1983.

Picault, Ch., and Murat, J.: A propos de trois cas de surélévation congénitale de l'omoplate traites par la technique de Woodward. Ann. Chir., 19:627, 1965.

Ross, D. M., and Cruess, R. L.: The surgical correction of congenital elevation of the scapula. Clin. Orthop., 125:17, 1977.

Woodward, J. W.: Congenital elevation of the scapula. Correction by release and transplantation of muscle origins. J. Bone Joint Surg., 43-A:219, 1961.

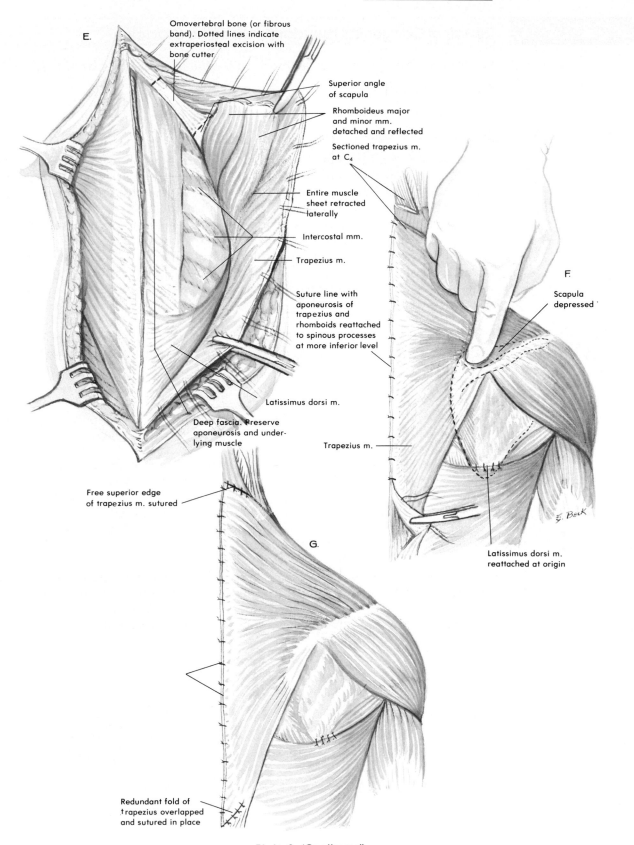

E.

Omovertebral bone (or fibrous band). Dotted lines indicate extraperiosteal excision with bone cutter

Superior angle of scapula

Rhomboideus major and minor mm. detached and reflected

Sectioned trapezius m. at C₄

Entire muscle sheet retracted laterally

Intercostal mm.

Trapezius m.

Suture line with aponeurosis of trapezius and rhomboids reattached to spinous processes at more inferior level

Latissimus dorsi m.

Deep fascia. Preserve aponeurosis and under-lying muscle

Scapula depressed

F.

Trapezius m.

Latissimus dorsi m. reattached at origin

Free superior edge of trapezius m. sutured

G.

Redundant fold of trapezius overlapped and sutured in place

Plate 3. (Continued)

PLATE 4   ## Repair of Congenital Pseudarthrosis of the Clavicle

Indications. Presence of pseudarthrosis in a child at least one year of age.

Blood for Transfusion. Yes.

Special Instrumentation. AO instrumentation.

Operative Technique

A. A horizontal incision 4 to 6 cm. long is made in line with the skin creases of the neck about 2 cm. above the clavicle. (It is best to mark the site of the skin incision when the patient is upright and not in supine position because the skin creases will move upward when the neck is hyperextended.) A direct incision over the clavicle is absolutely not recommended. The resultant scar and keloid will be very disfiguring. An arcuate skin incision low down over the second rib (recommended by Owen) avoids supraclavicular nerves, and any keloid can be hidden by clothing; however, it makes exposure of the pseudarthrosis difficult. The subcutaneous tissue is divided in line with the skin incision, and the wound is pulled down directly over the clavicle.

B. The fascia is divided. Any superficial veins are clamped and coagulated. The periosteum is divided over the anterior aspect of the sternal and clavicular segments of the clavicle. With a curved elevator, normal bone is exposed subperiosteally before getting to the pseudarthrosis site.

The periosteum is gently elevated circumferentially around the clavicle; small Chandler periosteal elevators are placed behind the clavicle to protect the subclavicular vessels and brachial plexus. The pseudarthrosis site is excised with an oscillating electric saw or bone cutter. Sclerotic bone is removed until healthy osseous tissue is exposed.

C. With a small curet, the sternal and acromial ends of the clavicle are cleaned of all sclerotic osseous tissue. Avoid bone splintering. A threaded Steinmann pin of appropriate size is gently drilled, preferably by electric drill, into the acromial segment of the clavicle until it protrudes from the skin lateral to the shoulder; the two segments are approximated snugly, and the pin is drilled retrograde into the sternal segment of the clavicle. Do not use a smooth Steinmann pin because it may migrate.

D. Cancellous autogenous bone for grafting is obtained from the ilium and packed around the pseudarthrosis site, and the periosteum is closed. The wound is closed in the usual fashion—skin closure should be subcuticular. The shoulder is immobilized in a Velpeau bandage, reinforced with a second layer of cast.

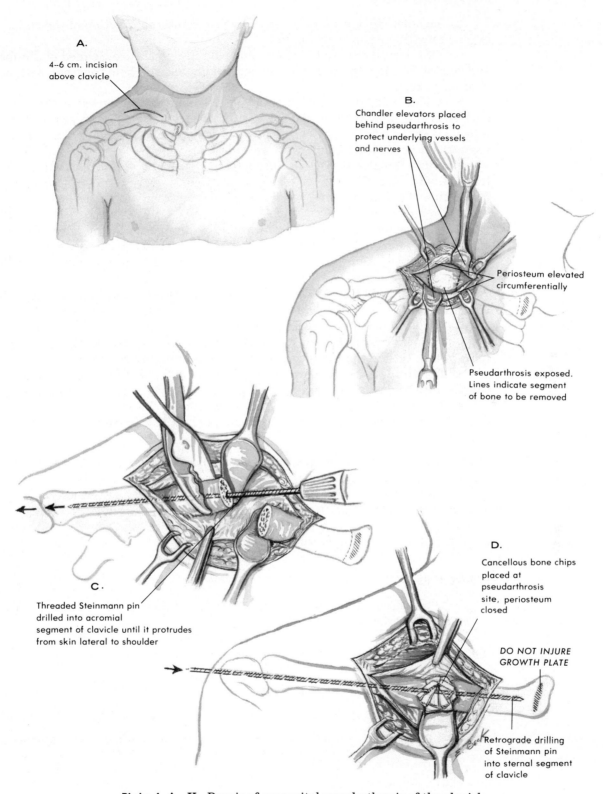

A.

4–6 cm. incision above clavicle

B.

Chandler elevators placed behind pseudarthrosis to protect underlying vessels and nerves

Periosteum elevated circumferentially

Pseudarthrosis exposed. Lines indicate segment of bone to be removed

C.

Threaded Steinmann pin drilled into acromial segment of clavicle until it protrudes from skin lateral to shoulder

D.

Cancellous bone chips placed at pseudarthrosis site, periosteum closed

DO NOT INJURE GROWTH PLATE

Retrograde drilling of Steinmann pin into sternal segment of clavicle

Plate 4. A.–K., Repair of congenital pseudarthrosis of the clavicle.

In the older child, some surgeons may prefer internal fixation of the clavicular segments with a compression plate.

E. After the sternal and acromial ends of the clavicle are cleaned of all fibrous and sclerotic tissue, the segments are approximated and held together with bone-holding forceps.

F. A four-hole, small semitubular or AO plate is contoured to the superior surface of the approximated clavicle. Chandler elevator retractors are used on the inferior surface of the clavicle to prevent inadvertent injury to the subclavian vessels and penetration of the drill into the thorax.

The first hole is drilled in the acromial segment of the clavicle near the fracture site. A drill guide is placed eccentrically away from the fracture site. Determine the length of the screw, then tap the screw hole and insert the first screw. Do *not* screw it home.

G. The second drill hole is again eccentrically placed in the sternal segment of the clavicle next to the fracture site. After the length and tapping are determined, the second screw is inserted. Do not tighten the heads into the plate holes. Note the gap at the fracture site.

H. The sternal screw is tightened and countersunk into the plate hole. Note that the head is pushed toward the fracture gap by the edge of the plate hole, taking bone fragment with it. The fracture gap narrows.

I. When the acromial screw is tightened and countersunk, the same action takes place, closing the fracture gap and compressing the segments.

J. The third and fourth screws are inserted after drilling and tapping. Cancellous autogenous bone is grafted and packed around the pseudarthrosis site.

K. The periosteum is closed, and the wound is closed in the usual fashion. Shoulder immobilization is with a Velpeau bandage reinforced with a second layer of cast.

Postoperative Care. The Velpeau cast is changed as necessary every three weeks. The union is usually solid in eight to ten weeks. At this time, the pin across the clavicle is removed, with the child under appropriate sedation (preferably, general anesthesia), and the child is gradually allowed to use the shoulder normally. When plate and screws are used for internal fixation, they are removed six to nine months following healing of the pseudarthrosis.

REFERENCES

Bargar, W. L., Marcus, R. E., and Ittleman, F. P.: Late thoracic outlet syndrome secondary to pseudarthrosis of the clavicle. J. Trauma, 24:857, 1984.

Gibson, D. A., and Carroll, N.: Congenital pseudarthrosis of the clavicle. J. Bone Joint Surg., 52-B:629, 1970.

Gulino, G., and Ragazzi, P. G.: Congenital pseudarthrosis of the clavicle. Considerations of surgical treatment. Chir. Organi. Mov., 65:701, 1979.

Jinkins, W. J.: Congenital pseudarthrosis of clavicle. Clin. Orthop., 62:183, 1969.

Marmor, L.: Repair of congenital pseudarthrosis of the clavicle: Report of three cases. A.J.R., 132:678, 1979.

Quinlan, W. R., Brady, P. G., and Regan, B. F.: Congenital pseudarthrosis of the clavicle. Acta Orthop. Scand., 51:489, 1980.

Schnall, S. B., King, J. D., and Marrero, G.: Congenital pseudarthrosis of the clavicle: A review of the literature and surgical results of six cases. J. Pediatr. Orthop., 8:316, 1988.

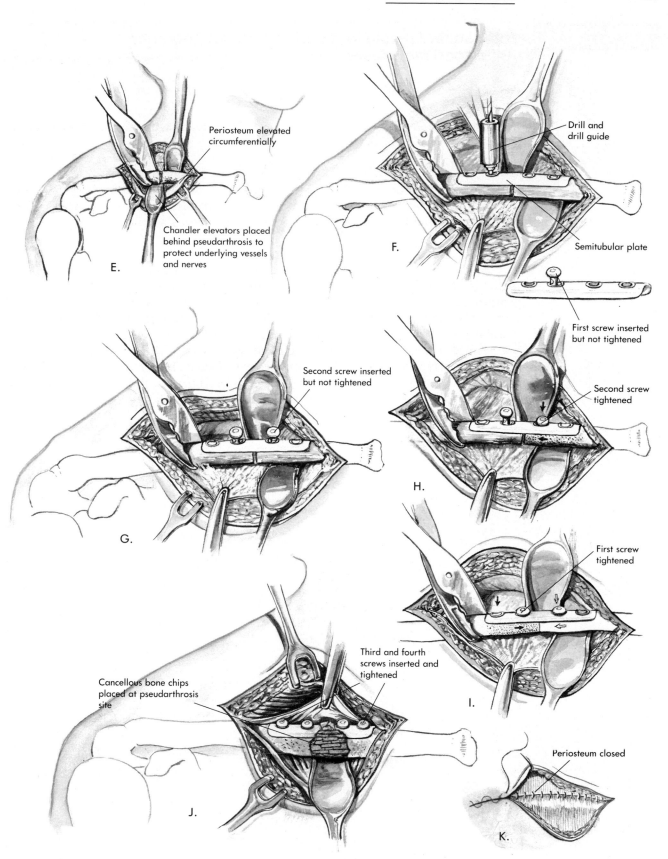

Periosteum elevated circumferentially

Chandler elevators placed behind pseudarthrosis to protect underlying vessels and nerves

E.

Drill and drill guide

Semitubular plate

First screw inserted but not tightened

F.

Second screw inserted but not tightened

G.

First screw inserted but not tightened

Second screw tightened

H.

First screw tightened

Third and fourth screws inserted and tightened

I.

Cancellous bone chips placed at pseudarthrosis site

J.

Periosteum closed

K.

Plate 4. (Continued)

PLATE 5

Forequarter Amputation from the Posterior Approach
(Littlewood Technique)

Indications. Malignant tumor of the scapula or humerus in which the limb cannot be salvaged.

Preoperative Measures. Arrangements should be made with a competent prosthetist for prosthetic fitting.

Blood for Transfusion. Yes.

Patient Position. The patient is placed in lateral position, and the neck, chest, and whole upper limb are prepared and draped. Blood loss is minimal, but adequate whole blood should be available for transfusion if necessary.

Operative Technique

A.–C. The cervicothoracic incision begins at the medial end of the clavicle and extends laterally along the anteroinferior border of the clavicle to the lateral protuberance of the acromion, where it curves posteriorly; then it is continued along the lateral border of the scapula to its inferior angle, where it curves medially to terminate 3 to 4 cm. lateral to the midline of the spine.

The pectoroaxillary incision begins at the center of the clavicle and extends inferolaterally along the deltopectoral groove; it then crosses the anterior axillary fold and joins the posterior incision at the lower third of the lateral border of the scapula. The subcutaneous tissue and fascia are divided in line with the skin incision, and the wound flaps are mobilized to expose the underlying muscles.

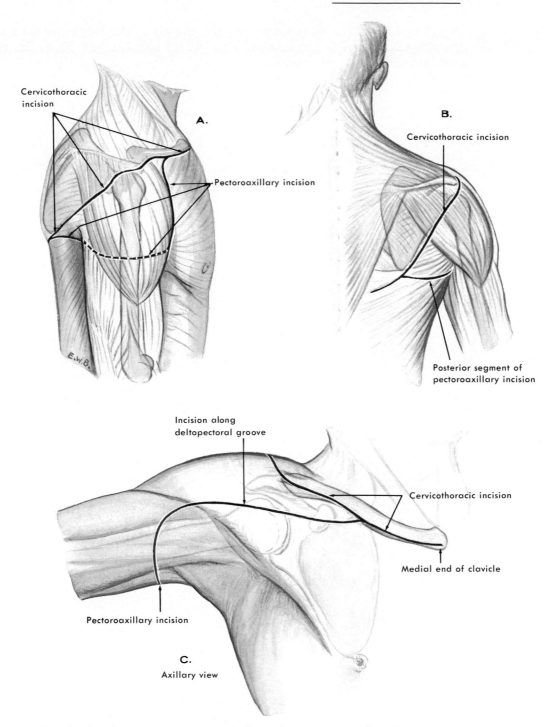

Plate 5. A.–R., Forequarter amputation from the posterior approach (Littlewood technique).

D. and **E.** The muscles connecting the scapula to the trunk are detached from the scapula in layers and marked with "whip" silk sutures. First, the trapezius and latissimus dorsi are divided.

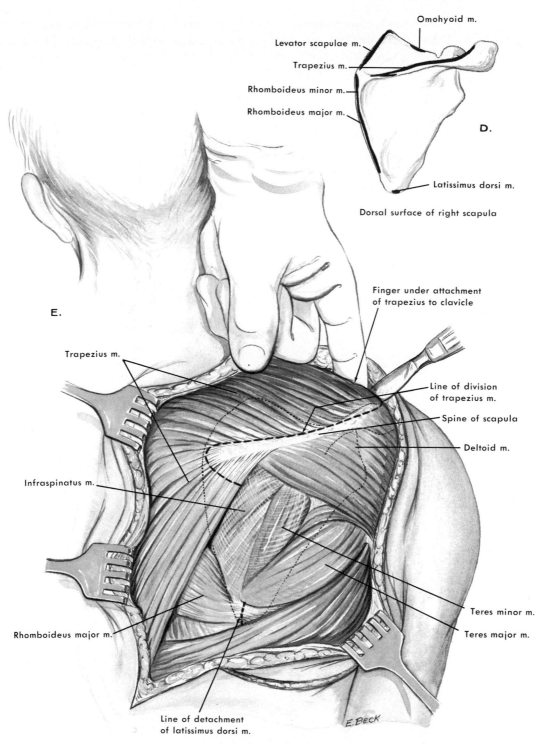

Omohyoid m.

Levator scapulae m.

Trapezius m.

Rhomboideus minor m.

Rhomboideus major m.

D.

Latissimus dorsi m.

Dorsal surface of right scapula

E.

Finger under attachment
of trapezius to clavicle

Trapezius m.

Line of division
of trapezius m.

Spine of scapula

Deltoid m.

Infraspinatus m.

Teres minor m.

Teres major m.

Rhomboideus major m.

E. BECK

Line of detachment
of latissimus dorsi m.

Plate 5. (Continued)

F. Next, the omohyoid, levator scapulae, and rhomboid muscles are detached. Transverse cervical and transverse scapular vessels are ligated and divided as dissection proceeds. The cords of the brachial plexus are sectioned with a very sharp scalpel near their origin.

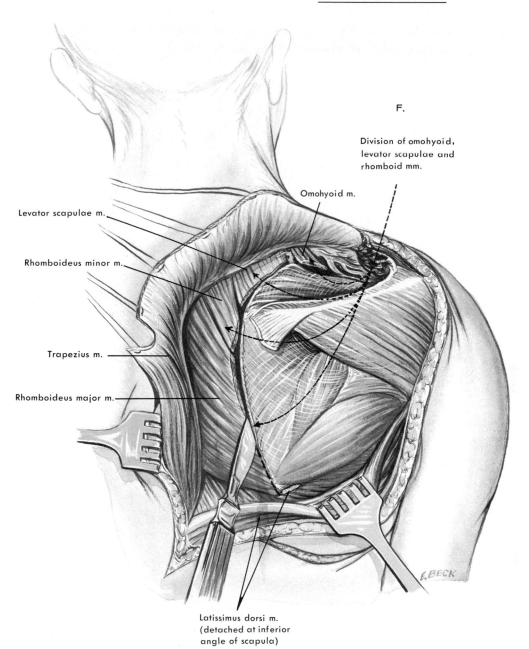

F.

Division of omohyoid,
levator scapulae and
rhomboid mm.

Omohyoid m.

Levator scapulae m.

Rhomboideus minor m.

Trapezius m.

Rhomboideus major m.

Latissimus dorsi m.
(detached at inferior
angle of scapula)

Plate 5. (Continued)

G. and **H.** The scapula is retracted forward, and the serratus anterior muscle is sectioned and detached from the scapula.

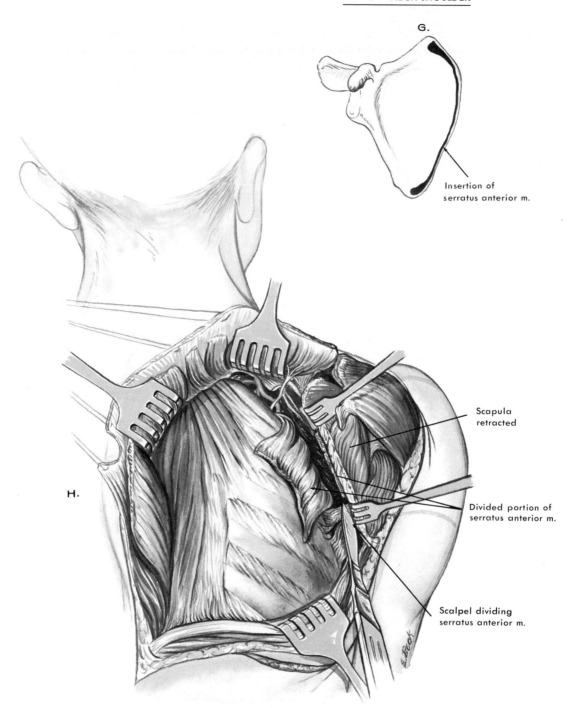

G.

Insertion of
serratus anterior m.

H.

Scapula
retracted

Divided portion of
serratus anterior m.

Scalpel dividing
serratus anterior m.

Plate 5. (Continued)

I.–K. The patient is turned on his or her back, and the medial end of the clavicle is subperiosteally exposed. Chandler periosteal elevators are placed deep to the clavicle to protect the underlying neurovascular structures. With bone-cutting forceps or a Gigli saw, the clavicle is sectioned near its sternal attachment. The subclavius muscle is divided next.

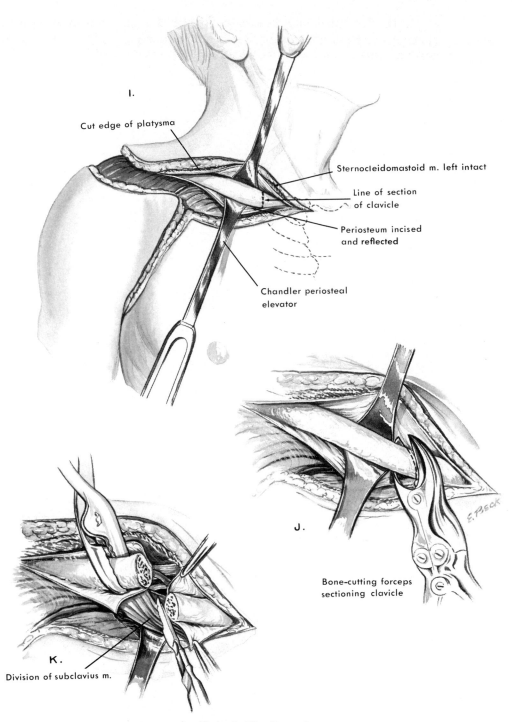

I.

Cut edge of platysma

Sternocleidomastoid m. left intact

Line of section
of clavicle

Periosteum incised
and reflected

Chandler periosteal
elevator

J.

Bone-cutting forceps
sectioning clavicle

K.

Division of subclavius m.

Plate 5. (Continued)

L.–N. The subclavian vessels and brachial plexus are exposed by allowing the upper limb to fall anteriorly. The subclavian artery and vein are isolated, individually clamped, doubly ligated with sutures, and divided.

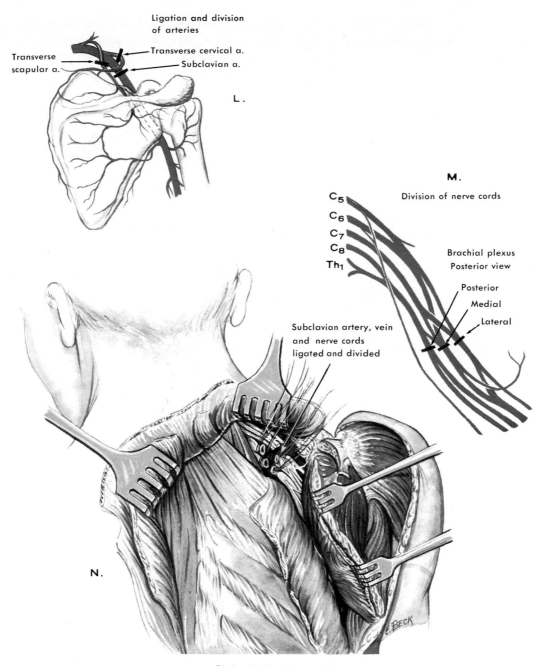

Ligation and division
of arteries

Transverse cervical a.

Transverse
scapular a.

Subclavian a.

L.

M.

C₅
C₆
C₇
C₈
Th₁

Division of nerve cords

Brachial plexus
Posterior view

Posterior
Medial
Lateral

Subclavian artery, vein
and nerve cords
ligated and divided

N.

Plate 5. (Continued)

O.–Q. The pectoralis major and minor, the short head of the biceps, coracobrachialis and latissimus dorsi are sectioned, completing ablation of the limb.

R. The wound flaps are approximated and sutured together. Closed suction catheters are inserted and connected to the Hemovac evacuator. A firm compression dressing is applied.

Postoperative Care. The patient is fitted with the appropriate upper limb prosthesis.

REFERENCES

Haggart, G. E.: The technic of interscapulothoracic amputation. Lahey Clin. Bull., 2:16, 1940.

Hardin, C. A.: Interscapulothoracic amputations for sarcomas of the upper extremity. Surgery, 49:355, 1961.

Knaggs, R. L.: Mr. Littlewood's method of performing the interscapulothoracic amputation (letter to the editor). Lancet, 1:1298, 1910.

Levinthal, D. H., and Grossman, A.: Interscapulothoracic amputations for malignant tumors of the shoulder region. Surg. Gynecol. Obstet., 60:234, 1939.

Linberg, B. E.: Interscapulo-thoracic resection for malignant tumors of the shoulder joint region. J. Bone Joint Surg., 10:344, 1928.

Littlewood, H.: Amputations at the shoulder and at the hip. Br. Med. J., 1:381, 1922.

Nadler, S. H., and Phelan, J. T.: A technique of interscapulothoracic amputation. Surg. Gynecol. Obstet., 122:359, 1966.

Pack, G. T., McNeer, G., and Coley, B. L.: Interscapulothoracic amputations for malignant tumors of the upper extremity: a report of thirty-one consecutive cases. Surg. Gynecol. Obstet., 74:161, 1942.

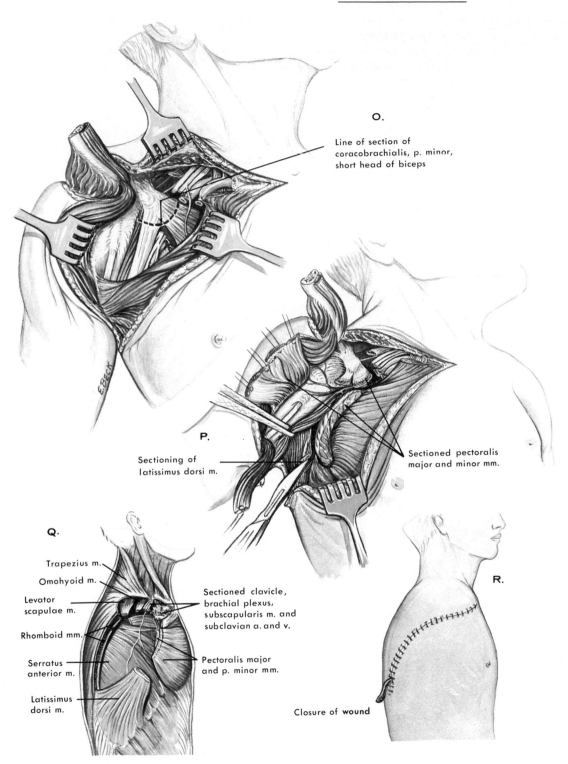

O.

Line of section of
coracobrachialis, p. minor,
short head of biceps

Sectioned pectoralis
major and minor mm.

P.

Sectioning of
latissimus dorsi m.

Q.

Trapezius m.
Omohyoid m.
Levator
scapulae m.
Rhomboid mm.
Serratus
anterior m.
Latissimus
dorsi m.

Sectioned clavicle,
brachial plexus,
subscapularis m. and
subclavian a. and v.

Pectoralis major
and p. minor mm.

R.

Closure of wound

Plate 5. (Continued)

PLATE 6 Scapulectomy

Indications. Malignant tumor of the scapula. Surgical stage I or IIA (intracompartmental).

Blood for Transfusion. Yes.

Patient Position. The patient is placed in prone position. The neck, chest, and whole upper limb are prepared and draped with the entire upper limb free so that it may be moved as required during the procedure.

Operative Technique

A. An elliptical skin incision is made, extending from the tip of the acromion process superolaterally to the lower tip of the scapula inferomedially. Subcutaneous tissue is divided in line with the skin incision, and the skin flaps are mobilized and raised.

B. and **C.** The superficial fascia is incised, and the trapezius muscle is exposed and retracted superiorly and medially. Expose and identify the supraspinatus, deltoid, infraspinatus, and teres minor and major, and latissimus dorsi.

The origin of the deltoid muscle is detached from the lateral margin of the acromion and the lower edge of the crest of the spine of the scapula as far as the smooth triangular surface at its end. The latissimus dorsi is detached in the inferior angle of the scapula.

D. The latissimus dorsi muscle is retracted inferiorly and the deltoid muscle superolaterally. The scapula is everted, and the rhomboideus major and minor and levator scapulae are detached.

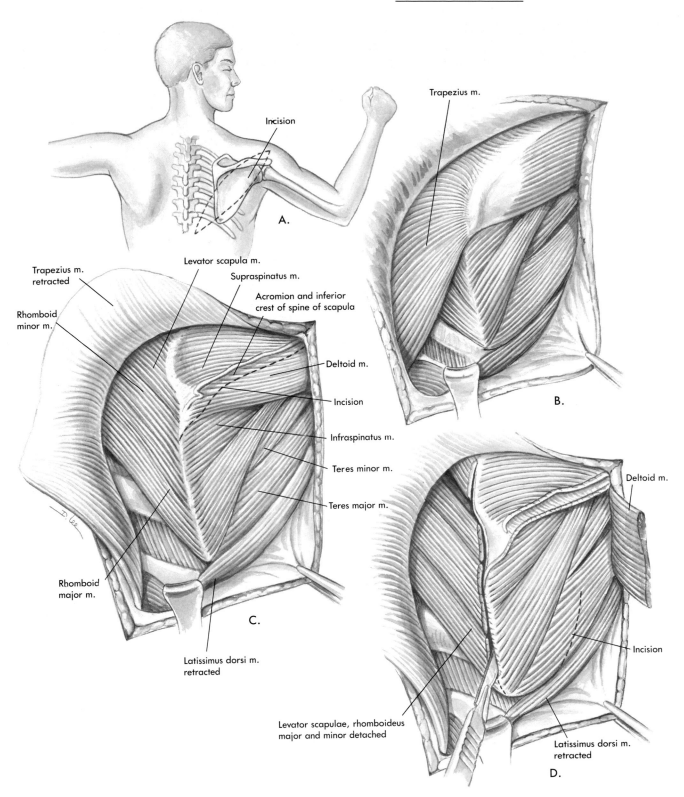

Incision

Trapezius m.

Levator scapula m.

Supraspinatus m.

Acromion and inferior
crest of spine of scapula

Trapezius m.
retracted

Rhomboid
minor m.

Deltoid m.

Incision

Infraspinatus m.

Teres minor m.

Teres major m.

Rhomboid
major m.

B.

Deltoid m.

Incision

Latissimus dorsi m.
retracted

Levator scapulae, rhomboideus
major and minor detached

Latissimus dorsi m.
retracted

D.

A.

C.

Plate 6. A.–J., Scapulectomy.

E. and **F.** The shoulder joint is abducted, and the axillary contents are retracted from the scapula. The following muscles are sectioned from their attachments to the scapula: teres major, teres minor, long head of triceps brachii, supraspinatus, infraspinatus, and serratus anterior.

G. and **H.** The shoulder joint is exposed posteriorly and superiorly. The scapular spine is sectioned near the acromion by a sharp osteotome or an oscillating saw.

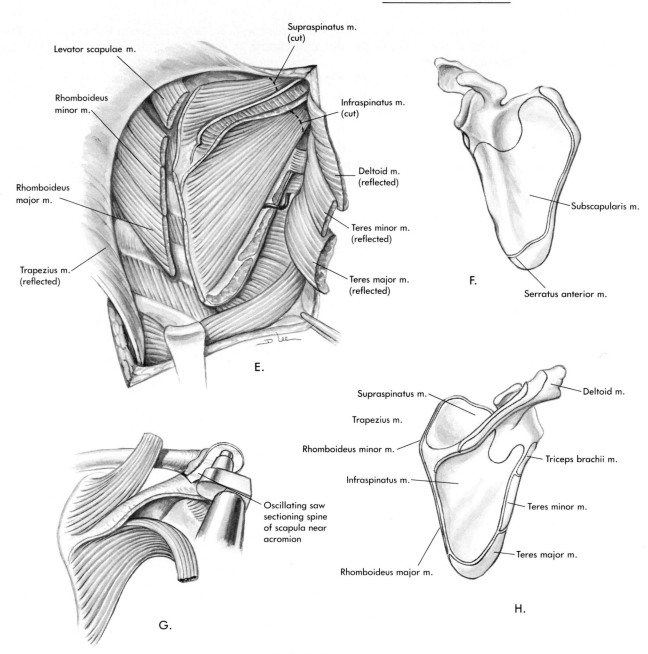

Levator scapulae m.

Rhomboideus
minor m.

Rhomboideus
major m.

Trapezius m.
(reflected)

Supraspinatus m.
(cut)

Infraspinatus m.
(cut)

Deltoid m.
(reflected)

Teres minor m.
(reflected)

Teres major m.
(reflected)

E.

Subscapularis m.

Serratus anterior m.

F.

Oscillating saw
sectioning spine
of scapula near
acromion

G.

Supraspinatus m.

Trapezius m.

Rhomboideus minor m.

Infraspinatus m.

Rhomboideus major m.

Deltoid m.

Triceps brachii m.

Teres minor m.

Teres major m.

H.

Plate 6. (Continued)

I. An electric saw or Gigli saw is passed around the neck of the scapula. The scapular neck is divided, and the scapula is removed. *Caution!* Do not enter the glenohumeral joint.

J. After complete hemostasis is obtained, the trapezius and deltoid muscles are sutured together and the teres major and minor muscles are sutured to the chest wall. Hemovac suction tubes are placed, and the wound is closed in the usual fashion. A Velpeau bandage is applied.

Postoperative Care. The Velpeau bandage and sutures are removed in two to three weeks, and a shoulder sling is applied. Active exercises are performed to develop range of motion of the shoulder joint and motor strength of the muscles.

REFERENCES

Das Gupta, T. K.: Scapulectomy: Indications and technique. Surgery, 67:601, 1970.

Ryerson, E. W.: Excision of the scapula: Report of case with excellent functional result. J.A.M.A., 113:1958, 1939.

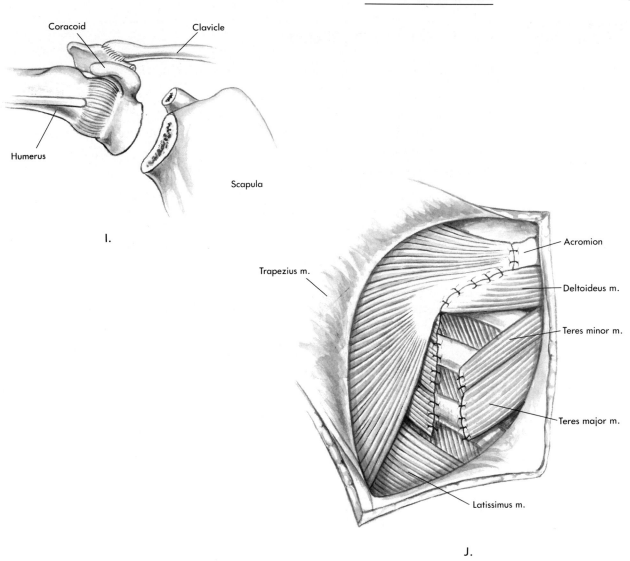

Coracoid

Clavicle

Humerus

Scapula

I.

Trapezius m.

Acromion

Deltoideus m.

Teres minor m.

Teres major m.

Latissimus m.

J.

Plate 6. (Continued)

PLATE 7   Disarticulation of the Shoulder

Indications. Malignant tumor of the arm in which the limb cannot be salvaged.

Blood for Transfusion. Yes.

Patient Position. The patient is placed in semilateral position so that the posterior aspect of the affected shoulder, scapula, axilla, and the entire upper limb can be prepared and draped sterile.

Operative Technique

A. The skin incision begins at the coracoid process and extends distally in the deltopectoral groove to the insertion of the deltoid muscle; it then is continued proximally along the posterior border of the deltoid muscle to terminate at the posterior axillary fold. A second incision in the axilla connects the anterior and posterior borders of the first incision.

B. In the deltopectoral groove, the cephalic vein is identified, ligated, and excised. The deltoid muscle is retracted laterally to expose the humeral attachment of the pectoralis major muscle, which is divided at its insertion and reflected medially. The coracobrachialis and short head of the biceps are divided at their origins from the coracoid process and are reflected distally.

Next, the deltoid muscle is detached from its insertion on the humerus and retracted proximally.

C. The axillary artery and vein and the thoracoacromial vessels are identified, isolated, doubly ligated with 0 Tycron or nonabsorbable suture, and divided. The thoracoacromial artery is a short trunk branching from the anterior surface of the axillary artery. Its origin is usually covered by the pectoralis minor muscle. The median, ulnar, musculocutaneous, and radial nerves are identified, isolated, pulled distally, and divided with a sharp knife, then allowed to retract beneath the pectoralis minor muscle.

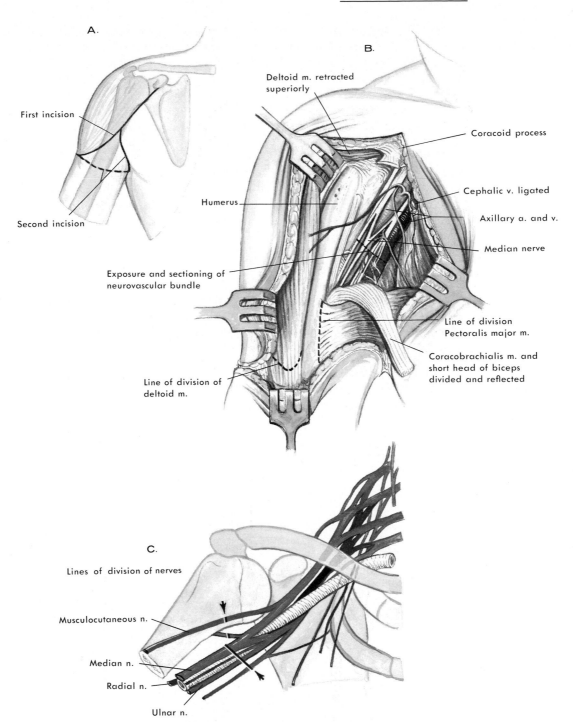

A.

First incision

Second incision

B.

Deltoid m. retracted
superiorly

Coracoid process

Humerus

Cephalic v. ligated

Axillary a. and v.

Median nerve

Exposure and sectioning of
neurovascular bundle

Line of division
Pectoralis major m.

Coracobrachialis m. and
short head of biceps
divided and reflected

Line of division of
deltoid m.

C.

Lines of division of nerves

Musculocutaneous n.

Median n.

Radial n.

Ulnar n.

Plate 7. A.–E., Disarticulation of the shoulder.

D. The capsule of the shoulder joint is exposed by retracting the deltoid muscle superiorly. Next, the arm is placed in marked external rotation. The subscapularis muscle, the long head of the biceps at its origin, and the anterior capsule of the shoulder joint are divided. The teres major and latissimus dorsi muscles are sectioned near their insertion to the intertubercular groove of the humerus. The acromion process is exposed extraperiosteally by elevating the origin of the deltoid muscle from its lateral border and superior surface. The acromion process is partially excised with an osteotome to give the shoulder a rounded smooth contour.

The arm is placed across the chest with the shoulder in marked internal rotation. The supraspinatus, infraspinatus, and teres minor muscles are divided at their insertion.

The capsule of the shoulder joint is divided superiorly and posteriorly. The long head of the triceps brachii is sectioned near its origin from the infraglenoid tuberosity of the scapula. The inferior capsule of the joint is divided, completing disarticulation of the shoulder. The hyaline articular cartilage of the glenoid cavity is curetted, exposing cancellous raw bleeding bone. The cut ends of the muscles are sutured to the glenoid fossa.

E. The deltoid muscle is sutured to the inferior aspect of the neck of the scapula. Suction catheters are placed deep to the deltoid muscle and connected to a Hemovac. The subcutaneous tissue and skin are closed in layers with interrupted sutures.

Postoperative Care. A shoulder prosthesis is fitted as soon as the wound is healed and the patient is comfortable.

REFERENCE

Slocum, D. B.: Atlas of Amputations. St. Louis: C. V. Mosby, 1949.

D.

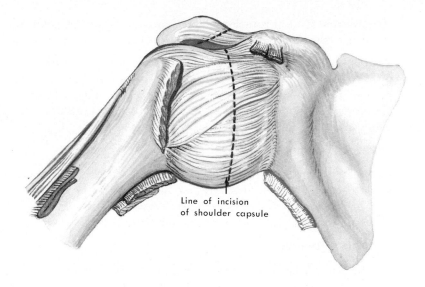

Line of incision
of shoulder capsule

E.

Skin closure with
interrupted sutures

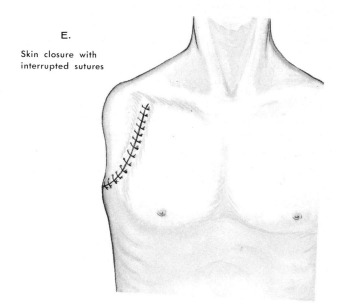

Plate 7. (Continued)

PLATE 8   Modified Sever-L'Episcopo Procedure (After Green)

Indications. Medial rotation adduction contracture of shoulder without joint deformity or dislocation.

Requisites. Normal or good motor function of the latissimus dorsi, teres major, and pectoralis major muscles. *Caution!* Weakness of medial rotation of shoulder may result. Perform Z-lengthening of pectoralis major first; it increases range of shoulder abduction as well as lateral rotation. Transfer only the latissimus dorsi or teres major. Preserve medial rotation strength.

Blood for Transfusion. Yes.

Patient Preparation. A sandbag is placed under the upper part of the chest for proper exposure. The entire upper limb, the front and back of the shoulder, and the lateral half of the chest are prepared and draped sterile. An adequate amount of whole blood should be available for transfusion.

Operative Technique

A. An anterior incision is made, beginning over the coracoid process and extending distally along the deltopectoral groove for 12 cm. When exposure of the acromion is indicated, the incision extends superiorly and laterally.

B. The cephalic vein is identified. It may be ligated or retracted out of the way with a few fibers of deltoid muscle. By blunt dissection, the interval between the pectoral and deltoid muscles is developed and the coracobrachialis, the short head of the biceps, the coracoid process, the insertion of the tendinous portion of the subscapularis, and the insertion of the pectoralis major are exposed by adequate retraction.

C. The coracobrachialis and short head of the biceps are detached from their origin from the coracoid process and reflected downward. In the distal part of the wound, the insertion of the pectoralis major is exposed at its humeral attachment. Both its anterior and posterior surfaces are well defined and separated from the adjacent tissues.

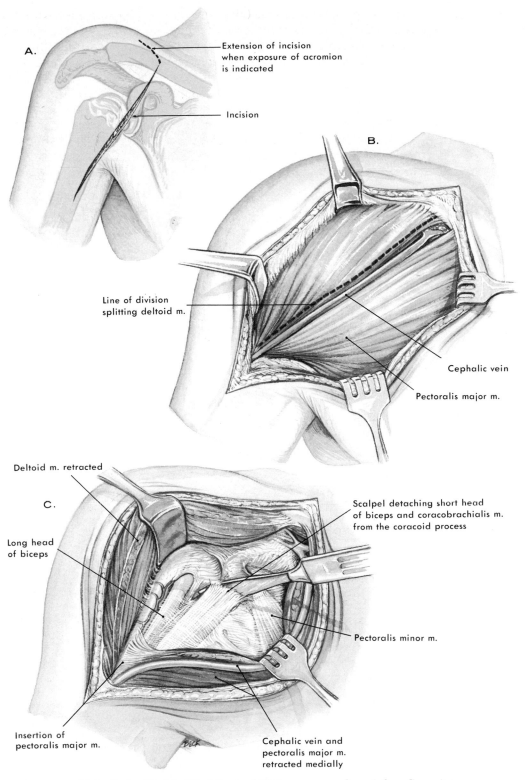

A. — Extension of incision when exposure of acromion is indicated

Incision

B.

Line of division splitting deltoid m.

Cephalic vein

Pectoralis major m.

Deltoid m. retracted

C.

Long head of biceps

Scalpel detaching short head of biceps and coracobrachialis m. from the coracoid process

Pectoralis minor m.

Insertion of pectoralis major m.

Cephalic vein and pectoralis major m. retracted medially

Plate 8. A.–Q., Modified Sever-L'Episcopo procedure (after Green).

D.–F. With a periosteal elevator, the muscle fibers of the pectoralis major are reflected medially in order to expose the tendinous portion of its insertion as much as possible. Z-lengthening is obtained by dividing the distal half of the tendinous insertion of the pectoralis major immediately on the humeral shaft. The upper half of the tendinous portion of the pectoralis major is divided as far medially as good aponeurotic tendinous material exists, usually 4 to 5 cm. from its insertion. Later, the distal tendon stump is to be attached to the proximal tendon left inserted on the humerus, thus providing further length to the pectoralis major. The reattachment of the tendon more proximally permits a greater degree of shoulder abduction but still allows rotary function. At this time, whip sutures are applied to the tendon still attached to the shaft and to the portion of the tendon attached to the muscle.

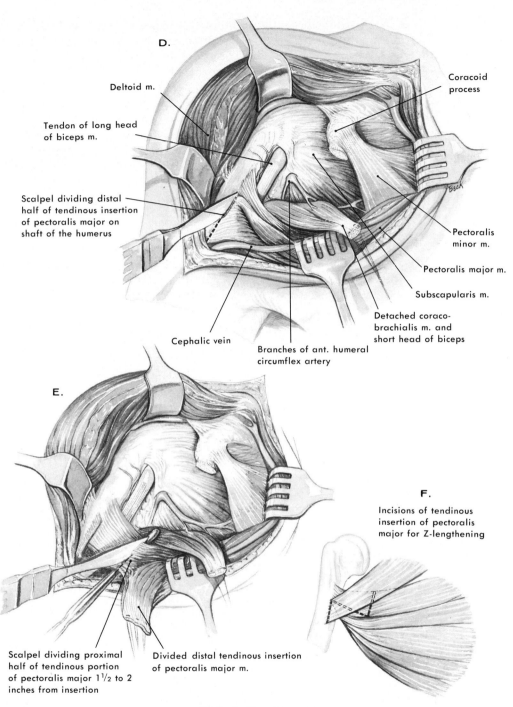

D.

Deltoid m.

Tendon of long head of biceps m.

Scalpel dividing distal half of tendinous insertion of pectoralis major on shaft of the humerus

Cephalic vein

Branches of ant. humeral circumflex artery

Coracoid process

Pectoralis minor m.

Pectoralis major m.

Subscapularis m.

Detached coraco-brachialis m. and short head of biceps

E.

F.

Incisions of tendinous insertion of pectoralis major for Z-lengthening

Scalpel dividing proximal half of tendinous portion of pectoralis major 1½ to 2 inches from insertion

Divided distal tendinous insertion of pectoralis major m.

Plate 8. (Continued)

G. Next, the subscapularis muscle is exposed over the head of the humerus. Starting medially with a blunt instrument, the subscapularis muscle is separated and elevated from the capsule. The shoulder capsule should not be opened; if it is incised inadvertently, it should be repaired.

H. With a knife, the subscapularis tendon is lengthened on the flat by an oblique cut starting medially, splitting the tendon into anterior and posterior halves, becoming more superficial laterally, and completing the division at the insertion of the subscapularis into the humerus. Again, meticulous care should be taken not to open the capsule. Ordinarily, once the subscapularis is divided, the shoulder joint will abduct and externally rotate freely. The coracoid process is excised to its base if it is elongated, and hooked downward and laterally if it limits lateral rotation. The acromion process is partially resected if it is beaked downward, obstructing shoulder abduction.

I. Next, the insertions of the latissimus dorsi and teres major are identified and exposed by separating them from adjacent tissues both anteriorly and posteriorly. The attachment of the latissimus dorsi is superior and anterior to that of the teres major. Both tendons are divided immediately on bone, and into each tendon 0 Tycron is sutured by a whip stitch.

MODIFIED SEVER—L'EPISCOPO PROCEDURE cont'd

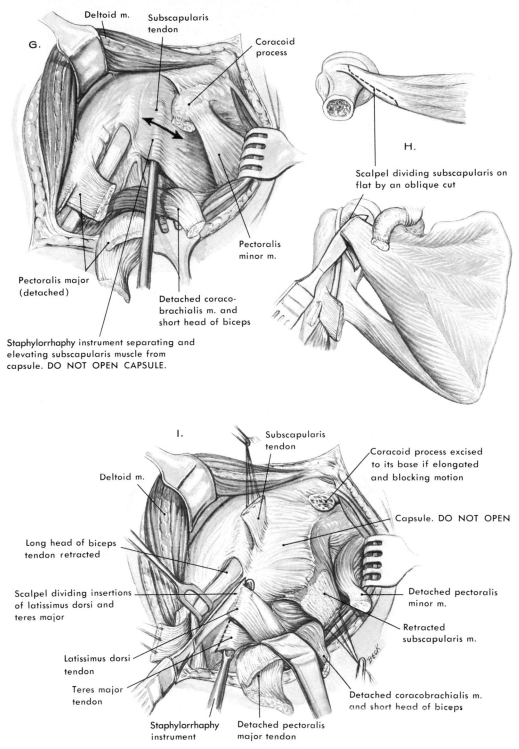

G.

Deltoid m.

Subscapularis tendon

Coracoid process

Pectoralis minor m.

Pectoralis major (detached)

Detached coraco-brachialis m. and short head of biceps

Staphylorrhaphy instrument separating and elevating subscapularis muscle from capsule. DO NOT OPEN CAPSULE.

H.

Scalpel dividing subscapularis on flat by an oblique cut

I.

Deltoid m.

Subscapularis tendon

Coracoid process excised to its base if elongated and blocking motion

Capsule. DO NOT OPEN

Long head of biceps tendon retracted

Scalpel dividing insertions of latissimus dorsi and teres major

Latissimus dorsi tendon

Teres major tendon

Staphylorrhaphy instrument

Detached pectoralis major tendon

Detached pectoralis minor m.

Retracted subscapularis m.

Detached coracobrachialis m. and short head of biceps

Plate 8. (Continued)

J. With the patient turned over on his or her side and the arm adducted across the chest, an incision 7 to 8 cm. long is made over the deltoid-triceps interval.

K. The deltoid muscle is retracted anteriorly and the long head of the triceps, posteriorly. One should be careful not to damage the radial and axillary nerves. The lateral surface of the proximal diaphysis of the humerus is subperiosteally exposed. A 5-cm.-long longitudinal cleft is made, using drills, osteotome, and curet.

L.–N. Four drill holes are made from the depth of the cleft coming out on the medial surface of the humeral shaft at the site of the former insertion of the teres major and latissimus dorsi muscles. The tendons of the latissimus dorsi and teres major are identified in the anterior wound and are delivered into the posterior incision so that their line of pull is straight from their origins to the proposed site of attachment on the lateral humerus. The latissimus dorsi and teres major tendons are drawn into the slot in the humerus and tied securely in position with 0 Tycron or nonabsorbable sutures anteriorly.

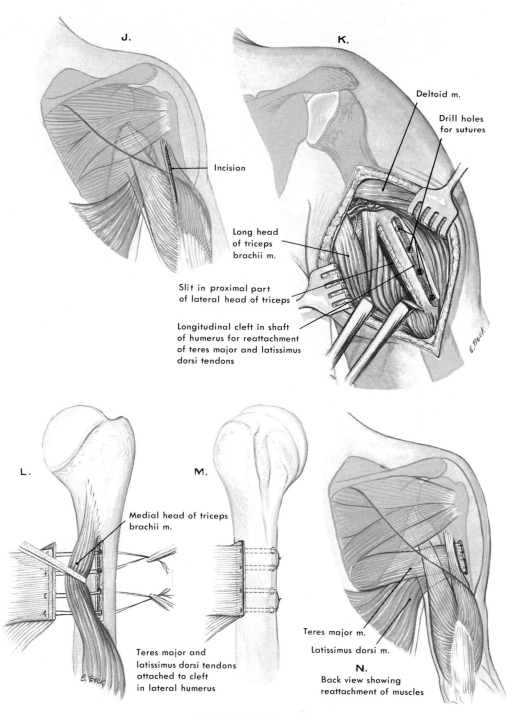

J.

Incision

K.

Deltoid m.

Drill holes for sutures

Long head of triceps brachii m.

Slit in proximal part of lateral head of triceps

Longitudinal cleft in shaft of humerus for reattachment of teres major and latissimus dorsi tendons

E. Beck

L.

Medial head of triceps brachii m.

M.

Teres major and latissimus dorsi tendons attached to cleft in lateral humerus

E. Beck

Teres major m.

Latissimus dorsi m.

N.
Back view showing reattachment of muscles

Plate 8. (Continued)

O.–Q. The subscapularis tendon, which is lengthened "on the flat," is sutured at its divided ends so as to provide maximal lengthening. The pectoralis major is reconstituted in a similar way. The coracobrachialis and short head of the biceps are reattached to the coracoid process at its base. If the coracobrachialis and short head of the biceps are short, they are lengthened at their musculotendinous junction. The lengthened muscles should be long enough to permit complete external rotation in abduction without undue tension. The wound is closed in the usual manner, and the upper limb is immobilized in a previously prepared bivalved shoulder spica cast that holds the shoulder in 90 degrees of abduction, 90 degrees of external rotation, and 20 degrees of forward flexion. The elbow is in 80 to 90 degrees of flexion. The forearm and hand are placed in a functional neutral position.

An alternate method is to use a single anterior incision. The teres major and latissimus dorsi tendons, after detachment at their insertion, are passed posteriorly about the humerus from the anterior incision and reattached to the humerus immediately lateral to the course of the long head of the biceps lateral to the bicipital groove. Another variation in technique is employed when the teres major is markedly contracted; in such an instance, the teres major tendon may be attached to the latissimus dorsi tendon in a recessed position, which, in turn, is attached to the humerus. This allows greater scapulohumeral motion.

Postoperative Care. Almost three weeks after surgery, exercises are begun to develop abduction and external rotation of the shoulder as well as shoulder adduction and internal rotation. Particular emphasis is given to developing function and strength of the transferred muscles. When the arm adducts satisfactorily, a sling is used during the day and the bivalved shoulder spica cast is used at night. The night support is continued for three to six more months. Exercises are performed for many months or years to preserve functional range of motion of the shoulder and to maintain muscle control.

REFERENCES

Green, W. T., and Tachdjian, M. O.: Correction of residual deformities of the shoulder in obstetrical palsy. J. Bone Joint Surg., 45-A:1544, 1963.

L'Episcopo, J. B.: Tendon transplantation in obstetrical paralysis. Am. J. Surg., 25:122, 1934.

L'Episcopo, J. B.: Restoration of muscle balance in the treatment of obstetrical paralysis. N.Y. J. Med., 39:357, 1939.

Zachary, R. B.: Transplantation of teres major and latissimus dorsi for loss of external rotation at the shoulder. Lancet, 2:757, 1947.

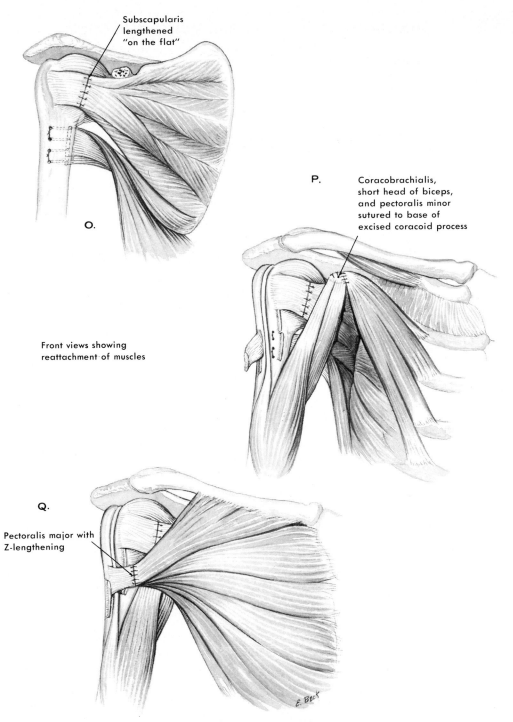

Subscapularis
lengthened
"on the flat"

O.

P.   Coracobrachialis,
short head of biceps,
and pectoralis minor
sutured to base of
excised coracoid process

Front views showing
reattachment of muscles

Q.

Pectoralis major with
Z-lengthening

E. Beck

Plate 8. (Continued)

PLATE 9   Recession of the Subscapularis Muscle at Its Origin

Indications. Medial rotation contracture of shoulder.

Carlioz, in 1976, reported the results of subscapularis recession at its origin in 31 patients with a maximum follow-up of five years. In two cases the results were poor; in one case there was incongruity of the shoulder joint and deformity of the humeral head and glenoid.

Radiograms of the shoulder, in the anteroposterior and lateral projections, should be thoroughly studied to rule out articular deformations. When indicated, arthrography of the shoulder joint is performed.

When the humeral head is flattened medially, advancement of the subscapularis muscle by recession at its origin is contraindicated; derotation osteotomy of the proximal humerus is performed in such cases.

The second case was a failure because of poor postoperative care. In the remaining 29 cases, the range of lateral rotation of the shoulder was maintained or improved.

Requisites. No contracture of pectoralis major and no limitation of shoulder abduction. Congruous glenohumeral joint with no fixed deformity or dislocation.

Patient Position. The patient is placed in supine position and the table is tilted 20 to 30 degrees lateral. The shoulder is flexed and adducted across the chest, with an assistant holding the arm in that position from the opposite side of the table.

Operative Technique

A. A posterior incision is made parallel to the axillary border of the scapula, extending from its inferior angle to the posterosuperior corner of the shoulder joint. (The surgical approach should allow simultaneous lateral transfer of the latissimus dorsi muscle, if necessary.)

B. The subcutaneous tissue and deep fascia are divided in line with the skin incision. The wound edges are retracted. The latissimus dorsi covers the lateral edge of the scapula, with its fibers originating from the inferior angle of the scapula. The latissimus dorsi is undermined by blunt dissection and retracted inferiorly.

C. The scapula is stabilized and pulled distally by placing a Tycron traction suture through its inferior angle, with the help of periosteal elevators. The subscapularis muscle is elevated from its origin, beginning inferiorly and going cephalad. All dissection should be extraperiosteal. There is no danger of injury to neurovascular structures, as they are kept out of the way.

D. The upper part of the subscapularis muscle near the posterior capsule of the shoulder joint is freed.

E. On external rotation of the shoulder, the subscapularis muscle will recess and advance, releasing the medial rotation contracture of the shoulder. Tubes for closed suction are placed, and the wound is closed in the usual fashion.

Postoperative Care. It is not necessary to immobilize the shoulder in abduction-lateral rotation. As soon as the patient is comfortable, guided active and passive exercises are performed to increase and maintain the range of shoulder motion. It is best to make a splint holding the shoulder in 30 to 40 degrees of lateral rotation with the arm in 20 degrees of abduction. The child wears the splint part of the day and at night for three to four weeks. Then the day-wearing is discontinued, and the splint is worn only at night for another six to eight weeks.

REFERENCE

Carlioz, H., and Brahimi, L.: La place de la désinsertion interne du sous-scapulaire dans le traitement de la paralysie obstétricale due membre supérieur chez l'enfant. Ann. Chir. Infant., 12:159, 1971.

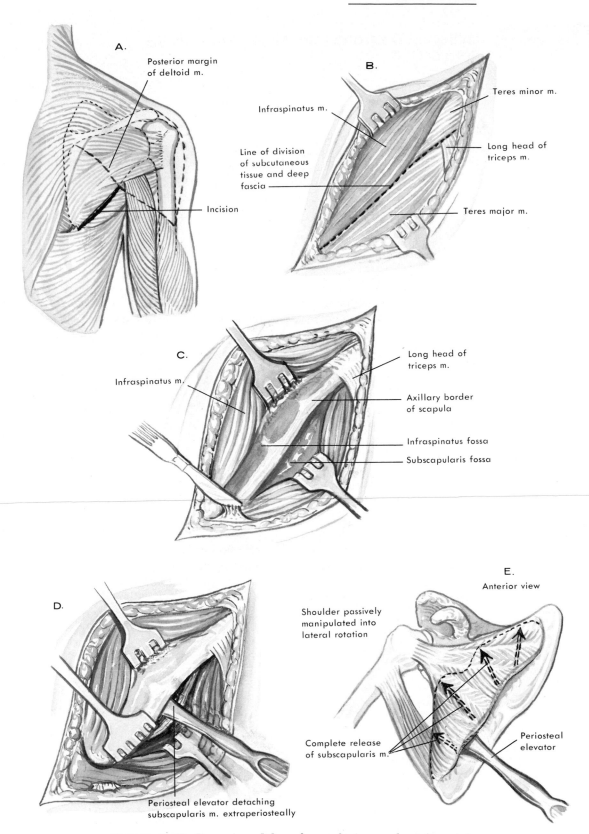

A.
Posterior margin of deltoid m.

Incision

B.
Infraspinatus m.

Line of division of subcutaneous tissue and deep fascia

Teres minor m.

Long head of triceps m.

Teres major m.

C.
Infraspinatus m.

Long head of triceps m.

Axillary border of scapula

Infraspinatus fossa

Subscapularis fossa

D.
Periosteal elevator detaching subscapularis m. extraperiosteally

E.
Anterior view

Shoulder passively manipulated into lateral rotation

Complete release of subscapularis m.

Periosteal elevator

Plate 9. A.–E., Recession of the subscapularis muscle at its origin.

PLATE 10 **Latissimus Dorsi and Teres Major Transfer to the Rotator Cuff**

Indications. Weakness of lateral rotators of the shoulder without adduction or medial rotation contracture of the shoulder.

Requisites

1. Concentrically reduced shoulder.
2. Normal passive range of shoulder motion.
3. Normal motor strength of teres major and latissimus dorsi.
4. Deltoid muscle should be fair or better in motor strength.
5. Motor function and sensation of the hand and pronation-supination of the forearm should be normal.

Contraindications. Poor function and sensation in the hand.

Blood for Transfusion. Yes.

Preoperative Measures. In order to save anesthesia time in the operating room, it is desirable to manufacture a bivalved shoulder spica cast with the shoulder and upper limb in appropriate position for postoperative immobilization. This is relatively simple in the cooperative patient.

Patient Position. The patient is positioned in side-lying lateral posture, and the paralyzed upper limb, shoulder, and neck are prepared and draped. The upper limb should be draped free, and the sterile area of preparation should extend to the midline anteriorly and posteriorly. If there is persistent adduction-medial rotation deformity of the shoulder, the pectoralis major is sectioned at its insertion through a short anterior axillary incision. This author prefers to lengthen and not section the pectoralis major (see Plate 8) because the cosmetic appearance is much more pleasing and it saves power of medial rotation of the shoulder.

Operative Technique

A. The arm is adducted across the chest, and a 7- to 8-cm.-long incision is made over the deltoid-triceps interval. The incision should be proximal enough to expose the rotator cuff. Retract the deltoid muscle anteriorly and the long head of the triceps posteriorly. Avoid injury to the radial and axillary nerves and posterior circumflex humeral vessels.

B. Next, the tendinous insertions of the latissimus dorsi and teres major are identified, sectioned at their insertions, and passed posterior to the long head of the triceps.

A.

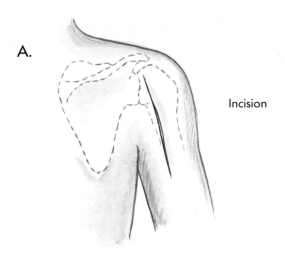

Incision

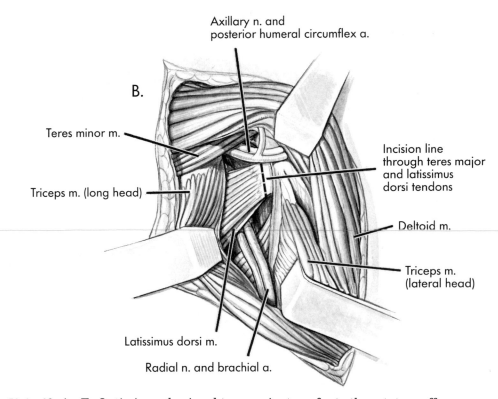

Axillary n. and
posterior humeral circumflex a.

B.

Teres minor m.

Incision line
through teres major
and latissimus
dorsi tendons

Triceps m. (long head)

Deltoid m.

Triceps m.
(lateral head)

Latissimus dorsi m.

Radial n. and brachial a.

Plate 10. A.–E., Latissimus dorsi and teres major transfer to the rotator cuff.

C.–E. The interval between the posterior border of the deltoid and rotator cuff is then developed by blunt dissection. The shoulder is maximally abducted and laterally rotated, and the tendons of latissimus dorsi and teres major are passed through two incisions in the rotator cuff and sutured to themselves. The transferred latissimus dorsi and teres major function as lateral rotators instead of medial rotators of the shoulder. The wounds are closed in the routine fashion. The preoperatively manufactured bivalved shoulder spica cast is applied for immobilization.

Postoperative Care. The spica cast is bivalved four weeks postoperatively, and the tendon transfer is trained as a lateral rotator. Shoulder abduction and medial rotation exercises are performed to mobilize the elbow, forearm, and wrist. Between exercise periods, the shoulder is maintained in abduction-lateral rotation until the transferred muscles are fair or better in motor strength. Thereafter, new shoulder splints are made, gradually adducting the shoulder. The shoulder splint is worn at night for a period of six months.

REFERENCES

Hoffer, M. M., Wickenden, R., and Roper, B.: Brachial plexus birth palsies. Results of tendon transfers to the rotator cuff. J. Bone Joint Surg., 60-A:691, 1978.

Roper, B.: A new operation to improve weakness of the abductors and external rotators of the shoulder. In: Orthopedic Seminars. Downey, Calif., Rancho Los Amigos Hospital, 4:347, 1971.

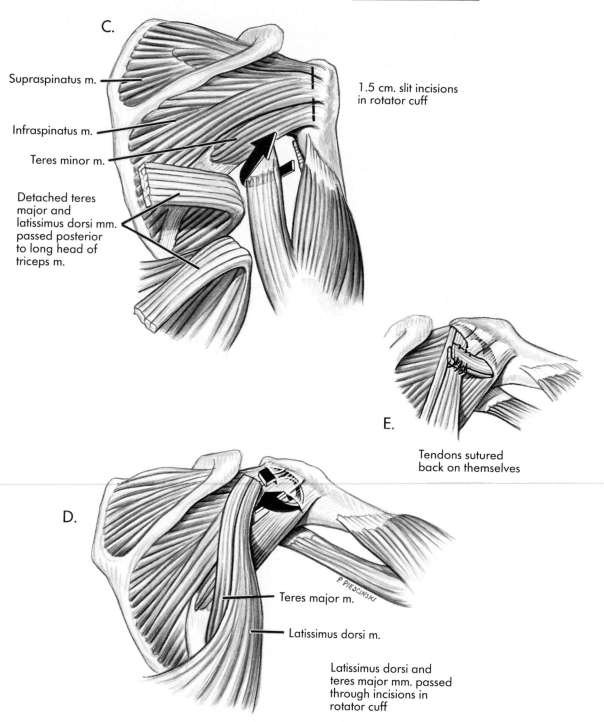

C.

Supraspinatus m.

Infraspinatus m.

Teres minor m.

Detached teres
major and
latissimus dorsi mm.
passed posterior
to long head of
triceps m.

1.5 cm. slit incisions
in rotator cuff

E.

Tendons sutured
back on themselves

D.

P. PIESCINSKI

Teres major m.

Latissimus dorsi m.

Latissimus dorsi and
teres major mm. passed
through incisions in
rotator cuff

Plate 10. (Continued)

PLATE 11   Lateral Rotation Osteotomy of the Proximal Humerus

Indications

1. Fixed medial rotation-adduction deformity of the shoulder with paralysis of teres major and latissimus dorsi (muscles not strong enough to transfer to function as lateral rotators of the shoulder).

2. Marked retrotorsion of the humerus (as demonstrated by CT scan).

3. Structural deformity of the glenohumeral joint with instability or posterior subluxation or dislocation.

4. Positive Putti sign on clinical examination.

Objective. To improve the posture and function of the arm by increasing range of lateral rotation and abduction of the shoulder).

Requisites. Patient at least three to four years of age.

Blood for Transfusion. Yes.

Operative Technique

A. The skin incision begins at the coracoid process, extends to the middle of the axilla, and then curves distally on the medial aspect of the arm, terminating at its upper third. Surgical exposure of the proximal humerus by this axillary approach results in minimal visibility of the operative scar.

B. The lateral skin margin is retracted laterally; with the shoulder in medial rotation, the upper humeral shaft is exposed. Avoid injury to the cephalic vein and anterior humeral circumflex vessels. Do not disturb the proximal humeral physis.

C. The level of osteotomy is distal to the insertion of the pectoralis major and proximal to that of the deltoid. The pectoralis major tendon is lengthened as described in Plate 8. This increases range of shoulder abduction and also facilitates exposure of the humeral shaft. This author recommends internal fixation with a four-hole or five-hole plate.

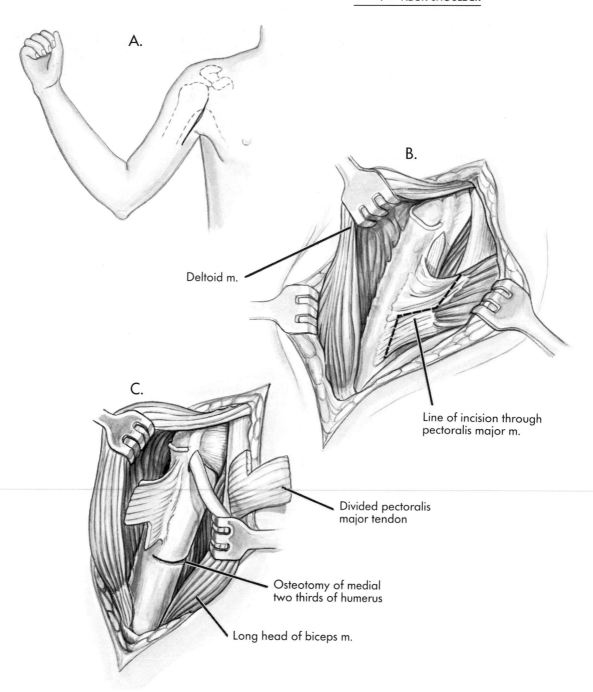

A.

B.

Deltoid m.

Line of incision through
pectoralis major m.

C.

Divided pectoralis
major tendon

Osteotomy of medial
two thirds of humerus

Long head of biceps m.

Plate 11. A.–F., Lateral rotation osteotomy of the proximal humerus.

D.–F. First, perform an incomplete osteotomy of the humeral diaphysis three fourths of the way through the anteromedial aspect. Second, fix the upper humeral segment to the plate by two screws (**D.**). Then complete the osteotomy with an electric saw, rotate the arm laterally to the desired degree, and temporarily fix with a bone-holding forceps (**E.**). Next, test passive range of shoulder rotation. The ideal position of the shoulder is complete lateral rotation of the shoulder in 90 degrees of abduction. Then, with the shoulder in abduction, the hand should touch the anterior abdomen without elevating the scapula. Avoid the pitfall of overcorrection, as it will produce lateral rotation-abduction contracture of the shoulder.

Finally, once the desired degree of lateral rotation is obtained, complete internal fixation of the osteotomy by insertion of the distal two or three screws (**F.**). The wound is closed as usual. The shoulder is immobilized in a shoulder spica cast. In order to save operating room time, the shoulder spica cast may be manufactured preoperatively, bivalved, and fitted at completion of surgery.

Postoperative Care. Six weeks following surgery, the cast is removed and range of motion exercises of the shoulder and elbow are performed.

The results of lateral rotation osteotomy of the humerus are very satisfactory; the improved rotational posture of the shoulder increases range of shoulder abduction.

REFERENCES

Chung, S. M. K., and Nissenbaum, M. M.: Obstetrical paralysis. Orthop. Clin. North Am., 6:393, 1975.
Rogers, M. H.: An operation for the correction of the deformity due to "obstetrical paralysis." Boston Med. Surg. J., 174:163, 1916.
Zancolli, E. A.: Classification and management of the shoulder in birth palsy. Orthop. Clin. North Am., 12:433, 1981.

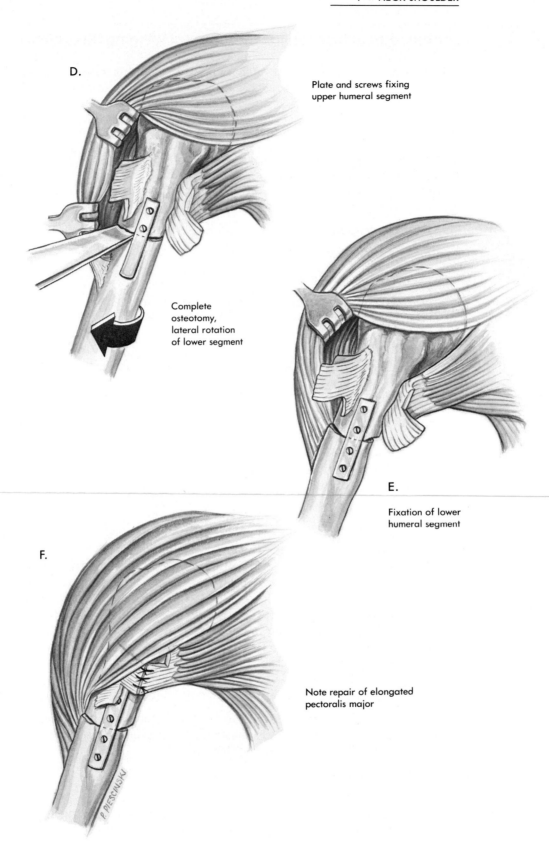

D.

Plate and screws fixing
upper humeral segment

Complete
osteotomy,
lateral rotation
of lower segment

E.

Fixation of lower
humeral segment

F.

Note repair of elongated
pectoralis major

Plate 11. (Continued)

PLATE 12   Scapulocostal Stabilization for Scapular Winging (Ketenjian)

Indications. Limited abduction of shoulder and scapular winging caused by paralysis of scapulocostal muscles, such as in facioscapulohumeral muscular dystrophy (Landouzy and Dejerine). Involvement is frequently bilateral. I recommend surgery on one shoulder at a time because of the potential complication of pneumothorax and difficulty with breathing and respiratory distress.

Requisites. Normal passive range of shoulder abduction and at least fair motor strength of abductors of the glenohumeral joint. It is desirable to prearrange for a thoracic surgeon to be available in the operating room suites in case the pleura is inadvertently punctured.

Blood for Transfusion. Yes.

Radiographic Control. Yes.

Special Instrumentation. Rib stripper.

Preoperative Determination. In winging of the scapula in facioscapulohumeral muscular dystrophy, the scapula is malrotated, with its longitudinal axis deviated medially and its inferomedial angle displaced toward the spinous processes of the vertebrae.

First, determine the position in which the scapula is to be fixed to the thoracic cage. This is done prior to surgery, with the patient standing and the surgeon behind the patient.

A. Between your thumb and fingers, hold the superomedial border of the scapula steady with one hand; with the thumb of your opposite hand, hook the inferior angle of the scapula with the palm and fingers grasping the thoracic cage laterally. The patient's arm hangs loosely at his or her side.

B. Laterally displace the inferior angle of the scapula until the medial border of the scapula is parallel with the longitudinal axis of the spinous processes of the vertebrae. With the scapula fixed on the thoracic cage, the patient actively abducts the shoulder and the degree of glenohumeral active abduction is measured. (In this illustration, active shoulder abduction is 80 degrees.)

C. Next, laterally displace the inferior angle of the scapula, thus laterally rotating the scapula in the coronal (scapular) plane. (In this illustration, the medial border of the scapula is tilted laterally 40 degrees in relation to the vertebral spine.) The patient is asked to actively abduct the shoulder, and the total range of thoracoglenohumeral abduction is measured and correlated with the scapuloaxial angle, i.e., the angle formed by the medial border of the scapula with the longitudinal line connecting the spinous processes of the vertebrae.

At surgery the scapula is fixed to the thoracic cage at the scapuloaxial angle obtained at the maximum desired position of shoulder abduction.

Patient Position. The operation is performed with the patient in prone position. The neck, entire thorax, and involved upper limb are prepared and carefully draped to allow free manipulation of the shoulder.

Operative Technique

D. With the scapula in position to be fixed to the thoracic cage, a longitudinal incision is made at its medial border. The subcutaneous tissue and superficial fascia are divided in line with the skin incision.

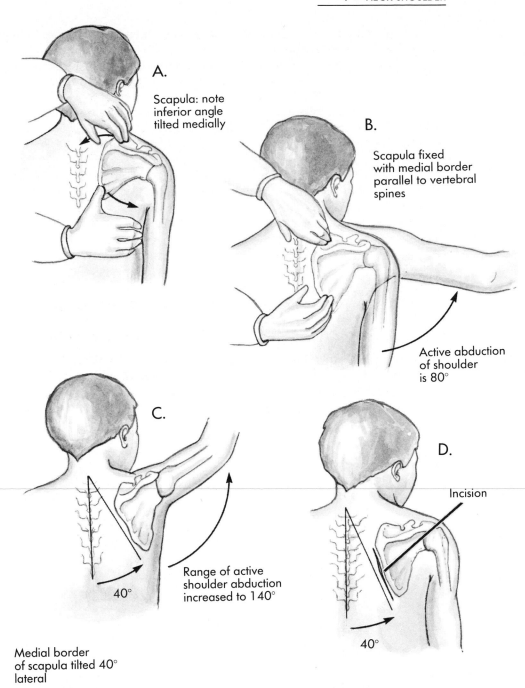

A. Scapula: note inferior angle tilted medially

B. Scapula fixed with medial border parallel to vertebral spines

Active abduction of shoulder is 80°

C. Range of active shoulder abduction increased to 140°

40°

Medial border of scapula tilted 40° lateral

D. Incision

40°

Plate 12. A.–H., Scapulocostal stabilization for scapular winging (Ketenjian).

E. The trapezius, levator scapulae, and rhomboids are sectioned from the medial border of the scapula; these muscles will be atrophic and replaced by fibrous or fibrofatty tissue. With a periosteal elevator, the supraspinatus, infraspinatus, and subscapularis are elevated for a distance of 2.5 cm. from the medial border of the scapula.

F. Next, make four drill holes 1.3 cm. from the medial border of the scapula at the levels of the adjacent ribs when the scapula is placed in the desired position for stabilization. The scapula is tilted to approximately 40 degrees of lateral rotation.

G. Expose the ribs underlying the drill holes in the scapula subperiosteally one rib at a time. *Caution!* Do not injure the intercostal vessels and nerves at the inferior margin of the ribs. Irrigate the operative area with normal saline, and ask the anesthesiologist to inflate the lungs. Look for air bubbles. If they are present, they indicate that the pleura is punctured by the periosteal elevator or the rib stripper. When such a complication develops, a thoracic surgeon is called in for consultation for insertion of a chest tube. Then pass Mersilene or fascia lata strips around the ribs.

H. Pass the strips through the drill holes and tie them snugly, with the scapula maintained at 40 degrees of lateral rotation. Then test the stability of fixation of the scapula to the rib cage. The wound is closed in the usual fashion.

Postoperative Care. The upper limb is supported in a sling. Several days postoperatively, active assisted and gentle passive range of motion exercises are performed several times a day. Codman pendulum exercises are begun seven days after surgery. The sling support is discontinued four to five weeks after operation.

REFERENCE

Ketenjian, A. Y.: Scapulocostal stabilization for scapula winging in facioscapulohumeral muscular dystrophy. J. Bone Joint Surg., 60-A:476, 1978.

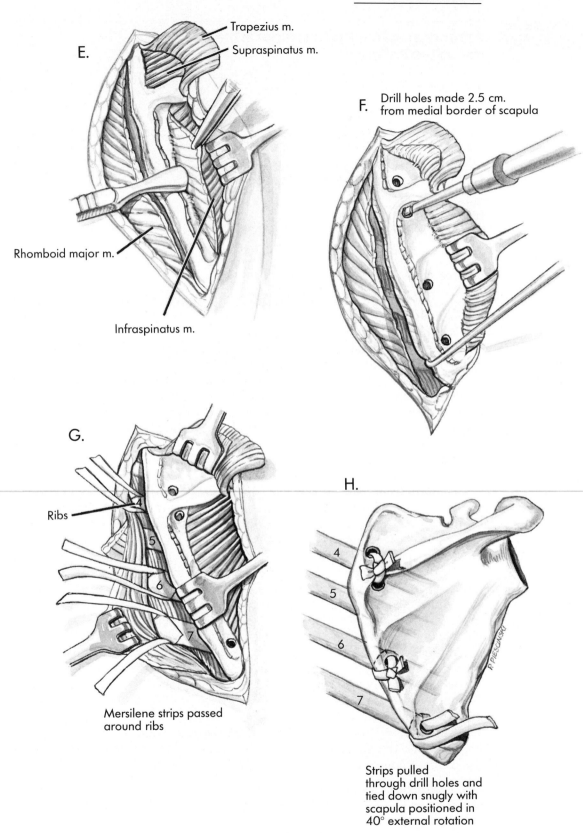

E.

Trapezius m.

Supraspinatus m.

Rhomboid major m.

Infraspinatus m.

F. Drill holes made 2.5 cm.
from medial border of scapula

G.

Ribs

4

5

6

7

Mersilene strips passed
around ribs

H.

4

5

6

7

Strips pulled
through drill holes and
tied down snugly with
scapula positioned in
40° external rotation

Plate 12. (Continued)

PLATE 13

Arthrodesis of the Flail Shoulder in the Skeletally Immature Patient

Indications. Flail shoulder.

Requisites

1. Normal to good motor strength of trapezius and scapulocostal muscles and scapular elevators.
2. A functional hand.
3. Patient at least ten years of age.

Blood for Transfusion. Yes.

Radiographic Control. Image intensifier.

Patient Position. The patient is supine.

Operative Technique

A. The anterior aspect of the shoulder joint and glenoid fossa are approached through an anterior deltoid incision.

B. The subscapularis muscle is sectioned near its insertion. The capsule of the shoulder joint is incised, and the paralyzed musculotendinous rotator cuff is divided at its insertion on the humerus.

C. Dislocate and totally expose the head of the humerus. With the help of osteotomes and rongeurs, totally denude the humeral head of all cartilage. In children the upper humeral epiphysis is covered by articular cartilage on its superomedial side and also on its superolateral side by the cartilage of the greater and lesser tuberosities. Remove the entire cartilage covering the humeral head and not just the articular cartilage. Do not disturb the proximal humeral growth plate, which bounds the humeral head distally.

D. With the help of a power drill, insert two smooth Steinmann pins of appropriate diameter retrograde in a proximal-distal direction; the pins penetrate the humeral head, pass through the proximal humeral physis along the humeral shaft, and exit through the skin at the upper third of the humeral diaphysis. Articular cartilage of the glenoid is curetted until raw cancellous bone is exposed.

E. With a power drill, the pins are drilled distally until their proximal tips are flush with the humeral head; the lateral ends protrude through the skin. The shoulder is abducted until the humeral head is fully apposed to the glenoid; it is then flexed 25 degrees and laterally rotated 25 degrees. Drill the pins into the glenoid and scapula for a distance of 2 to 3 cm. under image intensifier radiographic control. There should be complete bone-to-bone contact, with no remaining gap between the humeral head and the glenoid. Radiograms are made to ensure adequacy of fixation of the shoulder and the pins. The protruding ends of the Steinmann pins are shortened. Their tips are bent to prevent migration and are buried under the skin.

The wounds are closed in the usual fashion, and a shoulder spica cast is applied with the shoulder in the above position. In the skeletally mature child, use compression screws for internal fixation.

Postoperative Care. The pins are removed in four weeks, and another shoulder spica cast is applied for an additional three to five weeks until there is solid fusion.

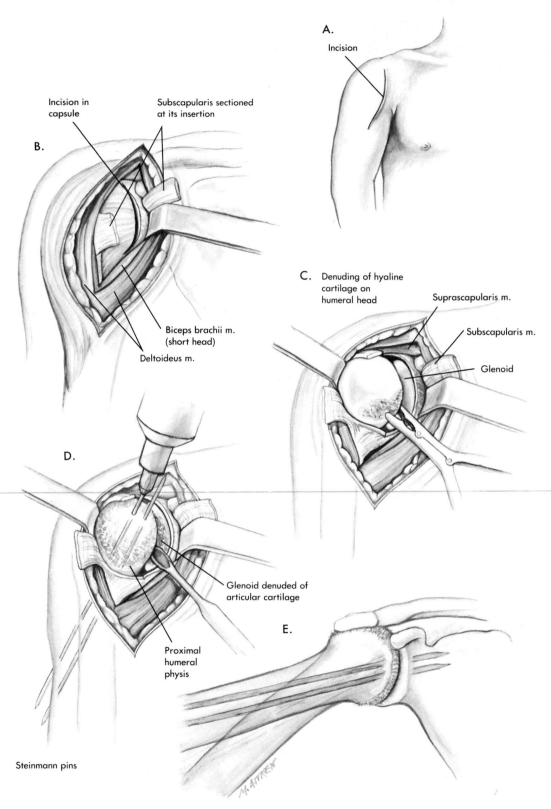

A.
Incision

B.
Incision in capsule
Subscapularis sectioned at its insertion
Biceps brachii m. (short head)
Deltoideus m.

C. Denuding of hyaline cartilage on humeral head
Suprascapularis m.
Subscapularis m.
Glenoid

D.
Glenoid denuded of articular cartilage
Proximal humeral physis

E.

Steinmann pins

Plate 13. A.–E., Arthrodesis of the flail shoulder joint in the skeletally immature patient.

REFERENCES

Mah, J. Y., and Hall, J. E.: Arthrodesis of the shoulder in children. J. Bone Joint Surg., 72-A:582, 1990.

Makin, M.: Early arthrodesis for flail shoulder in young children. J. Bone Joint Surg., 59-A:317, 1977.

Pruitt, D. L., Hulsey, R. E., Fink, B., and Manske, P. R.: Shoulder arthrodesis in pediatric patients. J. Pediatr. Orthop., 12:640, 1992.

Rowe, C. R.: Reevaluation of the position of the arm in arthrodesis of the shoulder in the adult. J. Bone Joint Surg., 56-A:913, 1974.

Saha, A, K.: Surgery of the paralysed and flail shoulder. Acta Orthop. Scand. Suppl., 97:13, 1967.

Tyazhelkova, P. I.: The remote results of arthrodesis of the shoulder in children and adolescents with poliomyelitis sequelae. Khirurgia (Moscow), 43:106, 1967.

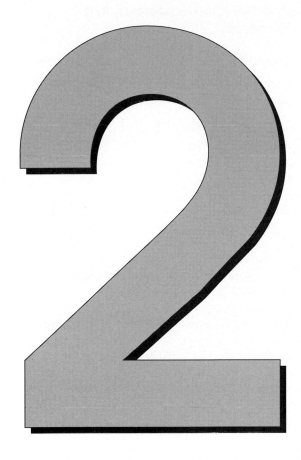

Arm

PLATE 14 **Aspiration and Injection of Depo-Medrol (Corticosteroid) in a Unicameral Bone Cyst (Proximal Humerus)**

Indications. Presence of a thin-walled unicameral bone cyst that is not multilocular.

Preoperative Measures. Assess the thickness of the cortex in anteroposterior, lateral, and oblique projections. Rule out bony septa in the cystic cavity.

Special Instrumentation. Power drill, drill guide, and 16- or 18-gauge lumbar puncture needle.

Radiographic Control. Image intensifier.

Operative Technique

The procedure is performed on an outpatient basis. General anesthesia is used under strict aseptic technique in the operating room. The entire limb and the cystic area are prepared and draped sterile, as in a formal surgical procedure.

A. Under image intensifier radiographic control, the cystic area is determined. If the cortex of the cystic cavity is thin, it is punctured by manual pressure with a 16- or 18-gauge lumbar puncture needle with a stylet inside. Do not break the point of the needle!

B. When the cortex is thick, use a drill guide and an electric drill to make a hole in the cortex.

C. Keep the drill guide in place to facilitate the location of the hole for the insertion of the needle with a stylet.

Caution! Be gentle; do not fracture the cortex and collapse the cystic cavity.

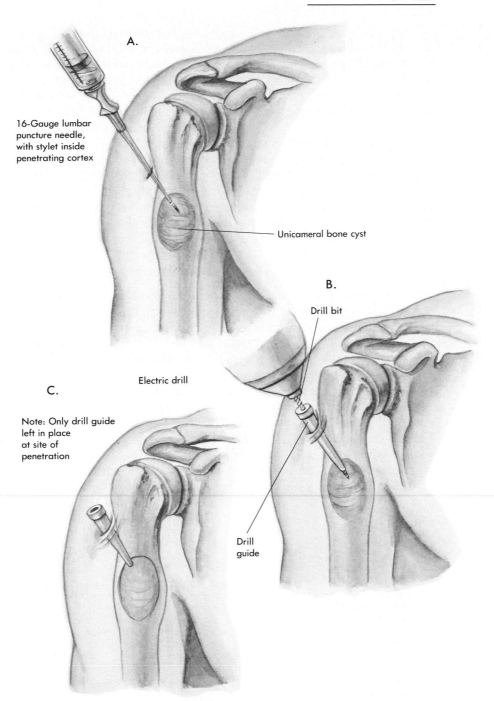

A.

16-Gauge lumbar
puncture needle,
with stylet inside
penetrating cortex

Unicameral bone cyst

B.

Drill bit

Electric drill

C.

Note: Only drill guide
left in place
at site of
penetration

Drill
guide

Plate 14. A.–F., Aspiration and injection of Depo-Medrol (corticosteroid) in a unicameral
bone cyst (proximal humerus).

D. A lumbar puncture needle is inserted through the drill guide. The contents of the cyst are aspirated, and the volume of the fluid obtained is measured.

E. and F. At the inferior part of the cystic cavity, another lumbar puncture needle with a stylet inside is inserted by manual pressure, if the cortex is thin, or through a drill hole, if the cortex is thick. The contents of the cystic cavity are aspirated, and irrigated with normal saline solution for five minutes.

If the upper needle and lower needle do not communicate, a contrast examination, with diatrizoate (Renografin) diluted 1:1 with normal saline, is performed to demonstrate the presence of intracystic fibrous or osseous septa and loculation. The presence of these septa is not necessarily related to previous fractures or surgical procedures. The septa prevent distribution of the injected methylprednisone, and the incidence of failure of healing increases. Therefore, it is important to inject the corticosteroid into each cystic cavity individually in multicameral bone cysts. Seal one needle with a stylet and instill methylprednisone acetate (Depo-Medrol), 40 mg./ml., into the cystic cavity or cavities as a milliliter-per-milliliter replacement of the aspirate, but never exceeding 3 ml. (120 mg.).

Postoperative Care. A simple compression dressing is applied. Immobilization of the limb is usually not required. Weight-bearing long bones of the lower limb are protected by the use of crutches. When the humerus is aspirated, partial support is provided by a sling for a period of two to three weeks. In the lower limb, the duration of crutch protection depends on the integrity of the regional cortex.

Radiographic changes usually are not noted in the first two to three months; therefore, barring the complication of a pathologic fracture, radiographic studies in this immediate post-injection period are generally not necessary. Radiograms to assess healing are made at two-month intervals. Radiographic signs of healing include diminution in the size of the cyst, cortical thickening, remodeling of the surrounding bone, and increased internal density due to calcification or new bone trabeculation. If there is no evidence of healing in three months, the injection is repeated using the same technique. Ordinarily, two or three injections of corticosteroids are sufficient; Scaglietti, however, recommends up to four injections, if necessary, to attain healing.

REFERENCES

Campanacci, M., De Sessa, L., and Bellando Randone, P.: Cisti ossea (rivisione di 275 osservazioni; risultati della cura chirurgica e primi risultati della cura incruenta con metilprednisolone acetato). Chir. Organi Mov., 62:471, 1975.

Capanna, R., Albisinni, U., Caroli, G. C., and Campanacci, M.: Contrast examination as a prognostic factor in the treatment of solitary bone cyst by cortisone injection. Skeletal Radiol., 12:97, 1984.

Capanna, R., Dal Monte, A., Gitelis, S., and Campanacci, M.: The natural history of unicameral bone cyst after steroid injection. Clin. Orthop., 166:204, 1982.

Fernbach, S. K., Blumenthal, D. H., Poznanski, A. K., Dias, L. S., and Tachdjian, M. O.: Radiographic changes in unicameral bone cysts following direct injection of steroids: A report of 12 cases. Radiology, 140:689, 1981.

Kohler, R.: Traitement des kystes essentiels des os par l'injection de corticoides. Lyon Chir., 78:158, 1982.

Oppenheim, W. L., and Galleno, H.: Operative treatment versus steroid injection in the management of unicameral bone cysts. J. Pediatr. Orthop., 4:1, 1984.

Scaglietti, O.: L'azione osteogenetica dell'acetato di metilprednisone. Bull. Sci. Med. (Bologna), 146:159, 1974.

Scaglietti, O., Marchetti, P. G., and Bartolozzi, P.: Sulla azione scheletro. Arch. Putti Chir. Organi Mov., 27:9, 1976.

Scaglietti, O., Marchetti, P. G., and Bartolozzi, P.: Risultati a distanza dell'azione topica dell'acetato di metilprednisolone in microcristalli in alcuni lesioni dell scheletro. Arch. Putti Chir. Organi Mov., 29:11, 1978.

Scaglietti, O., Marchetti, P. G., and Bartolozzi, P.: The effects of methylprednisolone acetate in the treatment of bone cysts: Results of three years follow-up. J. Bone Joint Surg., 61-B:200, 1979.

Scaglietti, O., Marchetti, P. G., and Bartolozzi, P.: Final results obtained in the treatment of bone cysts with methylprednisolone acetate (Depo-Medrol) and a discussion of results achieved in other bone lesions. Clin. Orthop., 165:33, 1982.

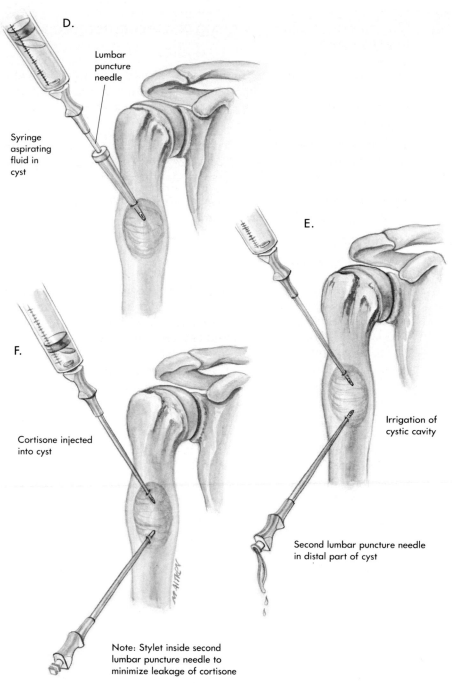

D.

Lumbar
puncture
needle

Syringe
aspirating
fluid in
cyst

E.

Irrigation of
cystic cavity

F.

Cortisone injected
into cyst

Second lumbar puncture needle
in distal part of cyst

Note: Stylet inside second
lumbar puncture needle to
minimize leakage of cortisone

Plate 14. (Continued)

PLATE 15 ## Curettage and Bone Grafting of a Unicameral Bone Cyst of the Humerus

Indications. Failure to heal following repeated local injections of corticosteroids. In the upper end of the femur, this procedure may be the initial method of treatment if the cortices of the femoral neck are thinned and if there is risk of pathologic fracture.

Special Instrumentation. When a cyst in the femoral neck is complicated by pathologic fracture, internal fixation with one or two cannulated screws or external fixator, such as Orthofix or Ilizarov, may be required.

Blood for Transfusion. Yes. When a tourniquet cannot be applied, such as on the upper end of the humerus or femur.

Patient Position. Supine.

Operative Technique

A. Begin the skin incision just below and 1 cm. medial to the superolateral corner of the axillary fold, and extend it distally for a distance of 10 to 12 cm. The subcutaneous tissue and deep fascia are divided along the line of the skin incision. The skin flaps are developed and retracted laterally and medially.

B. The cephalic vein is identified in the deltopectoral groove and retracted medially with a thin strip of deltoid muscle. Ramifications of the cephalic vein from the deltoid muscle are ligated or coagulated.

C. Expose the upper portion of the humerus and the tendon of the pectoralis major muscle by lateral retraction of the deltoid muscle. The long head of the biceps and the deltoid branches of the thoracoacromial artery are identified. It is best to ligate the vessels. The arm is medially rotated, and the periosteum is incised lateral to the long head of the biceps and the tendon of the pectoralis major muscle.

D. Gently elevate the periosteum, exposing the thinned "eggshell" cortical wall of the bone cyst.

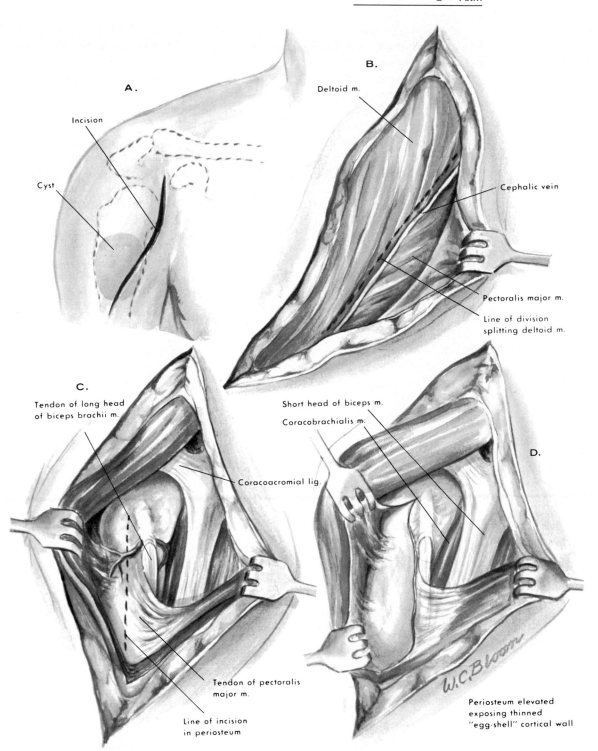

A.

Incision

Cyst

B.

Deltoid m.

Cephalic vein

Pectoralis major m.

Line of division
splitting deltoid m.

C.

Tendon of long head
of biceps brachii m.

Coracoacromial lig.

Tendon of pectoralis
major m.

Line of incision
in periosteum

Short head of biceps m.

Coracobrachialis m.

D.

Periosteum elevated
exposing thinned
"egg-shell" cortical wall

W.C.Bloom

Plate 15. A.–J., Curettage and bone grafting of a unicameral bone cyst of the humerus.

86   ARM • 2

E. Aspirate the cyst. A straw-colored or amber fluid is usually obtained; however, if there has been a recent fracture, the fluid may be hemorrhagic or serosanguineous.

F. Next, with drill holes and osteotomes, make a large rectangular window by removing the cyst wall.

G. Connective tissue membrane is thoroughly curetted from the wall of the cyst. Do not injure the proximal humeral physis.

H. Next, the cavity is tightly packed with autogenous bone grafts. If in doubt, take radiograms in the operating room to determine the extent of the cyst. Usually, the cyst is unilocular; however, repeated fractures may cause partition of the cavity by fibrous septa.

I. The window is closed with an outer plate of iliac bone graft.

J. The periosteum and the wound are closed in layers in the usual manner. Apply a Velpeau bandage, reinforced with a few layers of cast or plastic.

Postoperative Care. Sutures are removed in about two weeks, but immobilization in a cast-reinforced Velpeau bandage is continued for eight weeks until there is radiographic evidence of healing with incorporation of the grafts and obliteration of the cystic cavity.

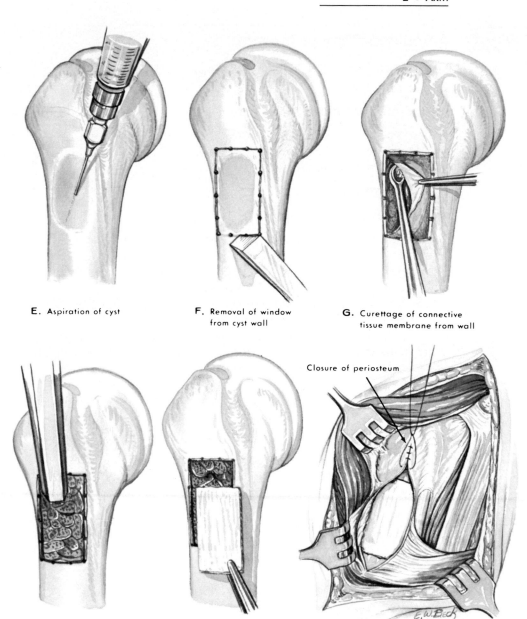

E. Aspiration of cyst

F. Removal of window from cyst wall

G. Curettage of connective tissue membrane from wall

H. Packing of cavity with bone grafts

I. Closing of window with outer plate of iliac bone

Closure of periosteum

J. Bone graft sealing tightly packed cavity

Plate 15. (Continued)

PLATE 16   ## Amputation Through the Arm

Indications. Malignant tumor of the forearm or elbow region in which the limb cannot be salvaged.

Preoperative Measures. Make arrangements with a competent prosthetist.

Patient Position. The patient is placed in supine position with a sandbag under the shoulder that is to be operated on. A sterile Esmarch tourniquet is applied on the axillary region for hemostasis.

Blood for Transfusion. Yes.

Operative Technique

   A. Anterior and posterior skin flaps are fashioned so that they are equal in length and 1 cm. longer than half the diameter of the arm at the intended level of amputation. The subcutaneous tissue and deep fascia are divided in line with the skin incision, and the wound flaps are retracted.

   B. and **C.** The brachial artery and vein are identified, doubly ligated, and divided. The median and ulnar nerves are isolated, pulled distally, sectioned with a sharp knife, and allowed to retract proximally. The muscles in the anterior compartment of the arm are divided 1.5 cm. distal to the site of bone division, and the muscle mass is beveled distally.

PLATE 16

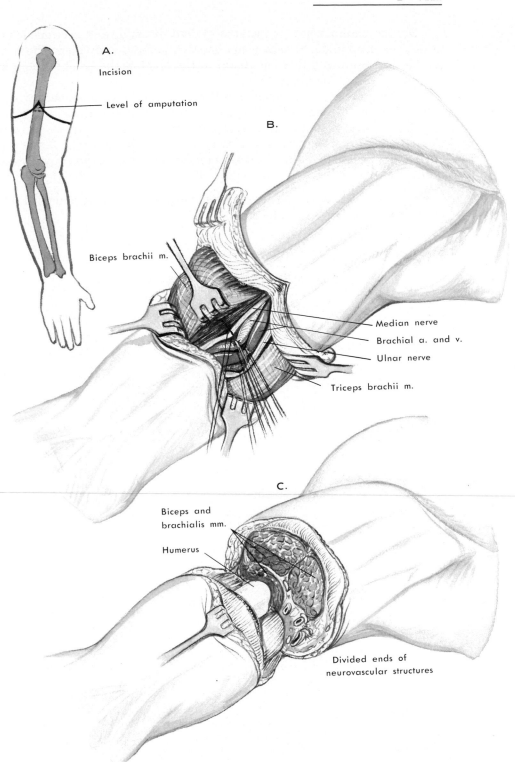

A.

Incision

Level of amputation

B.

Biceps brachii m.

Median nerve

Brachial a. and v.

Ulnar nerve

Triceps brachii m.

C.

Biceps and
brachialis mm.

Humerus

Divided ends of
neurovascular structures

Plate 16. A.–F., Amputation through the arm.

D. The radial nerve is isolated, pulled distally, and sectioned with a sharp knife. The deep brachial vessels are doubly ligated and divided. The triceps brachii muscle is sectioned 3 to 4 cm. distal to the level of the bone section, and beveled to form a musculotendinous flap.

E. The humerus is divided, and the bone end is made smooth with a rasp.

F. The distal end of the triceps muscle is brought anteriorly and sutured to the deep fascia of the anterior compartment muscles. Catheters are inserted for closed suction and the wound is closed in routine fashion. The fascia, muscles, and subcutaneous tissue are closed with interrupted sutures, the skin with subcuticular 00 nylon.

Postoperative Care. The patient is fitted with an appropriate upper limb prosthesis as soon as he or she is comfortable.

REFERENCE

Slocum, D. B.: Atlas of Amputations. St. Louis: C. V. Mosby, 1949.

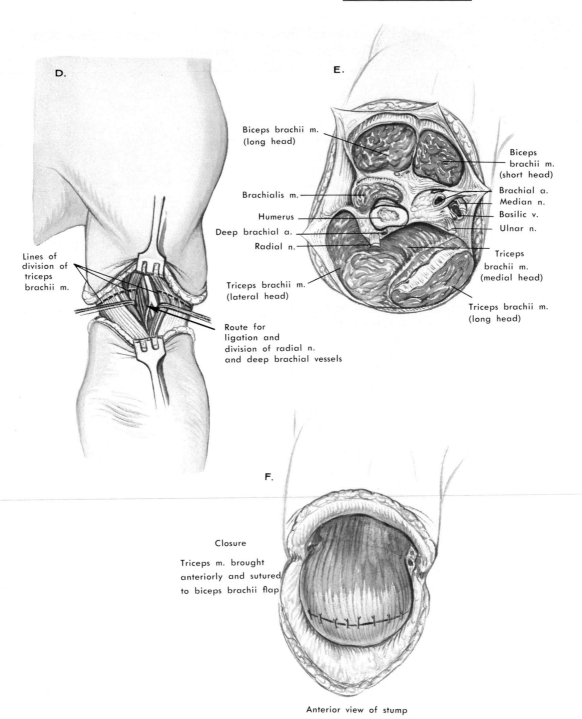

D.

Lines of
division of
triceps
brachii m.

Route for
ligation and
division of radial n.
and deep brachial vessels

E.

Biceps brachii m.
(long head)

Biceps
brachii m.
(short head)

Brachialis m.

Brachial a.
Median n.

Humerus

Basilic v.

Deep brachial a.

Ulnar n.

Radial n.

Triceps
brachii m.
(medial head)

Triceps brachii m.
(lateral head)

Triceps brachii m.
(long head)

F.

Closure

Triceps m. brought
anteriorly and sutured
to biceps brachii flap

Anterior view of stump

Plate 16. (Continued)

PLATE 17 ## Recession of the Deltoid Muscle at Its Insertion for Correction of Abduction Contracture of the Shoulder

Indications

1. Abduction contracture of the shoulder caused by spasticity of the deltoid muscle.

2. Failure to respond and correct by passive stretching exercises and splinting.

Requisites

1. Functional use of hand.

2. Voluntary control over elbow—flexion-extension and pronation-supination of the forearm.

Patient Position. Supine with a sandbag under the ipsilateral scapula and shoulder.

Operative Technique

A. A longitudinal incision is made beginning 2 cm. distal to the insertion of the deltoid muscle and extending proximally for a distance of 5 to 7 cm. The subcutaneous tissue and superficial fascia are divided in line with the skin incision. Wound margins are retracted, and the lower one half to one third of the deltoid muscle is exposed.

B. and **C.** The clavicular portion of the deltoid flexes and abducts the glenohumeral joint whenever the scapular portion extends and abducts the shoulder. By sharp and dull dissection, the anterior two thirds of the deltoid muscle are incised and detached from their insertion to the tuberosity of the humerus. The posterior one third of the deltoid is left intact.

Caution! Avoid injury to the radial nerve.

D. With the shoulder adducted 25 degrees across the chest, the clavicular and acromial portions of the deltoid are recessed proximally on the humerus. If necessary, the recessed muscle fibers may be sutured to the posterior deltoid at a more proximal position.

The wound is closed in the usual manner. The shoulder is immobilized in a Velpeau bandage that is reinforced by a plaster of Paris cast.

Postoperative Care. Three to four weeks postoperatively, the Velpeau bandage-cast is removed. Physical therapy, involving active and passive exercises, is performed several times a day to develop range of joint motion and motor strength of the shoulder abductors and extensors.

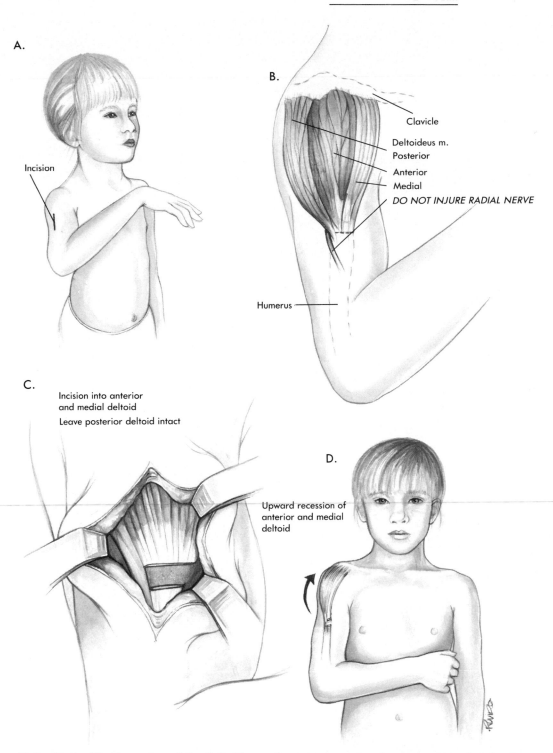

A.

Incision

B.

Clavicle

Deltoideus m.
Posterior
Anterior
Medial
DO NOT INJURE RADIAL NERVE

Humerus

C.

Incision into anterior
and medial deltoid

Leave posterior deltoid intact

D.

Upward recession of
anterior and medial
deltoid

Plate 17. A.–D., Recession of the deltoid muscle at its insertion for correction of abduction contracture of the shoulder.

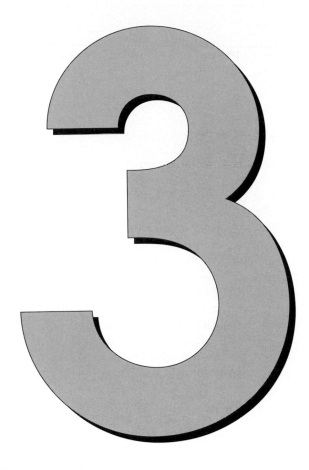

3

Elbow

PLATE 18   ## Disarticulation of the Elbow

Indications. Malignant tumor of the forearm in which the limb cannot be salvaged.

Blood for Transfusions. Yes. The procedure is performed with a sterile pneumatic tourniquet on the proximal arm, but hemorrhage can still be a problem.

Patient Position. Supine.

Operative Technique

A. The anterior and posterior skin flaps are fashioned equal in length to the medial and lateral epicondyles of the humerus, which serve as the medial and lateral proximal points. The lower margin of the posterior flap is 2.5 cm. distal to the tip of the olecranon; the distal margin of the anterior flap is immediately inferior to the insertion of the biceps tendon on the tuberosity of the radius.

B. The wound flaps are undermined and reflected 3 cm. proximal to the level of the epicondyles of the humerus. The lacertus fibrosus is sectioned. The common flexor muscles of the forearm are divided at their origin from the medial epicondyle of the humerus, elevated extraperiosteally, and reflected distally.

C. and D. The brachial vessels and the median nerve on the medial aspect of the biceps tendon are exposed. The brachial vessels are doubly ligated and divided proximal to the joint level. The median nerve is pulled distally, divided with a sharp knife, and allowed to retract proximally. The ulnar nerve is dissected free in its groove behind the medial epicondyle, drawn distally, and sharply sectioned. The biceps tendon is detached from its insertion on the radial tuberosity.

The radial nerve is isolated in the interval between the brachioradialis and brachialis muscles; the nerve is pulled distally and divided with a sharp knife; the brachialis muscle is divided at its insertion to the coronoid process.

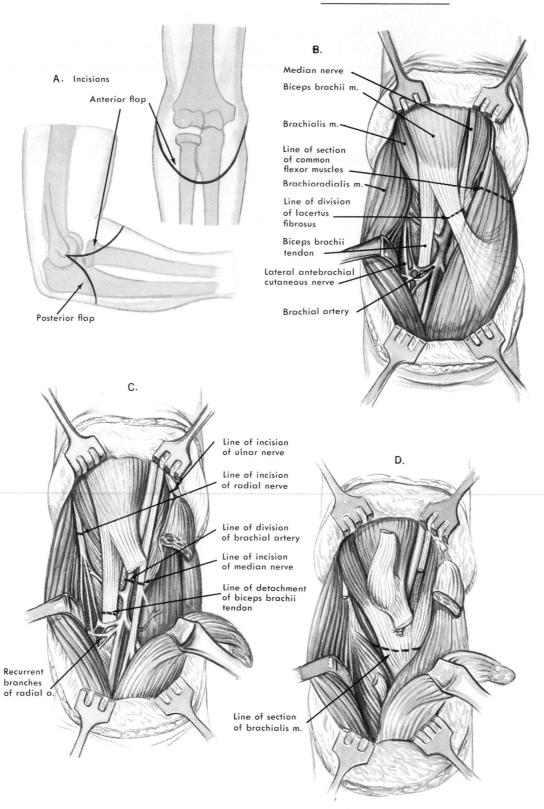

A. Incisions

Anterior flap

Posterior flap

B.

Median nerve

Biceps brachii m.

Brachialis m.

Line of section
of common
flexor muscles

Brachioradialis m.

Line of division
of lacertus
fibrosus

Biceps brachii
tendon

Lateral antebrachial
cutaneous nerve

Brachial artery

C.

Line of incision
of ulnar nerve

Line of incision
of radial nerve

Line of division
of brachial artery

Line of incision
of median nerve

Line of detachment
of biceps brachii
tendon

Recurrent
branches
of radial a.

D.

Line of section
of brachialis m.

Plate 18. A.–I., Disarticulation of the elbow.

E. and **F.** The brachioradialis and common extensor muscles are sectioned transversely about 4 to 5 cm. distal to the joint line. Following detachment of the triceps tendon at its insertion near the tip of the olecranon process, division of the common extensor muscles of the forearm is completed.

G. and **H.** The capsule and ligaments of the elbow joint are divided, and the forearm is removed. The tourniquet is released and complete hemostasis is obtained.

I. The triceps tendon is sutured to the brachialis and biceps tendons. The proximal segment of the extensor muscles of the forearm is brought laterally and sutured to the triceps tendon. The wound flaps are approximated with interrupted sutures. Catheters are placed in the wound for closed suction. The fascia, subcutaneous tissue, and skin are closed in routine fashion.

Postoperative Care. The patient is fitted with a prosthesis as soon as he or she is comfortable.

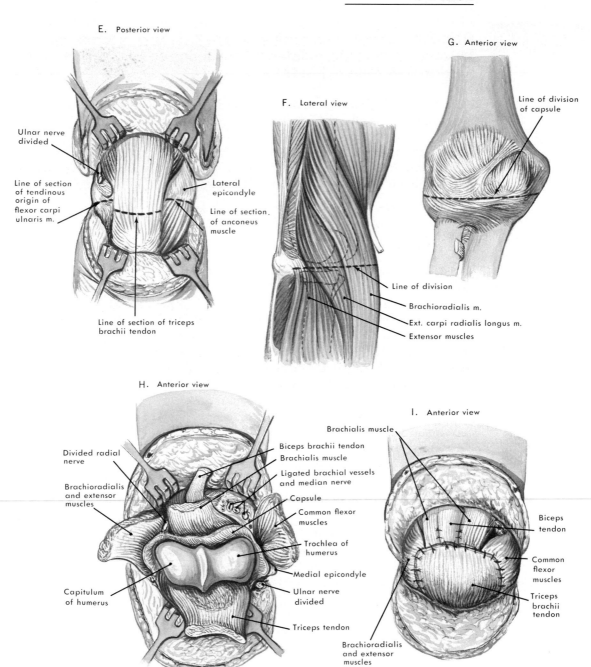

E. Posterior view

Ulnar nerve divided

Line of section of tendinous origin of flexor carpi ulnaris m.

Lateral epicondyle

Line of section of anconeus muscle

Line of section of triceps brachii tendon

F. Lateral view

Line of division

Brachioradialis m.

Ext. carpi radialis longus m.

Extensor muscles

G. Anterior view

Line of division of capsule

H. Anterior view

Divided radial nerve

Brachioradialis and extensor muscles

Capitulum of humerus

Biceps brachii tendon

Brachialis muscle

Ligated brachial vessels and median nerve

Capsule

Common flexor muscles

Trochlea of humerus

Medial epicondyle

Ulnar nerve divided

Triceps tendon

I. Anterior view

Brachialis muscle

Biceps tendon

Common flexor muscles

Triceps brachii tendon

Brachioradialis and extensor muscles

Plate 18. (Continued)

PLATE 19 — Fractional Lengthening of the Biceps Brachii and Brachialis Muscles at Their Musculotendinous Juncture for Correction of Flexion Deformity of the Elbow

Indications. Moderate or severe flexion deformity of the elbow not responding to nonsurgical measures of passive stretching exercises, splinting, or a stretching cast or serial casting. There should be significant functional handicap. Do not operate for cosmetic appearance.

Caution! Do not weaken strength of elbow flexion by overlengthening. Z-lengthening of the biceps tendon will weaken supination strength of the forearm.

Patient Position. The patient is supine. A pneumatic tourniquet, preferably sterile, is placed high on the upper arm.

Operative Technique

A. A skin incision is made on the anterolateral aspect of the lower arm. It begins 5 to 6 cm. above the flexion crease of the elbow joint and extends distally along the lateral margin of the biceps muscle. Avoid crossing the flexion crease of the elbow. The subcutaneous tissue is divided in line with the skin incision.

B. The superficial fascia is divided, with the brachioradialis muscle exposed laterally and the biceps and brachialis muscles exposed medially. A transverse incision is made in the biceps tendon, leaving its underlying muscles intact. A Z-lengthening of the biceps tendon is not recommended because it causes weakening of the supination action of the biceps muscle.

C. and D. Next, the brachialis muscle is exposed. Do not injure the musculocutaneous nerve. Identify and retract the musculotendinous nerve out of harm's way. Make two transverse incisions in the brachialis muscle. The elbow is extended, lengthening the brachialis and biceps brachii muscles.

The wound is closed in the usual manner, and an above-elbow cast is applied with the elbow in complete extension.

Postoperative Care. Two to three weeks after surgery, the cast is removed and passive and active assisted exercises are performed to develop range of elbow extension and flexion. A night splint holding the elbow in complete extension is worn for several months. In the older cooperative patient, part-time use of a Dynasplint elbow orthosis is recommended.

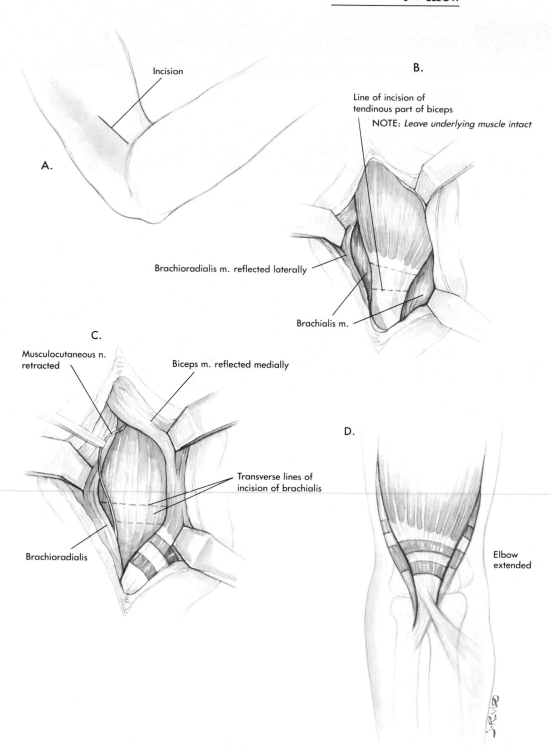

Incision

B.

Line of incision of
tendinous part of biceps

NOTE: *Leave underlying muscle intact*

A.

Brachioradialis m. reflected laterally

Brachialis m.

C.

Musculocutaneous n.
retracted

Biceps m. reflected medially

Transverse lines of
incision of brachialis

Brachioradialis

D.

Elbow
extended

Plate 19. A.–D., Fractional lengthening of the biceps brachii and brachialis muscles at their musculotendinous juncture for correction of flexion deformity of the elbow.

PLATE 20   Flexorplasty of the Elbow (Steindler Method)

Indications. Inability to flex the elbow against gravity.

Requisites

1. Functional range of passive elbow flexion, 100 to 130 degrees.
2. Fair or better motor strength of the triceps brachii.
3. Patient at least five to six years of age.
4. At least fair strength of supinators of the forearm.

Patient Position. Supine with upper limb on hand table.

Operative Technique

A. With the elbow in extension, a curved longitudinal incision is made over the anteromedial side of the elbow, beginning approximately 3 inches above the flexion crease of the elbow joint over the medial intermuscular septum and extending distally to the anterior aspect of the medial epicondyle. At the joint level it turns anterolaterally on the volar surface of the forearm along the course of the pronator teres muscle for a distance of approximately 5 to 7 cm.

B. The subcutaneous tissue and fascia are divided in line with the skin incision, and the wound flaps are widely mobilized and retracted. Next, the ulnar nerve is located posterior to the medial intermuscular septum and lying in a groove on the triceps muscle. It is isolated, and a moist hernia tape or Silastic tubing is passed around it for gentle handling. The ulnar nerve is traced distally to its groove between the posterior aspect of the medial epicondyle of the humerus and the olecranon process. The fascial roof over the ulnar nerve is carefully divided under direct vision over a Freer elevator.

C. The ulnar nerve is dissected free distally to the point where it passes between the two heads of the flexor carpi ulnaris muscle. Avoid inadvertent damage to the branches of the ulnar nerve to the flexor carpi ulnaris muscle. A second hernia tape is passed around the ulnar nerve in the distal part of the wound, and the nerve is retracted posteriorly.

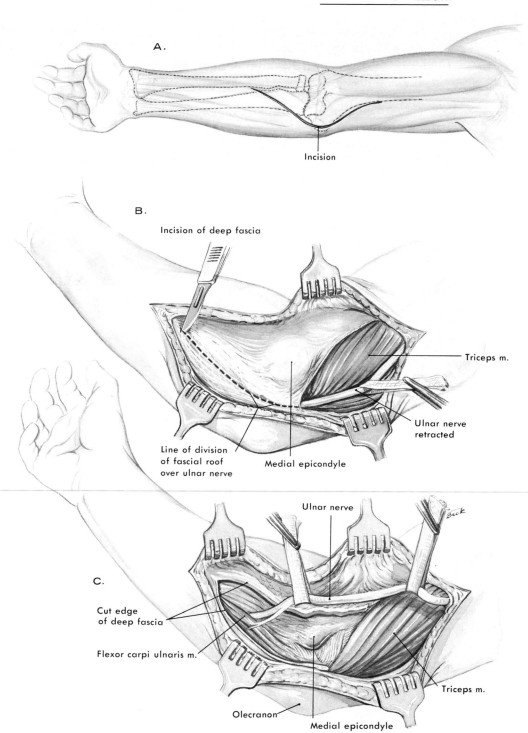

A.

Incision

B.

Incision of deep fascia

Triceps m.

Ulnar nerve
retracted

Line of division
of fascial roof
over ulnar nerve

Medial epicondyle

Ulnar nerve

C.

Cut edge
of deep fascia

Flexor carpi ulnaris m.

Triceps m.

Olecranon

Medial epicondyle

Plate 20. A.–J., Flexorplasty of the elbow (Steindler method).

D. The biceps tendon is identified over the anterior aspect of the elbow joint. The deep fascia and the lacertus fibrosus are divided along the medial aspect of the biceps tendon.

E. By digital palpation, the interval between the biceps and pronator teres muscle is developed. The brachial artery with its accompanying veins runs along the medial side of the biceps tendon. The median nerve, lying medial to the brachial artery, is dissected free of the surrounding tissues and gently retracted anteriorly with a moist hernia tape or Silastic tubing. The branches of the median nerve to the pronator teres muscle must be identified and protected from injury.

F. With an osteotome, the common flexor origin of the pronator teres, flexor carpi radialis, palmaris longus, flexor digitorum sublimis, and flexor carpi ulnaris is detached en bloc with a flake of bone from the medial epicondyle.

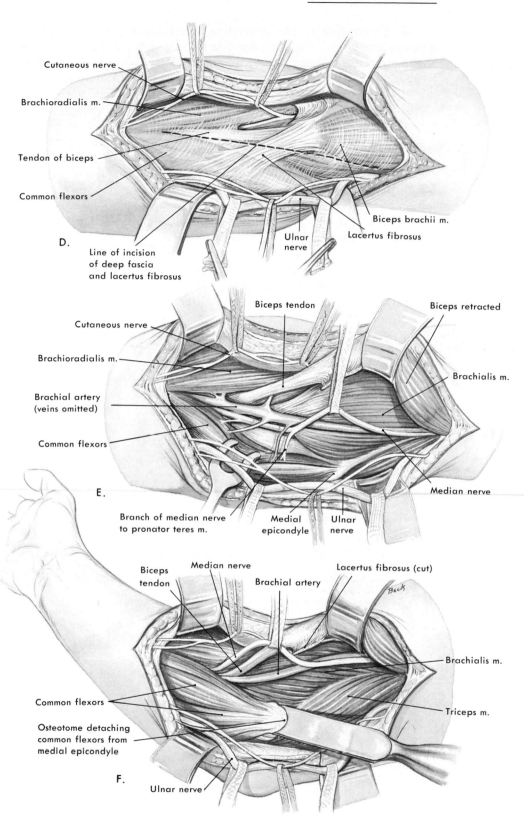

Cutaneous nerve

Brachioradialis m.

Tendon of biceps

Common flexors

Biceps brachii m.

Lacertus fibrosus

Ulnar nerve

D. Line of incision of deep fascia and lacertus fibrosus

Biceps tendon

Biceps retracted

Cutaneous nerve

Brachioradialis m.

Brachial artery (veins omitted)

Common flexors

Brachialis m.

Median nerve

E.

Branch of median nerve to pronator teres m.

Medial epicondyle

Ulnar nerve

Biceps tendon

Median nerve

Brachial artery

Lacertus fibrosus (cut)

Beck

Brachialis m.

Common flexors

Osteotome detaching common flexors from medial epicondyle

Triceps m.

F.

Ulnar nerve

Plate 20. (Continued)

G. By sharp and blunt dissection, the flexor muscle mass is freed and mobilized distally away from the joint capsule and the ulna as far as the motor branches of the median nerve and ulnar nerve will permit. A 0 or 00 Tycron (or nonabsorbable) whip suture is placed in the proximal end of the common flexors.

H. The biceps muscle, brachial vessels, and median nerve are retracted laterally, and the atrophied brachial muscle is split longitudinally. The periosteum is incised and stripped, exposing the anterior aspect of the distal humerus.

The elbow is then flexed to 120 degrees to determine the site of attachment of the transfer (usually 4 to 5 cm. proximal to the elbow). With a drill, make a hole on the anterior surface of the humerus. The opening is enlarged with progressively larger diamond-head hand drills and curet to receive the transferred muscle. The action of the transfer as a pronator of the forearm is decreased by transferring it laterally on the humerus. With smaller size drill points, two tunnels are created from the lateral and medial cortices of the humerus and are connected to the larger hole for passing the suture.

I. and **J.** Because the elbow will be immobilized in acute flexion, it is best to close the distal half of the wound before anchoring the transplant to the humerus. The ends of the whip suture are brought out through the tunnels, and the common flexors and the origin are firmly secured in the larger hole. The periosteum is closed with interrupted sutures over the transferred tendon, thus reinforcing its anchorage. A medium-sized Hemovac suction tube is inserted for drainage. The proximal half of the wound is closed, and an above-elbow cast is applied with the elbow in acute flexion and the forearm in full supination.

Postoperative Care. The cast is removed four weeks postoperatively, and active exercises are performed with gravity eliminated to obtain elbow flexion and extension. A plastic splint is made for night use to keep the elbow in flexion and the forearm in supination.

REFERENCES

Bunnell, S.: Restoring flexion to the paralytic elbow. J. Bone Joint Surg., 33-A:566, 1951.

Carroll, R. E., and Gartland, J. J.: Flexorplasty of the elbow. An evaluation of a method. J. Bone Joint Surg., 35-A:706, 1953.

Kettelkamp, D. B., and Larson, C. B.: Evaluation of the Steindler flexorplasty. J. Bone Joint Surg., 45-A:518, 1963.

Mayer, L., and Green, W.: Experience with the Steindler flexorplasty at the elbow. J. Bone Joint Surg., 36-A:775, 1954.

Steindler, A.: A muscle plasty for the relief of flail elbow in infantile paralysis. Interstate Med. J., 25:235, 1918.

Steindler, A.: Operative treatment of paralytic conditions of the upper extremity. J. Orthop. Surg., 1:608, 1919.

Steindler, A.: Muscle and tendon transplantation at the elbow. A.A.O.S. Instructional Course Lectures on Reconstruction Surgery. Ann Arbor, J. W. Edwards, 1944, p. 276.

Steindler, A.: Reconstruction of poliomyelitis upper extremity. Bull. Hosp. Joint Dis., 15:21, 1954.

STEINDLER FLEXORPLASTY OF THE ELBOW (cont'd)

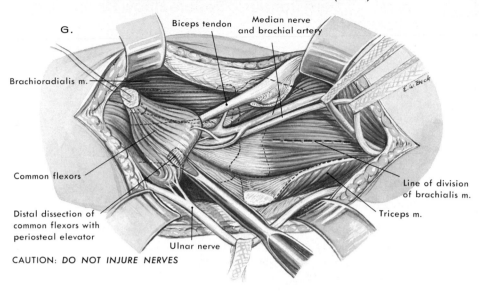

G.

Biceps tendon

Median nerve and brachial artery

Brachioradialis m.

E.W.Beck

Common flexors

Line of division of brachialis m.

Distal dissection of common flexors with periosteal elevator

Triceps m.

Ulnar nerve

CAUTION: *DO NOT INJURE NERVES*

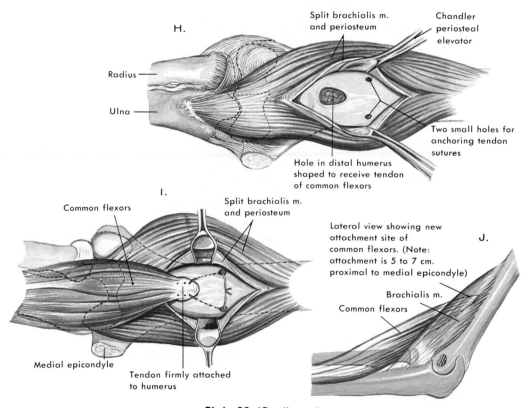

H.

Split brachialis m. and periosteum

Chandler periosteal elevator

Radius

Ulna

Two small holes for anchoring tendon sutures

Hole in distal humerus shaped to receive tendon of common flexors

I.

Common flexors

Split brachialis m. and periosteum

Lateral view showing new attachment site of common flexors. (Note: attachment is 5 to 7 cm. proximal to medial epicondyle)

J.

Brachialis m.

Common flexors

Medial epicondyle

Tendon firmly attached to humerus

Plate 20. (Continued)

PLATE 21
Latissimus Dorsi Transfer to Restore Elbow Flexion and Extension

Indications. Inability to flex the elbow against gravity when Steindler flexorplasty is not appropriate.

Requisites

1. Normal motor function of latissimus dorsi.
2. Good function of forearm and hand.
3. Functional range of passive elbow flexion, 100 to 130 degrees.
4. Fair or better motor strength of the triceps brachii.
5. Patient at least five to six years of age.

Blood for Transfusion. Yes.

Patient Position. It is lateral, with the involved upper limb upward. The entire upper limb, shoulder, ipsilateral chest, and upper abdomen are prepared and draped sterile so that the upper limb can be moved fully without contaminating the operative field.

Operative Technique

To Restore Elbow Flexion

A. The skin incision begins in the upper abdomen over the flank and extends cephalad along the lateral border of the latissimus dorsi to the posterior axillary fold; it then curves toward the medial aspect of the elbow along the medial surface of the arm. At the elbow joint, the skin incision extends anterolaterally and terminates on the lateral aspect of the insertion of the biceps tendon in the antecubital fossa.

B. The subcutaneous tissue is divided in line with the skin incision. The dorsal and lateral aspects of the latissimus dorsi are exposed; do not disturb its investing fascia. The origin of the latissimus dorsi muscle is mobilized by sectioning its musculofascial junction inferiorly and its muscle fibers superiorly. By blunt dissection, the latissimus dorsi muscle is gently freed from underlying abdominal and flank muscles.

C. Divide the four slips of the latissimus dorsi muscle that originate from the lower four ribs and the attachments of the muscle from the inferior angle of the scapula.

Carefully protect the neurovascular bundle that enters the superior third of the muscle. To prevent injury of the vessels to the latissimus dorsi, ligate their branches that anastomose with the lateral thoracic vessels. Identify and gently free the thoracodorsal nerve that supplies the muscle; its trunk is about 15 cm. long and runs from the apex of the axilla along the deep surface of the muscle belly.

A.

Incision

B.

Line of detachment of
origin of latissimus dorsi m.

Latissimus dorsi m.

C.

Thoracodorsal n.

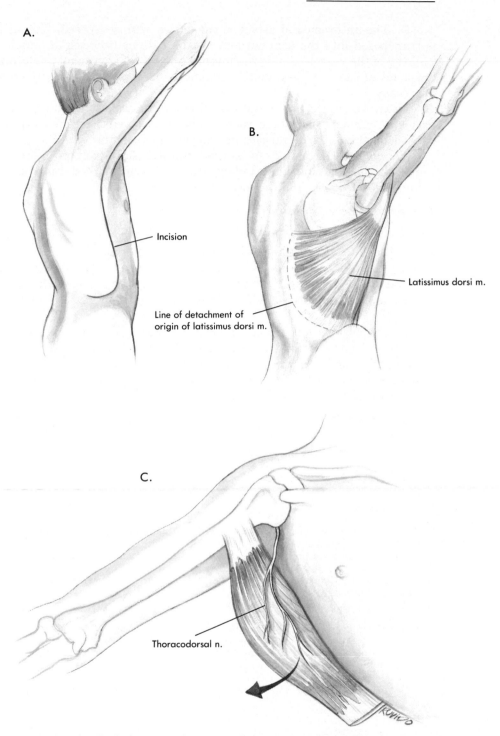

Plate 21. A.–F., Latissimus dorsi transfer to restore elbow flexion and extension.

D. The anteromedial aspect of the entire arm is exposed. The latissimus dorsi is transposed into the arm without twisting its neurovascular supply. To prevent kinking of the vessels, divide the intercostobrachial nerve and the lateral cutaneous branches of the third and fourth intercostal nerves; also free any fascial bands as necessary.

Next, suture the aponeurotic origin of the muscle to the biceps tendon and the periosteal tissues about the radial tuberosity, and the remaining origin to the sheaths of the forearm muscles and to the lacertus fibrosus.

The wound is closed in layers in the usual fashion. The upper arm is immobilized in a Velpeau bandage with the arm against the thorax, the elbow flexed to 90 degrees, and the forearm pronated.

To Restore Elbow Extension

E. The skin incision begins in the upper lumbar region, extending superiorly along the lateral margin of the latissimus dorsi to the posterior axillary fold, distally along the posteromedial aspect of the arm to the medial epicondyle, and then laterally to end over the posterior aspect of the ulnar shaft. The origin of the muscle is freed and elevated. Carefully preserve the nerve and blood supply to the muscle.

F. The posterior aspect of the entire arm and elbow is exposed. The latissimus dorsi is transposed distally, and its aponeurotic origin is sutured to the triceps tendon, the periosteum of the olecranon, and the connective tissue septa on the extensor surface of the forearm. Close the wound in layers, and bandage the limb to the side of the body with the elbow in extension.

Postoperative Care. While the cast is being worn, encourage finger, hand, and wrist movements. At three or four weeks, the bandage is removed and active and passive exercises are performed to restore range of motion of the elbow joint and to develop motor function of the transferred muscle as an elbow flexor or extensor.

REFERENCES

du Toit, G. T., and Levy, S. J.: Transposition of latissimus dorsi for paralysis of triceps brachii: Report of a case. J. Bone Joint Surg., 49-B:135, 1967.

Harmon, P. H.: Technic of utilizing latissimus dorsi muscle in transplantation for triceps palsy. J. Bone Joint Surg., 31-A:409, 1949.

Hovnanian, A. P.: Latissimus dorsi transplantation for loss of flexion or extension at the elbow. Ann. Surg., 143:493, 1956.

Schottstaedt, E. R., Larsen, L. G., and Bost, F. C.: Complete muscle transposition. J. Bone Joint Surg., 37-A:897, 1955.

Schottstaedt, E. R., Larsen, L. J., and Bost, F. C.: The surgical reconstruction of the upper extremity paralyzed by poliomyelitis. J. Bone Joint Surg., 40-A:633, 1958.

Zancolli, E., and Mitre, H.: Latissimus dorsi transfer to restore elbow flexion: An appraisal of eight patients. J. Bone Joint Surg., 55-A:1265, 1973.

D.

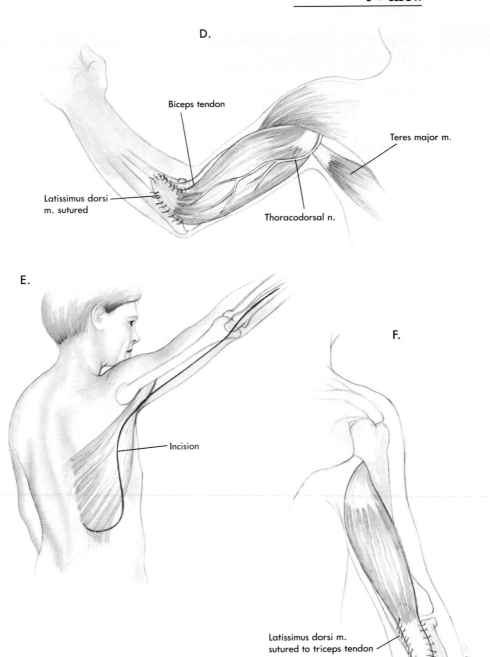

Biceps tendon

Teres major m.

Latissimus dorsi
m. sutured

Thoracodorsal n.

E.

Incision

F.

Latissimus dorsi m.
sutured to triceps tendon

Plate 21. (Continued)

PLATE 22 **Anterior Transfer of the Triceps Brachii (Carroll's Modification of Bunnell's Technique)**

Indications. Extension contracture of the elbow with an inability to flex the elbow against gravity and poor or trace motor strength of the biceps brachii and brachialis muscles.

Requisites

1. Functional range of passive elbow flexion, 100 to 130 degrees.
2. Fair or better motor strength of the triceps brachii.
3. Patient at least five to six years of age.
4. At least fair strength of supinators and pronators of the forearm with good function of the hand.

Patient Position. The patient is placed in lateral position.

Operative Technique

A. A midline incision is made on the posterior aspect of the arm, beginning in its middle half and extending distally to a point lateral to the olecranon process; then the incision is carried over the subcutaneous surface of the shaft of the ulna for a distance of 5 cm. The subcutaneous tissue is divided, and the wound flaps are mobilized.

B. The ulnar nerve is identified and mobilized medially to protect it from injury. The intermuscular septum is exposed laterally.

C. The triceps tendon is detached from its insertion with a long tail of periosteum.

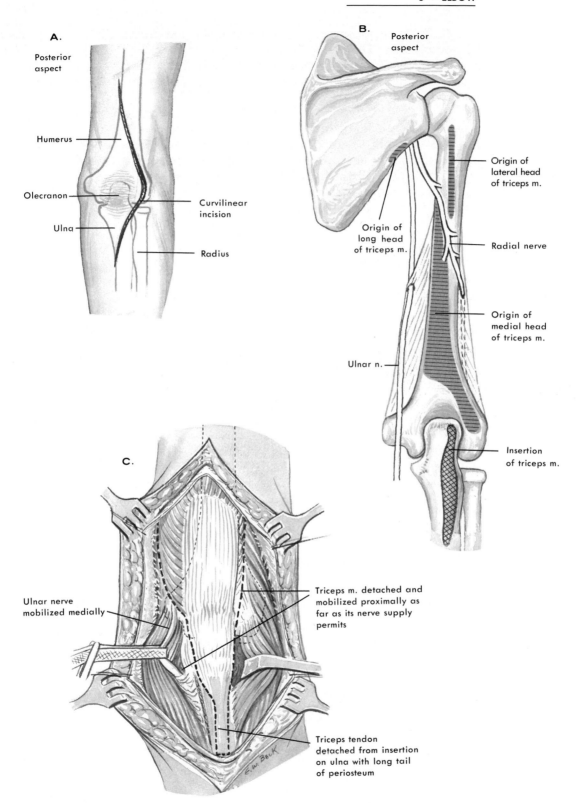

A.

Posterior
aspect

Humerus

Olecranon

Ulna

Curvilinear
incision

Radius

B.

Posterior
aspect

Origin of
lateral head
of triceps m.

Origin of
long head
of triceps m.

Radial nerve

Origin of
medial head
of triceps m.

Ulnar n.

Insertion
of triceps m.

C.

Ulnar nerve
mobilized medially

Triceps m. detached and
mobilized proximally as
far as its nerve supply
permits

Triceps tendon
detached from insertion
on ulna with long tail
of periosteum

Plate 22. A.–H., Anterior transfer of the triceps brachii (Carroll's modification of Bunnell's technique).

D. The triceps muscle is freed and mobilized proximally as far as its nerve supply permits. The motor branches of the radial nerve to the triceps enter the muscle in the interval between the lateral and medial heads as the radial nerve enters the musculospiral groove. The distal portion of the detached triceps is then sutured to itself to form a tube.

E. and **F.** Through a curvilinear incision in the antecubital fossa, the interval between the brachioradialis and the pronator teres is developed.

G. With an Ober tendon passer, the triceps tendon is passed into the anterior wound subcutaneously, superficial to the radial nerve.

H. With the elbow in 90 degrees of flexion and the forearm in full supination, the triceps tendon is either sutured to the biceps tendon or anchored to the radial tuberosity by a suture passed through a drill hole.

The wound is closed in routine fashion. An above-elbow cast is applied with the elbow in 90 degrees of flexion and full supination.

Postoperative Care. Four weeks after surgery, the cast is removed and active exercises are performed to develop elbow flexion. Gravity provides extension to the elbow.

REFERENCES

Carroll, R. E.: Restoration of flexion power in the flail elbow by transplantation of the triceps tendon. Surg. Gynecol. Obstet., 95:685, 1952.

Carroll, R. E., and Hill, N. A.: Triceps transfer to restore elbow flexion. J. Bone Joint Surg., 52-A:239, 1970.

Williams, P. F.: The elbow in arthrogryposis. J. Bone Joint Surg., 55-B:834, 1973.

Williams, P. F.: Management of upper limb problems in arthrogryposis. Clin. Orthop., 194:60, 1985.

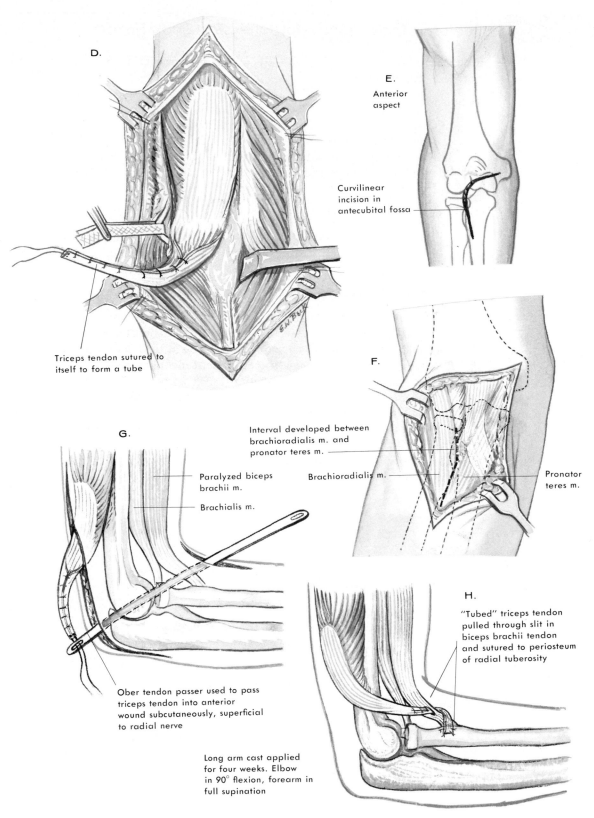

D.

Triceps tendon sutured to
itself to form a tube

E.
Anterior
aspect

Curvilinear
incision in
antecubital fossa

F.

Interval developed between
brachioradialis m. and
pronator teres m.

Brachioradialis m.

Pronator
teres m.

G.

Paralyzed biceps
brachii m.

Brachialis m.

Ober tendon passer used to pass
triceps tendon into anterior
wound subcutaneously, superficial
to radial nerve

Long arm cast applied
for four weeks. Elbow
in 90° flexion, forearm in
full supination

H.

"Tubed" triceps tendon
pulled through slit in
biceps brachii tendon
and sutured to periosteum
of radial tuberosity

Plate 22. (Continued)

| PLATE 23 | **Pectoralis Major Transfer for Paralysis of Elbow Flexors** |

Indications. Inability to flex the elbow against gravity in an upper limb with a normally functioning hand.

Requisites

1. Good or normal strength of pectoralis major.
2. Normal passive range of elbow flexion.
3. Functional use of hand and forearm.
4. Average intellect and ability to cooperate in postoperative care program.
5. Patient at least six to seven years of age.

Blood for Transfusion. Yes.

Patient Position. The patient is positioned supine with the upper limb supported on a hand table with the shoulder in 45 degrees of abduction and 30 degrees of lateral rotation.

Operative Technique

A. Two incisions are made, the first one following the deltopectoral groove extending from the clavicle down to the junction of the upper and middle thirds of the arm. The second incision is centered over the anteromedial aspect of the elbow.

B. Through the first incision, the subcutaneous tissue and deep fascia are divided, and the cephalic vein is ligated if necessary.

C. The pectoralis major tendon is identified and divided at its insertion, as close to the bone as possible. By blunt dissection, the muscle is mobilized from the chest wall toward the clavicle. The deltoid muscle is then retracted laterally, and the tendon of the long head of the biceps is exposed running upward toward the shoulder joint. It is severed at the upper end of the bicipital groove and pulled distally into the wound.

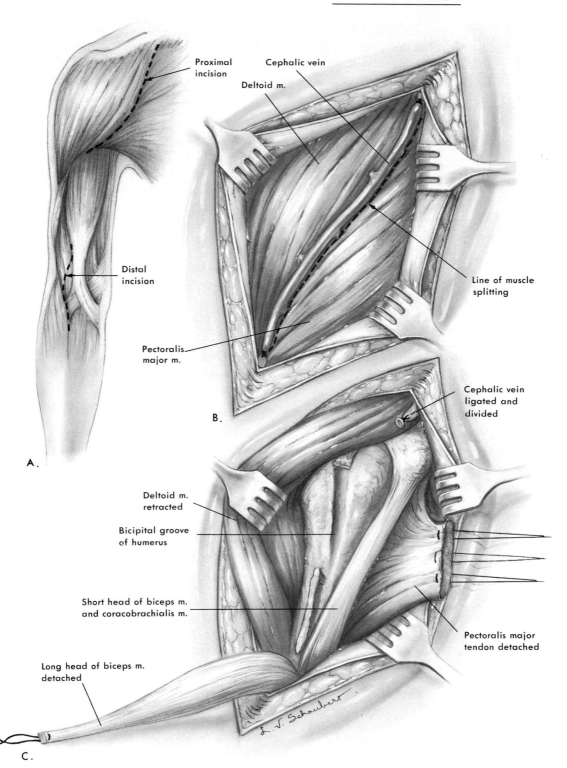

Proximal incision

Cephalic vein

Deltoid m.

Line of muscle splitting

Distal incision

Pectoralis major m.

A.

B.

Cephalic vein ligated and divided

Deltoid m. retracted

Bicipital groove of humerus

Short head of biceps m. and coracobrachialis m.

Pectoralis major tendon detached

Long head of biceps m. detached

C.

Plate 23. **A.–E.,** Pectoralis major transfer for paralysis of elbow flexors.

D. By blunt and sharp dissection, the muscle belly of the long head of the biceps is mobilized to the lowest third of the arm by freeing it from the short head. The vessels and nerves entering the muscle belly are divided and ligated as necessary. The tendon and muscle of the long head are delivered into the distal second incision and freed down to the tuberosity of the radius. Often, freeing the muscle from adhesions to the overlying fascia requires sharp dissection. After complete mobilization of the long head of the biceps by traction on its proximal end, one should be able to flex the elbow.

E. The long head of the biceps is pulled into the upper wound. Two slits are made in the tendon of the mobilized pectoralis major through which the tendon of the long head is passed, looped on itself, and brought down again into the distal wound. With the elbow acutely flexed, the proximal end of the tendon is sutured to its own tendon of insertion through a slit in the distal tendon. Tycron or nonabsorbable sutures are also inserted at the level of the tendon of the pectoralis major. The incisions are then closed in the routine manner. A plaster of Paris or plastic reinforced Velpeau bandage is applied with the elbow acutely flexed.

Postoperative Care. Plaster of Paris immobilization is continued for three weeks. At the end of this time, active flexion and extension exercises of the elbow are started, first with gravity eliminated and then against gravity. A sling is used to protect the transferred tendon from stretching. Care should be taken to extend the elbow gradually so that active flexion beyond the right-angle position is maintained. Extension of the elbow is regained slowly.

REFERENCES

Brooks, D. M., and Seddon, H. J.: Pectoral transplantation for paralysis of the flexor of the elbow. A new technique. J. Bone Joint Surg., 41-B:36, 1959.

Clark, J. M. P.: Reconstruction of biceps brachii by pectoral muscles transplantation. Br. J. Surg., 34:180, 1946.

Hohmann, G.: Eratz des gelahmten Biceps brachii durch den Pectoralis major. Munchen Med. Wochenschr., 65:1240, 1918.

Seddon, H. J.: Transplantation of pectoralis major for paralysis of the flexors of the elbow. Proc. R. Soc. Med., 42:837, 1949.

Segal, A., Seddon, H. J., and Brooks, D. M.: Treatment of paralysis of the flexors of the elbow. J. Bone Joint Surg., 41-B:44, 1959.

Spira, E.: The treatment of dropped shoulder: A new operative technique. J. Bone Joint Surg., 30-A:220, 1948.

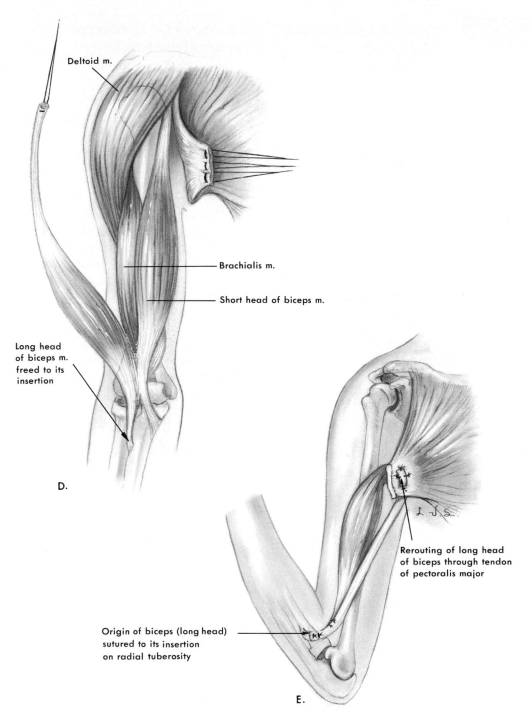

Deltoid m.

Brachialis m.

Short head of biceps m.

Long head
of biceps m.
freed to its
insertion

D.

Rerouting of long head
of biceps through tendon
of pectoralis major

Origin of biceps (long head)
sutured to its insertion
on radial tuberosity

E.

Plate 23. (Continued)

PLATE 24

Closed Reduction and Percutaneous Pin Fixation of a Displaced or Unstable Supracondylar Fracture of the Humerus

Indications. Unstable supracondylar fracture of the humerus.

Special Instrumentation. Power drill driver, drill guide, and Steinmann pins for percutaneous pin fixation.

Radiographic Control. Image intensifier.

Patient Position. General anesthesia is given. The child is completely relaxed and in a supine position. The prone position is preferred by some surgeons, particularly if there is a possibility of open reduction of a severely displaced fracture. The prone position provides ready anatomic accessibility of the medial epicondyle and lateral condyle of the humerus for pin insertion; however, visual orientation of the accuracy of reduction and proper orientation of the fragments with image intensification are more difficult than when the child is supine. I prefer the supine position for closed reduction and percutaneous pinning.

Operative Technique

A.–D. First, take further radiograms, if the preoperative films were not adequate, to delineate the degree and direction of the fracture and to determine whether the physis is involved. Rule out comminution of the cortices. The entire upper limb is prepared and draped sterile in the usual fashion.

During the making of the radiograms and the patient preparation, one surgeon should hold the upper limb in slight flexion while the assistant prepares and drapes.

Caution! To prevent further neurovascular injury, do not flex or hyperextend the elbow.

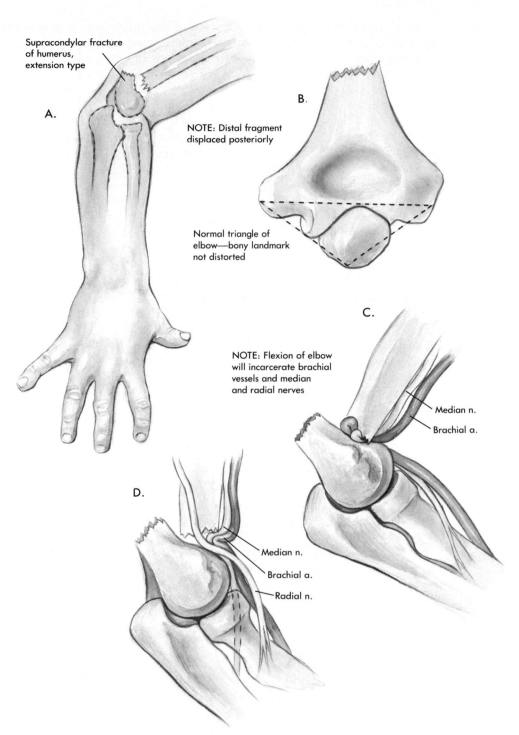

Supracondylar fracture of humerus, extension type

A.

B.

NOTE: Distal fragment displaced posteriorly

Normal triangle of elbow—bony landmark not distorted

C.

NOTE: Flexion of elbow will incarcerate brachial vessels and median and radial nerves

Median n.

Brachial a.

D.

Median n.

Brachial a.

Radial n.

Plate 24. A.–P., Closed reduction and percutaneous pin fixation of a displaced or unstable supracondylar fracture of the humerus.

E. The technique of closed reduction of the displaced, hyperextension type of supracondylar fracture of the humerus is performed as follows. Restore length first by traction and countertraction with the elbow in extension—but *not hyperextension*—to prevent pulling and injury of the brachial vessels.

F. Next, while maintaining traction (with the forearm pronated and the elbow in slight flexion), reduce posterior displacement of the distal fragment by lifting it anteriorly and by pushing the proximal fragment posteriorly.

G. Reduce lateral displacement by pushing the distal fragment medially; any rotation deformity is also corrected at this time.

H. The elbow is hyperflexed to 90 degrees to tighten the posterior hinge of the periosteum and to maintain the reduction.

In supracondylar fractures, the biceps brachii muscle loses its supinating action because of the break in continuity of the humerus. The unopposed action of the strong pronator teres muscle swings the proximal radioulnar joint into pronation. Because the joint is fixed by the pronators, varus deformity at the fracture site will result.

The direction of original displacement of the distal fragment is another consideration in deciding the position of the forearm when it is immobilized in the cast. If it was *displaced medially,* the forearm is *pronated* in order to tighten the medial hinge and to close the fracture line on the lateral side, thus preventing any cubitus varus deformity; if it was *displaced laterally, supination* of the forearm will tighten the lateral periosteal hinge and close the fracture line on the medial side, thus preventing cubitus valgus.

Next, make radiograms in the anteroposterior and lateral projections to determine the adequacy of reduction. *Any medial or lateral tilting of the distal fragment must be completely corrected;* if not corrected, cubitus varus or valgus deformity will result. Appositional malalignments are inconsequential, as they correct themselves spontaneously by extensive remodeling and have no effect on the carrying angle or final range of motion of the elbow. Rotation of the distal fragment is not corrected by remodeling and may look bizarre in the radiogram, but it will be compensated clinically by rotation at the shoulder. Posterior angulation of the distal fragment results in hyperextension at the elbow and anterior angulation in flexion deformity; however, these deformities are in the plane of motion of the elbow and spontaneously correct themselves.

Vigorous manipulations and remanipulations should be avoided, as they may cause further damage to vessels, nerves, and soft tissues.

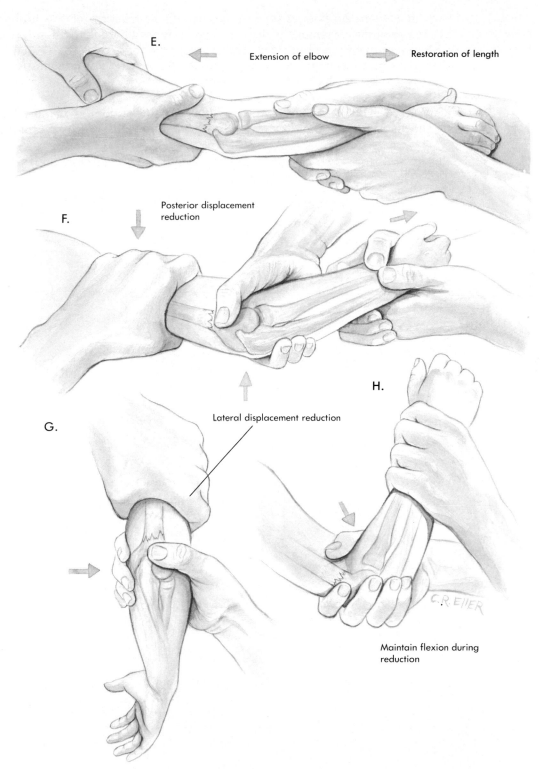

E. ← Extension of elbow   → Restoration of length

Posterior displacement reduction

F.

Lateral displacement reduction

G.

H.

Maintain flexion during reduction

Plate 24. (Continued)

I. and J. In the flexion type of supracondylar fracture of the humerus, note that the proximal fragment is displaced posteriorly whereas the distal fragment is displaced anteriorly and upward. The ulnar nerve tents over the posterior margin of the proximal fragment and is at high risk for injury. The brachial vessels may be kinked between the fracture fragments.

K. and L. Closed reduction is carried out by longitudinal traction with the elbow in extension to restore length. The proximal fragment is displaced anteriorly and the distal fragment posteriorly. Correct any lateral tilting by manual pressure.

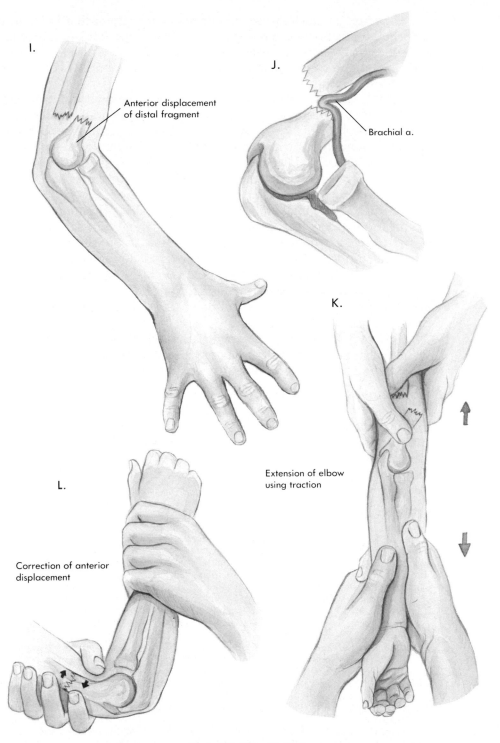

I.

Anterior displacement
of distal fragment

J.

Brachial a.

K.

Extension of elbow
using traction

L.

Correction of anterior
displacement

Plate 24. (Continued)

M. After satisfactory reduction, peripheral circulation is again assessed; if it is normal, percutaneous pinning is performed under image intensifier radiographic control. Smooth pins are used because they do not disturb growth. Make a stab wound over the medial epicondyle of the humerus and a second stab wound over the lateral epicondyle.

N. The stab wounds are enlarged and deepened with Metzenbaum scissors.

O. Use a drill guide to locate the lateral epicondyle under image intensifier radiographic control. With an electric power drill, a smooth Steinmann pin of adequate diameter is then drilled across the fracture site, engaging the opposite cortex of the proximal fragment of the distal humerus. Anteroposterior and lateral projections are made with image intensification to verify the position of the pin and the accuracy of reduction.

P. Then, following similar technique, a smooth Steinmann pin is drilled from the medial epicondyle, across the fracture site and into the opposite lateral cortex of the proximal fragment. Again, determine the position of the pins by image intensifier radiographic control. Criss-cross pins provide secure fixation. The tips of the pins are cut subcutaneously, and their tips are bent and buried in subcutaneous tissue in order to prevent migration. Some surgeons leave the tips of the pins protruding out of the skin. I don't like this method because of the probable risk of pin tract infection.

Apply an above-elbow cast with the elbow in 45 to 60 degrees of flexion and the forearm in 45 degrees of pronation. Extreme positions of the forearm and elbow are not required because of stability of fixation by the pins.

Postoperative Care. The patient is admitted to the hospital for observation of neurovascular function and possible development of compartment syndrome or Volkmann's ischemia. The pins are removed three to four weeks postoperatively. Another cast is applied for an additional two to three weeks, depending on the radiographic state of fracture healing. After removal of the cast, active assisted exercises are performed to restore range of motion of the elbow.

REFERENCES

Arino, V. L., Lluch, E. E., Ramirez, A. M., Ferrer, J., Rodriquez, L., and Baixault, F.: Percutaneous fixation of supracondylar fractures of the humerus in children. J. Bone Joint Surg., 59-A:914, 1977.

Aronson, D. D., and Prager, B. I.: Supracondylar fractures of the humerus in children: A modified technique for closed pinning. Clin. Orthop., 219:174, 1987.

Childress, H. M.: Transarticular pin fixation in supracondylar fractures at the elbow in children. A case report. J. Bone Joint Surg., 54-A:1548, 1972.

Flynn, J. C., Matthews, J. G., and Benoit, R. L.: Blind pinning of displaced supracondylar fractures of the humerus in children: Sixteen years' experience with long-term follow-up. J. Bone Joint Surg., 56-A:263, 1974.

Fowles, J. B., and Kassab, M. T.: Displaced supracondylar fractures of the elbow in children: Report on the fixation of extension and flexion fractures by two lateral percutaneous pins. J. Bone Joint Surg., 56-B:4590, 1974.

Haddad, R. J., Jr., Saer, J. K., and Riordan, D. C.: Percutaneous pinning of displaced supracondylar fractures of the elbow in children. Clin. Orthop., 71:112, 1970.

Jones, K. G.: Percutaneous pin fixation of fractures of the lower end of the humerus. Clin. Orthop., 50:53, 1967.

Kallio, P. E., Foster, B. K., and Paterson, D. C.: Difficult supracondylar elbow fractures in children. Analysis of percutaneous pinning technique. J. Pediatr. Orthop., 12:11, 1992.

Palmer, E. E., Niemann, K. M., Vesely, D., and Armstrong, J. H.: Supracondylar fracture of the humerus in children. J. Bone Joint Surg., 60-A:653, 1978.

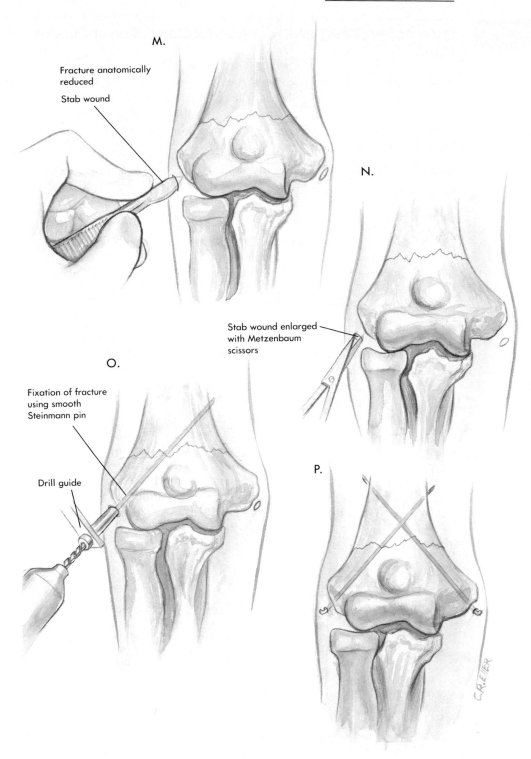

M.

Fracture anatomically reduced

Stab wound

N.

Stab wound enlarged with Metzenbaum scissors

O.

Fixation of fracture using smooth Steinmann pin

Drill guide

P.

Plate 24. (Continued)

PLATE 25

Osteotomy of the Distal Humerus for Correction of Cubitus Varus

Indications. Severe cubitus varus deformity that is cosmetically objectionable and is causing functional disability. On acute flexion of the elbow, the hand points lateral to the shoulder. *Caution!* Preoperatively, explain all of the vascular and neural complications to the patient and family. Volkmann's ischemia is a definite hazard, and nerve injury may occur.

Radiographic Control. Image intensifier.

Patient Position. Supine.

Operative Technique

A. A longitudinal incision is made over the anterolateral aspect of the distal third of the arm, with the anterior margin of the brachioradialis muscle serving as an anatomic landmark. The incision begins 1 cm. proximal and anterior to the lateral epicondyle of the humerus and extends proximally for a distance of approximately 7 cm.

B. The subcutaneous tissue and fascia are divided in line with the skin incision. The wound flaps are mobilized and retracted. The anterior margin of the brachioradialis muscle laterally and the lateral margin of the biceps muscle medially are identified, and by blunt dissection in the loose areolar tissue between these two muscles, the radial nerve is located. A moist hernia tape or Silastic tube is passed around the radial nerve for gentle handling and traction.

The biceps muscle is retracted medially, exposing the lateral half of the brachialis muscle beneath it. By blunt dissection with a periosteal elevator, the lateral one third to one half of the muscle fibers of the brachialis are raised, exposing the periosteum on the anterior aspect of the lower end of the humerus. The periosteum is incised longitudinally, as shown in the illustration, its distal end stopping 1 cm. proximal to the capsule of the elbow joint.

C. The periosteum is reflected with a periosteal elevator, and the lower end of the shaft of the humerus is exposed. It is essential not to disturb the growth of the distal humeral physis and to keep out of the elbow joint.

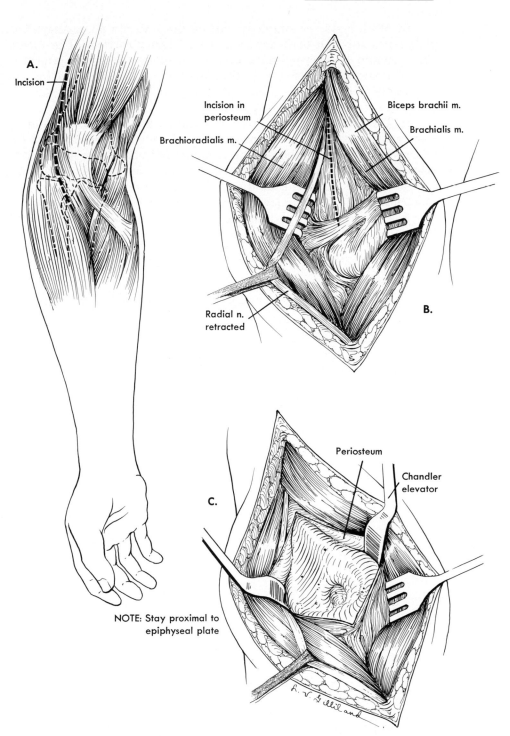

A.

Incision

Incision in
periosteum

Brachioradialis m.

Biceps brachii m.

Brachialis m.

Radial n.
retracted

B.

Periosteum

Chandler
elevator

C.

NOTE: Stay proximal to
epiphyseal plate

Plate 25. A.–K., Osteotomy of the distal humerus for correction of cubitus varus.

D. With a starter and drill, outline the line of a dome-shaped osteotomy with drill holes through both anterior and posterior cortices. The medial arch of the dome should be deeper and 1 to 1.5 cm. longer than the lateral arch, which is almost transverse. With sharp, thin osteotomes and/or oscillating electric saw, the osteotomy is completed, great care being taken not to split the medial cortex of the dome of the proximal fragment.

E. The bone fragments are manipulated, and angular and rotational deformities are corrected. If necessary, a wedge of bone may be removed from the lateral side of the distal fragment with a rongeur. The osteotomy fragments are fixed with criss-cross Steinmann pins inserted through stab wounds separate from the skin incision. Close the periosteum and the wound in the usual manner. It is vital to place a medium-size Hemovac closed suction tube for drainage.

F. The upper limb is immobilized in an above-elbow cast, with the elbow in 90 degrees of flexion and the forearm in 45 degrees of pronation.

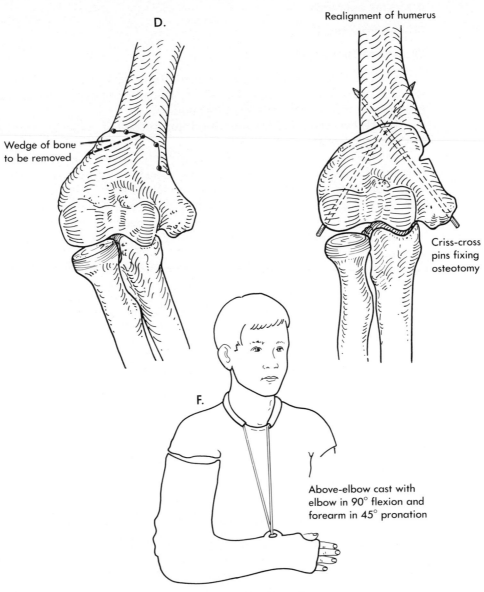

E.

Realignment of humerus

D.

Wedge of bone
to be removed

Criss-cross
pins fixing
osteotomy

F.

Above-elbow cast with
elbow in 90° flexion and
forearm in 45° pronation

Plate 25. (Continued)

An alternative method is to perform a closing-wedge osteotomy through the posterior approach.

Patient Position. Prone.

Operative Technique

G. The skin incision begins immediately above the tip of the olecranon and extends proximally for a distance of 7 to 10 cm. The subcutaneous tissue and fascia are opened in line with the skin incision.

H. The wound flaps are mobilized and retracted, exposing the lower one third of the tendon of triceps muscle.

I. The ulnar nerve is identified directly above the ulnar groove, dissected proximally, and retracted with silicone (Silastic) tubing posteriorly and inferiorly to protect it from injury. The triceps tendon is split longitudinally and each half is retracted, thus exposing the posterior surface of the humerus.

It is not necessary to expose the radial nerve as long as dissection does not extend more proximally than does the junction of the middle and distal thirds of the humerus.

Closing Wedge Osteotomy of Distal Humerus through
Posterior Approach for Correction of Cubitus Valgus

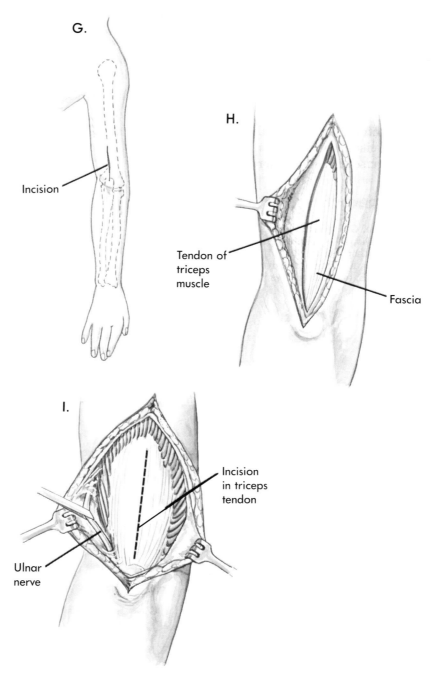

G.

Incision

H.

Tendon of
triceps
muscle

Fascia

I.

Incision
in triceps
tendon

Ulnar
nerve

Plate 25. (Continued)

144

| PLATE 28 | **Varus Angulation and Lateral Displacement Osteotomy of the Distal Humerus to Correct Cubitus Varus with Lateral Translocation of the Proximal Radius and Ulna** |

Indications. Cubitus valgus associated with lateral translocation of radial head and olecranon. Milch type B fracture pattern.

Radiographic Control. Image intensifier.

Patient Position. The patient is supine, with the shoulder abducted on an upper limb table. Use sterile tourniquet ischemia in order to visualize the alignment of the entire upper limb during surgery.

Operative Technique

A. The distal one third of the humerus is exposed by the anterolateral surgical approach, as described in steps **A.** to **E.** in Plate 26.

Under image intensifier radiographic control, the line of osteotomy is marked in the distal metaphysis of the humerus. It should be above the olecranon fossa.

B. With an oscillating electric saw, the osteotomy is made and the distal segment of the humerus is adducted into varus, opening up the osteotomy site.

C. Longitudinal traction is applied on the forearm, and the distal segment is translocated laterally, locking the medial spike of the distal humeral segment into the medullary cavity of the humeral shaft; thus, the longitudinal axis of the humerus is realigned with that of the forearm.

D. The osteotomized humeral segments are fixed with two or three criss-cross, threaded Steinmann pins, drilled through separate stab wounds over the humeral epicondyles.

E. Sometimes it may be necessary to use a plate and screws in addition to the pin fixation.

Insert Hemovac suction tubes, and close the wound in the usual fashion. Apply an above-elbow cast with the patient's elbow in 60 to 90 degrees of flexion.

Postoperative Care. Closely monitor neurovascular function. Make radiograms five to ten days postoperatively to check maintenance of alignment of the osteotomy. The cast is changed and the pins removed at four weeks. Another above-elbow cast is applied for an additional two to three weeks.

REFERENCE

Milch, H.: Fractures of the external humeral condyle. J.A.M.A., 166:220, 1958.

Closing Wedge Osteotomy of Distal Humerus through
Posterior Approach for Correction of Cubitus Valgus

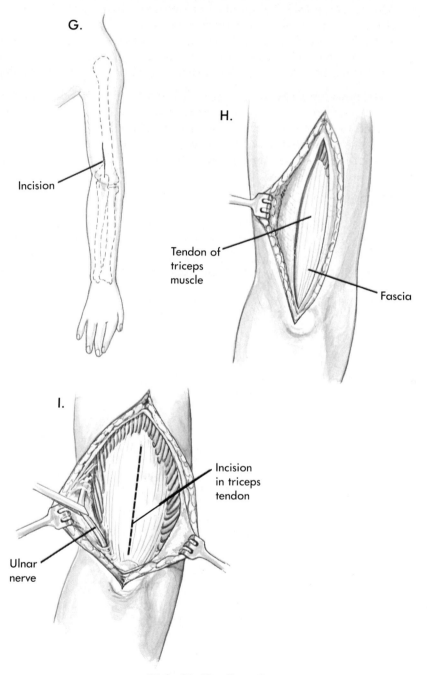

G.

Incision

H.

Tendon of
triceps
muscle

Fascia

I.

Incision
in triceps
tendon

Ulnar
nerve

Plate 25. (Continued)

J. and **K.** The periosteum on the posterior surface of the humerus is divided by a T-incision. Stay proximal to the olecranon fossa and distal humeral physis. A wedge osteotomy from the distal humeral methaphysis based laterally is resected. The osteotomized fragments are approximated and fixed internally with two or three criss-cross pins inserted through stab wounds separate from the skin incision. A medium-sized Hemovac suction tube is placed for closed suction.

The wound is closed in the usual fashion, and an above-elbow cast is applied, with the elbow in 90 degrees of flexion and the forearm in 45 degrees of pronation.

Postoperative Care. Radiograms are made after five days and again at two weeks to check maintenance of anatomic alignment of the fracture fragments. The osteotomy usually heals in six weeks. The cast and pins are removed, and *active* exercises are begun to restore range of motion of the elbow. Passive stretching exercises are *not* performed. Weights should not be lifted for two months.

REFERENCES

DeRosa, G. P., and Graziano, G. P.: A new osteotomy for cubitus varus. Clin. Orthop., 236:160, 1988.

Kanaujia, R. R., Ikuta, Y., and Muneshige, H.: Dome osteotomy for cubitus varus in children. Acta Orthop. Scand., 59:314, 1988.

Wilkins, K. E.: Supracondylar fractures of the humerus: In: Rockwood, C. H., Wilkins, K. E., and King, R. E. (eds.): Fractures in Children. Philadelphia, J. B. Lippincott, Co., 1984, p. 376.

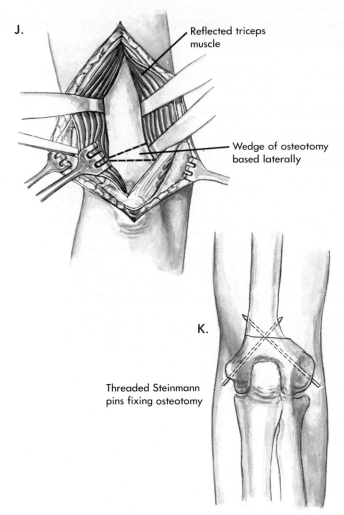

J.

Reflected triceps
muscle

Wedge of osteotomy
based laterally

K.

Threaded Steinmann
pins fixing osteotomy

Plate 25. (Continued)

| PLATE 26 | **Open Reduction and Internal Fixation of Fracture of the Lateral Condyle** |

Indications. Displaced fracture of the lateral condyle. Internally fix the minimally displaced fracture—it is the troublemaker!

Radiographic Control. Image intensifier.

Patient Position. Supine with upper limb on radiolucent hand table.

Operative Technique

A. The incision begins 5 to 7 cm. proximal to the lateral epicondyle of the humerus, extends distally over the epicondylar ridge of the lateral epicondyle, and continues distally and posteriorly over the interval between the anconeus and the extensor carpi ulnaris muscles for a distance of 2.5 cm.

B. The subcutaneous tissue and the deep fascia are opened in line with the skin incision. Working distally to proximally, develop the plane between the triceps muscle posteriorly and the brachioradialis muscle anteriorly. Frequently, there is a tear in the aponeurosis of the brachioradialis muscle, which leads directly to the fracture site. Avoid the radial nerve in the proximal end of the wound where it enters in the interval between the brachialis and brachioradialis muscles. The dissection is carried distally between the anconeus and the extensor carpi ulnaris muscles, exposing the joint capsule.

C. The periosteum is incised along the lateral epicondylar ridge and adjacent humerus, and the joint capsule is opened.

D. On exposure of the fracture site, the blood from the hematoma will flow out; the wound is irrigated with normal saline to remove small pieces of loose bone and to obtain clear visualization.

Caution! Do not dissect the fracture fragment, particularly its posterior aspect, where the only blood vessels supplying the lateral condylar apophysis enter; it will increase the risk of avascular necrosis.

It is vital to have a clear view of the fracture bed and the joint surface anteriorly and inferiorly. Insert a right-angled, long, narrow retractor (in pediatric surgery it is called an *infantile rectal retractor*) or a *Homan* retractor into the anterior aspect of the elbow, and visualize the radial head. To expose the joint surface, it may be necessary to incise a small amount of the capsule and synovium. With a Freer elevator, elevate the periosteum on the humeral shaft for a distance of 0.5 to 1.0 cm.; this measure provides a better definition of the fracture bed.

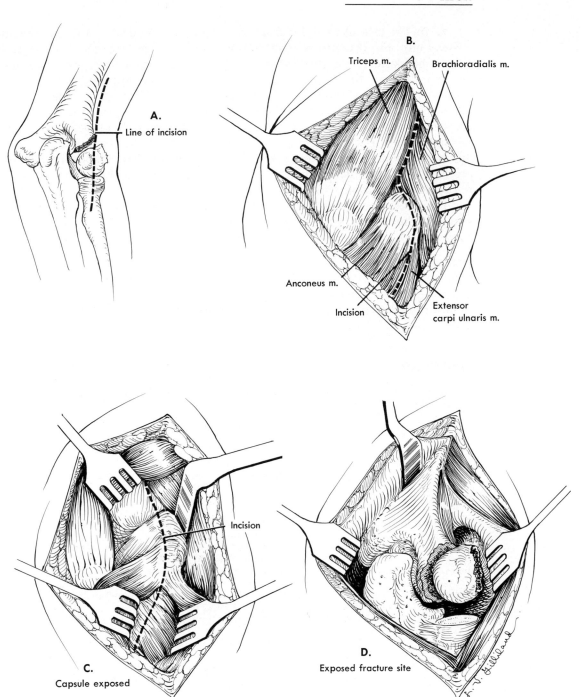

A.
Line of incision

B.
Triceps m.
Brachioradialis m.
Anconeus m.
Incision
Extensor carpi ulnaris m.

Incision

C.
Capsule exposed

D.
Exposed fracture site

Plate 26. A.–G., Open reduction and internal fixation of a displaced lateral condylar fracture of the humerus.

E. As the lateral condylar fracture fragment is held with a bone tenaculum or a towel clip, the fracture is reduced anatomically. The articular cartilage surface should be perfectly aligned; if it is not, delayed union and joint stiffness may develop. Inspect the lateral cortex of the humerus; apposition of the fracture fragments should be anatomic. Strive for perfection! Ordinarily, it is not necessary to detach the soft tissues from the lateral epicondyle. Two smooth Kirschner wires are drilled across the fracture site through stab wounds separate from the skin incision. The wires should engage the medial cortex of the humerus. The reduction and position of the wires are checked by radiograms. The distal ends of the wires are cut off but are left protruding slightly from the skin, and their ends are bent to prevent migration.

F. and **G.** The periosteum and the capsule of the joint are closed by interrupted sutures. The wound is closed, and the upper limb is immobilized in an above-elbow cast, with the elbow in 90 degrees of flexion and the forearm in neutral position.

Postoperative Care. In about three to four weeks, the pins are removed and another above-elbow cast is applied for an additional two to three weeks. Gentle, active exercises are performed to restore range of motion of the elbow joint. It is imperative to observe the patient for possible premature closure of the lateral portion of the distal humeral physis, cubitus valgus, or tardy ulnar nerve palsy.

REFERENCES

Blount, W. P.: Fractures of the lateral condyle of the humerus. In: Fractures in Children. Baltimore: Williams & Wilkins Co., 1954, pp. 43–45.

Flynn, J. C., and Richards, J. F.: Non-union of minimally displaced fractures of the lateral condyle of the humerus in children. J. Bone Joint Surg., 53-A:1096, 1971.

Flynn, J. C., Richards, J. F., Jr., and Saltzman, R. I.: Prevention and treatment of non-union of slightly displaced fractures of the lateral humeral condyle in children: An end-result study. J. Bone Joint Surg., 57-A:1087, 1975.

Fontanetta, P., MacKenzie, D. A., and Rosman, M.: Missed, maluniting, and malunited fractures of the lateral humeral condyle in children. J. Trauma, 18:329, 1978.

Foster, D. E., Sullivan, J. A., and Gross, R. H.: Lateral humeral condylar fractures in children. J. Pediatr. Orthop., 5:16, 1985.

Hardacre, J. A., Nahigian, S. H., Froimson, I., and Brown, J. E.: Fractures of the lateral condyle of the humerus in children. J. Bone Joint Surg., 53-A:1083, 1971.

Jakob, R., Fowles, J. B., Rang, M., and Kassab, M. T.: Observations concerning fractures of the lateral humeral condyle in children. J. Bone Joint Surg., 57-B:430, 1975.

Jones, K. G.: Percutaneous pin fixation of fractures of the lower end of the humerus. Clin. Orthop., 50:53, 1967.

Judet, H.: Fractures du Condyle Externe des L'humerus. In: Traite des Fractures des Mêmbres. 2nd ed. Paris: L'expansion Scientifique Français, 1922, pp. 139–146.

Maylahn, D. J., and Fahey, J. J.: Fractures of the elbow in children. Review of 300 consecutive cases. J.A.M.A., 166:220, 1958.

Milch, H.: Fractures of the external humeral condyle. J.A.M.A., 160:641, 1956.

Rang, M.: Fractures in Children. 2nd ed. Philadelphia: J. B. Lippincott Co., 1983, p. 178.

Walloe, A., Egund, N., and Eikelund, L.: Supracondylar fracture of the humerus in children: Review of closed and open reduction leading to a proposal for treatment. Injury, 16:296, 1985.

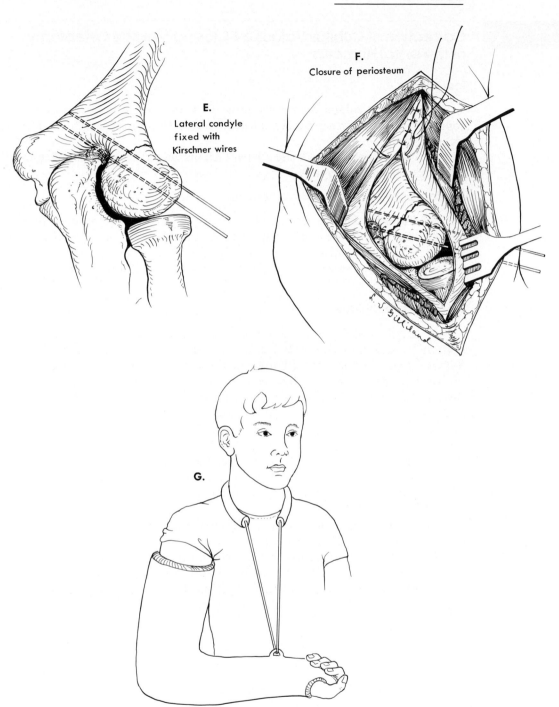

E.
Lateral condyle
fixed with
Kirschner wires

F.
Closure of periosteum

G.

Plate 26. (Continued)

PLATE 27 ## Correction of Cubitus Valgus by Closing-Wedge Osteotomy of the Distal Humerus

Indications

1. Cubitus valgus deformity caused by malunion or non-union of a lateral condylar fracture or asymmetrical growth due to premature physeal arrest of the lateral condyle.

2. Valgus deformity of the elbow with no lateral translation of the radial head or olecranon (Milch type A).

Radiographic Control. Image intensifier.

Patient Position. The patient is placed supine, with the shoulder abducted on an upper limb table. The entire upper limb and shoulder are prepared and draped sterile. A sterile tourniquet is used for ischemia; it is important to adequately visualize the upper arm in order to clinically determine the correction of the angular deformity.

Operative Technique

A. and **B.** The distal third of the humerus is exposed by anterolateral surgical approach. A skin incision 6 to 8 cm. long commences immediately above the elbow flexion crease at the lateral border of the biceps, extends proximally and slightly laterally over the groove between the biceps and brachioradialis muscles, and terminates at the desired point. The subcutaneous tissue and superficial fasciae are divided in line with the skin incision.

C. Locate the lateral margin of the biceps tendon, and retract the biceps muscle medially. It is vital to identify the lateral cutaneous nerve of the forearm; it traverses longitudinally between the biceps and brachialis, emerges from the lateral border of the biceps tendon, and pierces the deep fascia to enter the forearm. The lateral cutaneous nerve of the forearm is retracted laterally and kept out of harm's way.

Caution! Do not injure this nerve, as it supplies a large area of the skin over the radial aspect of the forearm.

D. With blunt retractors, retract the biceps muscle medially and the brachioradialis muscles laterally. Incise the deep fasciae over the interval between the brachioradialis and biceps distally and the brachioradialis and brachialis proximally.

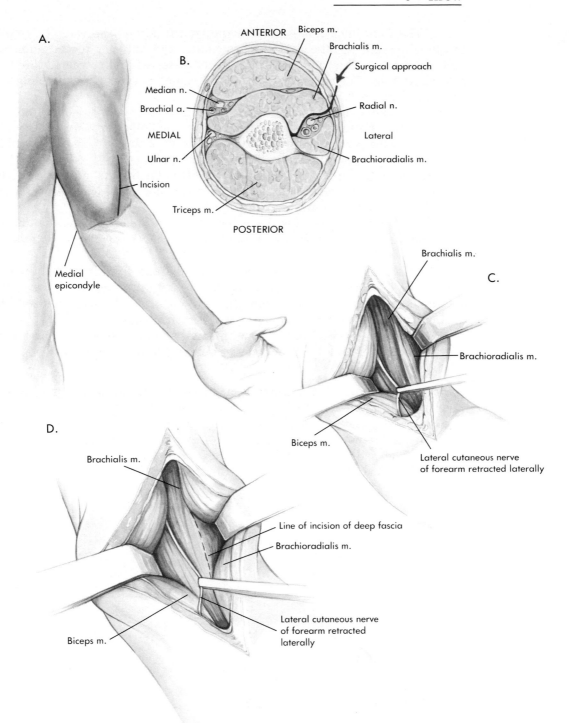

A.

B.

ANTERIOR

Biceps m.

Brachialis m.

Surgical approach

Median n.

Brachial a.

Radial n.

MEDIAL

Lateral

Ulnar n.

Brachioradialis m.

Incision

Triceps m.

POSTERIOR

Medial
epicondyle

Brachialis m.

C.

Brachioradialis m.

Biceps m.

Lateral cutaneous nerve
of forearm retracted laterally

D.

Brachialis m.

Line of incision of deep fascia

Brachioradialis m.

Lateral cutaneous nerve
of forearm retracted
laterally

Biceps m.

Plate 27. A.–H., Closing-up wedge osteotomy of the distal humerus to correct cubitus valgus.

E. The radial nerve is located in the lateral part of the wound, lying deep to the brachioradialis, lateral to the brachialis, and anterior to the humeral shaft and metaphysis. The radial nerve is gently dissected and retracted laterally with Silastic tubing. The motor branch of the radial nerve to the brachioradialis is identified and kept out of harm's way.

F. The radial border of the brachialis muscle is gently separated from the radial nerve. Retract the brachialis muscle medially, exposing the underlying bone. Incise the periosteum over the lateral third of the humeral shaft, and expose the humerus subperiosteally.

G. Insert Chandler retractors subperiosteally; on the medial side, exercise caution in order to prevent damaging the ulnar nerve, which lies posterior to the medial intermuscular septum at this level.

With an electric saw, a wedge osteotomy from the distal humeral metaphysis, based medially, is made. It is vital to keep proximal to the olecranon fossa and the distal humeral growth plate.

H. The osteotomized fragments are apposed and fixed internally with two or three criss-cross smooth pins inserted through stab wounds over the medial and lateral epicondyles separate from the skin incision. A medium-sized Hemovac suction tube is placed in the wound for closed drainage.

The wound is closed in the usual fashion and an above-elbow cast is applied, with the elbow in 60 to 70 degrees of flexion and the forearm in 45 degrees of pronation.

Postoperative Care. The patient is admitted to the hospital for observation of neurovascular function. Radiograms are made after five days and again at two weeks to verify maintenance of anatomic alignment of the osteotomized fragments. The pins are removed four weeks after surgery, and another above-elbow cast is applied. The osteotomy usually heals in six weeks, at which time the cast is removed and exercises are begun to restore range of motion of the elbow.

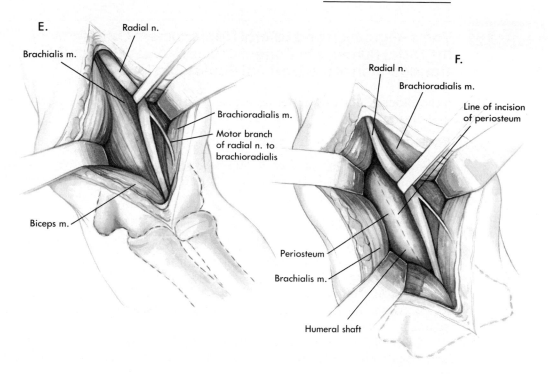

E.

Radial n.

Brachialis m.

Brachioradialis m.

Motor branch
of radial n. to
brachioradialis

Biceps m.

F.

Radial n.

Brachioradialis m.

Line of incision
of periosteum

Periosteum

Brachialis m.

Humeral shaft

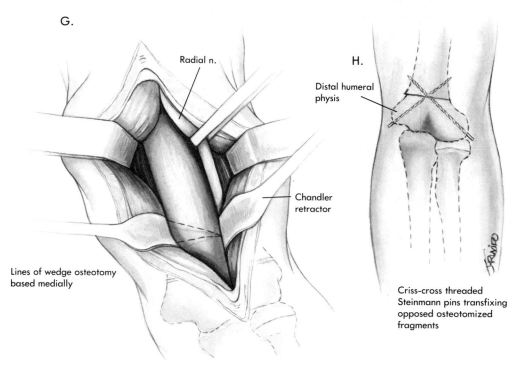

G.

Radial n.

Chandler
retractor

Lines of wedge osteotomy
based medially

H.

Distal humeral
physis

Criss-cross threaded
Steinmann pins transfixing
opposed osteotomized
fragments

Plate 27. (Continued)

PLATE 28 | **Varus Angulation and Lateral Displacement Osteotomy of the Distal Humerus to Correct Cubitus Varus with Lateral Translocation of the Proximal Radius and Ulna**

Indications. Cubitus valgus associated with lateral translocation of radial head and olecranon. Milch type B fracture pattern.

Radiographic Control. Image intensifier.

Patient Position. The patient is supine, with the shoulder abducted on an upper limb table. Use sterile tourniquet ischemia in order to visualize the alignment of the entire upper limb during surgery.

Operative Technique

A. The distal one third of the humerus is exposed by the anterolateral surgical approach, as described in steps **A.** to **E.** in Plate 26.

Under image intensifier radiographic control, the line of osteotomy is marked in the distal metaphysis of the humerus. It should be above the olecranon fossa.

B. With an oscillating electric saw, the osteotomy is made and the distal segment of the humerus is adducted into varus, opening up the osteotomy site.

C. Longitudinal traction is applied on the forearm, and the distal segment is translocated laterally, locking the medial spike of the distal humeral segment into the medullary cavity of the humeral shaft; thus, the longitudinal axis of the humerus is realigned with that of the forearm.

D. The osteotomized humeral segments are fixed with two or three criss-cross, threaded Steinmann pins, drilled through separate stab wounds over the humeral epicondyles.

E. Sometimes it may be necessary to use a plate and screws in addition to the pin fixation.

Insert Hemovac suction tubes, and close the wound in the usual fashion. Apply an above-elbow cast with the patient's elbow in 60 to 90 degrees of flexion.

Postoperative Care. Closely monitor neurovascular function. Make radiograms five to ten days postoperatively to check maintenance of alignment of the osteotomy. The cast is changed and the pins removed at four weeks. Another above-elbow cast is applied for an additional two to three weeks.

REFERENCE

Milch, H.: Fractures of the external humeral condyle. J.A.M.A., 166:220, 1958.

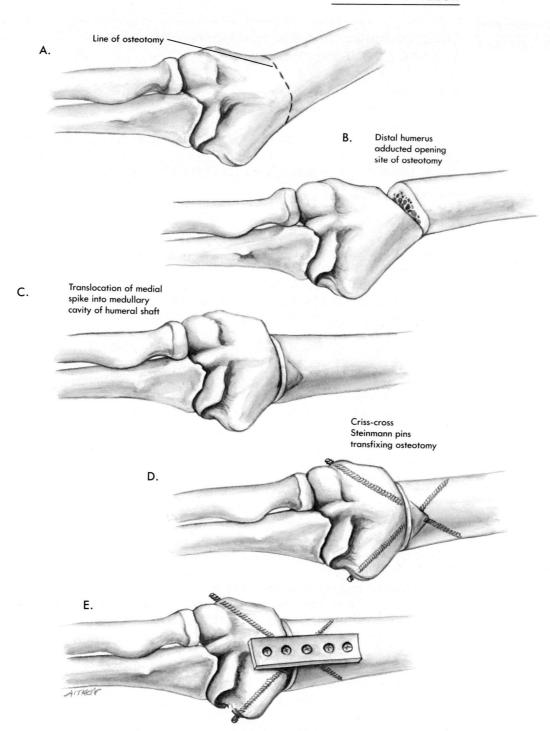

A. Line of osteotomy

B. Distal humerus adducted opening site of osteotomy

C. Translocation of medial spike into medullary cavity of humeral shaft

D. Criss-cross Steinmann pins transfixing osteotomy

E.

AITKEN

Plate 28. A.–E., Varus angulation and lateral displacement osteotomy of the distal humerus to correct cubitus varus and lateral translocation of the proximal radius and ulna.

PLATE 29 **Open Reduction and Internal Fixation of the Medial Epicondyle of the Humerus**

Indications

1. Markedly displaced medial epicondylar fracture, especially if the elbow joint is unstable.

2. Displaced fracture of the medial epicondyle in the skeletally immature patient.

3. Incarcerated medial epicondyle in the elbow joint.

Radiographic Control. Image intensifier.

Patient Position. The patient may be either supine or prone. I prefer the prone position. It is simpler to get to the medial epicondyle. When the patient is supine, the arm is abducted on an upper limb table and the shoulder is laterally rotated. When the patient is prone, the arm is extended and abducted at the shoulder. Do not hyperextend the shoulder when preparing and draping the patient. A pneumatic tourniquet should be placed as high as possible.

Operative Technique

A. A 5- to 7-cm. longitudinal incision is made over the medial aspect of the elbow joint. It begins about 1.5 to 2 cm. distal and anterior to the tip of the olecranon and extends proximally over the medial aspect of the arm parallel with the medial epicondylar ridge of the humerus.

B. The subcutaneous tissue and fascia are divided in line with the skin incision.

Identify the ulnar nerve in the ulnar groove and the fractured medial epicondyle. When anatomy is distorted as a result of marked displacement and soft tissue swelling and hemorrhage, the ulnar nerve is dissected free and retracted out of harm's way with Silastic tubing or moist hernia tape. The periosteum and the capsule are divided.

C. With a towel clip on the common tendon of the flexor muscles, the fractured medial epicondyle is repositioned to its bed and anatomically reduced.

D. Two smooth Kirschner wires or Steinmann pins are inserted with a power drill across the fracture site in a proximal and lateral direction. The pins should engage the lateral cortex. The position of the wires and the accuracy of reduction are verified by making radiograms of the elbow in the anteroposterior and lateral projections. The distal tips of the wires are bent into a hook and imbedded in the soft tissues deep to the skin to prevent migration. (Some surgeons may prefer to leave the ends protruding slightly through the skin for ease of removal.)

E. The periosteum and the capsule are repaired with interrupted sutures, giving further stability to the reduction of the fracture fragments. Close the wound in the usual fashion, and apply an above-elbow cast, immobilizing the patient's elbow in 90 degrees of flexion and the forearm in 45 degrees or full pronation.

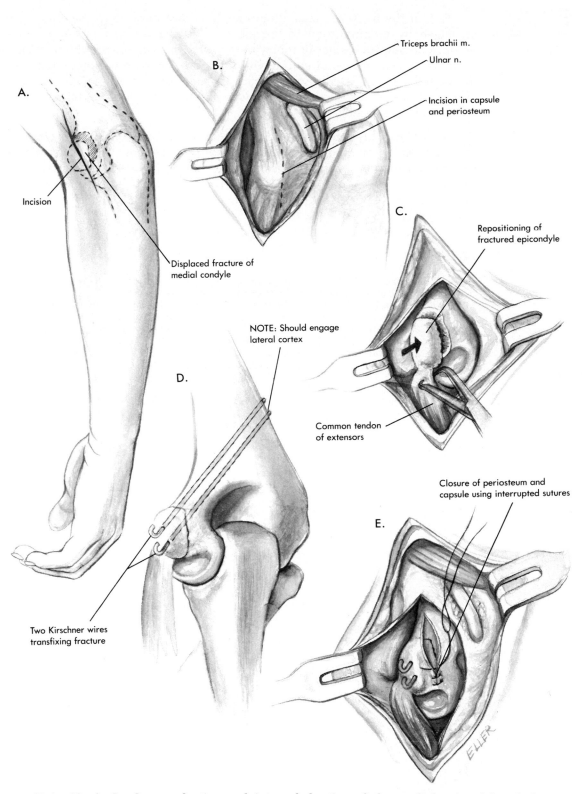

A.

Incision

Displaced fracture of medial condyle

B.

Triceps brachii m.

Ulnar n.

Incision in capsule and periosteum

C.

Repositioning of fractured epicondyle

Common tendon of extensors

D.

NOTE: Should engage lateral cortex

Two Kirschner wires transfixing fracture

E.

Closure of periosteum and capsule using interrupted sutures

ELLER

Plate 29. A.–I., Open reduction and internal fixation of the medial epicondyle of the humerus.

F.–I. If the fractured medial epicondyle is incarcerated in the elbow joint, it is dislodged by manipulation of the elbow. Closed reduction is not recommended because of definite danger of injury to the ulnar nerve, which may be incarcerated with the fractured medial epicondyle. After the incarcerated medial epicondyle is dislodged, it is pinned with two smooth Kirschner wires as shown in **D.** and **E.** Be sure that the elbow joint is not dislocated and that it is anatomically reduced. Make adequate radiograms.

Postoperative Care. In three to four weeks after surgery, the pins are removed and another above-elbow cast is applied with the elbow and forearm in similar position for an additional two weeks. After cast removal, active assisted exercises are performed to restore range of motion to the elbow joint. Inform the parents and child that it will take three to six months before normal range of elbow extension is restored.

REFERENCES

Balrov, G. A., and Gorely, I. V. V.: Transcutaneous temporary osteosynthesis of fractures of the inner supracondyle of the humerus in children. Ortop. Travmatol. Protez, 10:70, 1975.

Cataliotti, F., Giglio, A. L., and Salomone, G.: Percutaneous osteosynthesis in fracture-dislocation of the epitrochlea and of condylo-epicondyloid block in childhood. Minerva Med., 63:4256, 1972.

Dias, J. J., Johnson, G. V., Hoskinson, J., and Sulaiman, K.: Management of severely displaced medial epicondyle fractures. J. Orthop. Trauma, 1:59, 1987.

Fevre, M., and Roudiatis: La réduction non sanglante des fractures de l'epitrochlee avec interposition de ce fragment dans l'interlinge articulone du coude. Rev. Chir. Orthop., 20:300, 1933.

Hines, R. F., Herndon, W. A., and Evans, J. P.: Operative treatment of medial epicondyle fractures in children. Clin. Orthop., 223:170, 1987.

Woods, G. M., and Tullos, H. G.: Elbow instability and medial epicondyle fracture. Am. J. Sports Med., 5:23, 1977.

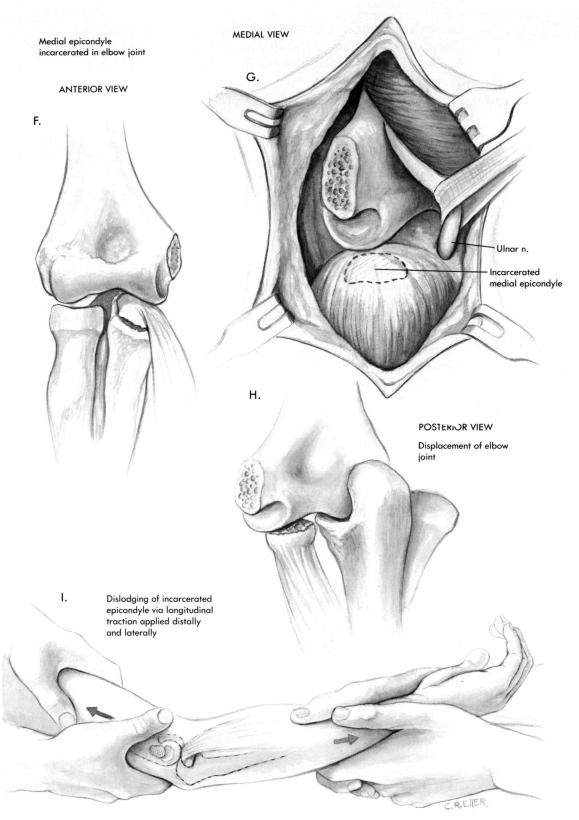

Medial epicondyle
incarcerated in elbow joint

MEDIAL VIEW

ANTERIOR VIEW

F.

G.

Ulnar n.

Incarcerated
medial epicondyle

H.

POSTERIOR VIEW

Displacement of elbow
joint

I.   Dislodging of incarcerated
epicondyle via longitudinal
traction applied distally
and laterally

C.R.EIIER

Plate 29. (Continued)

PLATE 30   ### Open Reduction and Repair of Non-union of a Lateral Condylar Fracture of the Humerus Through the Transarticular Approach with Osteotomy of the Olecranon Process

Indications. Non-union of lateral condylar fracture of the humerus.

Radiographic Control. Image intensifier.

Patient Position. The patient may be either prone or supine. I prefer the supine position, with the ipsilateral shoulder elevated with a sand bag. The entire upper limb is prepared and draped sterile in the usual orthopedic fashion. A sterile pneumatic tourniquet is applied as high on the arm as possible. The arm is adducted across the patient's chest, with an assistant on the opposite side of the patient holding the forearm.

Operative Technique

   A. The incision begins 5 cm. distal to the tip of the olecranon process over the subcutaneous border of the ulna, extends proximally along the lateral aspect of the olecranon process, and then extends proximally along the midline of the distal arm for the desired distance. The subcutaneous tissue is divided in line with the skin incision.

   B. The superficial fascia is incised, and the wound flaps are undercut and elevated as far as the medial and lateral epicondyle of the humerus. Identify the ulnar nerve; it lies posterior to the medial epicondyle of the humerus. To facilitate exposure of the nerve, identify the nerve in the upper part of the wound and then trace the nerve distally. It may be necessary to divide the medial intermuscular septum and retract the ulnar nerve out of harm's way. The radial nerve is well above the surgical incision, usually 8 to 10 cm. proximal to the lateral epicondyle of the humerus. It is not necessary to identify it, but its location and course should always be kept in mind.

   Identify the medial and lateral borders of the triceps tendon at its insertion, and mobilize the tendon first by making an incision on its lateral margin and dissecting it distally to the lateral epicondyle and then separating it from the anconeus muscles radially. Next, an incision is made along the medial margin of the triceps tendon, and it is freed distally to the medial epicondyle.

   C. Expose the olecranon process subperiosteally at the proposed level of osteotomy.

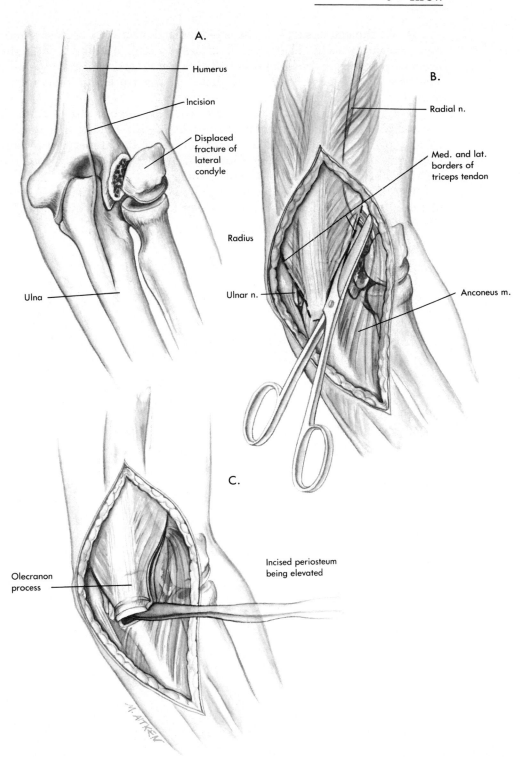

A.

Humerus

Incision

Displaced
fracture of
lateral
condyle

Ulna

Radius

B.

Radial n.

Med. and lat.
borders of
triceps tendon

Ulnar n.

Anconeus m.

C.

Olecranon
process

Incised periosteum
being elevated

M. AITKEN

Plate 30. A.–I., Open reduction and repair of non-union of a lateral condylar fracture of the
humerus through the transarticular approach with osteotomy of the olecranon process.

D. At the end of surgery, the osteotomized olecranon process should be rigidly and accurately fixed. Therefore, it is best to drill a hole through the olecranon process into the proximal shaft of the ulna for subsequent intramedullary fixation. The osteotomy line is 2 to 3 cm. distal to the tip of the olecranon in order to provide adequate intra-articular exposure.

E. With an oscillating electric saw, the olecranon is partially sectioned in the coronal plane and the osteotomy is completed with a sharp osteotome. Take great care not to damage the distal articular surface of the humerus. I recommend using radiographic image intensifier control in order to accurately determine the line and level of the osteotomy of the olecranon.

F. The osteotomized olecranon is pulled upward, and the capsule and synovium of the elbow joint are divided. The distal humeral shaft and articular surface of the distal humerus are exposed.

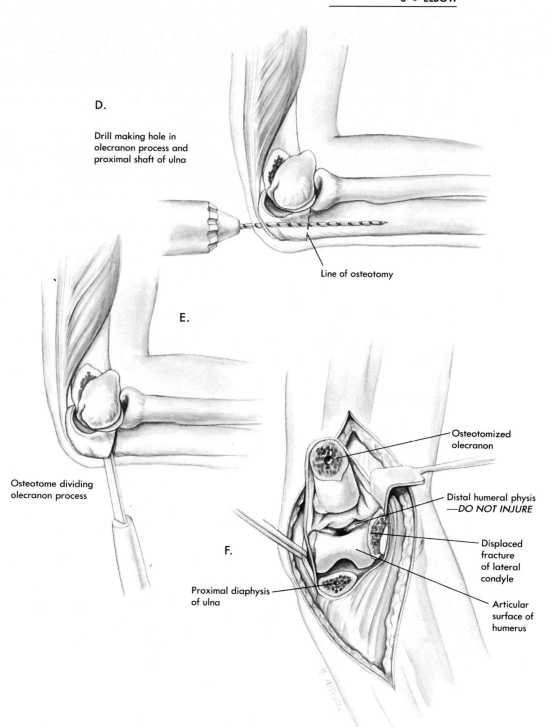

D.

Drill making hole in olecranon process and proximal shaft of ulna

Line of osteotomy

E.

Osteotome dividing olecranon process

F.

Proximal diaphysis of ulna

Osteotomized olecranon

Distal humeral physis —*DO NOT INJURE*

Displaced fracture of lateral condyle

Articular surface of humerus

Plate 30. (Continued)

G. Under image intensifier radiographic control, the physis of the lateral condyle and distal humerus are located by the use of Keith needles.

H. All fibrous tissue between the fracture fragments is meticulously excised, and the fracture fragment is reduced and fixed internally with two to three pins. It is important that the articular cartilage surface and the physis be anatomically aligned. Do not accept "step-off."

I. In the long-standing non-union, it is best to place autogenous fat between the repositioned lateral condyle and distal humeral physis as a spacer. First, with a dental bur and pituitary forceps, remove all soft tissue and bony remnants between the physes of the lateral condyle and the distal humerus and insert the autogenous fat to prevent osseous bridge formation. Suture the fat to surrounding tissues to prevent it from displacing.

The elbow joint is thoroughly irrigated. Be sure that the articular cartilage surface is congruous with no "step-off"; the olecranon fragment is fixed to the upper shaft of the ulna with a cancellous screw. The wound is closed in the usual fashion. An above-elbow cast is applied with the elbow in about 45 degrees of flexion.

Postoperative Care. About four to six weeks postoperatively, the cast is removed and radiograms are made. If there is adequate healing, gentle active assisted exercises are performed to restore range of motion of the elbow joint. The pins are removed when there is adequate healing of the bony segments.

REFERENCES

Bohler, L.: Fractures of the lateral condyle of the humerus in children. In: The Treatment of Fractures, Supplementary Volume to the 5th English edition, pp. 2490–2493. By L. and J. Bohler. Translated from the German edition by Alfred Wallner. New York and London: Grune & Stratton, 1966.

Fontanetta, P., MacKenzie, D. A., and Rosman, M.: Missed, maluniting, and malunited fractures of the lateral humeral condyle in children. J. Trauma, 18:329, 1978.

Hardacre, J. A., Nahigian, S. H., Froimson, I., and Brown, J. E.: Fractures of the lateral condyle of the humerus in children. J. Bone Joint Surg., 53-A:1083, 1971.

Jakob, R., Fowles, J. V., Rang, M., and Kassab, M. T.: Observations concerning fractures of the lateral humeral condyle in children. J. Bone Joint Surg., 57-B:430, 1975.

Jeffrey, C. C.: Non-union of the epiphysis of the lateral condyle of the humerus. J. Bone Joint Surg., 40-B:396, 1958.

Kalenak, A.: Ununited fractures of the lateral condyle of the humerus. A fifty year follow-up. Clin. Orthop., 124:181, 1977.

Maylahn, D. J., and Fahey, J. J.: Fractures of the elbow in children. Review of 300 consecutive cases. J.A.M.A., 166:220, 1958.

Roye, D. P., Bini, S. A., and Infosino, A.: Late surgical treatment of lateral condylar fractures in children. J. Pediatr. Orthop., 11:195, 1991.

Sarkar, S. D., and Bassett, C. A. L.: Healing of nonunion of a fractured lateral condyle of the humerus by pulsing electromagnetic induction. Contemp. Orthopaedics, 22:47, 1991.

Smith, F. M.: An eighty-four year follow-up on a patient with ununited fracture of the lateral condyle of the humerus: A case report. J. Bone Joint Surg., 55-A:378, 1973.

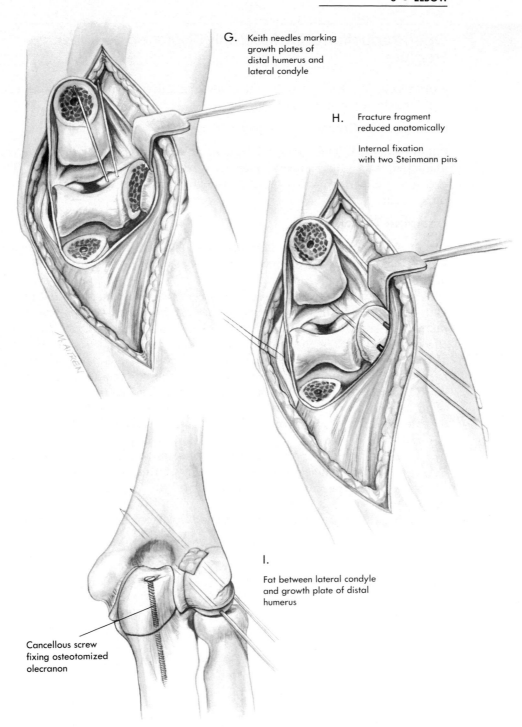

G. Keith needles marking
growth plates of
distal humerus and
lateral condyle

H. Fracture fragment
reduced anatomically

Internal fixation
with two Steinmann pins

I.
Fat between lateral condyle
and growth plate of distal
humerus

Cancellous screw
fixing osteotomized
olecranon

Plate 30. (Continued)

PLATE 31   Open Reduction of the Markedly Displaced Radial Neck Fracture

Indications. Markedly displaced radial neck fracture with 60 degrees of angulation and translocation greater than 4 mm.

Radiographic Control. Image intensifier.

Patient Position. The patient is placed in the supine position with the shoulder abducted, the elbow flexed, and the forearm in full pronation. The surgical procedure is performed with ischemia using a pneumatic tourniquet placed on the upper arm.

Operative Technique

A. An incision 5–6 cm. long is made, beginning 2 cm. distal to the head of the radius and extending proximally midway between the olecranon and lateral condyle of the humerus.

B. The subcutaneous tissue and superficial fascia are divided in line with the skin incision. The interval between the anconeus and triceps brachii is identified distally below the elbow joint, and these muscles are separated and retracted. In the proximal part of the wound, the triceps tendon and muscle fibers are spread. The anconeus muscle is retracted inferiorly, and the capsule of the elbow joint is exposed. A longitudinal incision is made in the posterolateral capsule.

C. and D. Do not injure the posterior interosseous nerve. The nerve originates from the radial nerve at the level of the lateral epicondyle of the humerus and spirals around the upper radius between the superficial and the deep parts of the supinator. With the forearm in pronation, the posterior osseous nerve moves anteromedially; with the forearm in supination, the nerve moves posterolaterally. When making the incision in the capsule, keep the child's forearm in full pronation, do not extend the capsular incision distal to the annular ligament, and stay posterior.

The radial head and the lateral condyle of the humerus are exposed.

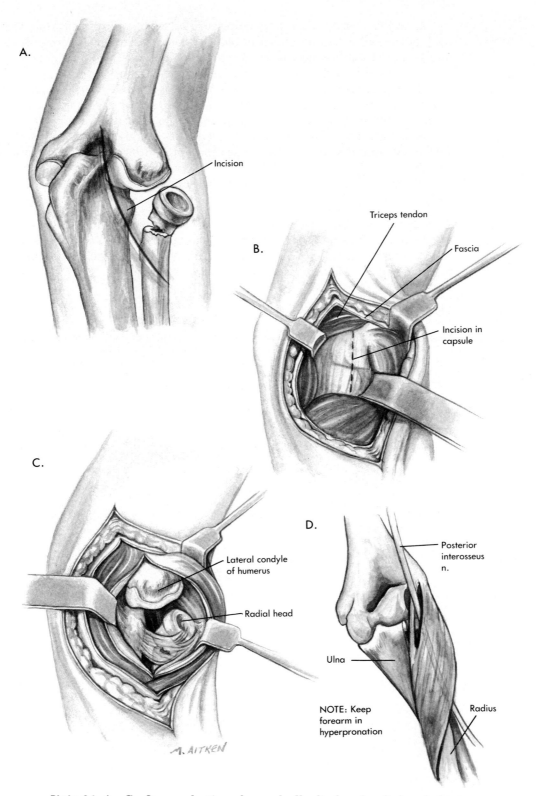

A. —Incision

B. Triceps tendon
Fascia
Incision in capsule

C. Lateral condyle of humerus
Radial head

D. Posterior interosseus n.
Ulna
Radius
NOTE: Keep forearm in hyperpronation

M. AITKEN

Plate 31. A.–G., Open reduction of a markedly displaced radial neck fracture.

E. and **F.** Gently, with finger pressure or with a blunt elevator, the fractured neck of the radius is anatomically reduced. Do not section the orbicularis ligament unless it is absolutely necessary to achieve reduction. The forearm is fully pronated and supinated to test the stability of reduction.

G. If reduction is unstable, fix the fracture internally with one or two threaded Kirschner wires (smooth wires tend to migrate and result in loss of reduction) inserted obliquely from distal to proximal from the radial neck into the head. Do not penetrate the elbow joint. This facilitates removal of the pins three to four weeks postoperatively. The pin ends are bent and left protruding distally through the skin.

The wound is closed in the usual fashion. An above-elbow cast is applied with the forearm in full supination.

Postoperative Care. The cast is removed three weeks after surgery, and the pins are removed. Another above-elbow cast is applied for two to three weeks, at which time the cast is removed and gentle, active-assisted range of motion exercises are performed to restore normal range of elbow motion.

REFERENCES

Fasol, P., and Schedl, R.: Percutaneous reduction of fractures of the neck of the radius in children by means of a Steinmann nail. Wien. Klin. Wochenschr., 88:135, 1976.

Fowles, J. B., and Kassab, M. T.: Observations concerning radial neck fractures in children. J. Pediatr. Orthop., 6:51, 1986.

Jeffrey, C. C.: Fractures of the neck of the radius in children. Mechanism of causation. J. Bone Joint Surg., 54-B:717, 1972.

Jones, E., and Esah, M.: Displaced fractures of the neck of the radius in children. J. Bone Joint Surg., 53-B:429, 1971.

O'Brien, P. I.: Injuries involving the proximal radial epiphysis. Clin. Orthop., 41:51, 1965.

Poulsen, O., and Tophoj, K.: Fracture of the head and neck of the radius. Follow-up on 61 patients. Acta Orthop. Scand., 45:66, 1974.

Scullion, J. E., and Miller, J. H.: Fracture of the neck of the radius in children: Prognostic factors and recommendations for management. J. Bone Joint Surg., 67-B:491, 1985.

Tibone, J. E., and Stoltz, M.: Fractures of the radial head and neck in children. A long term follow-up study of 43 cases. Acta Orthop. Trauma Surg., 99:167, 1982.

Wedge, J. H., and Robertson, D. E.: Displaced fractures of the neck of the radius. J. Bone Joint Surg., 64-B:256, 1982.

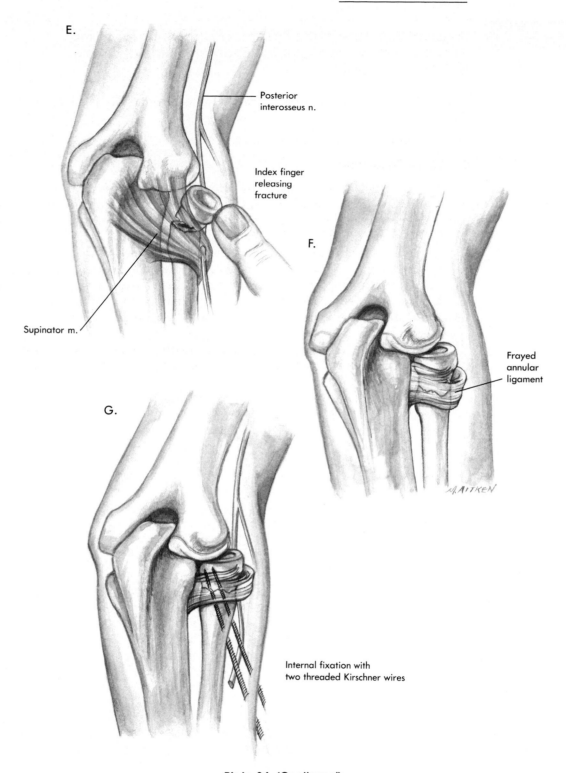

E.

Posterior
interosseus n.

Index finger
releasing
fracture

Supinator m.

F.

Frayed
annular
ligament

G.

Internal fixation with
two threaded Kirschner wires

Plate 31. (Continued)

PLATE 32 Surgical Exposure of the Proximal Radioulnar Joint and Repair of an Avulsed Annular Ligament in the Unstable Monteggia Fracture

Indications. Unstable Monteggia fracture-dislocation with avulsion of the orbicularis ligament.

Radiographic Control. Image intensifier.

Operative Technique

A. The incision begins over the lateral epicondyle of the humerus, extends distally and posteriorly along the interval between the anconeus and the extensor carpi ulnaris muscles, and ends medially at the subcutaneous margin of the upper one fourth of the ulna. The subcutaneous tissue and fascia are divided in line with the skin incision. The wound flaps are mobilized and retracted.

B. The interval between the anconeus and extensor carpi ulnaris muscles is developed, and dissection is extended down to the capsule of the elbow joint.

C. The anconeus muscle is detached partially to permit mobilization and facilitate further exposure of the joint. A longitudinal incision is made in the capsule.

D. The elbow joint is exposed, and the pathology is assessed. Note that the annular ligament is avulsed and interposed between the radial head and the radial notch of the ulna.

PLATE 32

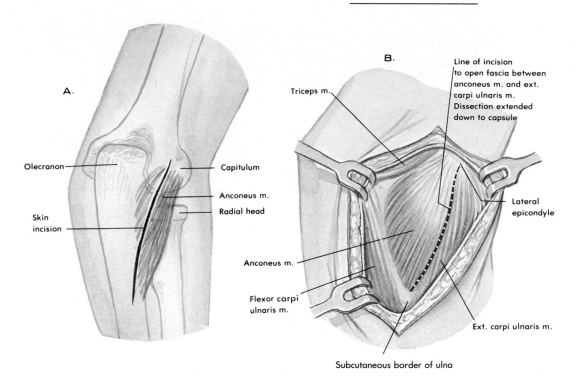

A.

Olecranon

Capitulum

Skin incision

Anconeus m.

Radial head

B.

Triceps m.

Line of incision to open fascia between anconeus m. and ext. carpi ulnaris m. Dissection extended down to capsule

Lateral epicondyle

Anconeus m.

Flexor carpi ulnaris m.

Ext. carpi ulnaris m.

Subcutaneous border of ulna

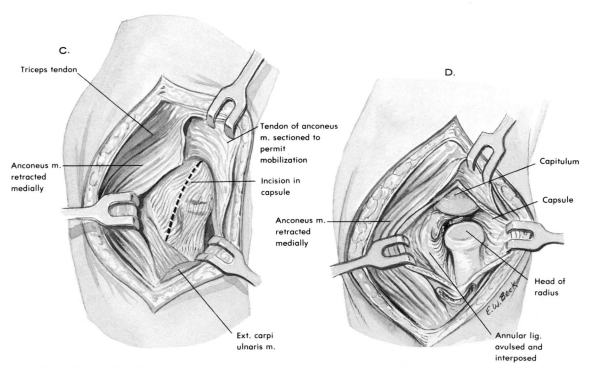

C.

Triceps tendon

Anconeus m. retracted medially

Tendon of anconeus m. sectioned to permit mobilization

Incision in capsule

Ext. carpi ulnaris m.

D.

Capitulum

Capsule

Anconeus m. retracted medially

Head of radius

Annular lig. avulsed and interposed

E. W. Beck

Plate 32. A.–G., Surgical exposure of the proximal radioulnar joint and repair of an avulsed annular ligament in the unstable Monteggia fracture.

E. If the annular ligament is torn, free the interposed segments with tissue forceps. The ends of the annular ligament are brought around the head of the radius and secured with interrupted sutures.

F. If the annular ligament is intact and interposed between the head of the radius and the radial notch of the ulna, use a Freer elevator to restore its position around the radial head.

G. If the annular ligament is intact but cannot be freed, make a vertical incision, bring the ends around the radial head, and join them with interrupted sutures.

The wound is closed in the usual fashion, and an above-elbow cast is applied, with the elbow in 90 degrees of flexion and the forearm in full supination.

Postoperative Care. The cast is removed in four to six weeks, and gentle, active-assisted exercises are performed to restore normal range of elbow motion.

REFERENCES

Boyd, H. B.: Surgical exposure of the ulna and proximal third of the radius through one incision. Surg. Gynecol. Obstet., 71:86, 1940.
Boyd, H. B.: Treatment of fractures of the ulna with dislocation of the radius. J.A.M.A., 115:1699, 1940.
Boyd, H. B., and Boals, J. C.: The Monteggia lesion: A review of 159 cases. Clin. Orthop., 66:94, 1969.

E.

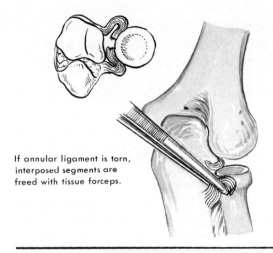

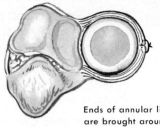

If annular ligament is torn,
interposed segments are
freed with tissue forceps.

Ends of annular ligament
are brought around head of
radius and secured with
interrupted sutures

F.

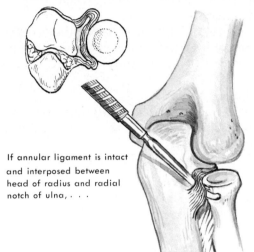

If annular ligament is intact
and interposed between
head of radius and radial
notch of ulna, . . .

. . . use Freer elevator to
restore position
around head

G.

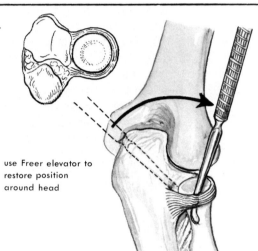

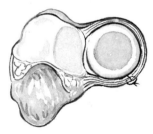

If annular ligament is intact but cannot be freed
intact from interposed position, make vertical
incision, bring ends around head of radius, and
join ends with interrupted sutures

Plate 32. (Continued)

PLATE 33

Open Reduction of Dislocation of the Radial Head in Monteggia Fracture-Dislocation and Reconstruction of the Annular Ligament with a Strip of Triceps Fascia

Indications. Monteggia fracture-dislocation in which annular ligament is torn and irreparable.

Radiographic Control. Image intensifier.

Patient Position. Supine with upper limb on radiolucent hand table.

Operative Technique

    A. The incision begins 5 to 7 cm. proximal to the tip of the olecranon, curving slightly laterally at the elbow joint toward the radial neck for a distance of 5 cm. The subcutaneous tissue and fascia are divided in line with the skin incision. The wound flaps are retracted, exposing the triceps tendon, flexor carpi ulnaris, anconeus, and extensor carpi ulnaris muscles.

    B. The fascia between the anconeus and extensor carpi ulnaris muscles is divided, and an incision is made over the insertion of the anconeus muscle.

    C. The anconeus muscle is freed from its lateral and medial attachments and elevated proximally.

    Caution! Preserve its nerve and blood supply.

    The extensor carpi ulnaris muscle is retracted laterally and the flexor carpi ulnaris muscle retracted medially so that the capsule of the elbow joint is exposed. A longitudinal incision is made in the capsule.

    D. The capsule is opened, and the dislocated radial head with the torn annular ligament is exposed.

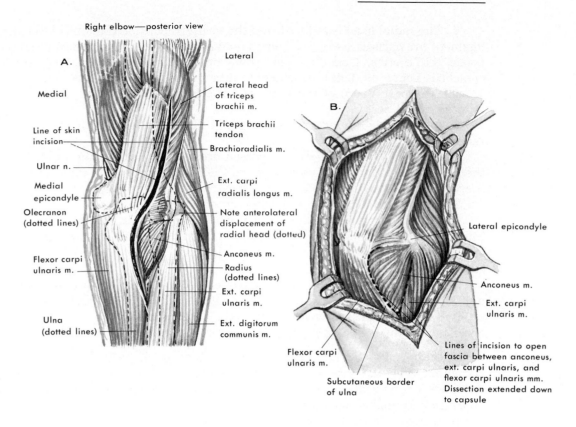

Right elbow—posterior view

A.

Lateral

Medial

Lateral head of triceps brachii m.

Line of skin incision

Triceps brachii tendon

Ulnar n.

Brachioradialis m.

Medial epicondyle

Ext. carpi radialis longus m.

Olecranon (dotted lines)

Note anterolateral displacement of radial head (dotted)

Anconeus m.

Flexor carpi ulnaris m.

Radius (dotted lines)

Ext. carpi ulnaris m.

Ulna (dotted lines)

Ext. digitorum communis m.

B.

Lateral epicondyle

Anconeus m.

Ext. carpi ulnaris m.

Flexor carpi ulnaris m.

Lines of incision to open fascia between anconeus, ext. carpi ulnaris, and flexor carpi ulnaris mm. Dissection extended down to capsule

Subcutaneous border of ulna

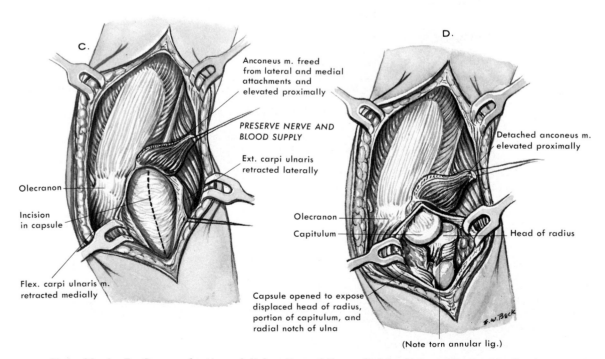

C.

Anconeus m. freed from lateral and medial attachments and elevated proximally

PRESERVE NERVE AND BLOOD SUPPLY

Ext. carpi ulnaris retracted laterally

Olecranon

Incision in capsule

Flex. carpi ulnaris m. retracted medially

D.

Detached anconeus m. elevated proximally

Olecranon

Capitulum

Head of radius

Capsule opened to expose displaced head of radius, portion of capitulum, and radial notch of ulna

(Note torn annular lig.)

f.w.Beck

Plate 33. A.–I., Open reduction of dislocation of the radial head in a Monteggia fracture. Dislocation and reconstruction of the annular ligament with a strip of triceps fascia.

E. The radial head is reduced, and the torn, irreparable remains of the annular ligament are excised. Next, the triceps tendon is cleared of surrounding connective tissue, and a strip, 1 cm. × 6 cm., from the lateral side of the triceps tendon is detached. Leave its distal attachments intact. The strip of triceps tendon should include the periosteum of the ulna, and the hinge should be at the level of the reduced radial neck.

F. A drill hole is made in the proximal ulna at a level with the neck of the radius.

G. The triceps tendon strip is passed around the neck of the radius through the drill hole in the ulna and sutured to the periosteum of the ulna and to itself; thereby, a new annular ligament is reconstructed.

H. The capsule is closed with interrupted sutures.

I. A stout, smooth Kirschner wire is drilled into the capitulum of the humerus into the center of the radial head and the proximal half of the radial shaft. The anconeus muscle is resutured to the periosteum of the ulna and fascia of the extensor carpi ulnaris.

The wound is closed, the tip of the Kirschner wire is bent to prevent migration, and an above elbow cast is applied, holding the elbow in 90 degrees of flexion. It is vital that the patient wear a sling and an Ace bandage around the chest in order to prevent breaking of the pin across the elbow joint.

Postoperative Care. The cast is removed four weeks after surgery, and the Kirschner wire is removed. Radiograms are made to assess concentricity of reduction of the radial head in the radial notch of the ulna, and another above-elbow cast is applied for an additional two weeks. The cast is then removed, and active-assisted exercises are performed to restore range of motion of the elbow joint.

REFERENCES

Bell Tawse, A. J. S.: The treatment of malunited anterior Monteggia fractures in children. J. Bone Joint Surg., 47-B:718, 1965.

Kalamchi, A.: Monteggia fracture-dislocation in children. Late treatment in two cases. J. Bone Joint Surg., 68-A:615, 1986.

Lloyd-Roberts, G. C., and Bucknil, T. M.: Anterior dislocation of the radial head in children. J. Bone Joint Surg., 59-B:402, 1977.

Stoll, T. M., Willis, R. B., and Paterson, D. C.: Treatment of the missed Monteggia fracture in the child. J. Bone Joint Surg., 74-B:436, 1992.

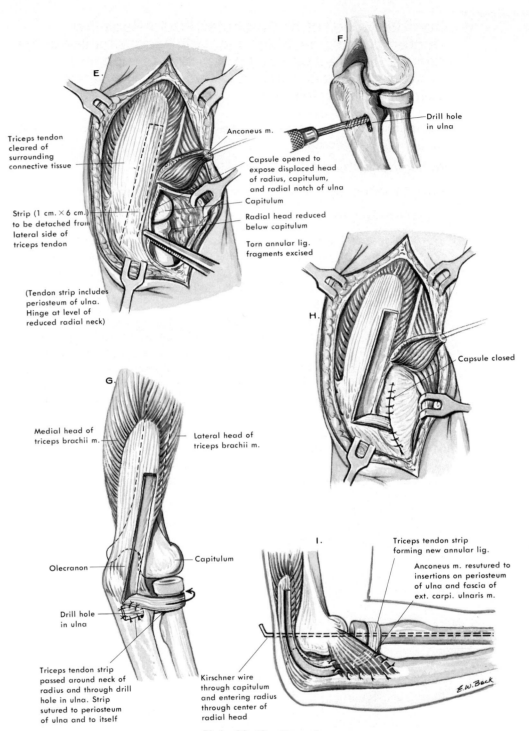

E.

Triceps tendon cleared of surrounding connective tissue

Strip (1 cm. × 6 cm.) to be detached from lateral side of triceps tendon

(Tendon strip includes periosteum of ulna. Hinge at level of reduced radial neck)

Anconeus m.

Capsule opened to expose displaced head of radius, capitulum, and radial notch of ulna

Capitulum

Radial head reduced below capitulum

Torn annular lig. fragments excised

F.

Drill hole in ulna

H.

Capsule closed

G.

Medial head of triceps brachii m.

Lateral head of triceps brachii m.

Olecranon

Capitulum

Drill hole in ulna

Triceps tendon strip passed around neck of radius and through drill hole in ulna. Strip sutured to periosteum of ulna and to itself

I.

Triceps tendon strip forming new annular lig.

Anconeus m. resutured to insertions on periosteum of ulna and fascia of ext. carpi. ulnaris m.

Kirschner wire through capitulum and entering radius through center of radial head

E.W. Back

Plate 33. (Continued)

PLATE 34   **Open Reduction of the Dislocated Radial Head in a Monteggia Fracture-Dislocation with Reconstruction of the Annular Ligament with a Strip of Triceps Tendon and Shortening of the Radius and Osteotomy of the Ulna to Correct Angular Deformity**

Indications. Old Monteggia fracture-dislocation that cannot be reduced without shortening of the radius.

Radiographic Control. Image intensifier.

Patient Position. Supine with upper limb on radiolucent hand table.

Operative Technique

A. The incision is made 7 cm. above the lateral epicondyle of the humerus and extended distally to the lateral epicondyle, where it is curved posteriorly and medially toward the ulna and terminates at the middle of the ulnar shaft. The subcutaneous tissue and fascia are divided in line with the skin incision. The wound flaps are retracted.

B. The triceps tendon, anconeus, flexor carpi ulnaris, and extensor carpi ulnaris muscles are exposed. Incisions are made between the fascia of anconeus and extensor carpi ulnaris and between the anconeus and flexor carpi ulnaris muscles. Dissection is extended to the capsule of the elbow joint.

C. The anconeus muscle is detached from its lateral and medial insertions and is retracted proximally. The supinator muscle is divided from its insertion to the ulna and radius.

Caution! Preserve the nerve supply to the anconeus muscle, and do not injure the posterior interosseous nerve.

D. Assess the pathology of the proximal radioulnar joint. Often the orbicularis ligament is shredded to pieces and the interosseous ligament is torn and scarred.

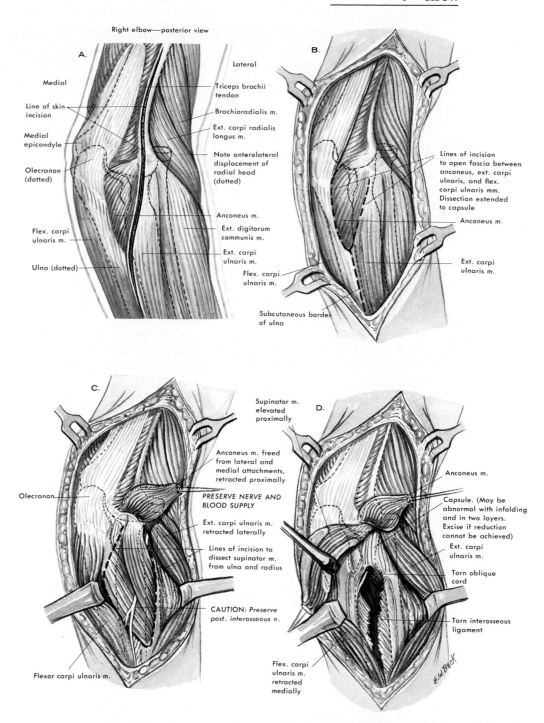

Right elbow—posterior view

A.

Lateral

Medial

Triceps brachii tendon

Line of skin incision

Brachioradialis m.

Medial epicondyle

Ext. carpi radialis longus m.

Olecranon (dotted)

Note anterolateral displacement of radial head (dotted)

Anconeus m.

Flex. carpi ulnaris m.

Ext. digitorum communis m.

Ext. carpi ulnaris m.

Ulna (dotted)

Flex. carpi ulnaris m.

B.

Lines of incision to open fascia between anconeus, ext. carpi ulnaris, and flex. carpi ulnaris mm. Dissection extended to capsule

Anconeus m.

Ext. carpi ulnaris m.

Subcutaneous border of ulna

C.

Supinator m. elevated proximally

Anconeus m. freed from lateral and medial attachments, retracted proximally

Olecranon

PRESERVE NERVE AND BLOOD SUPPLY

Ext. carpi ulnaris m. retracted laterally

Lines of incision to dissect supinator m. from ulna and radius

CAUTION: *Preserve post. interosseous n.*

Flexor carpi ulnaris m.

D.

Anconeus m.

Capsule. (May be abnormal with infolding and in two layers. Excise if reduction cannot be achieved)

Ext. carpi ulnaris m.

Torn oblique cord

Torn interosseous ligament

Flex. carpi ulnaris m. retracted medially

E.W.BECK

Plate 34. A.–I., Open reduction of a dislocated radial head in a Monteggia fracture-dislocation with reconstruction of the annular ligament with a strip of triceps tendon and shortening of the radius and osteotomy of the ulna to correct an angular deformity.

E. Prior to reconstructing an annular ligament, inspect and assess the deformation of the ulna and radius. The angular deformity of the malunited ulna should be corrected first by osteotomy and internal fixation with a four-hole plate or an intramedullary Steinmann pin. If the radius is relatively long in relation to the ulna, one has two options: (1) instantaneous elongation of the ulna with simultaneous correction of the angular deformity, or (2) shortening of the radius. I recommend shortening of the radius at its mid diaphysis through a separate incision; internal fixation is with a four-hole or six-hole AO plate.

F. In this illustration, the shortening of the radius is at its proximal third and through the same incision. After the radius is shortened, the radial head is easily reduced in its anatomic position. Reconstruction of the annular ligament with a strip of triceps fascia is similar to that described in Plate 33. Fixation is accomplished with a Kirschner wire, which is introduced retrograde through the osteotomy site of the midshaft of the radius and inserted into the radial head to its articular surface.

G. At this stage, loop the strip of triceps tendon around the radial neck, from medial to lateral; pass it through a drill hole in the ulna, and suture it to itself.

H. and **I.** After the anatomic reduction of the radial head is checked, the pin is drilled through the capitulum of the humerus out through the skin. The shortened segment of the radius in its mid diaphysis is then aligned, and the Kirschner wire is drilled into the distal segment of the radial shaft. Sometimes, in the adolescent, I have found it simpler to fix the shortened radius at its midshaft with a four-hole plate and to fix the radius to the capitulum separately by a percutaneous pin. In my experience, shortening of the radius has increased the range of pronation and supination of the forearm.

The wound is closed in the usual fashion, and an above-elbow cast is applied, with the elbow in 90 degrees of flexion and the forearm in full supination.

Postoperative Care. The capitulum-radius transfixation pin is removed in three to four weeks postoperatively, and the elbow is immobilized for an additional two weeks. Then active-assisted exercises are performed to restore range of motion of the elbow and forearm.

REFERENCE

Freedman, L., Luk., K., and Leong, J. C. Y.: Radial head reduction after missed Monteggia fracture: Brief report. J. Bone Joint Surg., 70-B:846, 1988.

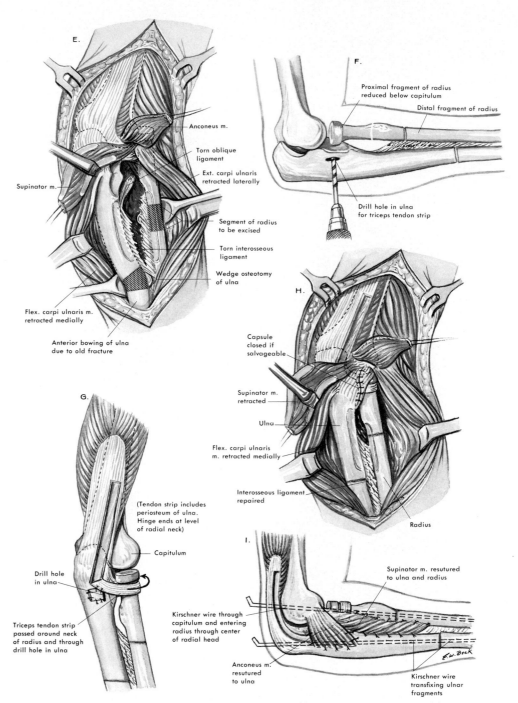

E.

Anconeus m.

Torn oblique
ligament

Ext. carpi ulnaris
retracted laterally

Supinator m.

Segment of radius
to be excised

Torn interosseous
ligament

Wedge osteotomy
of ulna

Flex. carpi ulnaris m.
retracted medially

Anterior bowing of ulna
due to old fracture

F.

Proximal fragment of radius
reduced below capitulum

Distal fragment of radius

Drill hole in ulna
for triceps tendon strip

H.

Capsule
closed if
salvageable

Supinator m.
retracted

Ulna

Flex. carpi ulnaris
m. retracted medially

Interosseous ligament
repaired

Radius

G.

(Tendon strip includes
periosteum of ulna.
Hinge ends at level
of radial neck)

Capitulum

Drill hole
in ulna

Triceps tendon strip
passed around neck
of radius and through
drill hole in ulna

I.

Supinator m. resutured
to ulna and radius

Kirschner wire through
capitulum and entering
radius through center
of radial head

Anconeus m.
resutured
to ulna

Kirschner wire
transfixing ulnar
fragments

E.W.Beck

Plate 34. (Continued)

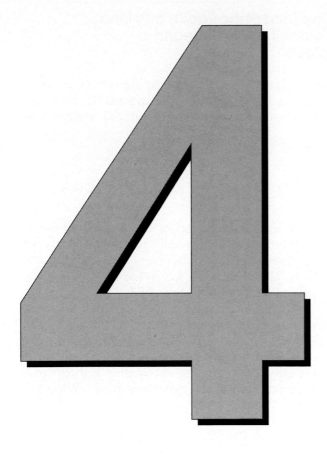

Forearm-Wrist

| PLATE 35 | Osteotomy of the Proximal One Third of the Radius and Ulna to Correct Hyperpronation Deformity of the Forearm in Congenital Radioulnar Synostosis |

Indications. Hyperpronation deformity of the forearm caused by congenital radioulnar synostosis. Proximal derotation osteotomy through the synostotic mass decreases the tension on neurovascular structures when the distal segment is derotated into supination.

Requisites. Functional hand.

Radiographic Control. Image intensifier.

Operative Technique

A. Make a longitudinal incision on the radial aspect of the posterior margin of the ulna beginning 2.5 cm. distal to the olecranon tip and extending distally for a distance of 6 to 8 cm., depending on the size of the patient. Subcutaneous tissue is divided in line with the skin incision. The deep fascia is divided in line with the skin incision, and the wound flaps are undermined and retracted.

B. The anconeus and extensor carpi ulnaris muscles are identified dorsolaterally, and the flexor carpi ulnaris muscle is identified medially and volar. The periosteum is incised longitudinally. Do not disturb the apophyseal growth plate of the olecranon.

C. Determine the level of osteotomy under image intensifier radiographic control. It should be through the distal one half of the synostotic mass. With fine drill holes, mark the osteotomy line.

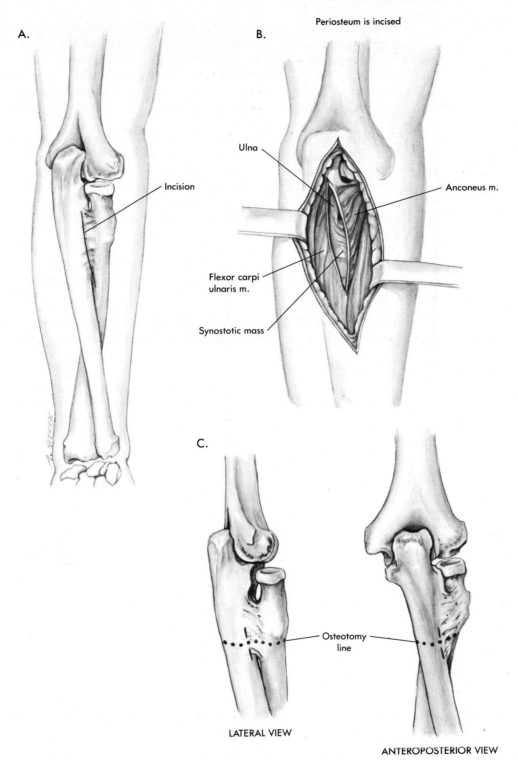

A.

Incision

B.

Periosteum is incised

Ulna

Anconeus m.

Flexor carpi
ulnaris m.

Synostotic mass

C.

Osteotomy
line

LATERAL VIEW

ANTEROPOSTERIOR VIEW

Plate 35. A.–G., Osteotomy of the proximal one third of the radius and ulna to correct hyperpronation deformity of the forearm in congenital radioulnar synostosis.

D. Mark the ulna on either side of the osteotomy line to determine the degree of rotation by the marks as well as by the position of the hand and forearm. Perform the osteotomy with the help of sharp AO osteotomes.

E. Under image intensifier radiographic control, insert a smooth Steinmann pin from the tip of the olecranon into the ulnar shaft stopping short of the osteotomy. Rotate the distal mass and forearm into the desired degree of supination, which is usually 20 to 45 degrees.

F. Drill the Steinmann pin further distally into the proximal half of the ulnar shaft. Usually, this type of internal fixation is satisfactory and the osteotomy is stable.

G. However, if control of rotation by the intramedullary Steinmann pin is not adequate, one or two criss-cross Kirschner wires can be inserted to control rotation. This author has not found it to be necessary to use any external fixation device. The tip of the Steinmann pin is left protruding at the olecranon process. It is bent to prevent migration.

The wound is closed in the usual fashion, and an above-elbow cast is applied, with the elbow in about 60 degrees of flexion and the forearm in the desired degree of supination.

Postoperative Care. The above-elbow cast and the pins are removed four weeks postoperatively. Another cast is applied for an additional two weeks.

REFERENCES

Green, W. T., and Mital, M. A.: Congenital radioulnar synostosis: Surgical treatment. J. Bone Joint Surg., 61–A:738, 1979.

Griffet, J., Berard, J., Michel, C. R., and Caton, J.: Les synostoses congénitales radio-cubitales supérieures. Int. Orthop., 10:265, 1986.

Judet, J., and Judet, H.: Synostose radio-cubitale congénitale. In: Techniques Chirurgicales Fractures et Orthopédie de l'Enfant. Paris, Maloine, 1974.

D.

Osteotomy
of synostotic
mass

E.

Smooth
Steinmann
pin

F.

Steinmann pin
drilled further
to proximal
ulna

G.

Criss-cross
Kirschner
wires

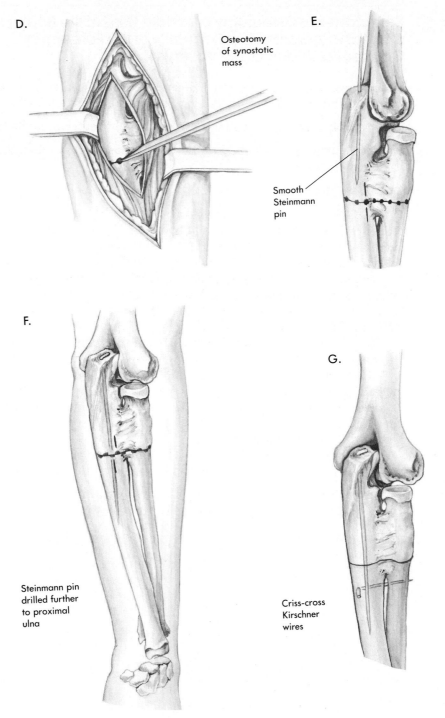

Plate 35. (Continued)

PLATE 36

Percutaneous Osteotomy of Middle Third of the Radius to Correct Hyperpronation Deformity of the Forearm in Congenital Radioulnar Synostosis

Indications. Rigid hyperpronation deformity of the forearm in congenital radioulnar synostosis when less than 60 degrees of derotation is required.

Radiographic Control. Image intensifier is used to determine the level of osteotomy.

Patient Position. The patient is in the supine position; the shoulder is abducted and the elbow extended.

Operative Technique

A. A 3-cm. longitudinal incision is made at the center of the middle one third of the radius. Subcutaneous tissue is divided in line with the skin incision. With the help of Metzenbaum scissors, the radius is exposed.

B. The periosteum is incised longitudinally. With the help of a Freer elevator, the radial shaft is exposed subperiosteally and Homan retractors are inserted subperiosteally to expose the radial shaft. The line of osteotomy is delineated; it is transverse. Do not perform it obliquely because on derotation the bone fragments will angulate.

C. Drill holes are made in the cortex of the radius circumferentially, and with the help of a small, sharp AO osteotome, a corticotomy of the radius is performed.

D. and **E.** By forceful manipulation, the radius is broken and the forearm is supinated to neutral position. Internal fixation is not necessary. The tourniquet is released, complete hemostasis is achieved, and a medium Hemovac is placed in the wound if there is bleeding from the bone. The periosteum is closed with 00 Tycron interrupted sutures.

The wound is closed in the usual fashion, and an above-elbow cast is applied with the elbow flexed 90 degrees and the forearm in neutral position.

Postoperative Care. The osteotomy usually heals in about 6 weeks, and the cast is removed. Ordinarily, no special physical therapy is required.

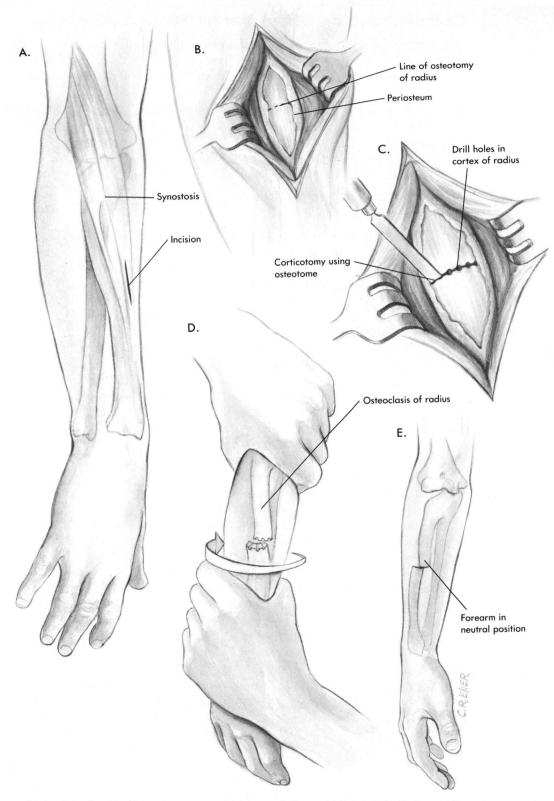

A.

B.
Line of osteotomy
of radius

Periosteum

C.
Drill holes in
cortex of radius

Synostosis

Incision

Corticotomy using
osteotome

D.

Osteoclasis of radius

E.

Forearm in
neutral position

C. R. Eller

Plate 36. A.–E., Percutaneous osteotomy of the middle third of the radius to correct hyperpronation deformity of the forearm in congenital radioulnar synostosis.

PLATE 37 ## Centralization of the Carpus over the Distal End of the Ulna

Indications. Unstable carpus with progressive radial drifting of the hand over the distal end of the ulna with total or partial absence of the radius. (Perform the procedure early; the child should preferably be between the ages of six and 12 months.)

Requisites. There should be functional range of elbow flexion. Be sure that radial deviation and flexion of the wrist are not required to bring the hand into feeding position.

Caution! Rule out hypoplastic or aplastic anemia, thrombocytopenia, and other associated anomalies.

Patient Position. Supine with the upper limb on a hand table.

Operative Technique

A. The skin incision begins on the dorsum of the hand on the radial border of the distal third of the second metacarpal; it extends proximally and ulnarward toward the prominence of the ulnar head, where it deviates radially and proximally to terminate at the proximal third of the volar surface of the forearm at its radial border. This approach permits an extensive view of the dorsal, radial, and volar aspects of the hand, wrist, and forearm. Subcutaneous tissue is divided in line with the skin incision. Avoid damage to the veins.

B. Next, the deep fascia is split widely in the forearm, and the median nerve with its peripheral distribution is identified. The median nerve is thicker than normal and almost invariably aberrant. About 6 to 7 cm. proximal to the wrist, it may divide into two large terminal branches, one passing to the volar surface of the forearm and wrist and through the carpal tunnel and the second continuing along the radial side of the forearm and wrist, supplying the innervator normally provided by the radial nerve. It is very easy to divide the radial branch inadvertently; it should be isolated and protected.

The median nerve is always preaxial, acting as a bowstring to the radially deviated forearm and wrist. Its course may vary in a number of ways. It may traverse superficially along the radial margin of the brachioradialis muscle until it enters the palm; it may lie beneath the palmaris longus and flexor digitorum sublimis; it may traverse along the radial edge of the flexor digitorum sublimis; or it may emerge superficially beneath the flexors at the middle of the forearm and course distally between the brachioradialis and the extensor digitorum communis. The median nerve can withstand a great deal of stretching and still provide sensory and motor conduction but cannot tolerate external compression by taut fascia and fibrous bands. Therefore, it is crucial to relieve it of all constricting bands and perform a thorough release of the deep fascia.

Caution! The median nerve is radial in its course and lies immediately beneath the deep fascia.

C. and **D.** The incision is developed to the level of the tendons on the dorsal, ulnar, and volar surfaces of the distal ulna. The *dorsal sensory branch of the ulnar nerve* is identified and gently retracted. The extensor carpi ulnaris tendon is identified, detached at its insertion, marked with 00 Tycron suture, and reflected proximally and medially (later to be advanced distally on the fifth metacarpal as tautly as possible). The flexor carpi ulnaris tendon is identified next by blunt dissection. (Avoid injury to the ulnar artery, the major blood supply to the hand; identify, isolate, and protect the ulnar vessels and nerve from injury.) The tendon is detached at its insertion to the pisiform bone; later on, along with the extensor carpi ulnaris, it will be sutured as snugly as possible to the dorsal and radial aspect of the fifth metacarpal.

E. Next, identify the distal end of the ulna and develop the interval between its borders and the carpus. Stay extraperiosteal! *Do not damage growth of the distal ulnar physis!* There will be a thickened false joint capsule covering the distal end of the ulna; carefully and gently section it, dissect it, and elevate it distally,

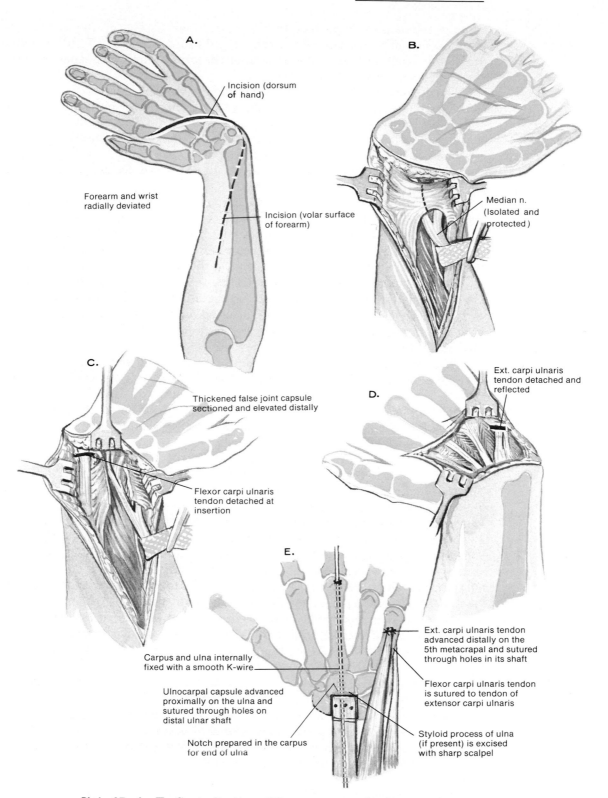

A.

Incision (dorsum of hand)

Forearm and wrist radially deviated

Incision (volar surface of forearm)

B.

Median n. (Isolated and protected)

C.

Thickened false joint capsule sectioned and elevated distally

Flexor carpi ulnaris tendon detached at insertion

D.

Ext. carpi ulnaris tendon detached and reflected

E.

Carpus and ulna internally fixed with a smooth K-wire

Ulnocarpal capsule advanced proximally on the ulna and sutured through holes on distal ulnar shaft

Notch prepared in the carpus for end of ulna

Ext. carpi ulnaris tendon advanced distally on the 5th metacrapal and sutured through holes in its shaft

Flexor carpi ulnaris tendon is sutured to tendon of extensor carpi ulnaris

Styloid process of ulna (if present) is excised with sharp scalpel

Plate 37. A.–E., Centralization of the carpus over the distal end of the ulna.

leaving the capsule attached to the dorsoulnar aspect of the carpus. (After implantation of the carpus, the distally based ulnocarpal capsule will be advanced proximally and sutured to the dorsum of the ulna.) The wrist tendons will have aberrant insertions to the capsule.

The flexor carpi radialis and brachioradialis tendons insert to the radial aspect of the carpus and joint capsule, acting as a strong radial tethering force. When sectioning the constricted fibrotic tendons, be sure not to buttonhole and weaken the capsule. To maintain alignment, the capsule must be tautly reefed. It is sectioned on the radial and volar surfaces of the wrist.

Caution! Any fibrous anlage of the radius is excised. Do not injure the median nerve and anterior interosseous vessels.

Measurements for the notch in the carpus for insertion of the distal end of the ulna are made on the radiograms. The sides of the slot should be as long as the diameter of the end of the ulna, the insertion being mechanically stable only when its depth is at least equal to its diameter—a vital basic biomechanical principle. Specific carpal bones are difficult to identify; the trapezium and navicular are often absent. The entire capitate bone is frequently excised to achieve stability. An adequate buttress of carpal wall must be maintained on the radial side.

The styloid process of the ulna is excised, and its cartilage is slightly shaved with a sharp scalpel. *Use no osteotomes, no hammering! Do not impair growth of the distal ulnar physis!*

With the elbow flexed, the carpus is reduced over the end of the ulna. Avoid excessive force. The fit must be easy but snug. The shaft of the third metacarpal should be perpendicular to the distal growth plate of the ulna. A single-bone forearm will have no rotation and no radioulnar deviation. With functional range of elbow and shoulder motion, it is best to place the distal ulna into the carpus in a position of 30 to 45 degrees of pronation.

Next, the carpus and ulna are internally fixed with a smooth Kirschner wire inserted proximally to distally through the shaft of the third metacarpal and out through its head. Be sure that it is not volar. The pin is drilled proximally through the center of the distal ulnar epiphysis and up the medullary cavity. If the ulna is markedly bowed, wedge osteotomy of its shaft is performed to correct the curvature.

After internal fixation, the tourniquet is deflated and complete hemostasis is obtained. Circulation in the hand is assessed. First, the distally based ulnocarpal capsule is advanced proximally on the ulna and sutured through holes on the distal ulnar shaft. Second, the *extensor carpi ulnaris tendon* is advanced distally on the fifth metacarpal as tautly as possible and sutured through holes in the bone's shaft. It is best to make the holes with an electric drill. Third, the *flexor carpi ulnaris tendon* is sutured to the extensor carpi ulnaris tendon as far dorsally and distally as possible. Thus, the hand is balanced dynamically over the distal end of the ulna.

A closed-suction Hemovac drainage tube is inserted in the wound, and the skin incisions are closed in the usual fashion.

An above-elbow cast is applied, with the elbow flexed 90 degrees and the hand in neutral position. The metacarpophalangeal and interphalangeal joints are left free for active and passive exercises to correct extension contracture of the metacarpophalangeal joints and flexion contracture of the proximal interphalangeal joints.

Some surgeons (and sometimes this author) prefer to apply a fluffy compression dressing with a dorsal plaster of Paris slab holding the elbow in 90 degrees of flexion. The hand is elevated for several days to minimize postoperative swelling, which usually subsides within a week. Then a new circular plaster of Paris above-elbow cast that extends distally to the metacarpal heads is applied.

Postoperative Care. The cast and sutures are removed in four weeks. A new above-elbow cast is worn for an additional four weeks, by which time a simultaneously

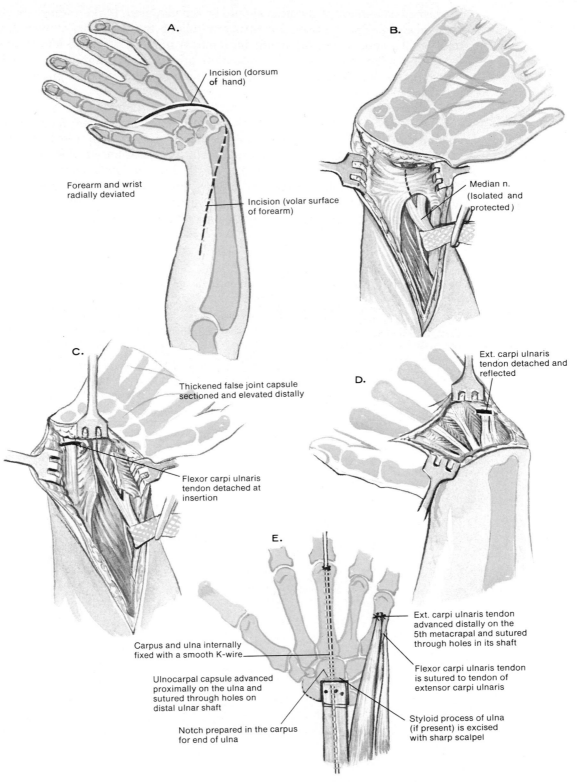

A.

Incision (dorsum of hand)

Forearm and wrist radially deviated

Incision (volar surface of forearm)

B.

Median n. (Isolated and protected)

C.

Thickened false joint capsule sectioned and elevated distally

Flexor carpi ulnaris tendon detached at insertion

D.

Ext. carpi ulnaris tendon detached and reflected

E.

Carpus and ulna internally fixed with a smooth K-wire

Ulnocarpal capsule advanced proximally on the ulna and sutured through holes on distal ulnar shaft

Notch prepared in the carpus for end of ulna

Ext. carpi ulnaris tendon advanced distally on the 5th metacrapal and sutured through holes in its shaft

Flexor carpi ulnaris tendon is sutured to tendon of extensor carpi ulnaris

Styloid process of ulna (if present) is excised with sharp scalpel

Plate 37. (Continued)

performed osteotomy of the ulna should be consolidated. Make radiograms to verify bone healing. There is some controversy about the duration of Kirschner wire fixation. This author recommends its removal in eight weeks, when the final cast is taken off. This allows some wrist motion, prevents potential damage to the distal ulnar physis, and obviates breakage of the wire at the wrist or pin extrusion and pin tract infection.

After pin and cast removal, a plastic dorsal hand orthosis is made; the splint should extend proximally to just below the elbow for proper lever support and should support the wrist in a few degrees of ulnar deviation and 10 to 20 degrees of dorsiflexion. Leaving the volar aspect relatively free encourages prehension and hand function. Initially, the orthosis is worn day and night. Several times a day, the splint is removed, and passive and active exercises are performed to develop wrist motion. Day use of the splint is discontinued when the child is two to three years of age, but night use is continued for an additional two years.

REFERENCES

Bora, F. W., Jr., Nicholson, J. T., and Cheema, H. M.: Radial meromelia: The deformity and its treatment. J. Bone Joint Surg., 52–A:966, 1970.

Bora, F. W., Osterman, A. L., Kaneda, R. R., and Esterhai, J.: Radial club-hand deformity. Long-term follow-up. J. Bone Joint Surg., 63–A:741, 1981.

Flatt, A.: The Care of Congenital Hand Anomalies. St. Louis, C. V. Mosby, 1977, pp. 286–327.

Lamb, D. W.: Radial club hand, a continuing study of sixty-eight patients with one hundred and seventeen club hands. J. Bone Joint Surg., 59–A:1, 1977.

Lidge, R.: Congenital radial deficient club hand. J. Bone Joint Surg., 51–A:1041, 1969.

Sayre, R. H.: A contribution to the study of club-hand. Trans. Am. Orthop. Assoc., 6:208, 1893.

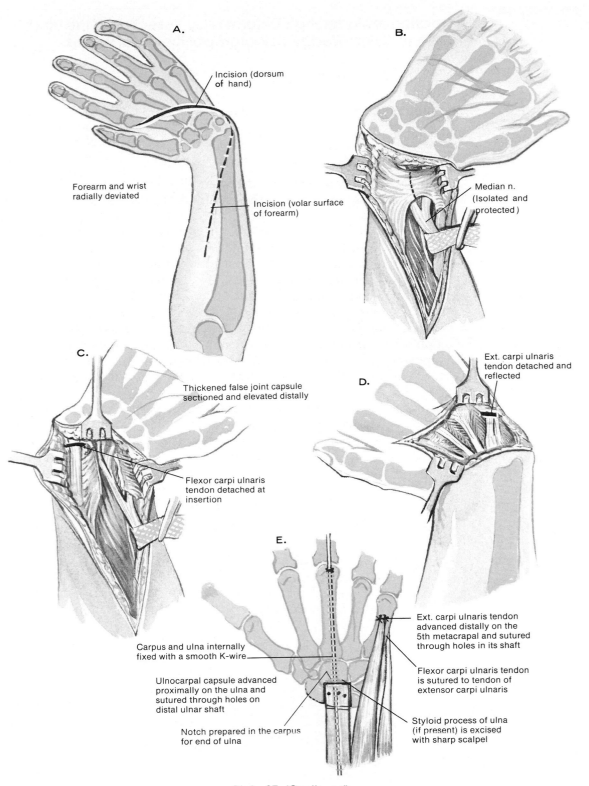

A.

Incision (dorsum of hand)

Forearm and wrist radially deviated

Incision (volar surface of forearm)

B.

Median n. (Isolated and protected)

C.

Thickened false joint capsule sectioned and elevated distally

Flexor carpi ulnaris tendon detached at insertion

D.

Ext. carpi ulnaris tendon detached and reflected

E.

Carpus and ulna internally fixed with a smooth K-wire

Ulnocarpal capsule advanced proximally on the ulna and sutured through holes on distal ulnar shaft

Notch prepared in the carpus for end of ulna

Ext. carpi ulnaris tendon advanced distally on the 5th metacrapal and sutured through holes in its shaft

Flexor carpi ulnaris tendon is sutured to tendon of extensor carpi ulnaris

Styloid process of ulna (if present) is excised with sharp scalpel

Plate 37. (Continued)

PLATE 38 ## Correction of Madelung's Deformity by Resection of the Ulnar Head and Open-Wedge Osteotomy of the Distal Radius

Indications. Pain and severe deformity of the wrist that is cosmetically objectionable in the patient 11 years and older.

Radiographic Control. Image intensifier.

Patient Position. Supine with upper limb on radiolucent hand table.

Operative Technique

A. Two longitudinal incisions are made. The first, on the dorsoulnar aspect of the wrist and forearm, begins on the dorsum of the base of the fourth metacarpal and extends proximally to the wrist where, at the dorsal crease, it traverses ulnarward immediately above the prominent distal ulnar head and then extends proximally for a distance of 5 to 7 cm. The second longitudinal incision is 7 cm. long on the radial margin of the volar surface of the wrist, beginning at the radial styloid process. The subcutaneous tissues are divided in line with the skin incisions. Avoid injury to dorsal veins and branches of sensory nerves.

B. The extensor retinaculum is divided and reflected ulnarward. The extensor carpi ulnaris is retracted radially. With an oscillating saw, perform an oblique resection of the distal ulna. The dorsal and radial part of the ulnar head, including its epiphysis, is removed. The osteotomy begins 3 cm. proximal to the distal articular surface of the ulna on its dorsoradial aspect and slants ulnarward. The resected ulnar head is kept sterile for bone graft.

C. Next, the extensor carpi ulnaris tendon is split into halves. A tunnel is made with an electric drill through the lower end of the ulnar shaft, and the free split half of the extensor carpi ulnaris tendon is passed through it and sutured to the continuous other half of the tendon.

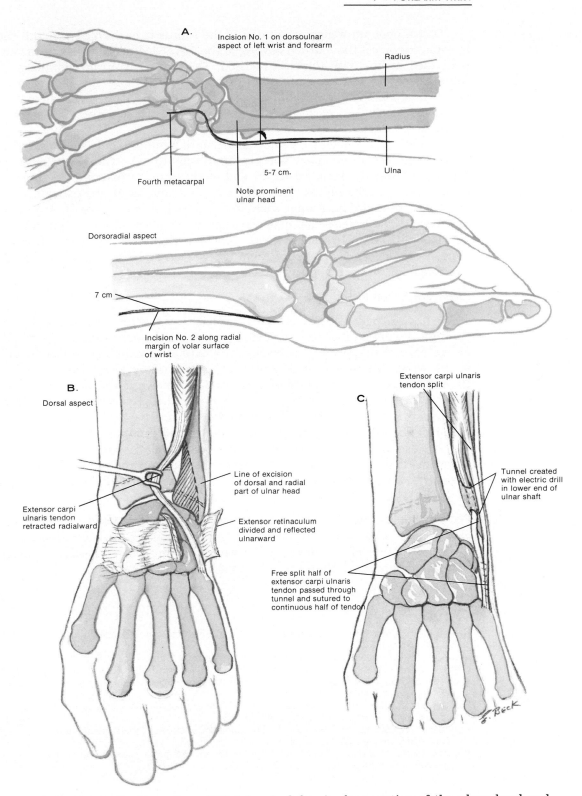

A.

Incision No. 1 on dorsoulnar
aspect of left wrist and forearm

Radius

Fourth metacarpal

5-7 cm.

Ulna

Note prominent
ulnar head

Dorsoradial aspect

7 cm

Incision No. 2 along radial
margin of volar surface
of wrist

B.

Dorsal aspect

Line of excision
of dorsal and radial
part of ulnar head

Extensor carpi
ulnaris tendon
retracted radialward

Extensor retinaculum
divided and reflected
ulnarward

C.

Extensor carpi ulnaris
tendon split

Tunnel created
with electric drill
in lower end of
ulnar shaft

Free split half of
extensor carpi ulnaris
tendon passed through
tunnel and sutured to
continuous half of tendon

Plate 38. A.–G., Correction of Madelung's deformity by resection of the ulnar head and
open-wedge osteotomy of the distal radius.

D. An open-up wedge osteotomy of the radius is performed through the volar incision to correct the marked bowing of the distal radius. The subcutaneous tissue is divided in line with the skin incision. The flexor carpi radialis along with the radial artery is retracted ulnarward. The distal shaft of the radius is exposed; avoid injury to the distal radial physis. With an oscillating saw, osteotomy of the distal radial shaft is performed on its volar and ulnar aspects. The dorsoradial cortex is left intact.

E. With a periosteal elevator and small laminar bone spreader, the distal radial segment is elevated dorsally and radially. A triangular piece of bone fashioned from the resected distal end of the ulna is inserted on the volar and ulnar aspects of the radius. The osteotomy and bone graft are transfixed with two criss-cross threaded Kirschner wires inserted with an electric drill. Anteroposterior and lateral radiograms are made to ensure adequacy of correction and internal fixation with the Kirschner wires. The tourniquet is released; after complete hemostasis, a Hemovac suction tube is inserted and the wound is closed in the usual fashion. An above-elbow cast is applied.

Alternate Procedure

F. and **G.** Some surgeons prefer to perform the osteotomy of the distal radius through the dorsal incision. In such an instance, the skin incision begins dorsally at the base of the second metacarpal and extends proximally to the dorsal crease of the wrist, where it swings ulnarward immediately above the ulnar head and then continues longitudinally upward for a distance of 5 to 7 cm. The distal radial shaft is exposed by developing a plane between the extensor carpi radialis and the extensor digitorum longus. The pronator quadratus is elevated and retracted distally. The osteotomy of the radius is performed from its ulnar side.

A close-up biplane osteotomy of the distal radial shaft is preferred by some surgeons. The base of the wedge to be resected is dorsal and radial. The osteotomized segments are apposed and anteromedially fixed internally with two criss-cross, threaded wires.

Postoperative Care. The osteotomy usually heals in six to eight weeks. The cast is changed as necessary. The two pins are removed. Passive exercises, to restore range of motion of the wrist, and active and progressive resistive exercises, to increase motor strength of the wrist and hand, are begun.

REFERENCES

Kelikian, H.: Congenital Deformities of the Hand and Forearm. Philadelphia, W. B. Saunders Co., 1974, pp. 753–779.

Matev, I., and Karagancheva, S.: The Madelung deformity. Hand, 7:152, 1975.

Milch, H.: Cuff resection of the ulna for malunited Colles' fracture. J. Bone Joint Surg., 23:311, 1941.

Nielsen, J. B.: Madelung's deformity: A follow-up study of 26 cases and a review of the literature. Acta Orthop. Scand., 48:379, 1977.

Ranawat, C. S., DeFiore, J., and Straub, L. R.: Madelung's deformity: An end-result study of surgical treatment. J. Bone Joint Surg., 57–A:772, 1975.

Rigault, P., Kipfer, M., and Beneux, J.: Treatment of so-called Madelung's deformity of the forearm. Rev. Chir. Orthop., 48:341, 1972.

Vickers, D. W.: Premature incomplete fusion of the growth plate. Causes and treatment by resection (physolysis) in fifteen cases. Aust. N. Z. J. Surg., 50:393, 1980.

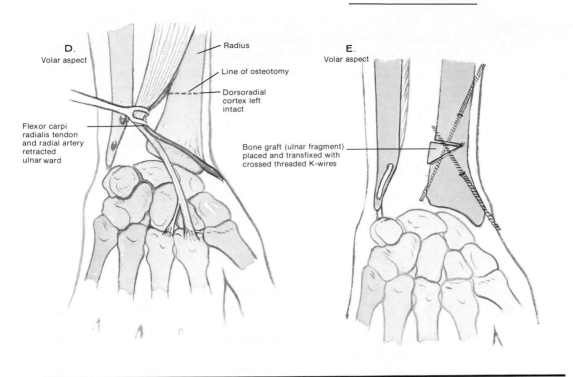

D.
Volar aspect

Radius

Line of osteotomy

Dorsoradial
cortex left
intact

Flexor carpi
radialis tendon
and radial artery
retracted
ulnar ward

E.
Volar aspect

Bone graft (ulnar fragment)
placed and transfixed with
crossed threaded K-wires

Alternate procedure

Correction with closing wedge bi-plane
osteotomy and distal ulnar resection
(shaded areas)

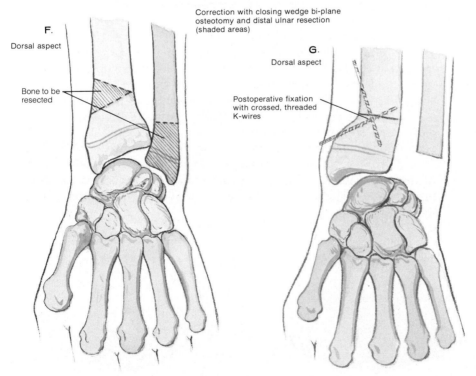

F.
Dorsal aspect

Bone to be
resected

G.
Dorsal aspect

Postoperative fixation
with crossed, threaded
K-wires

Plate 38. (Continued)

PLATE 39   **Excision of the Prematurely Fused Volar Ulnar Half of the Distal Radial Physis and Interposition of Fat (Langenskiöld Procedure) As Described by Vickers for Treatment of Madelung's Deformity**

Indications. Pain at wrist and severe deformity that is cosmetically objectionable.

Requisites. The patient should be ten years of age or younger.

Operative Technique

A. A volar surgical approach is used to expose the distal radius. A transverse incision is made into the proximal flexion crease of the wrist beginning at the tendon of flexor carpi ulnaris and extending to the interval between the tendons of brachioradialis laterally and flexor carpi ulnaris tendon medially. At this lateral point, the incision curves proximally in the interval between the two tendons for a distance of 4 to 5 cm. The subcutaneous tissue is divided in line with the skin incision. The skin margins are elevated with double-prong skin hooks; the skin flaps are developed and retracted. Avoid injury to the underlying neurovascular structures.

B. Next, the deep fascia of the forearm is incised. *Caution!* Do not inadvertently injure the radial vessels or the median nerve.

The brachioradialis tendon is identified and retracted dorsally and radially; the flexor carpi radialis tendon is pulled toward the ulna. The radial vessels are identified and dissected by blunt scissors or hemostat, mobilized, and protected with red silicone (Silastic) tubing.

C. The flexor carpi radialis tendon is retracted radially and the palmaris longus tendon medially, exposing the flexor digitorum sublimis muscle. The radial margin of the flexor digitorum sublimis is elevated by blunt dissection. The median nerve and its accompanying artery are exposed deep to the flexor digitorum sublimis; yellow Silastic tubing is passed around the median nerve.

D. The flexor digitorum profundus tendon is exposed by retracting the flexor digitorum sublimis ulnarward. It should be noted that the flexor digitorum profundus tendon traverses over the pronator quadriceps muscle and lies primarily in the front of the distal ulna and adjacent interosseous membrane. Next, the flexor carpi radialis tendon is retracted medially, exposing the flexor pollicis longus muscle and tendon, which lie in front of the radius and adjacent interosseous membrane.

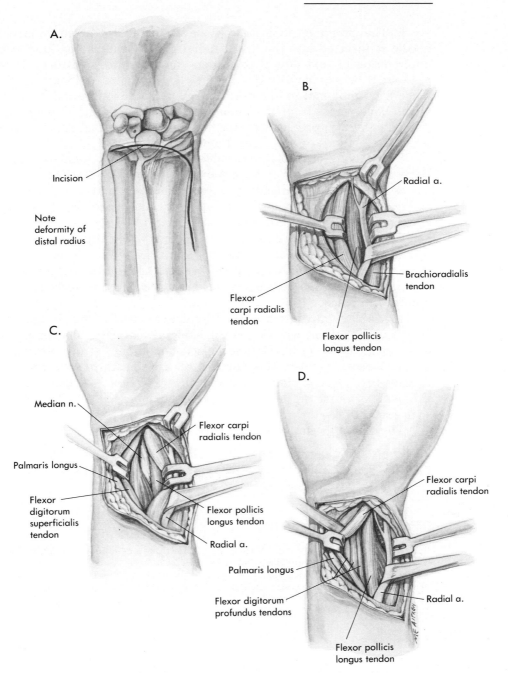

A.

Incision

Note
deformity of
distal radius

B.

Radial a.

Brachioradialis
tendon

Flexor
carpi radialis
tendon

Flexor pollicis
longus tendon

C.

Median n.

Flexor carpi
radialis tendon

Palmaris longus

Flexor
digitorum
superficialis
tendon

Flexor pollicis
longus tendon

Radial a.

D.

Flexor carpi
radialis tendon

Palmaris longus

Flexor digitorum
profundus tendons

Radial a.

Flexor pollicis
longus tendon

Plate 39. A.–G. Correction of Madelung's deformity by resection of the osseous bridge on the volar ulnar aspect of the distal radius.

E. The pronator quadratus is elevated and retracted ulnarward. A Keith needle is inserted into the distal radial physis, and radiograms are made in the anteroposterior and lateral projections for accurate identification of the growth plate. It is best to identify the distal radioulnar joint. A longitudinal osteotomy is made from proximal to distal in the radius approximately one third of the width of the bone across from the radioulnar joint. A triangle of bone and cartilage is incised carefully, preserving what remains of the distal radioulnar joint and the articular cartilage on the distal radius.

F. A wavy growth plate is visible just proximal to a narrowed bony epiphysis. Bone is removed with a fine rongeur until a healthy cartilaginous physis is seen across the bone. Magnification is recommended. A dental burr is then used to excise a little more bone on the metaphyseal side of the physis so that the cartilage stands up well clear of the bone.

G. After the cavity has been washed out with saline, a small amount of bone wax may be applied to the trough on both sides of the physis. A generous free fat graft is then inserted into the space between the reflected triangular ulnar segment of the radius and the physis. The fat graft is sutured to surrounding structures to secure it in place.

In the skeletally immature child, epiphyseodesis of the distal ulna is performed. In the older patient who is nearing skeletal maturity, shortening of the ulna by excision of its distal physis and adjacent metaphysis and internal fixation with staples is recommended. These procedures are done through a separate longitudinal dorsal-ulnar incision simultaneously with excision of the bony bridge of the distal radius. Shortening of the ulna improves the appearance and function of the radius with further growth.

The wound is closed in routine fashion.

Postoperative Care. A well-padded, above-elbow cast is applied with some compression of the radius toward the ulna. After three weeks, the cast is shortened to below the elbow for an additional three weeks.

REFERENCES

Ranawat, C. S., DeFiore, J., and Straub, L. R.: Madelung's deformity: An end-result study of surgical treatment. J. Bone Joint Surg., 57–A:772, 1975.

Vickers, D. W.: Premature incomplete fusion of the growth plate: Causes and treatment by resection (physolysis) in fifteen cases. Aust. N. Z. J. Surg., 50:393, 1980.

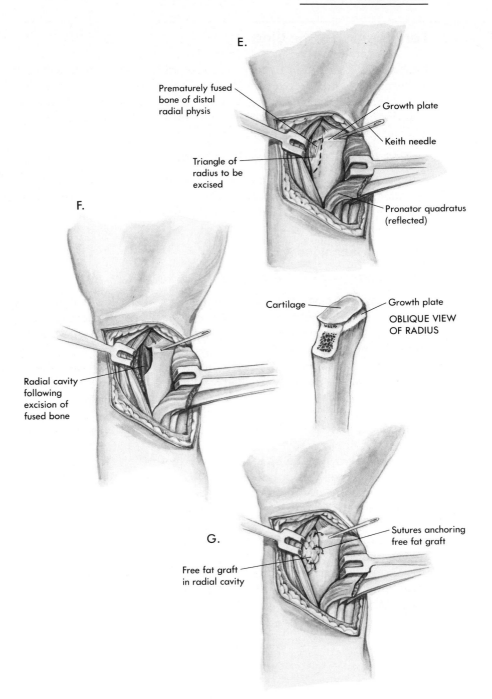

E.

Prematurely fused bone of distal radial physis

Growth plate

Keith needle

Triangle of radius to be excised

Pronator quadratus (reflected)

F.

Cartilage

Growth plate

OBLIQUE VIEW OF RADIUS

Radial cavity following excision of fused bone

G.

Sutures anchoring free fat graft

Free fat graft in radial cavity

Plate 39. (Continued)

PLATE 40   ## Lengthening of the Ulna

Indications. Short ulna in relation to the radius with progressive ulnar subluxation of the carpus and subluxation of the radial head with bowing of the radius. Perform instantaneous Z-lengthening if total length desired is 2 cm. or less. If greater lengthening is required, perform instantaneous proximal lengthening with bone graft or gradual lengthening.

Radiographic Control. Image intensifier.

Patient Position. The patient is supine with the upper limb resting on a hand operating table. A pneumatic tourniquet is applied on the proximal arm. After routine preparation and draping of the upper limb, the posterolateral aspect of the ulna is exposed.

Operative Technique

Instantaneous Z-step Cut Lengthening (A.–F.)

A. Make a posterior incision beginning at the lower end of the shortened ulna and extending proximally along its subcutaneous margin to terminate at the apophysis of the olecranon. Divide the subcutaneous tissue and fascia in line with the skin incision.

B. The periosteum is divided longitudinally, and the ulnar shaft is exposed subperiosteally. The extensor carpi ulnaris with its tendon is retracted anteriorly. Depending on the type of lengthening desired (Wagner, Orthofix or AO), under image intensifier radiographic control insert two threaded pins proximally and two pins distally. In this illustration, the small Wagner lengthening device is used; one small Schanz screw is drilled into the proximal ulnar shaft immediately distal to the apophysis of the olecranon, and another screw is drilled into the olecranon. Use the Wagner drill guide for correct placement of the second screw. The distal pair of Schanz screws should be parallel and in the same plane as the proximal pair so that the Wagner lengthening device can be easily applied.

With a small drill bit or Kirschner wire, drill the Z-step cut osteotomy line in the mediolateral plane. There should be adequate overlap of bone in the center for secure fixation.

C. Apply the lengthening device firmly to the screws. Perform the longitudinal osteotomy with a small oscillating saw. With a small AO osteotome, make the transverse cuts.

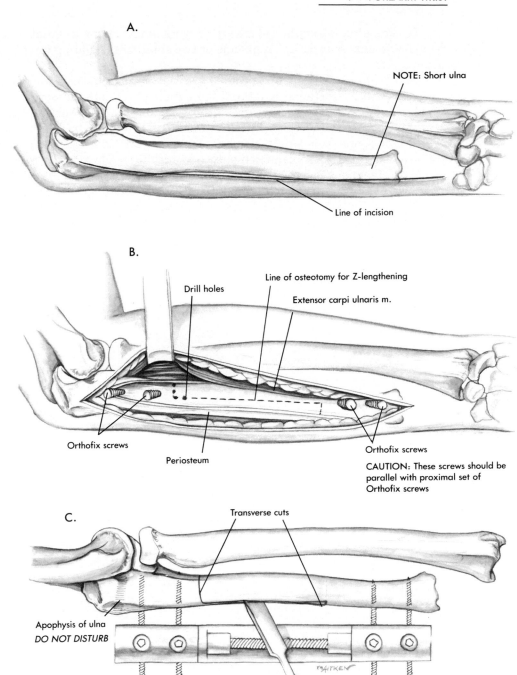

A.

NOTE: Short ulna

Line of incision

B.

Line of osteotomy for Z-lengthening

Drill holes

Extensor carpi ulnaris m.

Orthofix screws

Periosteum

Orthofix screws

CAUTION: These screws should be parallel with proximal set of Orthofix screws

C.

Transverse cuts

Apophysis of ulna
DO NOT DISTURB

AO osteotome

Plate 40. A.–N., Lengthening of the ulna. **A.–F.,** Instantaneous Z-step cut lengthening. **G.–N.,** Instantaneous lengthening of the ulna at its proximal one third with autogenous bone graft from the ilium and internal fixation with an intramedullary pin.

D. The ulna is lengthened slowly. During lengthening, angulation of the ulnar bone fragments may occur. Apply one or two small bone-holding forceps and control alignment.

Sometimes soft tissues, especially the flexor carpi ulnaris and extensor carpi ulnaris, require fractional lengthening at their musculotendinous junction.

E. Make anteroposterior and lateral radiograms to ensure that adequate lengthening is obtained. Be cautious—the distal ulna may fracture. The maximum lengthening one can safely achieve by this technique is about 2.5 cm. The osteotomized fragments are fixed with a semitubular plate and screws.

F. Autogenous bone is taken from the ilium and inserted into the space of the elongated sites both proximally and distally. Final radiograms are made.

The tourniquet is released, and complete hemostasis is achieved. The wound is closed in routine fashion, and a posterior above-elbow splint is applied.

D.   LATERAL VIEW

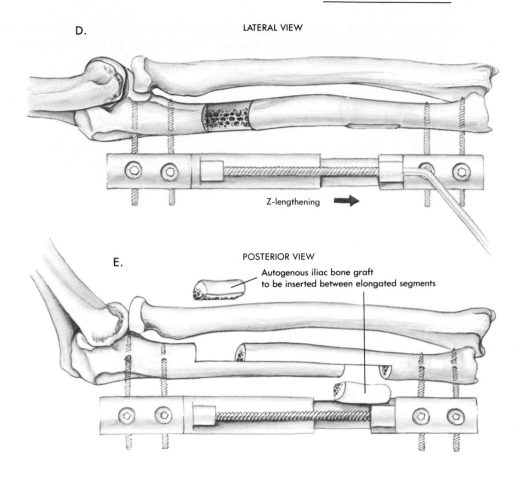

Z-lengthening ➡

E.

POSTERIOR VIEW

Autogenous iliac bone graft
to be inserted between elongated segments

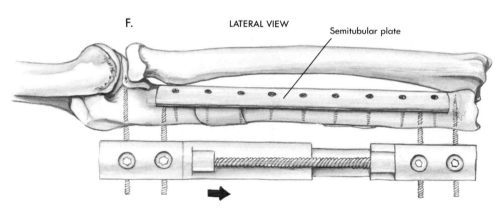

F.   LATERAL VIEW   Semitubular plate

➡

Plate 40. (Continued)

Instantaneous Lengthening of the Ulna at Its Proximal One Third with Autogenous Bone Graft from the Ilium and Internal Fixation with an Intramedullary Pin (G.–N.)

G. A posterior incision is made beginning at the tip of the olecranon and extending distally to the juncture of the proximal two thirds and distal one fourth of the ulna. Subcutaneous tissue is divided in line with the skin incision, and superficial fascia is incised. Do not disturb the apophyseal growth plate of the olecranon.

H. The periosteum is divided, and the proximal ulnar shaft is exposed periosteally. Retract the extensor carpi ulnaris anteriorly. Depending on the age of the patient, use the Orthofix (mini or small) or small Wagner lengthening device.

I. Insert one pin with an electric drill into the proximal ulnar metaphysis, and with the mini-Orthofix guide introduce another pin into the olecranon proximal to the apophysis. Insert two pins parallel to the first into the middle one third of the ulna, and connect the Orthofix apparatus to the pins.

J. A corticotomy of the ulna, 2 cm. distal to the growth plate of the olecranon, is performed.

G.

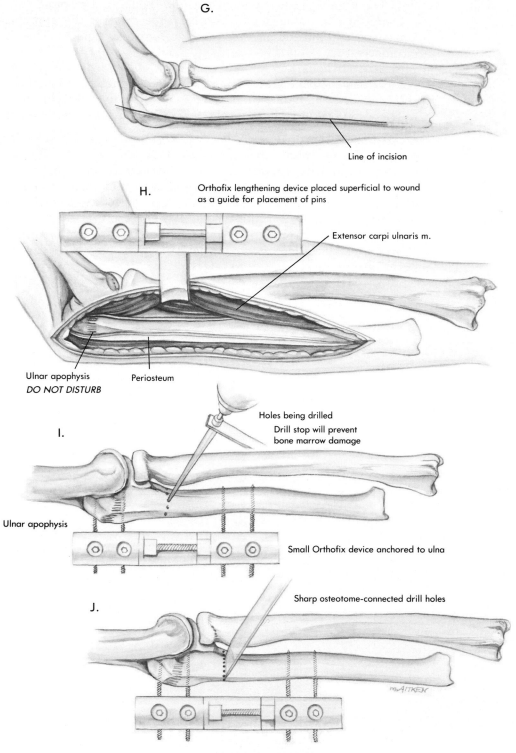

Line of incision

H.

Orthofix lengthening device placed superficial to wound
as a guide for placement of pins

Extensor carpi ulnaris m.

Ulnar apophysis
DO NOT DISTURB

Periosteum

I.

Holes being drilled
Drill stop will prevent
bone marrow damage

Ulnar apophysis

Small Orthofix device anchored to ulna

J.

Sharp osteotome-connected drill holes

Plate 40. (Continued)

K. The ulna is gradually lengthened to the desired amount.

L. and **M.** An autogenous bicortical bone graft of the appropriate length is taken from the ilium and inserted into the elongated segment. The ulnar fragments are compressed.

N. The Orthofix screws are removed, and the proximal and distal ulnar segments and the bone graft in the elongated segment are internally fixed with a small Rush or Steinmann pin, depending on the size of the patient.

The wound is closed in the usual fashion, and an above-elbow splint is applied.

Postoperative Care. In a few days, when the swelling has subsided, remove the posterior plaster splint and apply an above-elbow cast. Change the cast as necessary; ordinarily, the graft is well incorporated in eight weeks and there is adequate healing to remove the cast and start mobilization of the elbow, wrist, and fingers. A splint is made, and exercises are performed to restore range of elbow and wrist motion. Discontinue the splint when there is adequate strength of the ulna. The Steinmann pin is removed, usually six to twelve months after surgery.

When Z-step cut lengthening is performed, the plate is removed nine to twelve months after surgery.

K.   Ulna being lengthened

L.

Autogenous bicortical bone graft from ilium

M.

Compression of graft

N.

Internal fixation by intramedullary
Rush pin or Steinmann pin

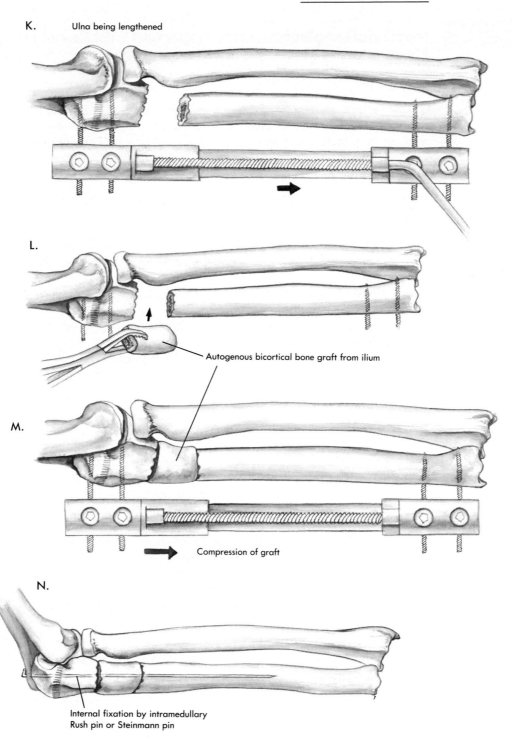

Plate 40. (Continued)

PLATE 41 ## Fractional Lengthening of the Finger and Wrist Flexors in the Forearm at the Musculotendinous Junction

Indications

1. Flexion deformity of the fingers and thumb at the metacarpophalangeal and interphalangeal joints caused by spasticity and myostatic contracture of the flexor digitorum sublimis and profundus and the flexor pollicis longus muscle.

2. Failure to respond to nonsurgical measures of passive stretching, splinting, and stretching cast.

Contraindications. Diffuse marked hypotonia of the upper limb.

Requisites

1. Difficulty in extending the fingers and thumb with the wrist in neutral position but ability to extend and flex the fingers and thumb with the wrist in acute flexion.

2. Presence of cerebral control over finger flexors and extensors with the wrist in hyperflexion.

3. Flexion deformity of the digits increased on wrist extension and diminished in hyperflexion of wrist.

4. Absence of fixed flexion contracture of joints.

Patient Position. Supine with upper limb on hand table.

Operative Technique

A. A midline longitudinal incision is made in the middle three fourths of the volar surface of the forearm. The subcutaneous tissue and deep fascia are divided in line with the skin incision. The wound flaps are undermined, elevated, and retracted with four-prong rake retractors to expose the superficial groups of muscles. On the radial side of the flexor carpi ulnaris tendon, the ulnar vessels and nerves are identified and protected from injury; similarly, on the radial side of the flexor carpi radialis tendon, the radial vessels and nerve are isolated to protect them from inadvertent damage. Sliding lengthening of the flexor carpi radialis and flexor carpi ulnaris muscles is performed at the musculotendinous junction by making two incisions of their tendinous fibers, about 1.5 cm. apart, without disturbing underlying muscle tissue. The proximal incision is transverse, and the distal one is oblique. The palmaris longus and flexor digitorum muscles are lengthened by only one transverse incision in each.

B. The wrist and the fingers are passively hyperextended. The tendinous parts will separate while the intact underlying muscle fibers will maintain continuity of the muscles.

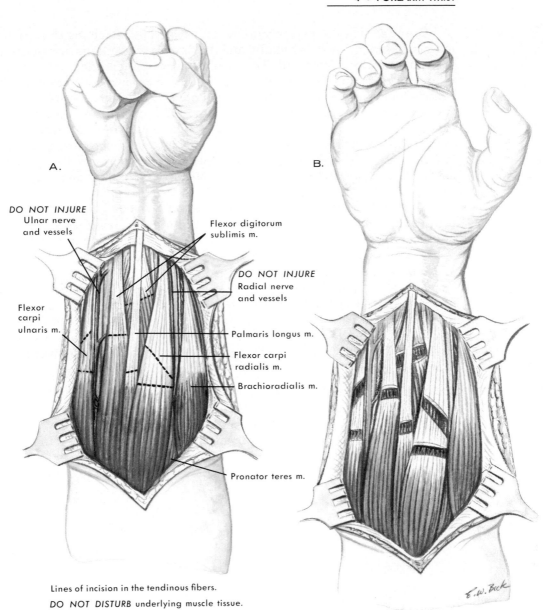

A.

DO NOT INJURE
Ulnar nerve
and vessels

Flexor digitorum
sublimis m.

DO NOT INJURE
Radial nerve
and vessels

Flexor
carpi
ulnaris m.

Palmaris longus m.

Flexor carpi
radialis m.

Brachioradialis m.

Pronator teres m.

Lines of incision in the tendinous fibers.
DO NOT DISTURB underlying muscle tissue.

B.

E.W. Beck

Separation of tendinous parts on extension
of wrist and digits

Plate 41. A.–D., Fractional lengthening of the finger and wrist flexors in the forearm at the musculotendinous junction.

C. and **D.** The deep volar muscles are exposed by retracting the brachioradialis muscle and radial vessels radially and the flexor carpi radialis and flexor digitorum sublimis muscles ulnarward. The median nerve is identified and protected from injury by retracting it medially with the flexor carpi radialis muscle. The flexor pollicis longus and flexor digitorum profundus muscles are lengthened by making two incisions in their tendinous parts and sliding them in the same manner as that described for the superficial volar forearm muscles. Continuity of muscles is maintained by gentle handling of tissues and by taking care that there is adequate muscle substance underlying the divided tendinous parts. Sliding lengthening is achieved by separating the tendinous fibers by slow but firm extension of the thumb and four ulnar digits.

Next, the range of passive supination of the forearm is tested. If there is pronation contracture, the pronator teres muscle is lengthened by two oblique incisions, 1.5 cm. apart, of its tendinous fibers. Again, do not disturb underlying muscle tissue. The forearm is forcibly supinated; the tendinous segments will slide and separate, elongating the muscle.

The tourniquet is released, and complete hemostasis is obtained. The deep fascia is not closed. The subcutaneous tissue and skin are approximated by interrupted sutures. An above-elbow cast that includes all the fingers and the thumb is applied to immobilize the forearm in full supination, the elbow in 90 degrees of flexion, the wrist in 50 degrees of extension, and the fingers and thumb in neutral extension.

Postoperative Care. Four weeks following surgery, the cast is removed and active exercises are started to develop motor power in the elongated muscle. Squeezing soft balls of varying sizes and other functional exercises are carried out several times a day. An aggressive occupational therapy program is essential. The corrected position is maintained in a plastic splint. As motor function develops in the elongated muscle and its antagonists, the periods out of the splint are gradually increased.

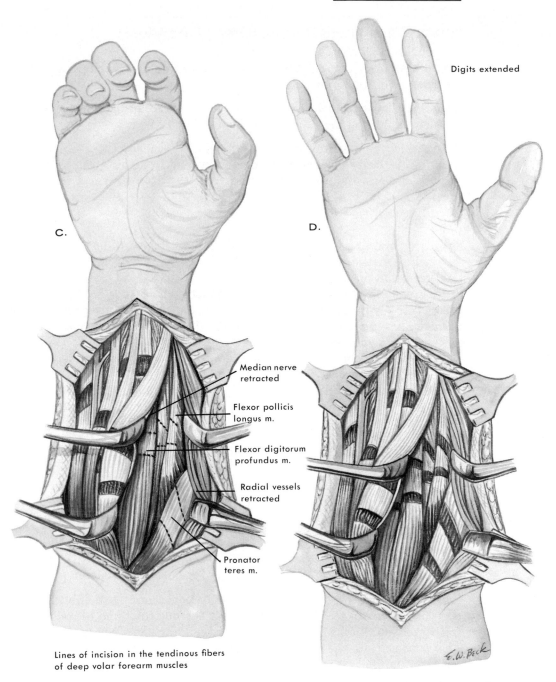

Digits extended

C.

D.

Median nerve
retracted

Flexor pollicis
longus m.

Flexor digitorum
profundus m.

Radial vessels
retracted

Pronator
teres m.

E. W. Beck

Lines of incision in the tendinous fibers
of deep volar forearm muscles

Note the sliding lengthening by separation
of tendinous fibers

Plate 41. (Continued)

PLATE 42 ## Flexor Carpi Ulnaris Transfer (Green Procedure)

Indications. Flexion and ulnar deviation deformity of the wrist and pronation contracture of the forearm.

Objective. To provide active extension of the wrist and supination of the forearm, thereby improving the function of the hand and fingers.

Principle. To remove the deforming force of the flexor carpi ulnaris, which pulls the hand into flexion and ulnar deviation, and to reroute the tendon around the medial border of the ulna, transferring it to the extensor carpi radialis longus and brevis.

Requisites

1. Normal or good motor power of the flexor carpi ulnaris.

2. Full range of passive supination of the forearm, dorsiflexion of the wrist, and extension of the fingers.

Caution! Any fixed, contractural deformity that is present should be corrected preoperatively by passive stretching exercises, splinting, or stretching casts. If the patient fails to respond to the preceding measures, a soft tissue release should be performed preoperatively.

3. Voluntary motor control of fingers with the wrist in neutral extension; the patient should be able to actively extend the fingers.

4. Voluntary control of the muscles of the hand, wrist, forearm, and elbow. Normal hand placement test results; i.e., the patient should be able to place an object on the examination table, knee, or head.

5. Adequate sensory function in the hand.

6. Sufficient intellect so that the patient is cooperative with the postoperative habilitation program.

7. The child must be old enough to comply with the postoperative habilitation program. Delay surgery until the child is six or seven years of age.

8. Absence of athetosis. Any extrapyramidal tract involvement may result in extension deformity of the wrist and may be more disabling than the original deformity.

Special Instrumentation. Ober or another type of tendon passer.

Patient Position. The operation is usually performed with the patient in supine position; some surgeons, however, prefer the patient to be in prone position, as it facilitates manipulating the forearm and holding the wrist in dorsiflexed position. The author uses the prone position when there is pronation deformity of the forearm and medial rotation contracture of the shoulder.

Operative Technique

A. An anteromedial incision is made over the flexor carpi ulnaris tendon. It starts at the flexor crease of the wrist and extends proximally and somewhat ulnarward over the belly of the muscle to the junction of the middle and upper thirds of the forearm (Green and Banks make two incisions, one distal and the other proximal).

B. and C. The subcutaneous tissue is divided, and the tendon of the flexor carpi ulnaris is exposed. The ulnar nerve, lying immediately posterior to the tendon, is visualized and protected from injury. The tendon is detached at its insertion to the pisiform bone and is mobilized proximally. The muscle fibers of the flexor carpi ulnaris take their origin from the ulna quite distally; they are stripped extraperiosteally from the underlying bone by sharp and dull dissection. The muscle is freed proximally as far as possible without disturbing its nerve supply from the ulnar nerve (which is the limiting factor of proximal dissection).

FLEXOR CARPI ULNARIS TRANSFER (GREEN)

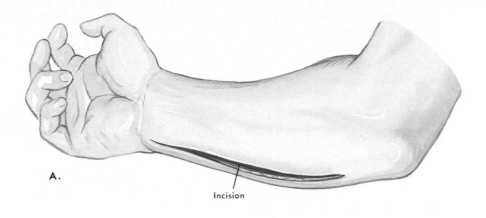

A.

Incision

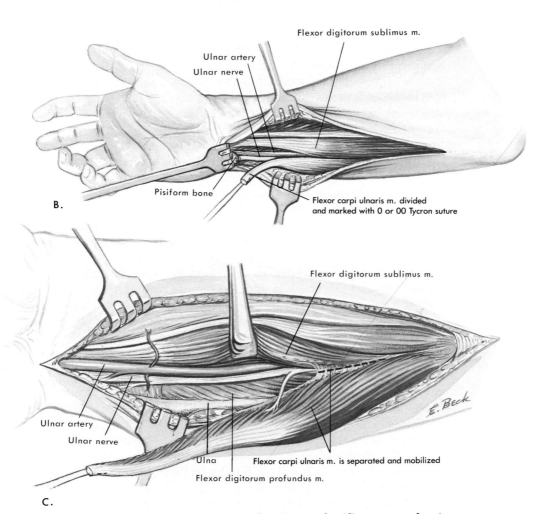

Flexor digitorum sublimus m.

Ulnar artery

Ulnar nerve

Pisiform bone

B.

Flexor carpi ulnaris m. divided
and marked with 0 or 00 Tycron suture

Flexor digitorum sublimus m.

Ulnar artery

Ulnar nerve

Ulna

Flexor digitorum profundus m.

Flexor carpi ulnaris m. is separated and mobilized

E. Beck

C.

Plate 42. A.–I., Flexor carpi ulnaris transfer (Green procedure).

The mobilization of the flexor carpi ulnaris should be high enough to allow its passage in a straight line from its origin to the dorsum of the wrist. The extensor compartment of the forearm is entered by excising a segment of the intermuscular septum at the medial margin of the ulna.

D. A longitudinal incision is made on the dorsum of the wrist over the extensor carpi radialis longus and brevis tendons. It starts at the distal end of the radius immediately above the transverse crease and extends proximally for a distance of 3 cm.

E. and **F.** The incision is carried through the subcutaneous tissue and fascia. The extensor carpi radialis longus (in line with the second metacarpal) and the extensor carpi radialis brevis (in line with the third metacarpal) tendons are identified and isolated.

An Ober tendon passer is inserted from the proximal portion of the ulnar incision to the wound on the dorsum of the wrist. The flexor carpi ulnaris tendon is passed around the ulna through the channel created by the Ober tendon passer. The line of pull of the tendon should be as straight as possible. On the dorsum of the wrist and forearm, the ulnaris tendon should be along the extensor communis tendons.

G. and **H.** With a No. 11 blade knife, a buttonhole is made in the extensor carpi radialis longus or brevis tendon. When there is ulnar deviation of the wrist, the ulnaris tendon is attached to the longus; when the wrist is in neutral posture, it is inserted into the radialis longus and brevis tendons. In the original description by Green, when there was ulnar deviation of the wrist, the ulnaris tendon was attached to the longus.

With the forearm in full supination and the wrist in 25 degrees of dorsiflexion, the ulnaris tendon is sutured to the extensor tendon. The tension on the ulnaris tendon should be such that the wrist can be passively palmar flexed 40 degrees, but when the tension is released, it should resume a position of 20 to 30 degrees of dorsiflexion. The method of suturing is not important. The author prefers that the ulnaris tendon pass through the buttonhole and be sutured to itself. In addition, three interrupted sutures are used to transfix the ulnaris and radialis tendons securely.

I. The wound is closed in layers as an assistant holds the forearm in full supination and the wrist in marked dorsiflexion. An above-elbow cast is applied with the forearm in full supination, the wrist in 30 to 45 degrees of dorsiflexion, the thumb in abduction, the metacarpophalangeal joint in 15 degrees of flexion, and the interphalangeal joint in neutral extension.

Postoperative Care. About three to four weeks after operation, the cast is bivalved and physical therapy is started in order to develop function in the transferred muscle. In the beginning, therapy consists of guided active exercises, attempting ulnar deviation and dorsiflexion of the wrist and supination of the forearm. Exercises are performed three to four times a day under supervision by the therapist and later by the parents (after thorough instruction by the therapist). The limb is maintained in the bivalved cast or plastic splint in the desired position except for the exercise periods for the following three weeks. The time out of the splint is then gradually increased.

When out of the splint and not exercising, the patient wears a light short arm orthosis or plastic splint, which holds the wrist in 30 degrees of dorsiflexion and the thumb in maximal abduction and opposition. Be sure that the metacarpophalangeal joint of the thumb does not subluxate! The support is discontinued when the flexor carpi ulnaris muscle is fair in motor strength and the wrist can be maintained in dorsiflexed functional position.

If there is a tendency for the wrist to drop into flexion, the support with the dorsiflexion orthosis is continued part time during the day. The use of a night splint is continued until good function has developed and there is no tendency for recurrence of the original deformity. This may take many months or even several

FLEXOR CARPI ULNARIS TRANSFER (GREEN)

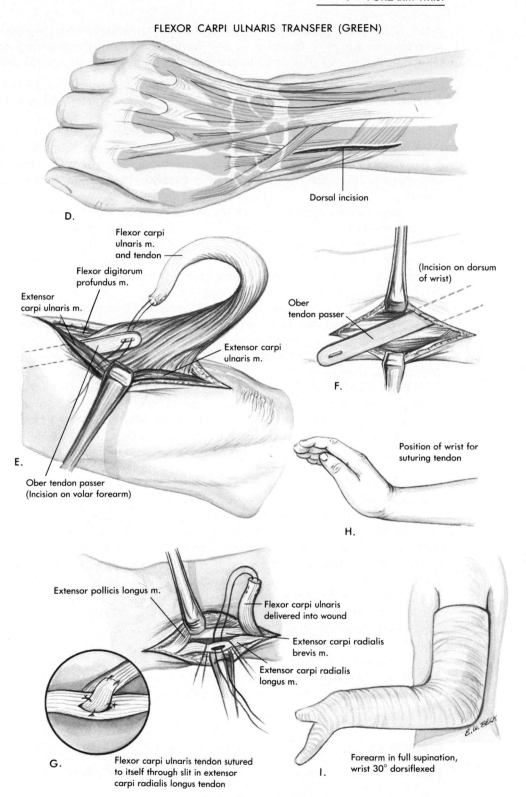

Dorsal incision

D.

Flexor carpi
ulnaris m.
and tendon

Flexor digitorum
profundus m.

Extensor
carpi ulnaris m.

Extensor carpi
ulnaris m.

Ober tendon passer
(Incision on volar forearm)

E.

(Incision on dorsum
of wrist)

Ober
tendon passer

F.

Position of wrist for
suturing tendon

H.

Extensor pollicis longus m.

Flexor carpi ulnaris
delivered into wound

Extensor carpi radialis
brevis m.

Extensor carpi radialis
longus m.

G.

Flexor carpi ulnaris tendon sutured
to itself through slit in extensor
carpi radialis longus tendon

Forearm in full supination,
wrist 30° dorsiflexed

I.

Plate 42. (Continued)

years. During the growth period, exercises are continued, with emphasis on active exercises to improve function of the hand and passive stretching exercises to maintain range of motion and to prevent recurrence of contractural deformity.

Complications. The reverse deformity of dorsiflexion contracture of the wrist may develop because of taut suturing of the flexor carpi ulnaris tendon with the wrist in 40 to 50 degrees of dorsiflexion. It is vital that the wrist be in only 25 degrees of dorsiflexion and that the wrist can be passively palmar flexed 40 degrees. Dorsiflexion deformity also may occur when the operation is performed in mixed cerebral palsy patients with spasticity and tension athetosis. The presence of extrapyramidal tract involvement is a contraindication to flexor carpi ulnaris transfer.

If dorsiflexion contracture of the wrist develops in the postoperative period, passive stretching casts are applied to correct, following which the wrist is supported part time in palmar flexed posture and exercises are performed to develop wrist flexion. If such nonoperative measures fail, the deformity is corrected by recessing the attachment of flexor carpi ulnaris near its insertion to extensor carpi radialis tendons.

Supination contracture is another complication that is often due to total release of the pronator teres performed simultaneously with flexor carpi ulnaris transfer. It is vital to lengthen and not totally release the pronator teres. Again, beware of the patient with tension athetoid type of cerebral palsy because reverse deformity may follow.

When there is flexion deformity of the wrist and pronation contracture of the forearm and the grasp is good, but there is poor release due to the weak finger flexors, the flexor carpi ulnaris should be transferred to the extensor digitorum communis. The dynamic electromyographic (EMG) studies of Hoffer et al. have shown that difficulty with a spastic hand is more that of weak release than that of weak grasp. To reiterate, the flexor carpi ulnaris is transferred to the finger extensors to improve finger extension, and flexor carpi ulnaris is transferred to extensor carpi radialis tendon to increase wrist extension alone.

Hoffer et al. recommend the following: Flexor carpi ulnaris is transferred to flexor digitorum communis when (1) release is weak, (2) grasp is adequate, and (3) EMG studies show that flexor carpi ulnaris is active. They recommend transfer of flexor carpi ulnaris to extensor carpi radialis tendons when (1) the grasp is weak with wrist flexion, (2) the release is adequate, and (3) dynamic EMG studies show that the flexor carpi ulnaris is active with flexor digitorum pollicis. When deforming muscles are active throughout both phases of the grasp-release cycle, it is best to fractionally lengthen these muscles at the musculotendinous junction rather than transfer them.

This author concurs with Hoffer et al.; however, when the finger and wrist flexors are lengthened fractionally at their musculotendinous juncture, extensor tenodesis or shortening of the wrist extensors is advised to provide some static support.

REFERENCES

Green, W. T.: Tendon transplantation of the flexor carpi ulnaris for pronation-flexion deformity of the wrist. Surg. Gynecol. Obstet., 75:337, 1942.

Green, W. T., and Banks, H. H.: Flexor carpi ulnaris transplant and its use in cerebral palsy. J. Bone Joint Surg., 44–A:1343, 1962.

Hoffer, M. M., Perry, J., and Melkonian, G. J.: Dynamic electromyography and decision-making for surgery in the upper extremity of patients with cerebral palsy. J. Hand Surg., 4:424, 1979.

Thometz, J. G., and Tachdjian, M. O.: Long-term follow-up of the flexor carpi ulnaris transfer in spastic hemiplegia children. J. Pediatr. Orthop., 8:407, 1988.

Thuilleux, G., and Tachdjian, M. O.: Traitement de la flexion pronation du poignet chez l'enfant hemiplegique. Rev. Chir. Orthop., 62:419, 1976.

FLEXOR CARPI ULNARIS TRANSFER (GREEN)

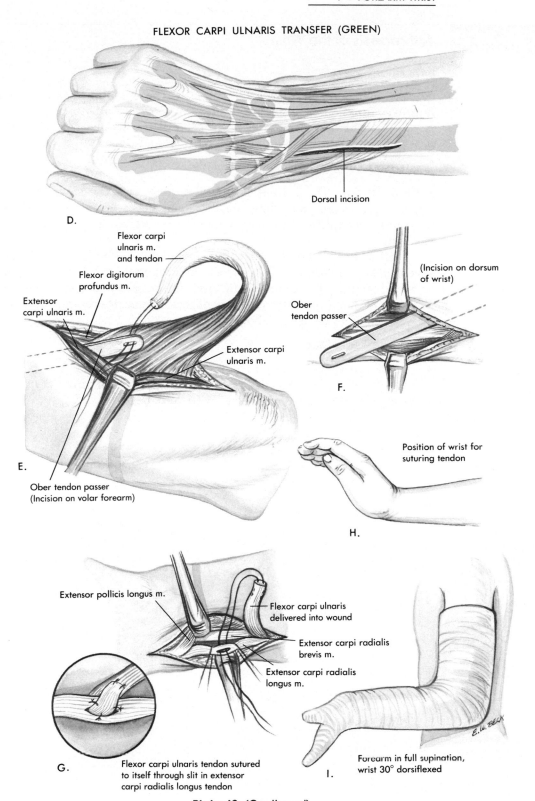

Dorsal incision

D.

Flexor carpi
ulnaris m.
and tendon

Flexor digitorum
profundus m.

Extensor
carpi ulnaris m.

Extensor carpi
ulnaris m.

E.

Ober tendon passer
(Incision on volar forearm)

(Incision on dorsum
of wrist)

Ober
tendon passer

F.

Position of wrist for
suturing tendon

H.

Extensor pollicis longus m.

Flexor carpi ulnaris
delivered into wound

Extensor carpi radialis
brevis m.

Extensor carpi radialis
longus m.

G.

Flexor carpi ulnaris tendon sutured
to itself through slit in extensor
carpi radialis longus tendon

Forearm in full supination,
wrist 30° dorsiflexed

I.

Plate 42. (Continued)

PLATE 43   Arthrodesis of the Wrist

Indications. Rare.

　　1. The completely flail wrist. In such a case, stabilization in neutral position improves function as an assisting post and provides a better-appearing hand.

　　2. In athetoid patients. Stabilization of the wrist in functional position improves finger control, enabling active grasp and release.

Radiographic Control. Image Intensifier.

Patient Position. The patient is placed supine with the shoulder abducted on an upper limb table, the elbow flexed, and the forearm pronated. A pneumatic tourniquet is applied on the upper arm. The procedure is performed with tourniquet ischemia.

　　Ordinarily, in the patient with cerebral palsy who has a flail hand-wrist with severe flexion deformity of the wrist, the proximal carpal row is resected to obtain relative length of the finger flexors; the resected carpal bones are used for autogenous bone graft to supplement the fusion; therefore, often the iliac crest does not need to be used as bone graft.

Operative Technique

　　A. Cross-section through the distal radial metaphysis.

　　B. Cross-section through the distal carpal row depicting the anatomic relationships of the bones, tendons, nerves, and vessels.

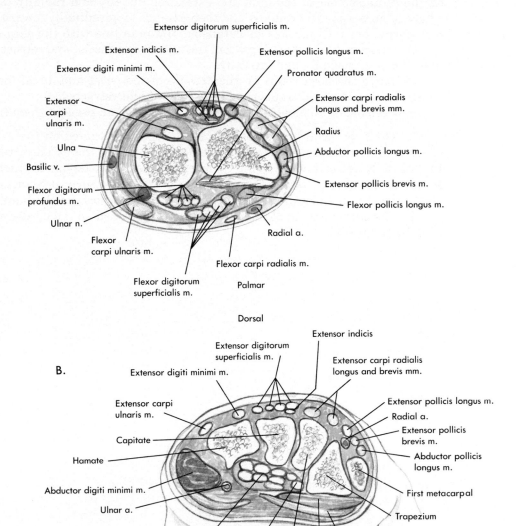

A.

Dorsal

Extensor digitorum superficialis m.

Extensor indicis m.

Extensor digiti minimi m.

Extensor pollicis longus m.

Pronator quadratus m.

Extensor carpi ulnaris m.

Extensor carpi radialis longus and brevis mm.

Radius

Ulna

Abductor pollicis longus m.

Basilic v.

Extensor pollicis brevis m.

Flexor digitorum profundus m.

Flexor pollicis longus m.

Ulnar n.

Radial a.

Flexor carpi ulnaris m.

Flexor carpi radialis m.

Flexor digitorum superficialis m.

Palmar

B.

Dorsal

Extensor indicis

Extensor digitorum superficialis m.

Extensor digiti minimi m.

Extensor carpi radialis longus and brevis mm.

Extensor carpi ulnaris m.

Extensor pollicis longus m.

Radial a.

Capitate

Extensor pollicis brevis m.

Hamate

Abductor pollicis longus m.

Abductor digiti minimi m.

First metacarpal

Ulnar a.

Trapezium

Flexor digitorum superficialis and profundus mm.

Flexor pollicis longus

Trapezoid

Abductor pollicis brevis m.

Opponens pollicis m.

Palmar

Plate 43. A.–J., Arthrodesis of the wrist.

C. Make a dorsal oblique incision beginning 6 to 8 cm. proximal to the wrist on the radial border of the ulna and extending distally and radially to the wrist, where it curves slightly radially and then extends longitudinally toward the second metacarpal head. Divide the subcutaneous tissue in line with the skin incision.

D. Undermine the skin flaps from the underlying fascia, and retract the wound margins both medially and laterally.

Preserve the large veins on the dorsum of the wrist and distal forearm. The veins crossing the field transversely are ligated and retracted.

It is important to identify the cutaneous nerves and prevent them from injury:

1. The superficial branch of the radial nerve is situated on the radial aspect of the lower radius, lying over the first compartment of the extensor retinaculum. Immediately above the wrist joint, it emerges beneath the tendon of brachioradialis. At the radial styloid, this cutaneous nerve divides into several branches that run longitudinally and distally to supply the dorsoradial aspect of the hand.

2. The dorsal branch of the ulnar nerve is identified on the border of the distal ulna by blunt dissection.

C.

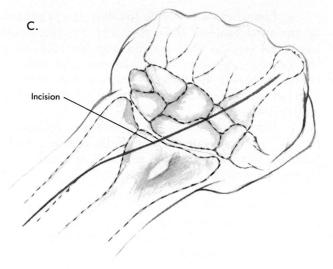

Incision

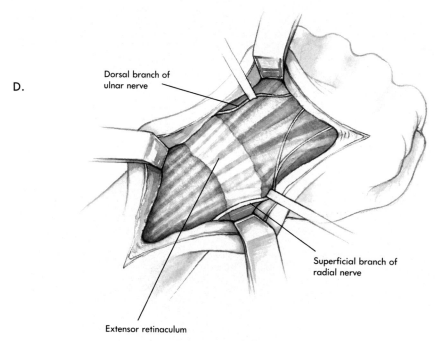

D.

Dorsal branch of
ulnar nerve

Superficial branch of
radial nerve

Extensor retinaculum

Plate 43. (Continued)

E. Longitudinally divide the deep fascia proximally, the extensor retinaculum on the ulnar side of the wrist, and the deep fascia on the dorsum of the hand. Incise the vertical fibrous septa from the extensor retinaculum, and mobilize all of the extensor tendons of the fingers and wrist that lie deep to the extensor retinaculum. In the proximal part of the wound, make a separate longitudinal incision in the fascial septa to mobilize the abductor pollicis longus and extensor pollicis brevis.

F. Retract the tendons of extensor pollicis longus, extensor carpi radialis longus, and extensor carpi radialis brevis, which are located radial to Lister's tubercle, toward the thumb side with the fascial flap of the extensor retinaculum. Retract the tendons of the long finger extensors and extensor carpi ulnaris ulnarward.

The capsule of the wrist joint is identified, sectioned from its attachment to the distal lip of the radius, and reflected as a distally based flap. This method of exposure of the distal radius and carpal bones is chosen when intramedullary pins are used for internal fixation.

G. An alternate method is to divide the capsule by a longitudinal incision and by sharp dissection elevate and reflect it from the distal radius and the underlying proximal carpal bones, i.e., the navicular, lunate, and capitate.

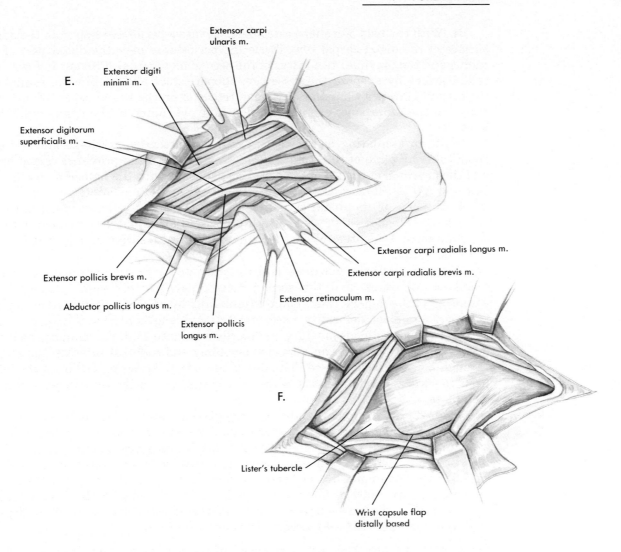

E.

Extensor carpi
ulnaris m.

Extensor digiti
minimi m.

Extensor digitorum
superficialis m.

Extensor pollicis brevis m.

Abductor pollicis longus m.

Extensor pollicis
longus m.

Extensor retinaculum m.

Extensor carpi radialis longus m.

Extensor carpi radialis brevis m.

F.

Lister's tubercle

Wrist capsule flap
distally based

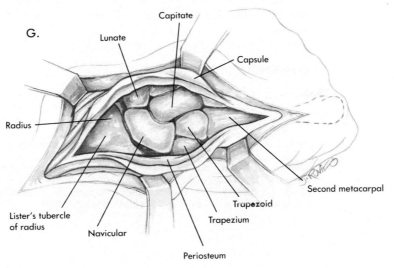

G.

Capitate

Lunate

Capsule

Radius

Second metacarpal

Lister's tubercle
of radius

Navicular

Periosteum

Trapezium

Trapezoid

Plate 43. (Continued)

H. With the help of a sharp osteotome, elevate a periosteal flap from the dorsal surface of the distal carpal row. Incise the periosteum over the distal part of the radius and the proximal two thirds of the second metacarpal. Prevent injury to the radial artery by keeping the dissection subperiosteal and within the confines of the capsule. Insert a Chandler or Homan retractor on the radial aspect of the wrist joint. On the ulnar side, exercise caution to avoid injury to the distal radioulnar joint.

With an oscillating electric saw, excise the articular cartilage and the subchondral bony plate of the distal radius. Next, remove the proximal carpal bones and the proximal one third of the distal carpal bones with the help of an oscillating saw and AO osteotomes. Do not injure the distal radioulnar joint.

I. The base of the distal carpal bones and the distal radius are apposed, and criss-cross, threaded Steinmann pins are inserted for temporary fixation with the wrist in about 10 degrees of dorsiflexion and neutral position as far as radial and ulnar deviation.

J. Use a small six-hole or seven-hole AO plate for fixation of the distal radius, distal carpal bones, and the second metacarpal. At this point, double check extension of the fingers; they should extend fully by passive manipulation. If there is persisting flexion deformity, perform fractional lengthening of the finger flexors at the musculotendinous juncture, as described in Plate 41. If the thumb is adducted across the palm, perform an adductor myotomy and a dorsal interosseous release through a dorsal incision (see Plate 60). If there is no active extension of the digits prior to surgery, perform flexor carpi ulnaris transfer on the long finger extensors (see Plate 42).

Radiograms are made in the anteroposterior, lateral, and oblique planes to double-check the position of the screws and the plate. The wound is irrigated, and a compression dressing is applied. The pneumatic tourniquet is released. Complete hemostasis is achieved, and the wound is closed in layers, the capsule and the extensor retinaculum with 00 Tycron sutures, the superficial fascia and subcutaneous tissue with 000 or 0000 Vicryl sutures, and the skin with 00 subcuticular nylon sutures. An above-elbow cast is applied, with the elbow in about 35 degrees of flexion and the wrist and forearm in neutral rotation.

Postoperative Care. The cast is removed in three to four weeks, and all sutures are removed. Another above-elbow cast is applied for an additional two to three weeks.

REFERENCES

Butler, A. A.: Arthrodesis of the wrist joint: Graft from inner table of the ilium. Am. J. Surg., 78:625, 1949.

Clendenin, M. B., and Green, D. P.: Arthrodesis of the wrist: Complications and their management. J. Hand Surg., 6:253, 1981.

Dick, H.: Wrist arthrodesis. In: Green, D. P.: Operative Hand Surgery. 2nd ed. New York, Churchill Livingstone, 1988, pp. 155–166.

Epstein, S.: Arthrodesis for flail wrist. Am. J. Surg., 8:621, 1930.

Evans, D. L.: Wedge arthrodesis of the wrist. J. Bone Joint Surg., 37–B:126, 1955.

Heim, U., and Pfeiffer, K. M.: Small Fragment Set Manual. Technique Recommended by the ASIF Group. 2nd ed. New York, Springer-Verlag, 1982.

Segment of carpal bones to be excised

H.

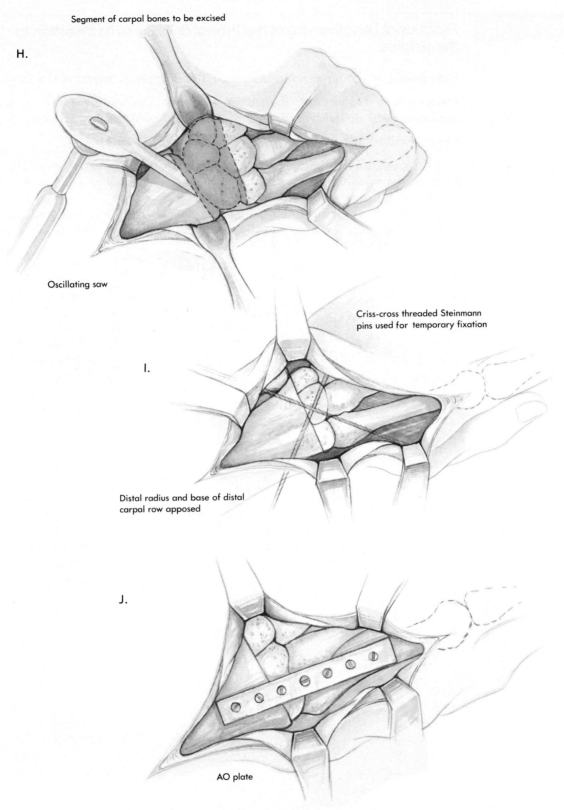

Oscillating saw

Criss-cross threaded Steinmann
pins used for temporary fixation

I.

Distal radius and base of distal
carpal row apposed

J.

AO plate

Plate 43. (Continued)

PLATE 44 **Fractional Lengthening of the Pronator Teres at Its Insertion to the Radius**

Indications. Fixed pronation contracture (30 degrees or more) of the forearm.

Preoperative Assessment. Radiograms of both elbows. Rule out posterolateral subluxation or dislocation of the radial head. Muscle testing. Dynamic EMG.

Operative Technique

   A. Make a longitudinal incision 4 to 5 cm. over the insertion of the pronator teres at the middle third of the radius. Subcutaneous tissue and fascia are divided in line with the incision.

   B. Retract the brachioradialis and radial vessels ulnarward and the extensor carpi radialis longus dorsolaterally, exposing the tendon and muscle fibers of the pronator teres.

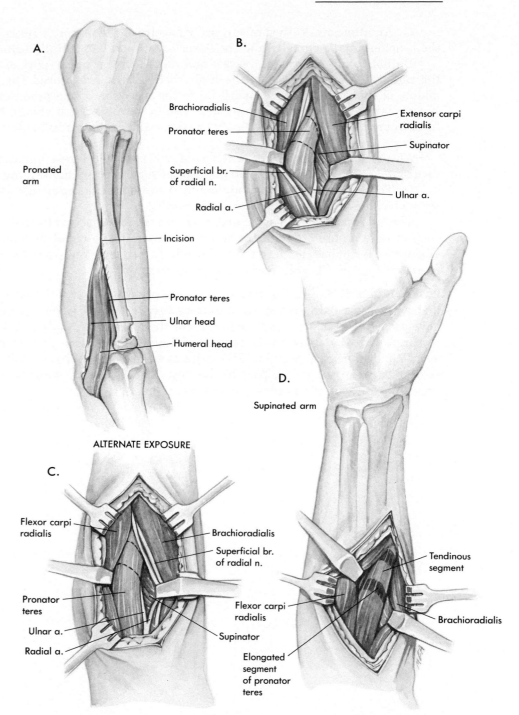

A. Pronated arm

Incision

Pronator teres

Ulnar head

Humeral head

B.

Brachioradialis

Pronator teres

Superficial br. of radial n.

Radial a.

Extensor carpi radialis

Supinator

Ulnar a.

D. Supinated arm

ALTERNATE EXPOSURE

C.

Flexor carpi radialis

Pronator teres

Ulnar a.

Radial a.

Brachioradialis

Superficial br. of radial n.

Supinator

Tendinous segment

Flexor carpi radialis

Brachioradialis

Elongated segment of pronator teres

Plate 44. A.–D., Fractional lengthening of the pronator teres at its insertion to the radius.

C. An alternate method of surgical exposure of the pronator teres is to retract the brachioradialis dorsally and the flexor carpi radialis medially (ulnarward).

Do not injure the radial vessels and nerve. In the upper part of the wound, the radial nerve is covered by the fleshy belly of the brachioradialis, and in the middle of the wound, it lies superficial to the insertion of the pronator teres. The superficial branch of the radial nerve is also in harm's way; it should be protected from injury. It lies behind the brachioradialis and on the radial side of the radial artery.

At the musculotendinous junction of the pronator teres, make two oblique incisions 1 to 1.5 cm. apart. Do not disturb the muscle fibers underlying the tendon.

D. The forearm is forcibly supinated. The tendinous segments will slide and separate, elongating the pronator teres muscle.

The tourniquet is released, and complete hemostasis is achieved. A Hemovac suction tube is inserted, and the wound is closed in the usual fashion. An above-elbow cast is applied, holding the forearm in full supination, wrist-hand in neutral position, and the elbow in 60 to 70 degrees of flexion.

Postoperative Care. At three to four weeks postoperatively, the cast is removed and active assisted and passive exercises are performed several times a day to develop active pronation and supination of the forearm. A plastic splint is manufactured with the elbow in 60 degrees of flexion, forearm in full supination, and wrist-hand in neutral position. The splint is worn at night. In the initial weeks, it is best to wear the splint part of the day. An aggressive occupational therapy program is crucial to improve function of the hand.

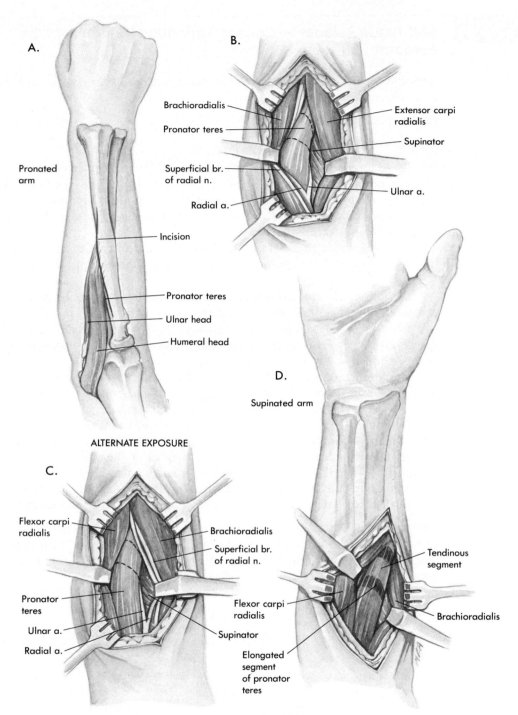

A.

Pronated arm

Incision

Pronator teres

Ulnar head

Humeral head

B.

Brachioradialis

Pronator teres

Superficial br. of radial n.

Radial a.

Extensor carpi radialis

Supinator

Ulnar a.

ALTERNATE EXPOSURE

C.

Flexor carpi radialis

Brachioradialis

Superficial br. of radial n.

Pronator teres

Ulnar a.

Radial a.

Supinator

Flexor carpi radialis

D.

Supinated arm

Tendinous segment

Flexor carpi radialis

Brachioradialis

Elongated segment of pronator teres

Plate 44. (Continued)

PLATE 45   ## Soft-Tissue Release to Correct Supination Deformity of the Forearm

Indications. Fixed supination contracture of the forearm with no bony deformity blocking rotation of forearm.

Radiographic Control. No.

Operative Technique

A. A longitudinal dorsal incision is made midway between the radius and ulna; it begins at the radial head and terminates at the distal one fourth of the forearm. When release of the dorsal distal radioulnar ligament is indicated, the incision is extended to the wrist. The subcutaneous tissue and fascia are divided in line with the skin incision.

B. The interosseous nerve is protected by radially retracting the dorsal muscles of the forearm. The interosseous membrane and oblique descending band are exposed.

C. The contracted interosseous membrane and the oblique descending band are sectioned near their ulnar attachment.

Check passive range of pronation of the forearm; if it is not full, by gentle dissection expose the interosseous nerve and release the supinator brevis muscle near its ulnar insertion.

Range of passive pronation of the forearm is tested again; if hyperpronation of the forearm is not achieved, section the dorsal ligaments of the distal radioulnar joint. If necessary, also divide the pronator quadratus.

D. and **E.** If there is still a supination contracture and the radial head is subluxating anteriorly, perform a Z-plasty of the biceps tendon. Reroute the distal segment of the biceps tendon around the neck of the radius, passing it mediolaterally. Resuture the divided biceps tendon segments side to side at the length that will maintain full pronation of the forearm and extension of the elbow.

Suture the proximal segment of the biceps tendon to the brachialis tendon.

Postoperative Care. An above-elbow cast is applied, with the elbow in 60 degrees of flexion, the forearm in full pronation, and the wrist-hand in functional position. The cast is removed in three to four weeks, and range-of-motion exercises are commenced.

REFERENCE

Zancolli, E. A.: Paralytic supination contracture of the forearm. J. Bone Joint Surg., 49–A:1275, 1967.

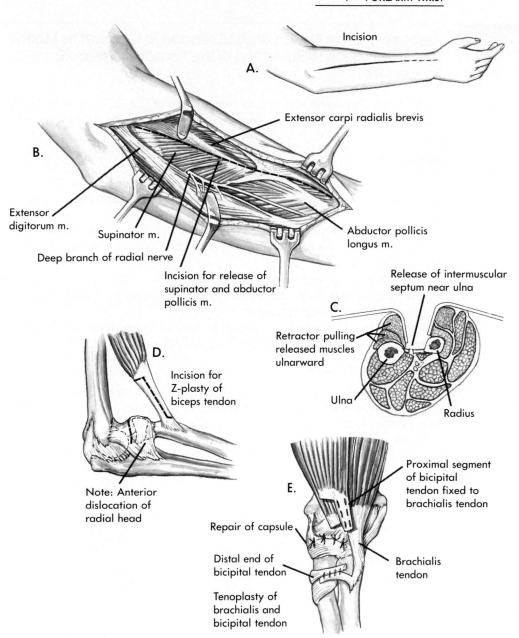

A. Incision

B.

Extensor carpi radialis brevis

Extensor digitorum m.

Supinator m.

Deep branch of radial nerve

Incision for release of supinator and abductor pollicis m.

Abductor pollicis longus m.

C.

Release of intermuscular septum near ulna

Retractor pulling released muscles ulnarward

Ulna

Radius

D.

Incision for Z-plasty of biceps tendon

Note: Anterior dislocation of radial head

E.

Proximal segment of bicipital tendon fixed to brachialis tendon

Repair of capsule

Distal end of bicipital tendon

Brachialis tendon

Tenoplasty of brachialis and bicipital tendon

Plate 45. **A.–E.,** Soft-tissue release to correct supination deformity of the forearm.

| PLATE 46 | **Rerouting of the Biceps Brachii Tendon to Convert Its Motion from Supination to Pronation of the Forearm (Zancolli Procedure)** |

Indications. Paralytic supination contracture of the forearm with the biceps brachii muscle normal or good in motor function and the pronators of the forearm paralyzed.

Requisites

1. Full range of passive pronation and supination of the forearm. If fixed supination deformity is present, correct by stretching casts or soft tissue release first.

2. Normal anatomic relationship of the proximal and distal radioulnar joints. If there is anterior dislocation of the radial head or dorsal displacement of the distal ulna, reduce it first.

3. No bowing of the anatomic configuration of the radius. If a deformed radius is blocking pronation of the forearm, correct it first by osteotomy.

4. Adequate hand function.

5. Child old enough to cooperate and to be motivated. This tendon transfer necessitates meticulous postoperative training.

Operative Technique

A. An S-shaped incision is made on the volar surface of the elbow. Begin 3 to 5 cm. above the elbow joint and extend to the antecubital crease, then laterally to the radial head and distally into the forearm for a distance of 5 cm. The subcutaneous tissue and deep fascia are divided in line with the skin incision.

B. Expose the biceps tendon, and trace it distally to its insertion to the bicipital tuberosity of the radius. Identify and trace brachial vessels and median nerve.

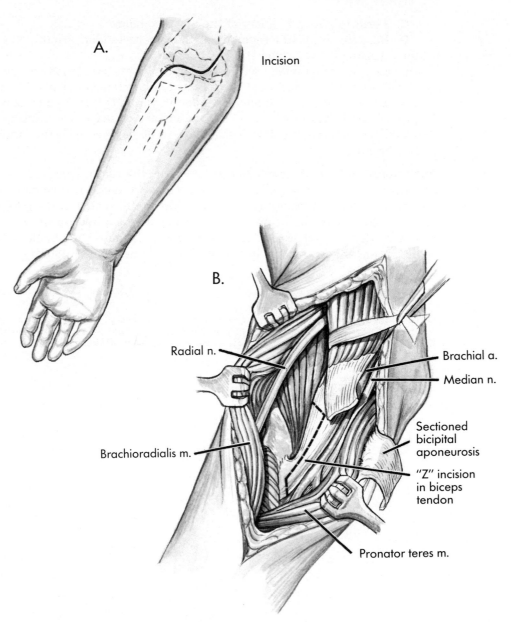

A.

Incision

B.

Radial n.

Brachioradialis m.

Brachial a.

Median n.

Sectioned
bicipital
aponeurosis

"Z" incision
in biceps
tendon

Pronator teres m.

Plate 46. **A.–E.,** Rerouting of the biceps brachii tendon to convert its motion from supination to pronation of the forearm (Zancolli procedure).

C. Perform a long Z-plasty of the biceps tendon.

D. Reroute the distal segment of the biceps tendon around the neck of the radius, passing it mediolaterally.

E. Resuture the divided biceps tendon segments side to side at the length that will maintain full pronation of the forearm and extension of the elbow.

Avoid excessive tension on the tendon in young children and when the forearm is hyperflexible into pronation. The wounds are closed in the routine fashion. An above-elbow cast is applied with the elbow in 30 degrees of flexion and the forearm in full pronation.

Postoperative Care. Four weeks after surgery, the cast is removed. Active assisted exercises are performed three to four times a day to develop pronation and supination of the forearm and elbow flexion-extension. Gentle passive exercises are carried out to maintain full pronation and supination of the forearm and complete flexion and extension of the elbow. At night a plastic splint is worn, maintaining the forearm in full pronation and the elbow in 30 degrees of flexion.

REFERENCES

Owings, R., Wickstrom, J., Perry, J., and Nickel, V. L.: Biceps brachii rerouting in treatment of paralytic supination contracture of the forearm. J. Bone Joint Surg., 53–A:137, 1971.

Zancolli, E. A.: Paralytic supination contracture of the forearm. J. Bone Joint Surg., 40–A:1275, 1967.

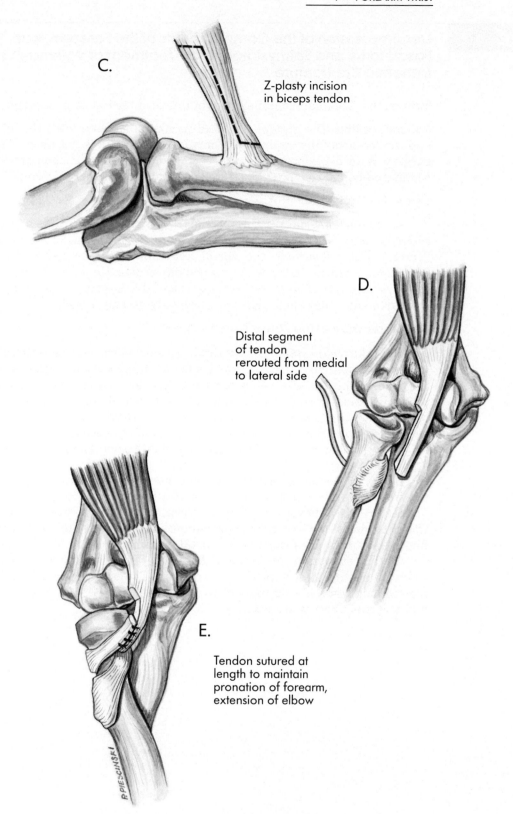

C.

Z-plasty incision
in biceps tendon

D.

Distal segment
of tendon
rerouted from medial
to lateral side

E.

Tendon sutured at
length to maintain
pronation of forearm,
extension of elbow

R. PIESCINSKI

Plate 46. (Continued)

PLATE 47

Decompression of the Compartments of the Forearm, with Fasciotomy and Epimysiotomy, for Treatment of Volkmann's Ischemic Contracture

Indications. Volkmann's ischemia. Obtain consultation as necessary.

Patient Position. The patient is placed in supine position with the elbow extended and the forearm fully supinated. Tourniquet ischemia is not used. The objective of surgery is to decompress the superficial and deep flexor compartments and the radial and dorsal compartments, if necessary, and the carpal tunnel.

Operative Technique

A. In the forearm are three compartments: flexor, radial, and dorsal. These compartments are interconnected. Fasciotomy of the flexor compartment may decrease the pressure in the dorsal and radial compartments. Decompress the flexor compartment first; however, when physical findings and direct measurements show persistence of high intracompartmental pressure in the radial and dorsal compartments, they should also be surgically decompressed.

Decompression of the Flexor Compartment

B. Make a curvilinear longitudinal incision on the volar surface of the forearm. It begins proximally at the flexor crease of the elbow and extends distally along the medial third of the volar surface of the forearm to the flexor crease of the wrist. Proximally the incision may be extended along the medial border of the biceps brachii to expose the brachial artery without crossing the flexor crease. Distally the incision may extend into the palm to decompress the carpal tunnel. At the wrist, between the flexor creases, the incision should be zigzag, with wide angles.

Caution! Do not extend the skin incision perpendicular to the flexor crease of the wrist because it will result in a painful hypertrophic scar.

At the distal flexor crease of the wrist, the incision extends distally along the radial border of the hypothenar prominence in line with the metacarpal of the ring finger and terminates short of the distal palmar crease.

C. The subcutaneous tissue is divided in line with the skin incision, and the wound flaps are undermined and retracted. The superficial and deep fasciae are incised longitudinally throughout their entire length. At the elbow, the deep fascia and lacertus fibrosus are divided.

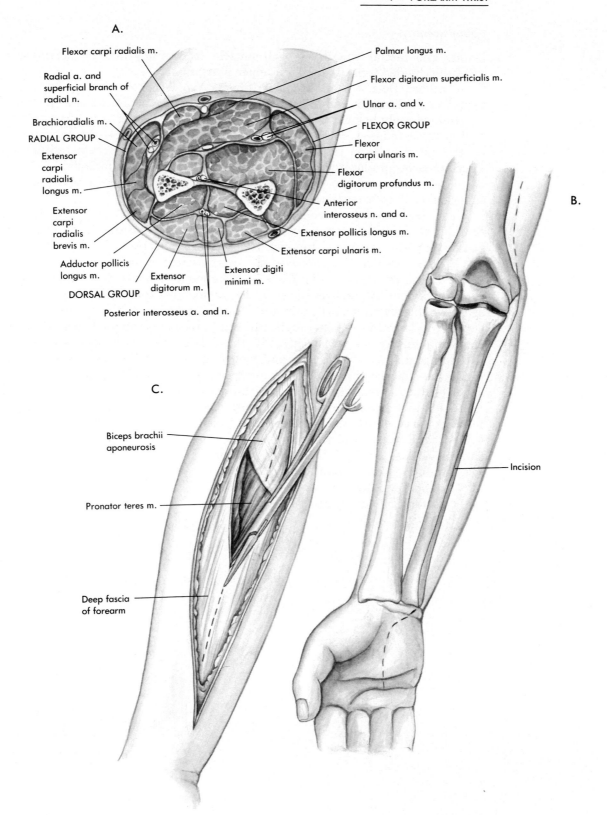

A.

Flexor carpi radialis m.

Radial a. and superficial branch of radial n.

Brachioradialis m.
RADIAL GROUP

Extensor carpi radialis longus m.

Extensor carpi radialis brevis m.

Adductor pollicis longus m.

DORSAL GROUP

Extensor digitorum m.

Posterior interosseus a. and n.

Palmar longus m.

Flexor digitorum superficialis m.

Ulnar a. and v.

FLEXOR GROUP

Flexor carpi ulnaris m.

Flexor digitorum profundus m.

Anterior interosseus n. and a.

Extensor pollicis longus m.

Extensor carpi ulnaris m.

Extensor digiti minimi m.

B.

Incision

C.

Biceps brachii aponeurosis

Pronator teres m.

Deep fascia of forearm

Plate 47. A.–N., Technique of decompression of the compartments of the forearm, with fasciotomy and epimysiotomy, for treatment of Volkmann's ischemic contracture.

Epimysiotomy

D. The fascial sheath of each muscle (the epimysium or perimysium) is carefully divided from its lower to upper margin.

Caution! Do not section muscle fibers. Avoid inadvertent injury to sensory nerves of the forearm and to any nerve branches that penetrate the epimysium.

Immediately below the lateral epicondyle of the humerus lies Henry's mobile wad of three muscles. From anterior to posterior they are (1) the brachioradialis, (2) the extensor carpi radialis longus, and (3) the extensor carpi radialis brevis. These muscles are located in the radial compartment of the forearm.

The muscles in the flexor compartment are arranged in three layers: (1) superficial, (2) intermediate, and (3) deep.

The *superficial layer* consists of the oblique pronator teres, the flexor carpi radialis, the palmaris longus (which may be absent), and the flexor carpi ulnaris. Carefully perform epimysiotomy of each of these muscles.

E. Next, expose the *intermediate layer,* which consists of one muscle—the flexor digitorum superficialis. Distally its tendons traverse deep to the transverse carpal ligament. It behooves the surgeon to remember the two-layered arrangement of flexor digitorum superficialis and its close relation to the median nerve. The superficial layer of the flexor digitorum sublimis forms the tendons of the long and ring fingers. At the wrist, identify these two anteriorly situated tendons by extending and flexing the ring and long fingers and trace them cephalad. Proximally the superficial part of flexor digitorum sublimis consists of a relatively thin sheet of muscle that slants from the humerus to the radius either at an inferior level, distal to pronator teres or, more superiorly, deep to pronator teres. The median nerve enters the forearm deep to this bridge (or arch), which is double-layered and consists of the pronator teres and flexor digitorum sublimis. When the superficial part of the flexor digitorum sublimis is situated at a lower level, the pronator teres and sublimis are separated by a gap. Divide the epimysium of the superficial layer of sublimis.

Caution! Do not injure the median nerve.

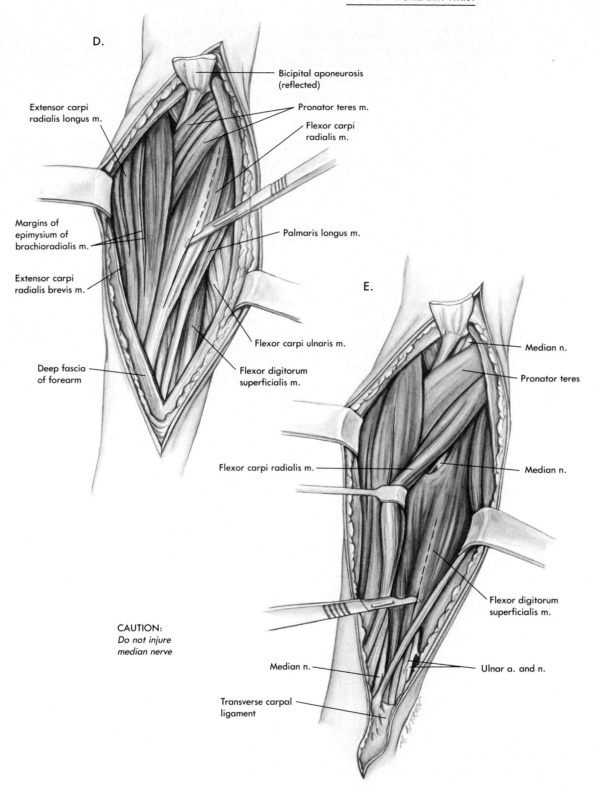

D.

Bicipital aponeurosis (reflected)

Extensor carpi radialis longus m.

Pronator teres m.

Flexor carpi radialis m.

Margins of epimysium of brachioradialis m.

Palmaris longus m.

Extensor carpi radialis brevis m.

Flexor carpi ulnaris m.

Deep fascia of forearm

Flexor digitorum superficialis m.

CAUTION:
Do not injure median nerve

E.

Median n.

Pronator teres

Flexor carpi radialis m.

Median n.

Flexor digitorum superficialis m.

Median n.

Ulnar a. and n.

Transverse carpal ligament

Plate 47. (Continued)

F. Next, expose the deep part of flexor digitorum superficialis, a trigastric muscle. The proximal belly takes its origin from the medial epicondyle of the humerus, and the distal two bellies provide tendons to the index and little fingers. Note at the wrist the flexor digitorum sublimis tendon of the index and little fingers lie posterior to those of the long and ring fingers. With a sharp scalpel, carefully divide the epimysium of the three muscle bellies of the deep layer of flexor digitorum superficialis.

G. The *deep layer* of muscles in the flexor compartment consists of (1) the flexor pollicis longus (which lies on the radius), (2) the flexor digitorum profundus (which lies on the ulna with its tendons spread in a single layer, unlike the two-layer arrangement of the tendons of flexor digitorum superficialis), (3) the pronator quadratus, distally, and (4) the supinator brevis, near the elbow. Carefully decompress the flexor pollicis longus and flexor digitorum profundus. Ordinarily, epimysiotomy of the quadratus and supinator is not required.

Following decompression there will be dramatic return of circulation. If the vascular supply does not improve, explore the brachial artery. The muscles, however, will be edematous of varying degree. Occasionally, especially in late cases, parts of the muscles may be grossly gangrenous.

H. The next step is exploration and decompression of the major nerves; of particular importance is decompression of the median nerve as it passes beneath the humeral and ulnar heads of pronator teres.

At the antecubital fossa, locate the biceps tendon. The brachial artery lies immediately ulnar to the biceps tendon, runs deep to the bicipital aponeurosis, and at the elbow joint divides into the radial and ulnar arteries. The median nerve lies ulnar to the brachial artery. Identify the median nerve proximal to pronator teres, gently dissect it free, and pass Silastic tubing around it. Retract the humeral head of the pronator teres ulnarward and mobilize the median nerve traversing between its ulnar and humeral heads; do not injure the branches of the median nerve to pronator teres. By blunt dissection, delineate and develop the interval between the flexor carpi radialis and humeral head of pronator teres.

Next, begin the dissection distally where the tendons of these two muscles diverge widely and then proceed proximally. With a moist sponge held in your index fingers, separate the muscle bellies of pronator teres (radially) and flexor carpi radialis (ulnarward). In the interval between these two muscles, the median nerve runs vertically and passes deep to the proximal fibrous arch of flexor digitorum superficialis.

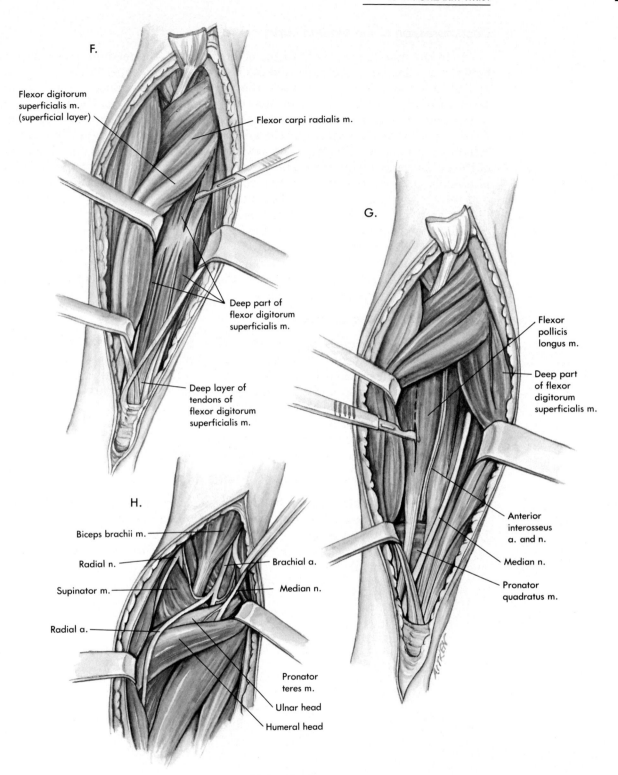

F.

Flexor digitorum
superficialis m.
(superficial layer)

Flexor carpi radialis m.

Deep part of
flexor digitorum
superficialis m.

Deep layer of
tendons of
flexor digitorum
superficialis m.

G.

Flexor
pollicis
longus m.

Deep part
of flexor
digitorum
superficialis m.

Anterior
interosseus
a. and n.

Median n.

Pronator
quadratus m.

H.

Biceps brachii m.

Radial n.

Supinator m.

Radial a.

Brachial a.

Median n.

Pronator
teres m.

Ulnar head

Humeral head

Plate 47. (Continued)

Decompression of the Median Nerve

I. In the middle and distal thirds of the forearm, the median nerve is exposed between the flexor carpi ulnaris and the flexor digitorum superficialis. At the wrist and at the distal forearm, identify the palmaris longus muscle and retract its tendon toward the ulna. In about one third of cases, however, the nerve is ulnar to the tendon, and in 10 per cent the tendon is absent. The median nerve lies in front of the flexor digitorum superficialis tendon of the long finger. This is a more reliable anatomic relationship. The flexor retinaculum is incised on the ulnar side of the palmaris longus tendon. The epimysium of the flexor digitorum superficialis is already incised; dissect the ulnar border of the flexor digitorum superficialis, and retract the muscle radially. The median nerve is mobilized proximally to the fibrous arch of the flexor digitorum superficialis.

Identify the palmar cutaneous branch of the median nerve, which branches from the median nerve approximately 5 cm. proximal to the distal crease of the wrist. Do not injure it. In the lower forearm, the palmar cutaneous branch traverses distally in a fibrous tunnel formed from the antecubital fascia between the flexor carpi radialis and the palmaris longus.

Decompression of the Ulnar Nerve

J. By dull dissection, mobilize the radial border of the flexor carpi ulnaris from the flexor digitorum superficialis and flexor digitorum profundus (the latter lies deep to the flexor digitorum superficialis and the flexor carpi ulnaris). Retract the flexor carpi ulnaris medially and identify the ulnar nerve, which enters the forearm between the two heads of the flexor carpi ulnaris. Identify the dorsal sensory branch of the ulnar nerve, which originates in the distal one third of the forearm deep to the flexor carpi ulnaris. Locate the ulnar vessels and divide any fascial bands or muscles compressing the ulnar vessels and nerves.

Decompression of the Carpal Tunnel

K. The flexor tendons of the fingers, the median nerve, and the flexor pollicis longus traverse through the carpal tunnel. The tunnel is a fibro-osseous canal bounded anteriorly by the flexor retinaculum, which attaches from the tubercle of the navicular and the ridge of the trapezium radially to the hook of the hamate and pisiform on the ulnar side.

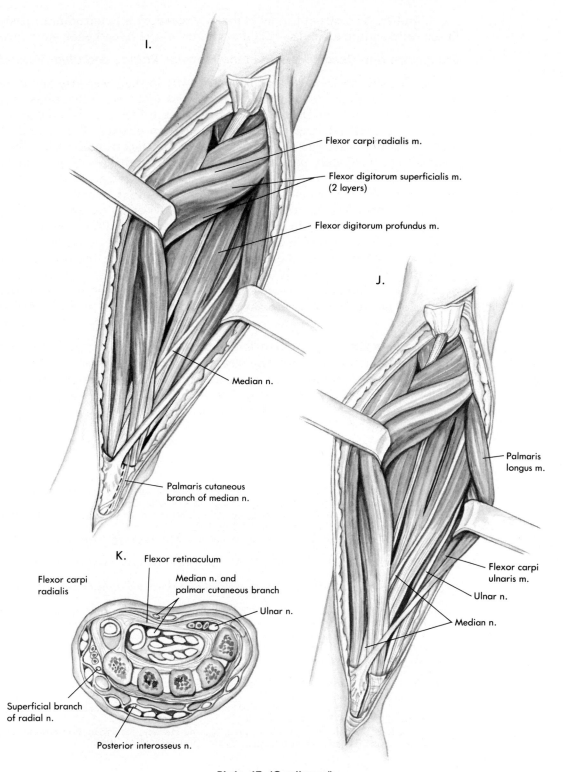

I.

Flexor carpi radialis m.

Flexor digitorum superficialis m. (2 layers)

Flexor digitorum profundus m.

Median n.

Palmaris cutaneous branch of median n.

J.

Palmaris longus m.

Flexor carpi ulnaris m.

Ulnar n.

Median n.

K.   Flexor retinaculum

Flexor carpi radialis

Median n. and palmar cutaneous branch

Ulnar n.

Superficial branch of radial n.

Posterior interosseus n.

Plate 47. (Continued)

L. and **M.** The carpal tunnel is decompressed by a longitudinal incision of the flexor retinaculum along the radial boundary of the hypothenar eminence.

Exploration and Decompression of the Brachial, Radial, and Ulnar Vessels

N. The skin incision is extended proximally in the lower arm along the medial border of the biceps tendon for the required distance. Subcutaneous tissue is divided in line with the skin incision, and the skin flaps are elevated and reflected. Incise the superficial fascia in line with the skin incision. Ligate and divide the median cubital vein. Incise the deep fascia and lacertus fibrosus. The brachial vessels lie immediately medial to biceps tendon, and the artery is lateral to the median nerve. The humeral head of pronator teres is retracted ulnarward, and the brachial vessel is traced distally to its radial and ulnar branches.

In the upper forearm, the radial artery is exposed by sectioning of the pronator teres at its insertion and by retracting its humeral and ulnar heads medially. The brachioradialis is identified and retracted laterally. The radial vessels cross deep to the biceps tendon and then traverse distally between the brachioradialis and supinator. The ulnar vessels are readily identified, as they are larger, and pass deep to the median nerve. Do not close the wound. The nerves are covered by soft tissue. Do not leave them bare. Apply layers of nonadhesive sterile dressings and bandages.

Postoperative Care. The patient is taken back to the operating room on the third day after decompression, and the wound is inspected. Excise any necrotic tissue, and apply sterile saline-soaked gauze dressings to the wound. Recheck the wound on the seventh and tenth days after fasciotomy. Following subsidence of the edema, secondary closure of the wound may be performed or a split-thickness skin graft is applied.

REFERENCES

Cohn, B. T., Shall, J., and Berkowitz, M.: Forearm fasciotomy for acute compartment syndrome: A new technique for delayed primary closure. Orthopedics, 9:1243, 1986.

Eaton, R. G., and Green, W. T.: Epimysiotomy and fasciotomy in the treatment of Volkmann's ischemic contracture. Orthop. Clin. North Am., 3:175, 1972.

Eaton, R. G., and Green, W. T.: Volkmann's ischaemia: A volar compartment syndrome of the forearm. Clin. Orthop., 113:58, 1975.

Eaton, R. G., Green, W. T., and Stark, H. A.: Volkmann's ischemic contracture. J. Bone Joint Surg., 47–A:1289, 1965.

Geary, N.: Late surgical decompression for compartment syndrome of the forearm. J. Bone Joint Surg., 66–B:745, 1984.

Matsen, F. A. III, Mubarak, S. J., and Rorabeck, C. H.: A practical approach to compartmental syndromes. In: Instructional Course Lectures, A.A.O.S., 32:88, 1983. St. Louis, C.V. Mosby Co.

Matsen, F. A. III, Winquist, R. A., and Krugmire, R. B., Jr.: Diagnosis and management of compartmental syndromes. J. Bone Joint Surg., 62–A:286, 1980.

Mubarak, S. J., and Carroll, N. C.: Volkmann's contracture in children: Aetiology and prevention. J. Bone Joint Surg., 61–B:285, 1979.

Mubarak, S. J., and Hargens, A. R.: Compartment Syndromes and Volkmann's Contracture. Philadelphia, W. B. Saunders Co., 1981.

Sheridan, G. W., and Matsen, F. A. III: Fasciotomy in the treatment of acute compartment syndrome. J. Bone Joint Surg., 58–A:112, 1976.

Whitesides, T. E., Jr., Haney, T. C., Morimoto, K., and Harada, H.: Tissue pressure measurements as a determinant for the need of fasciotomy. Clin. Orthop., 113:43, 1975.

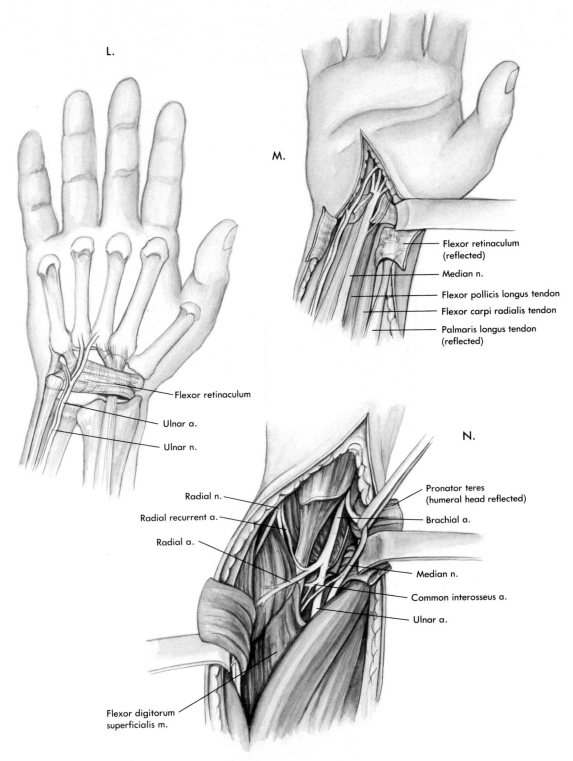

L.

M.

Flexor retinaculum
(reflected)

Median n.

Flexor pollicis longus tendon

Flexor carpi radialis tendon

Palmaris longus tendon
(reflected)

Flexor retinaculum

Ulnar a.

Ulnar n.

N.

Radial n.

Radial recurrent a.

Radial a.

Flexor digitorum
superficialis m.

Pronator teres
(humeral head reflected)

Brachial a.

Median n.

Common interosseus a.

Ulnar a.

Plate 47. (Continued)

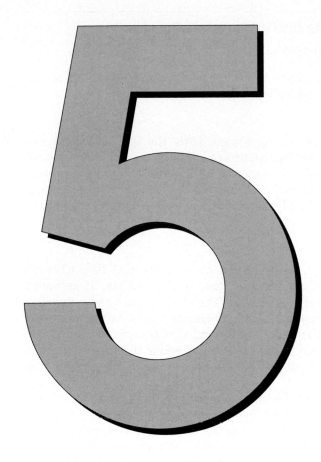

Hand

PLATE 48   Separation of Simple Complete and Incomplete Syndactyly Between the Ring and Long Fingers

Indications. Presence of webbing of digits interfering with normal spread of the fingers and impairment of function. Objectionable cosmetic appearance.

Requisites. Normal circulation.

Operative Technique. The operation is performed with the aid of tourniquet ischemia. To save tourniquet time, the incisions are planned and outlined before the tourniquet is applied. It is crucial to release the tourniquet before skin closure to obtain hemostasis and also at the end of the operation before a compression dressing is applied. If a finger is blue and congested or pale, the sutures at its base are removed.

Complete Simple Syndactyly

A. First, raise a commissural flap. Make an incision shaped like a broad horseshoe on the dorsum of the hand between the webbed digits. It is based proximally, beginning from the distal one fourth of the metacarpals and extending distally at least two thirds of the way from the metacarpal heads to the proximal interphalangeal joints. This dorsal flap should be broad in order to provide adequate width to the commissure; its proximal base is somewhat wider than its distal end. Flatt recommends sloping the end of the dorsal flap so that the first dorsal interdigital flap has a wider base.

Because the skin of the dorsum of the hand is mobile and thin, the dorsal flap is made thicker as it is elevated proximally toward its base in order to provide it with adequate circulation. This maneuver also gives the newly constructed commissure a dorsopalmar slope similar to that of the normal interdigital web, increasing the length of the palm as compared with the dorsum of the hand. The proximal placement of the dorsal flap and the resultant deeper commissure is in anticipation of the distal advancement of the interdigital web consequent to the child's growth. Utilization of two triangular flaps, one dorsal and the other palmar, is not recommended because the reconstructed interdigital commissure will be narrow and V-shaped.

B.–E. Next, make a palmar transverse incision, which will mark the palmar margin of the web space. As children grow, the interdigital web advances distally; therefore, make the commissure deeper by placing the palmar incision 5 to 6 mm. proximal to the normal level of that web. In the palm, the normal interdigital webs between the long and ring fingers and between the ring and little fingers incline from distal-radial to proximal-ulnar. In placing the incisions, pay attention to this detail.

Separate the syndactylized fingers by two interdigital undulating or zigzag longitudinal incisions. There is always insufficient skin, and it is difficult to cover the two digits totally with flaps. It is best not to favor one finger by providing greater flap size. Because the interdigital groove in the web is usually present on the dorsum but not on the palmar aspect of the conjoined fingers, the dorsal interdigital incision is made first, the apices of its flaps corresponding to the midpoint of the base of the palmar interdigital flap. From these apices, straight needles are inserted to emerge on the palmar aspect to serve as guideposts for the bases of the palmar interdigital flaps. If the base of the flap release incision on the dorsum includes the crease of the proximal interphalangeal joint, the crease on the palmar aspect should be at the apex of the palmar flap. The bases and apices of the flaps should extend approximately to the midlines of the digits. The palmar incisions should not cross the interphalangeal flexion creases.

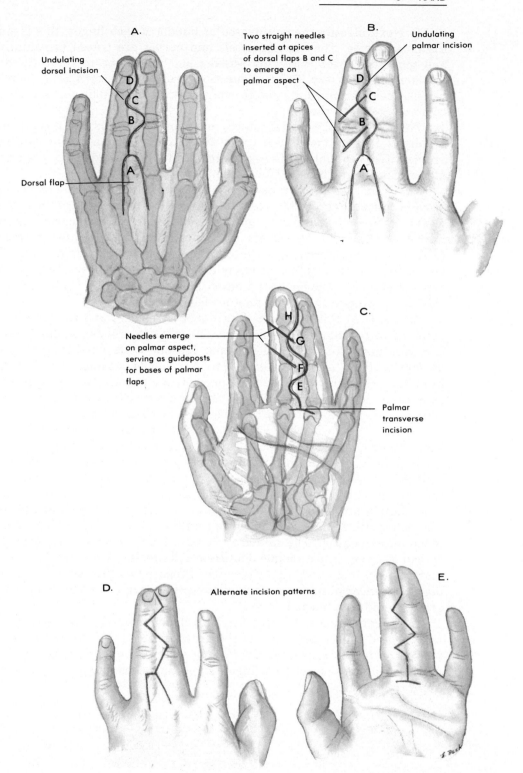

Plate 48. A.–O., Separation of simple complete and incomplete syndactyly between the ring and long fingers.

F. Next, identify the neurovascular bundle of each finger; this is simpler from the palmar side. The digital vessels and nerves are traced proximally by sharp and blunt dissection with tiny scissors and fine probe to the bifurcation of the common digital artery. The configuration, branching pattern, and size of the digital vessels are determined. In simple syndactyly there is usually no crossing of vessels or nerves between the fingers.

Next, release the fascial interconnections. If there is any bony union between the digits, it is sectioned with a very sharp scalpel. The adjacent flaps of the digits are defatted, especially if they are abnormally contoured. Take care not to injure digital vessels and nerves. Check the span of the palm.

G. Often the deep transverse metacarpal ligament has to be sectioned to provide adequate spread between the fingers. The bifurcation of the common digital vessels is retracted palmarly, and the deep transverse metacarpal ligament, lying immediately behind the vessels, is divided. Should one ligate an arterial branch to one of the conjoined fingers to allow a more proximal commissure? This author recommends it in simple syndactyly and in complex syndactyly provided preoperative studies by Doppler examination and arteriography show that the opposite side of the webbed finger has another feeder artery.

H. and I. At this stage, the tourniquet is released and complete hemostasis is obtained by coagulating the bleeders. The commissural dorsal flap is pulled toward the palm and sutured into the palmar incision with nonabsorbable sutures such as 000 or 0000 nylon. Kelikian prefers No. 34 stainless steel suture; in his procedure, the threads of the steel are not tied but are twisted together until the skin edges are brought together. The unabsorbable nylon or wire sutures are supplemented by 00000 absorbable sutures (such as Vicryl).

J. Next, cut a pattern exactly the size and shape of the defect and with a sharp scalpel, obtain an elliptical full-thickness skin graft of appropriate size from the hairless area of the groin. It is not necessary to use a dermatome or very thick split-thickness graft. The hairless area of the inguinal region is preferable to either the medial aspect of the upper arm, the volar surface of the upper forearm immediately distal to the cubital crease, or the inner aspect of the upper thigh. The donor site at the groin heals well and cosmetically is hidden, and the scar is much more pleasing. The skin graft removed is turned with its raw side up and is spread by tying it to a tongue depressor. All areolar tissue and fat are scraped off, and the skin is serrated like a piecrust. Prepare two such skin grafts, one for each digit. By undermining and immobilizing the margins of the donor site, close the groin wound as a linear incision.

The temptation is to close the skin flaps primarily, but often this results in tension and causes deformity of the growing fingers. *There should be no lines of tension on the reconstructed sides of the separated fingers.* It is best to graft skin on the adjacent sides of *both* fingers. It is time-consuming, but results justify the extra time spent.

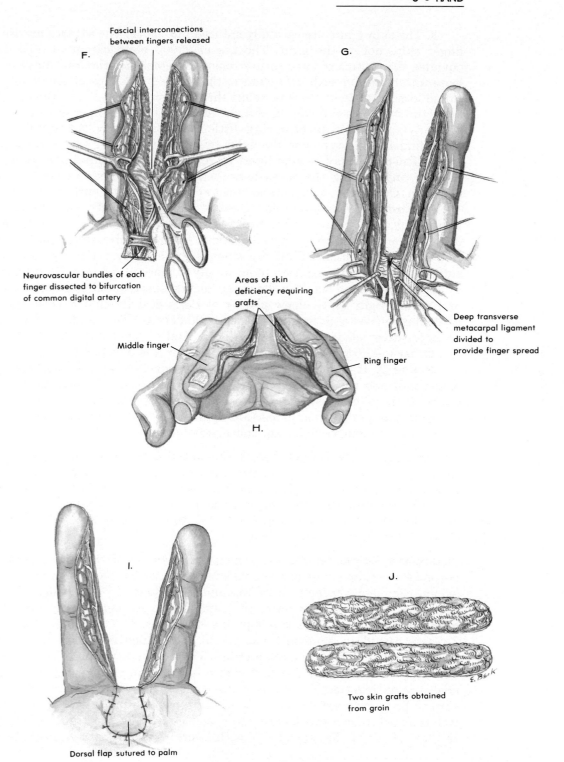

F.

Fascial interconnections
between fingers released

G.

Neurovascular bundles of each
finger dissected to bifurcation
of common digital artery

Areas of skin
deficiency requiring
grafts

Middle finger

Ring finger

Deep transverse
metacarpal ligament
divided to
provide finger spread

H.

I.

J.

Two skin grafts obtained
from groin

Dorsal flap sutured to palm

E. Beck

Plate 48. (Continued)

K. The skin grafts are carefully sutured into place. The sutures are tied on the finger skin, not on the graft. The use of 00000 plain catgut or Vicryl sutures obviates the trauma of later suture removal. Sometimes the interdigital webs are loose and broad; in such an instance, the interdigital flaps of one finger may be closed loosely, without tension. Select the "dominant" finger, i.e., the one that will carry the flap. As a rule, the "dominant" digit is the ring finger in ring–long finger syndactyly, the little finger in ring–little finger syndactyly, the thumb in thumb–index finger syndactyly, and the index finger in index–long finger syndactyly.

L. The digits may be kept apart by introducing fine Kirschner wires subcutaneously and holding the wires apart with a spreader bar as recommended by Kelikian. Ordinarily, this method is not employed by this author.

M. *Postoperative bandaging* should be simple but effective in immobilizing the upper limb. The separated fingers are spread apart widely, and sterile wet cotton dressings are placed in the space between them (wet dressings can be molded to the web configuration). Fluff dressings are placed over the wet dressing with sufficient pressure to maintain them snugly in place in the interdigital space. Fluff dressings are placed between the other fingers, sheet-wadding is rolled over them, and a very light above-elbow plaster of Paris cast is applied with the wrist in neutral extension and the elbow flexed to 90 degrees. The small child is active and uncooperative; adequate immobilization is vital.

Other methods used are Xeroform gauze or fine mesh gauze.

N. and O. If the nails are conjoined in syndactyly, excise a sufficient amount of the nail and nail bed to provide lateral wall closure. The subjacent fibrofatty tissue of the digital pad may have to be partially excised. This management of adjacent nail borders is an important detail. Any osseous connections distal to the metacarpal phalangeal joint are sharply divided.

Postoperative Care. Do not disturb the initial dressing for three weeks; at that time, there is usually adequate healing. Remove nonabsorbable sutures over the dorsal commissural flap. Crustings over the incision and grafts are left alone. Another glovelike soft dressing is applied for an additional five to seven days. Following this, all dressings are removed, the wound is exposed to air, and the child is allowed to use the hand fully.

Incomplete Simple Syndactyly. Incomplete webbing of the fingers that extends beyond the proximal interphalangeal joint is treated by the same surgical technique as for complete syndactyly. In incomplete syndactyly that stops short of the proximal interphalangeal joint, the commissure is deepened by an interdigital butterfly flap that utilizes two opposing Z-plasties. The two dorsal halves of each Z-plasty provide a common broad dorsal flap, which is turned palmarward and proximally to create a deep commissure. There are two possibilities for the palmar halves of each Z-plasty. The first choice is to create a wide-angle V. The second choice is an inverted Y—this is utilized when the web is abundant. It provides skin to be transferred on each side of the separated fingers. Thumb–index finger web contracture can be widened and deepened by four-flap Z-plasty, as illustrated in Plate 49, or by the central V-Y with lateral Z-plasties shown in Plate 50.

REFERENCES

Flatt, A. E.: The Care of Congenital Anomalies of the Hand. St. Louis, C.V. Mosby, 1977, p. 170.
Flatt, A. E.: Practical factors in the treatment of syndactyly. In: Littler, J. W., Cramer, L. M., and Smith, J. W. (eds.): Symposium on Reconstructive Hand Surgery. St. Louis, C.V. Mosby, 1974, pp. 144–156.
Iselin, F.: Traitement chirurgical des syndactylies congénitales. Résultats d'àpres 42 observations. Rev. Prat., 10:2611, 1960.
Kelikian, H.: Congenital Deformities of the Hand and Forearm. Philadelphia, W. B. Saunders Co., 1974, pp. 331–407.

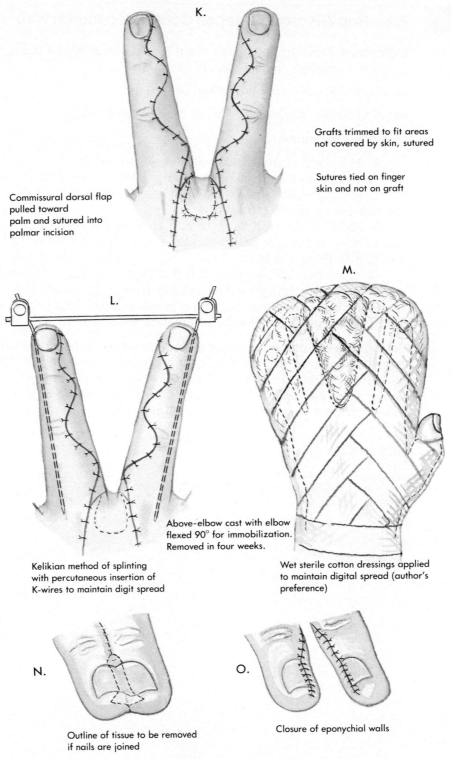

K.

Commissural dorsal flap
pulled toward
palm and sutured into
palmar incision

Grafts trimmed to fit areas
not covered by skin, sutured

Sutures tied on finger
skin and not on graft

L.

M.

Kelikian method of splinting
with percutaneous insertion of
K-wires to maintain digit spread

Above-elbow cast with elbow
flexed 90° for immobilization.
Removed in four weeks.

Wet sterile cotton dressings applied
to maintain digital spread (author's
preference)

N.

Outline of tissue to be removed
if nails are joined

O.

Closure of eponychial walls

Plate 48. (Continued)

PLATE 49   Four-Flap Z-Plasty to Deepen Contracted Thumb Web

Indications. Contracture of web space between thumb and index finger restricting range of abduction and function of thumb.

Requisites. Normal circulation and sensation.

Patient Position. Supine with upper limb on hand table.

Operative Technique

A. Make a Z-plasty incision in the contracted skin web as illustrated. Divide the subcutaneous tissue and contracted fasciae in line with the skin incision.

Caution! Do not injure the digital vessels and nerves. Release the tourniquet, and achieve complete hemostasis.

B. Mobilize the skin flaps; bring flap C into the gap between the base of the index finger and flap A, and bring flap B to the gap between the base of the thumb and flap D. Bring the point of flap D into the apex between flaps A and B.

C. Close the skin margins with interrupted sutures. If the deformity is severe, use a smooth pin through the thumb into the carpus to hold the thumb in complete abduction and opposition. Apply a compression dressing and an above-elbow cast, with the patient's thumb held in complete abduction and opposition.

Postoperative Care. Change the cast as necessary. The pin is removed two to three weeks postoperatively, at which time sutures are removed. Use an abduction-opposition splint part-time to keep the thumb in the corrected position. Passive skin stretching exercises are performed several times a day, and active exercises are carried out to develop function in the thumb.

REFERENCE

Strickland, J. W.: Thumb reconstruction. In: Green, D. P. (ed.): Operative Hand Surgery. 2nd ed. New York, Churchill Livingstone, 1988, pp. 2191–2192.

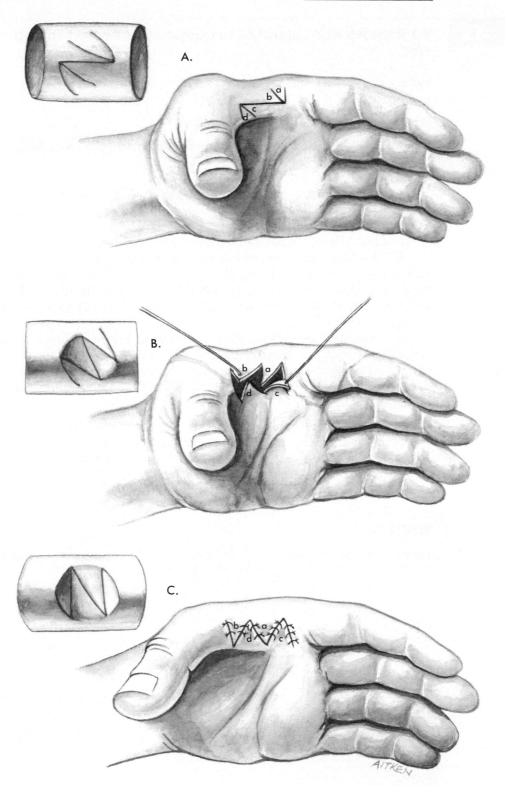

Plate 49. A.–C., Four-flap Z-plasty to deepen contracted thumb web.

| PLATE 50 | V-Y Release with Lateral Z's to Deepen Contracted Thumb Web |

Indications. Severe web space contracture of the thumb restricting range of motion and abduction.

Radiographic Control. Image intensifier.

Patient Position. Supine with upper limb supported on a hand table.

Operative Technique

A. Mark the skin incisions with a thin indelible pencil as illustrated. Make the incisions, and divide the subcutaneous tissue in line with the skin incisions. Section all fibrotic contractures.

Caution! Do not injure the digital vessels and nerves.

B. The skin flaps are mobilized, the tourniquet is released, and complete hemostasis is achieved. Bring the apex of the V-flap E into end of the Y, i.e., between C and A. Criss-cross the Z flaps by bringing the apex of flap B between A and the base of the index finger and the apex of flap D between the base of the thumb and flap C.

C. Close the skin flaps with interrupted sutures. Under image intensifier radiographic control, transfix the thumb with a smooth Steinmann pin into the carpus, with the thumb in complete abduction and opposition. Apply a compression dressing and above-elbow cast, with the patient's thumb held in complete abduction and opposition.

Postoperative Care. Change the cast as necessary. The pin is removed two to three weeks postoperatively, at which time sutures are removed; an abduction-opposition splint is used part-time to keep the thumb in the corrected position. Passive skin stretching exercises are performed several times a day, and active exercises are carried out to develop function in the thumb.

REFERENCE

Brown, P. W.: Adduction-flexion contracture of the thumb. Correction with dorsal rotation flap and release of contracture. Clin. Orthop., 88:161, 1972.

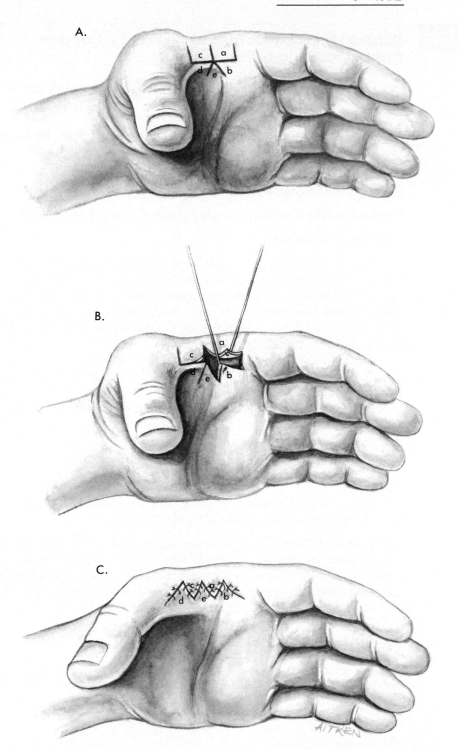

Plate 50. A.–C., V-Y release with lateral Z's to deepen contracted thumb web.

PLATE 51   Rotation Flap from Dorsum of the Hand to Deepen Contracted Thumb Web

Indications. Severe web space contracture between the thumb and index finger.

Requisites

1. Normal skin covering over the dorsal aspect of the index metacarpal and metacarpophalangeal joint.
2. Normal circulation.

Radiographic Control. Image intensifier.

Patient Position. Supine with upper limb supported on a hand table.

Operative Technique

A. and **B.** The skin incision begins on the dorsum of the index metacarpal at the juncture of the proximal and middle one third. It extends distally to the index metacarpal head, where it curves palmarward to the center of the index metacarpal neck. At this point, it extends proximally toward the third metacarpal and distally for 1 to 2 cm. Divide subcutaneous tissue in line with the skin incision. Elevate and undermine the wound flaps.

Caution! Do not injure digital vessels and nerves.

C. Divide interosseous fascia and contracted soft tissue between the index and first metacarpals to obtain complete abduction of the thumb.

D. Bring the point of the dorsal skin at the distal angle palmarward, and delineate the location and direction of the incision for the palmar limb of the Z-plasty. Interchange the skin angles with the thumb completely abducted, and suture the skin with interrupted 0000 nylon sutures.

E. Cover the remaining skin defect with a full-thickness skin graft taken from the groin.

Apply a compression dressing and an above-elbow cast with the patient's thumb held in complete abduction and opposition.

Postoperative Care. Change the cast as necessary. The pin is removed two to three weeks postoperatively, at which time sutures are removed and an abduction-opposition splint is used part-time to keep the thumb in corrected position. Passive skin stretching exercises are performed several times a day, and active exercises are carried out to develop function in the thumb.

REFERENCES

Chase, R. A.: Atlas of Hand Surgery. Vol. 2. Philadelphia, W. B. Saunders Co., 1984.
Strickland, J. W.: Thumb reconstruction. In: Green, D. P. (ed.): Operative Hand Surgery. 2nd ed. New York, Churchill Livingstone, 1988, pp. 2193–2194.

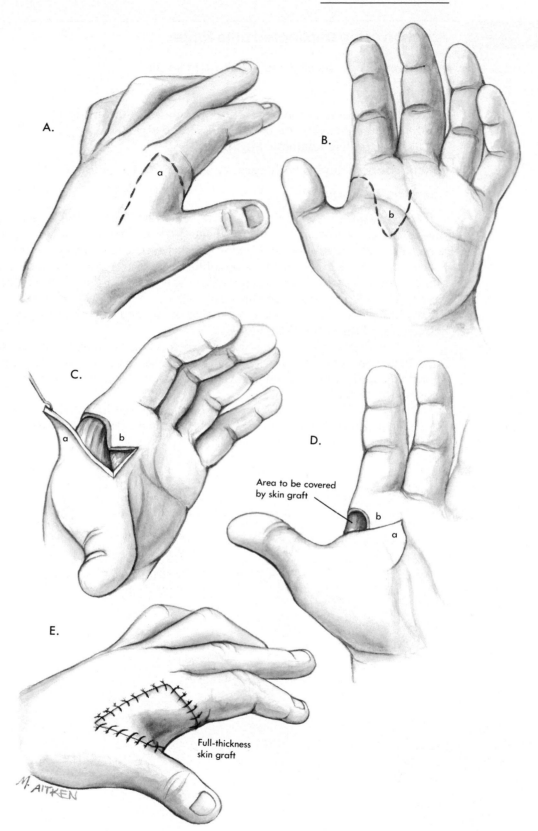

Area to be covered by skin graft

Full-thickness skin graft

M. AITKEN

Plate 51. A.–E., Rotation flap from the dorsum of the hand to deepen contracted thumb web.

PLATE 52 **Ablation of the Duplicated Little Finger**

Indications. Presence of a duplicated little finger.

Objectives

1. To maintain size and stability of remaining little finger.
2. To provide adequate motor control and strength.
3. To establish anatomic alignment.

Patient Position. Supine with upper limb supported on a hand table.

Operative Technique

A. A racquet incision is made. The solid lines are on the dorsal surface, and the dotted lines are on the volar surface. Avoid longitudinal straight scars. Be generous and err on the safe side. Excess skin can always be trimmed later. Preserve volar skin as much as possible because it is thicker and more durable and has better two-point discrimination than the thin dorsal skin. Subcutaneous tissue is divided in line with the skin incision. Next, make a midline incision on the radial aspect of the extra little finger for exposure of the long flexor and extensor tendons of the little finger.

B. The digital nerves and vessels are carefully isolated and protected. The hypothenar muscles are dissected off their insertions to the extra digit and the long flexor and extensor tendons are identified, divided distally, and dissected and reflected proximally.

C. The collateral ligaments are dissected, leaving their insertions to the metacarpal intact. Next, the extra digit is excised by division of the capsule at the metacarpophalangeal joint.

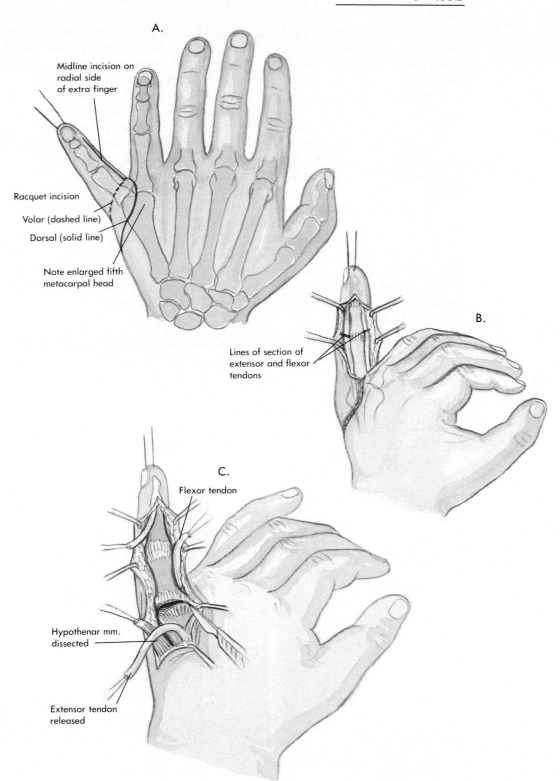

A.

Midline incision on
radial side
of extra finger

Racquet incision

Volar (dashed line)

Dorsal (solid line)

Note enlarged fifth
metacarpal head

Lines of section of
extensor and flexor
tendons

B.

C.

Flexor tendon

Hypothenar mm.
dissected

Extensor tendon
released

Plate 52. A.–F., Ablation of the duplicated little finger.

D. The fifth metacarpal head is usually enlarged, with a ridge separating the individual articular surfaces of the duplicated little fingers. The portion of the metacarpal head for the extra digit with a part of the subjacent thickened metacarpal shaft is removed with a thin sharp osteotome or a small oscillating saw. The cut is made parallel to the ridge on the articular surface of the metacarpal head. If the fifth metacarpal is angulated ulnarward, it may be necessary to perform an osteotomy of the metacarpal shaft for proper anatomic alignment.

E. The long flexor and extensor tendons of the ablated digit are transferred to the adjoining remaining little finger. The collateral ligament and hypothenar muscles are reattached to the base of the remaining proximal phalanx on its ulnar aspect.

Avoid injury to the growth plate. The capsule of the metacarpophalangeal joint is repaired with interrupted sutures.

F. A smooth Kirschner wire is used for internal fixation; it extends from the tip of the little finger to the base of the fifth metacarpal. It protects the repair of the collateral ligament and holds the metacarpophalangeal joint and the osteotomized metacarpal shaft in proper alignment. The tourniquet is removed, and after complete hemostasis, the wound is closed in routine fashion. An above-elbow cast or splint is applied.

Postoperative Care. In four weeks, the cast and Kirschner wire are removed and the infant is allowed to use the hand.

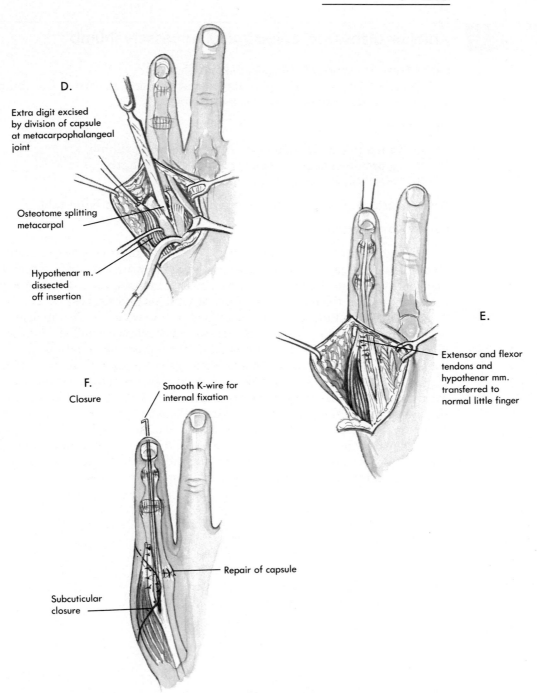

D.

Extra digit excised
by division of capsule
at metacarpophalangeal
joint

Osteotome splitting
metacarpal

Hypothenar m.
dissected
off insertion

E.

Extensor and flexor
tendons and
hypothenar mm.
transferred to
normal little finger

F.
Closure

Smooth K-wire for
internal fixation

Repair of capsule

Subcuticular
closure

Plate 52. (Continued)

PLATE 53 ## Ablation of the Duplicated Radial Accessory Thumb

Indications. Presence of a duplicated thumb.

Caution! Forewarn the parents that at skeletal maturity the thumb will be smaller than the contralateral normal thumb.

Objectives

1. To maintain size and stability of remaining thumb.
2. To provide adequate motor control and strength.
3. To establish anatomic alignment.

Patient Position. Supine with upper limb supported on a hand table.

Operative Technique.

A. and **B.** Make a racquet incision over the base of the radial thumb to be ablated as illustrated. The dorsal incision is shown by a solid line and the volar incision by a dashed line. A midline incision is made on the radial aspect of the accessory thumb to facilitate exposure of tendons and nerves.

C. The subcutaneous tissue is divided in line with the skin incision. Take care not to injure digital vessels and nerves. The extensor pollicis longus tendon is identified and sectioned over the middle of the proximal phalanx of the accessory thumb. The flexor pollicis longus tendon of the accessory thumb is identified and sectioned near its insertion. The long flexor and extensor tendons are reflected proximally. The thenar muscles are transected at their insertions. The capsule of the metacarpophalangeal joint is identified and divided by a transverse incision. The nerves and vessels of the ulnar thumb are identified, and if they are present and adequate, the digital vessels of the radial thumb are divided and ligated, and the digital nerve of the radial thumb is divided with a sharp scalpel and allowed to retract (formation of a neuroma is ordinarily not a problem).

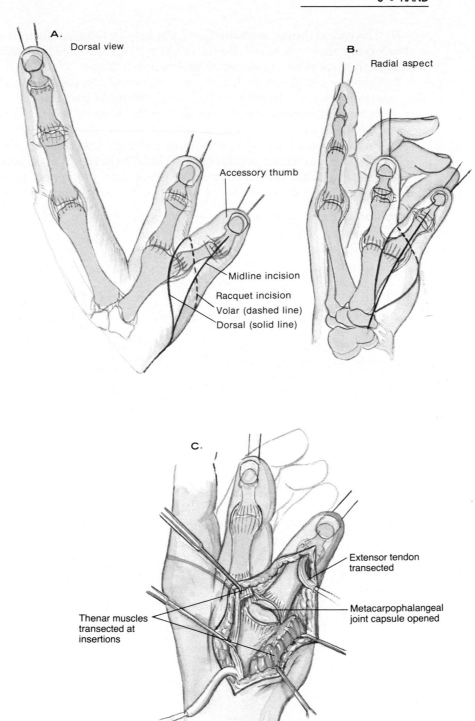

A.
Dorsal view

B.
Radial aspect

Accessory thumb

Midline incision

Racquet incision
Volar (dashed line)
Dorsal (solid line)

C.

Extensor tendon
transected

Metacarpophalangeal
joint capsule opened

Thenar muscles
transected at
insertions

Plate 53. **A.–F.,** Ablation of the duplicated radial accessory thumb.

D. The radial thumb is ablated, and the first metacarpal head is exposed. With a sharp osteotome or a small oscillating saw, trim the enlarged metacarpal head (the growth plate of the first metacarpal is proximal).

E. Transfer the flexor pollicis longus and extensor pollicis longus to those of the remaining thumb. Repair the collateral ligament and the capsule with interrupted sutures. Reattach thenar muscles to the base of the proximal phalanx of the remaining thumb.

F. Use a smooth Kirschner wire to transfix the metacarpophalangeal joint of the thumb. The tourniquet is released, and after hemostasis is obtained, the wound is closed in the usual fashion. An above-elbow cast is applied, incorporating the thumb. A cap is put over the thumb portion of the cast to protect the pin.

Postoperative Care. Remove the cast and pin in four to six weeks. Exercises are begun to restore function.

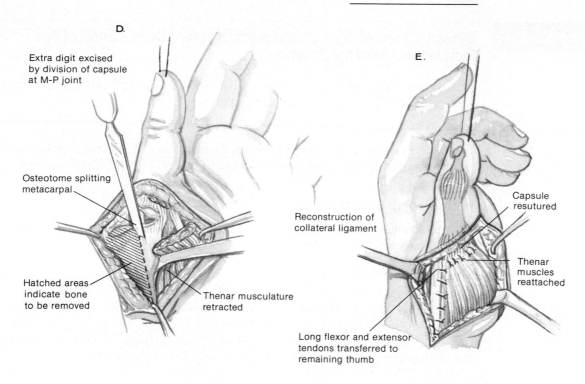

D.

Extra digit excised
by division of capsule
at M-P joint

Osteotome splitting
metacarpal

Hatched areas
indicate bone
to be removed

Thenar musculature
retracted

E.

Reconstruction of
collateral ligament

Capsule
resutured

Thenar
muscles
reattached

Long flexor and extensor
tendons transferred to
remaining thumb

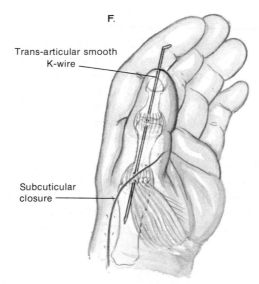

F.

Trans-articular smooth
K-wire

Subcuticular
closure

Plate 53. (Continued)

PLATE 54   **Bilhaut-Cloquet Operation for Incomplete Duplication of the Distal Phalanx of the Thumb**

Indications. Duplication of the distal phalanx of the thumb with both components diverging equally from the longitudinal axis.

Objectives

1. Formation of one distal phalanx by excision of a central triangular wedge.
2. Coaptation and fusion of the redundant parts of the distal segments in the midline.

Radiographic Control. Image intensifier.

Patient Position. With the patient supine and the shoulder abducted, the upper limb is positioned on the hand table.

Operative Technique

A. First, with a marking pen, outline the triangular wedges of skin that are to be excised on the dorsal and palmar aspects of the thumb. The apex of the triangular wedge should be at the distal one fourth of the proximal phalanx, and the distal end of the incision at the base of the triangles should be bisecting the duplicated distal phalanges. Incise the triangular wedge of skin with the adjoining nail bed. With the help of a sharp knife, excise the skin and nail on both the palmar and dorsal surfaces. Split and retract the extensor pollicis longus tendon on the ulnar and radial sides.

B. With the help of sharp AO osteotomes or an oscillating saw, slit the duplicated distal phalanges into two halves.

C. and D. The central wedge of bone is removed, and the lateral and medial halves of the remaining phalanges are approximated and fixed internally with the help of two threaded Steinmann pins that are inserted transversely. It is crucial that the growth plates be anatomically aligned with no "step-off." Reconstruct a single nail by bringing the nail beds and matrices together in the midline.

Close the wound in the usual fashion, and apply a below-elbow cast for immobilization.

Postoperative Care. Remove the pins when bony fusion has taken place, ordinarily in a matter of 6 weeks.

The problems with this operation include the split nail on the dorsum and the midline scar on the volar surface of the thumb and the difficulty of accurate approximation of the distal phalanges and their growth plates.

REFERENCES

Bilhaut, M.: Guerison d'un pouce bifide par un nouveau procède opératoire. Congr. Fr. Chir., 4:576, 1890.
Kelikian, H.: Congenital Deformities of the Hand and Forearm. Philadelphia, W. B. Saunders Co., 1974, pp. 408–456.

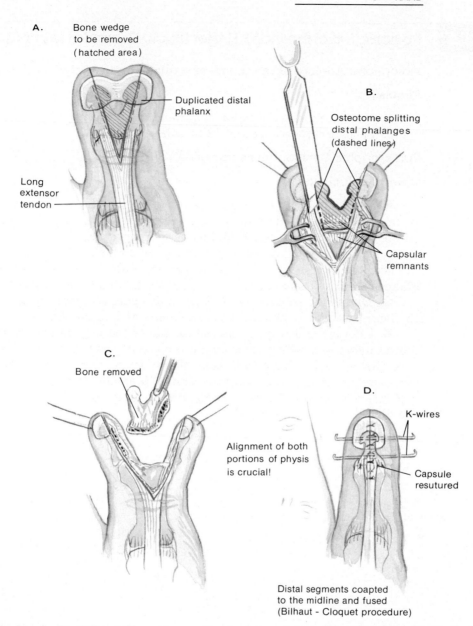

A. Bone wedge to be removed (hatched area)

Duplicated distal phalanx

Long extensor tendon

B.

Osteotome splitting distal phalanges (dashed lines)

Capsular remnants

C.

Bone removed

Alignment of both portions of physis is crucial!

D.

K-wires

Capsule resutured

Distal segments coapted to the midline and fused (Bilhaut - Cloquet procedure)

Plate 54. A.–D., Bilhaut-Cloquet operation for incomplete duplication of the distal phalanx of the thumb.

PLATE 55 Pollicization of the Index Finger (Buck-Gramcko Technique)

Indications. Absence of the thumb or a functionless, hypoplastic, floating thumb.

Requisites

1. Normal function of index finger and other digits.
2. Patient between six and 12 months of age.

Radiographic Control. Image intensifier.

Operative Technique

A. and **B.** Make a lazy S–shaped incision on the radial side of the palmar surface of the hand, beginning on the volar aspect of the index finger near its base and terminating at the wrist. Make another curvilinear incision across the base of the index finger at right angles and connected to the distal end of the first incision. Connect the two ends of the incision on the dorsum of the hand as shown in **B.** Make the third incision on the dorsum of the proximal phalanx of the index finger.

C. Divide the transverse fascicles of the palmar aponeurosis to gain access to the neurovascular bundle between the index and middle fingers.

D. Ligate the artery to the radial side of the long finger. Next, the common digital nerve is carefully separated into its component parts for the index and the long fingers. It is important that there be no tension on the neurovascular structures when the index finger is rotated. If an anomalous neural ring is present, it is sectioned so that there is no angulation of the digital artery. It is crucial that the digital veins be preserved.

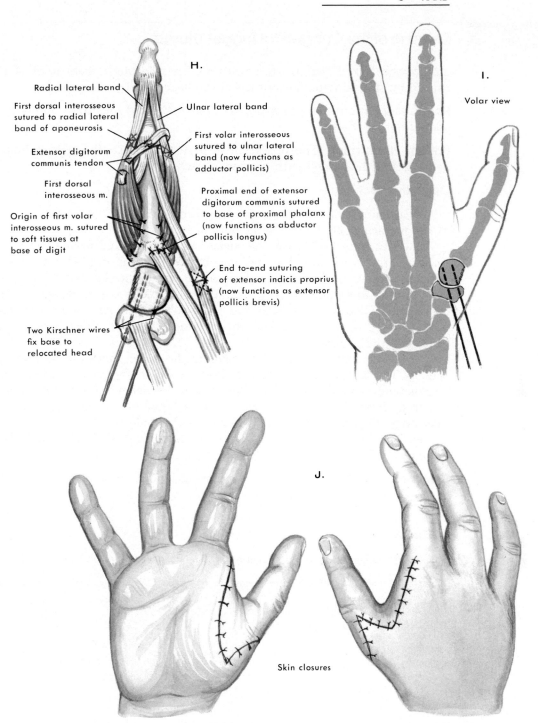

H.

Radial lateral band

First dorsal interosseous sutured to radial lateral band of aponeurosis

Ulnar lateral band

First volar interosseous sutured to ulnar lateral band (now functions as adductor pollicis)

Extensor digitorum communis tendon

First dorsal interosseous m.

Proximal end of extensor digitorum communis sutured to base of proximal phalanx (now functions as abductor pollicis longus)

Origin of first volar interosseous m. sutured to soft tissues at base of digit

End to-end suturing of extensor indicis proprius (now functions as extensor pollicis brevis)

Two Kirschner wires fix base to relocated head

I.

Volar view

J.

Skin closures

Plate 55. (Continued)

PLATE 56   Release of the Congenital Trigger Thumb

Indications. Fixed flexion contracture of the interphalangeal joint of the thumb caused by stenosing tendovaginitis of the flexor pollicis longus.

Requisites. Patient two years of age or older. Steroid injections do not succeed and should not be tried.

Patient Preparation. The operation is performed with the patient supine under general anesthesia and with tourniquet ischemia.

Operative Technique

A. A transverse incision 2 cm. long is made on the volar surface of the thumb at the metacarpophalangeal joint but not in the flexion crease.

B. With skin hooks, lift the incised skin edges and divide the subcutaneous tissue in line with the skin incision. Do not cut the digital nerves and vessels, which are close to the undersurface of the very thin skin. By blunt dissection in the longitudinal plane, the neurovascular structures are retracted to either side of the tendon. The flexor sheath and the tendon with its nodule are exposed. On flexion or extension of the thumb, the thickened and constricted sheath blocks gliding of the nodule.

C. A longitudinal incision is made in the flexor sheath in line with the flexor tendon. The thickened sheath is excised; inadvertent division of the flexor pollicis longus tendon must be avoided. Flexion and extension of the thumb should be fully restored. Partial excision of the thickened nodule of the flexor tendon is not necessary. Resist the temptation to reduce the nodule.

D. The tourniquet is released, and after hemostasis is obtained, the wound is closed with 00 subcuticular nylon sutures.

Postoperative Care. A simple soft dressing is applied. The child is encouraged to move the thumb freely. Bow-stringing of the tendon is not a problem.

REFERENCES

Fahey, J. J., and Bollinger, J. A.: Trigger-finger in adults and children. J. Bone Joint Surg., 36–A:1200, 1954.
Flatt, A. E.: The Care of Congenital Anomalies. St. Louis, C.V. Mosby, 1977, pp. 58–60.

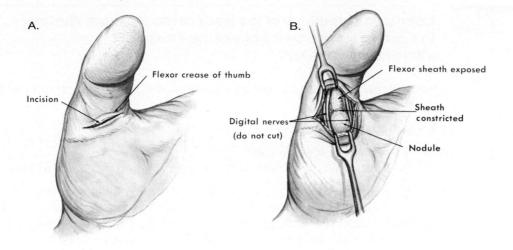

A.

Flexor crease of thumb

Incision

B.

Flexor sheath exposed

Digital nerves
(do not cut)

Sheath
constricted

Nodule

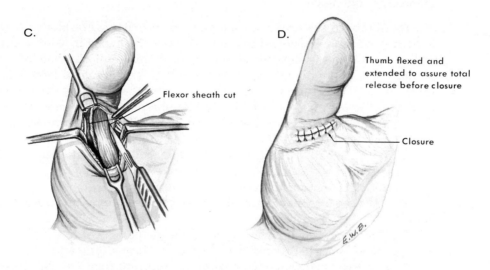

C.

Flexor sheath cut

D.

Thumb flexed and
extended to assure total
release before closure

Closure

E.W.B.

Plate 56. A.–D., Release of the congenital trigger thumb.

PLATE 57

Extension Osteotomy of the Neck of the Proximal Phalanx to Correct Flexion Deformity of the Proximal Interphalangeal Joint

Indications. Moderate flexion deformity of the proximal interphalangeal joint of the little finger.

Requisites

1. Skeletally mature hand.
2. Functional arc of flexion of the proximal interphalangeal joint.

Caution! Forewarn the patient and parents that the procedure does not improve the total range of motion but that the arc of motion will be different. Some degree of diminution of the ulnar grasp is the price for a straighter-appearing little finger; that is, there will be some degree of diminution of the strength of the ulnar grasp, but the finger will appear straighter.

Patient Position. The patient is supine.

Operative Technique

A. Approach the proximal phalanx and proximal interphalangeal joint of the little finger through a dorsal incision. Make an S-shaped incision beginning on the radial aspect of the dorsum of the little finger from the base of the proximal phalanx extending distally to the proximal interphalangeal joint where it curves laterally over the transverse dorsal crease and then distally over the dorsal ulnar border of the proximal half of the middle phalanx. Divide subcutaneous tissue in line with the skin incision. Neurovascular bundles are identified and kept out of harm's way.

B. With a small drill bit, make multiple drill holes outlining the dorsal wedge to be excised from the neck of the proximal phalanx.

Caution! Do not violate the volar periosteum.

C. With small osteotomes, complete the osteotomy and resect the wedge of bone.

D. The bone ends are then apposed on the periosteal hinge.

Caution! Be sure to maintain normal rotatory alignment.

E. Use two small Kirschner wires for internal fixation. The tips of the wires are left out percutaneously, and their ends are bent to prevent migration. The wound is closed in routine fashion.

Postoperative Care. Apply a below-elbow cast to provide immobilization for six weeks, at which time the cast and wires are removed and active, assisted and passive range of motion exercises are performed to restore motion of the proximal interphalangeal joint.

REFERENCES

Flatt, A. E.: The Care of Congenital Hand Anomalies. St. Louis, C.V. Mosby, 1977, pp. 147–154.
Oldfield, M. C.: Dupuytren's contracture (abridged). Proc. R. Soc. Med., 47:361, 1954.
Oldfield, M. C.: Camptodactyly: Flexor contractures of the fingers in young girls. Br. J. Plast. Surg., 8:312, 1956.

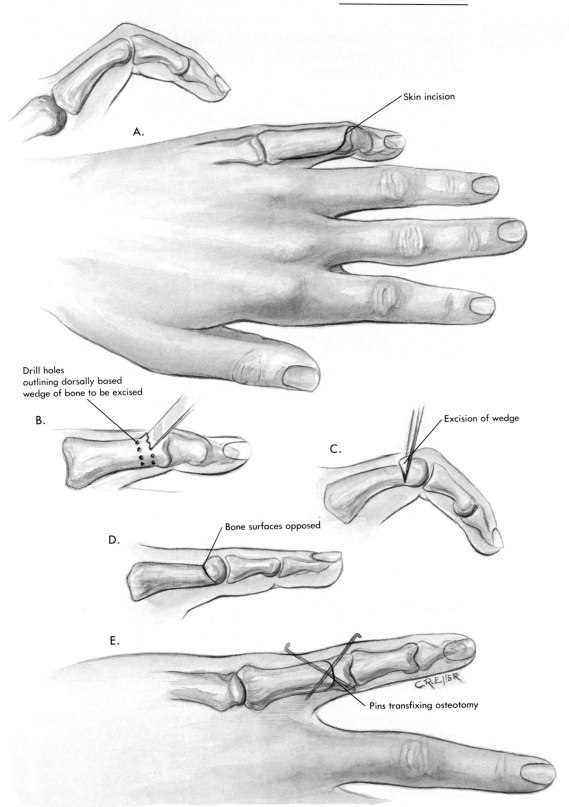

Skin incision

Drill holes
outlining dorsally based
wedge of bone to be excised

B.

C. Excision of wedge

D. Bone surfaces opposed

E. Pins transfixing osteotomy

C.RELIER

Plate 57. A.–E., Extension osteotomy of the neck of the proximal phalanx to correct flexion deformity of the proximal interphalangeal joint.

PLATE 58

Correction of Clinodactyly of the Little Finger by Closing-Wedge or Opening-Wedge Osteotomy of Its Middle Phalanx

Indications. Angular deformity of the little finger or another digit in which the deformed digit overlaps its neighbor when the patient makes a fist.

Patient Position. Supine.

Operative Technique

A. Make a midlateral longitudinal incision beginning 1 cm. distal to the distal interphalangeal joint and extending proximally to the proximal interphalangeal joint. Divide subcutaneous tissue in line with the skin incision. Retract the skin margins with skin hooks. The digital vessels and nerves are gently dissected, isolated free, and kept out of harm's way.

An alternate surgical approach is through a mid-dorsal incision.

B. The phalanx immediately proximal to the affected joint is exposed subperiosteally. In the little finger (the digit most commonly affected), the wedge is usually taken from the middle phalanx. Do not disturb the growth plate of the phalanx, which is proximal. The base of the wedge is located on the convex side (the side toward which correction is intended); in the little finger it is usually ulnar. With an oscillating electric saw, perform the wedge osteotomy. Leave the apex of the wedge on the concave side partly intact.

C. Remove the wedge of bone with a Freer elevator. The bone surfaces are apposed; the periosteal hinge on the concave side provides stability to the closing osteotomy.

Two criss-cross, threaded Kirschner wires are inserted obliquely with an electric drill from the ulnar side. Avoid injury to the dorsal extensor mechanism and to the physis of the phalanx.

D. Perform an opening wedge osteotomy when the middle phalanx is hypoplastic. The skin on the concave side is usually contracted; it is released and elongated by Z-plasty.

When the skin on the concave side is not contracted, the middle phalanx is exposed subperiosteally through a mid-dorsal incision. When the skin is contracted, a Z-incision is made on the concave side as illustrated.

E. Perform an osteotomy of the middle phalanx with an electric saw. Leave the cortex on the convex side intact.

F. A wedge of cortical bone graft of appropriate size is taken from the iliac crest. The osteotomy site is opened up, and the wedge of bone is inserted into it.

G. The opening osteotomy with the wedge of bone is transfixed with two criss-cross, threaded Kirschner wires.

The tourniquet is released, and complete hemostasis is obtained. The Z-plasty skin flaps are transposed and sutured with interrupted sutures.

Apply a below-elbow cast for immobilization, incorporating the patient's little and ring fingers.

Postoperative Care. The osteotomy usually heals in four to six weeks, at which time the cast and Kirschner wires are removed. The digit may be protected in an aluminum or plastic splint for an additional two weeks.

REFERENCES

Barsky, A. J.: Congenital Anomalies of the Hand and Their Surgical Treatment. Springfield, Ill., Charles C Thomas, 1958.

Flatt, A. E.: The Care of Congenital Hand Anomalies. St. Louis, C.V. Mosby, 1977, pp. 146–155.

Wood, V. E.: Clinodactyly. In: Green, D. P. (ed.): Operative Hand Surgery. 2nd ed. New York, Churchill Livingstone, 1988, pp. 422–424.

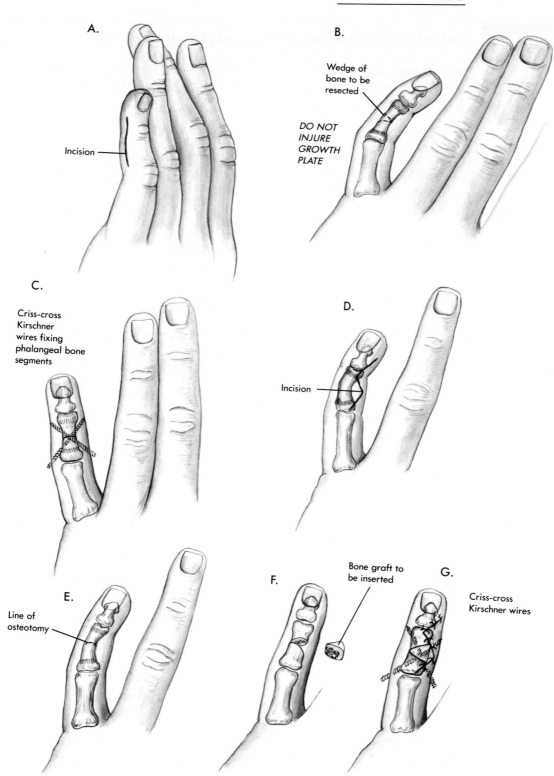

A.

Incision

B.

Wedge of
bone to be
resected

*DO NOT
INJURE
GROWTH
PLATE*

C.

Criss-cross
Kirschner
wires fixing
phalangeal bone
segments

D.

Incision

E.

Line of
osteotomy

F.

Bone graft to
be inserted

G.

Criss-cross
Kirschner
wires

Plate 58. A.–G., Correction of clinodactyly of the little finger by closing-wedge or opening-wedge osteotomy at its middle phalanx.

| PLATE 59 | **Release of the Adductor Pollicis Muscle in the Palm** |

Indications. Adduction contracture of the thumb interfering with function. This procedure preserves some degree of function of the thumb adductor.

Patient Position. Supine.

Operative Technique

 A. Make a skin incision in the palm beginning at the lateral border of the proximal palmar crease and extended proximally to the wrist. Subcutaneous tissue is divided in line with the skin incision.

 B. The palmar aponeurosis is divided, with due care taken not to injure the digital vessels and nerves.

 C. The digital branches of the median nerve are visualized and kept out of harm's way. The second lumbrical muscle is retracted ulnarward, the flexor tendons of the index finger are retracted radially, and adductor pollicis muscle is visualized in the palm.

 D. An incision is made at the origin of the adductor pollicis from the third metacarpal, and with periosteal elevators it is reflected radially and distally.

 The tourniquet is released, and after complete hemostasis a small Hemovac drain is used for closed suction. Subcutaneous tissue and the skin are closed in the usual fashion, and a below-elbow cast is applied, holding the thumb in maximal abduction.

Postoperative Care. Remove the cast three weeks following surgery. A splint is manufactured for night use, holding the thumb in maximal abduction; another splint is made for day use. Prescribe a physical therapy regimen consisting of active and passive exercises to elongate the adductor pollicis and develop functional use for activities of daily living.

REFERENCES

Hoffer, M. M., Perry, J., Garcia, M., and Bullock, D.: Adduction contracture of the thumb in cerebral palsy. J. Bone Joint Surg., 65–A:755, 1983.

House, J. H., Gwathmey, F. W., and Fidler, M. O.: A dynamic approach to the thumb-in-palm deformity in cerebral palsy. J. Bone Joint Surg., 63–A:216, 1981.

Zancolli, E. A., and Zancolli, E. A., Jr.: Surgical management of the hemiplegic spastic hand in cerebral palsy. Surg. Clin. North Am., 61:395, 1981.

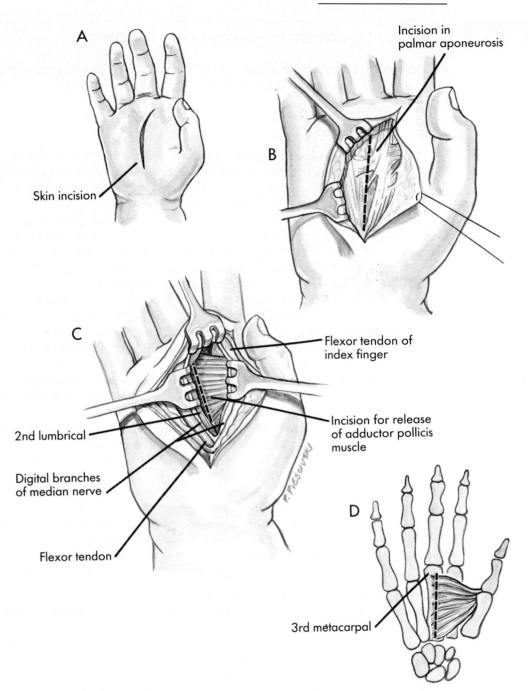

A

Skin incision

Incision in
palmar aponeurosis

B

C

Flexor tendon of
index finger

Incision for release
of adductor pollicis
muscle

2nd lumbrical

Digital branches
of median nerve

Flexor tendon

D

3rd metacarpal

Plate 59. A.–D., Release of the adductor pollicis muscle in the palm.

PLATE 60   Adductor Myotomy of the Thumb at Its Insertion

Indications. Adduction contracture of the thumb. *Note:* The procedure is technically simple, but it does not preserve function of the thumb adductor.

Patient Position. Supine.

Operative Technique

A. and **B.** An oblique incision 2 to 3 cm. long is made over the dorsum of the hand. It begins at the ulnar border of the first metacarpal head, extends proximally to the middle third of the metacarpal, and then swings ulnarward toward the base of the second metacarpal. Avoid the distal margin of the thumb web, as the cicatrix may cause contracture of the web. This surgical approach permits stripping of the first dorsal interosseous muscle if necessary. When only an adductor tenotomy is to be done, an alternate approach is a 1.5- to 2-cm.-long transverse incision immediately proximal to the flexor crease of the thumb. Again, the ulnar border of the incision should stop short of the distal margin of the thumb web. (When a Z-plasty of the contracted thumb web is indicated, a transverse skin incision is made at the distal border of the web, extending between the ulnar border of the proximal flexion crease of the thumb and the radial border of the proximal transverse crease of the palm, and two oblique cuts at a 45- to 60-degree angle are made for Z-lengthening.)

C. Divide the subcutaneous tissue. The first dorsal interosseous muscle is retracted proximally, and the tendon of the adductor pollicis is identified near its insertion.

D. With a staphylorrhaphy elevator, the adductor pollicis longus tendon is lifted dorsally and 1 cm. of the adductor tendon is excised near its insertion. Care should be exercised not to disturb the tendon mechanism of the extensors and the abductors of the thumb.

If the first dorsal interosseous muscle is contracted, it is stripped from the metacarpal with a periosteal elevator through the same incision.

The wound is closed in routine manner. A well-molded, above-elbow cast is applied to hold the thumb metacarpal in maximal abduction, the metacarpophalangeal joint in neutral extension, and the interphalangeal joint in 10 degrees of flexion. The elbow should be in slight flexion with the forearm in full supination.

Postoperative Care. Three weeks after surgery, the cast is bivalved and an opponens splint is made to hold the thumb in a position of maximal abduction and functional opposition. Active exercises are begun to develop active motion of the thumb in all directions—adduction, abduction, opposition, flexion, and extension. Passive exercises are also performed to maintain maximal range of motion. In the beginning two weeks, the opponens splint is worn continuously, except during the exercise periods; later the use of the splint is gradually decreased and an aggressive regimen of occupational therapy is instituted to develop function.

REFERENCE

Hoffer, M. M., Perry, J., Garcia, M., and Bullock, D.: Adduction contracture of the thumb in cerebral palsy. J. Bone Joint Surg., 65–A:755, 1983.

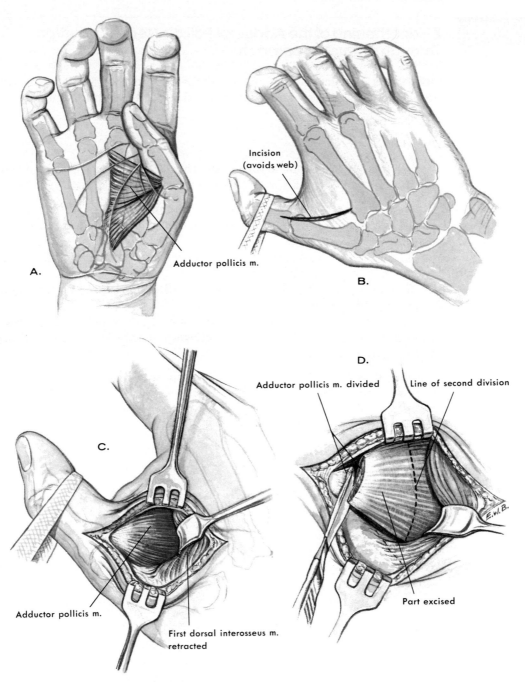

A.

Adductor pollicis m.

B.

Incision
(avoids web)

C.

Adductor pollicis m.

First dorsal interosseus m.
retracted

D.

Adductor pollicis m. divided   Line of second division

Part excised

E.W.B.

Plate 60. A.–D., Adductor myotomy of the thumb at its insertion.

PLATE 61 **Z-Lengthening of the Adductor Pollicis Near Its Insertion Through a Dorsal Approach**

Indications. Adduction contracture of the thumb interfering with function. This procedure preserves some degree of function of the thumb adductor.

Patient Position. Supine.

Operative Technique

When adduction contracture of the thumb is not severe, this author prefers Z-lengthening of the adductor pollicis tendon through a dorsal incision.

A. A skin incision is made on the dorsum of the hand between the index and thumb metacarpals. The subcutaneous tissue is divided in line with the skin incision.

B. Adductor pollicis muscle is exposed and gently elevated from its underlying tendon. A Z-incision is made in the tendon.

C. Close the two ends of the tendon with interrupted sutures elongating the adductor pollicis muscle.

The wound is closed in the usual fashion, and a below-elbow cast is applied, holding the wrist in 20 degrees of dorsiflexion and the thumb in maximal abduction and neutral extension.

Postoperative Care. The cast is removed three weeks following surgery. A splint is manufactured for night use, holding the thumb in maximal abduction; another splint is made for day use. A physical therapy regimen consisting of active and passive exercises is prescribed.

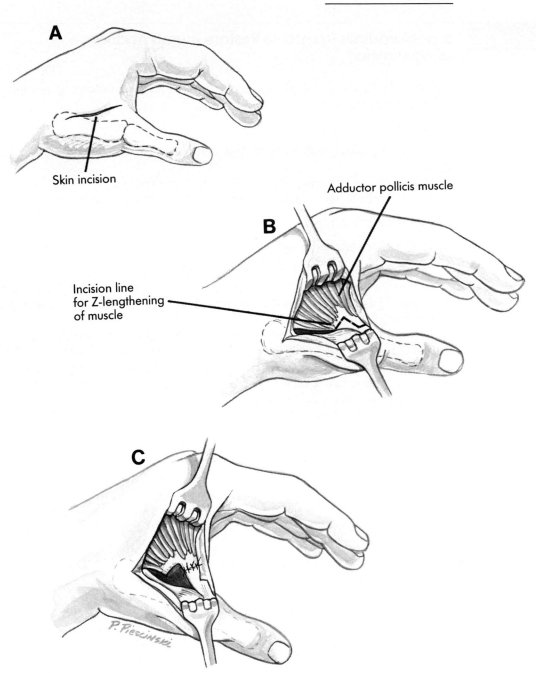

A Skin incision

B Adductor pollicis muscle

Incision line for Z-lengthening of muscle

C

P. Pieszinski

Plate 61. A.–C., Z-lengthening of the adductor pollicis near its insertion through a dorsal approach.

PLATE 62 ## Brachioradialis Transfer to Restore Thumb Abduction and Extension

Indications. Lack of thumb abduction and extension following release of thumb adduction contracture.

Requisites

1. Full passive abduction of first metacarpal and full passive extension of the thumb.
2. Stable metacarpophalangeal joint of the thumb.
3. Normal or good motor strength of the brachioradialis.

Patient Position. Supine.

Operative Technique

A. A long dorsoradial incision is made, beginning at the radial styloid process and extending proximally to a point 2 cm. distal to the lateral epicondyle of the humerus. Subcutaneous tissue is divided, and the wound edges are undermined and retracted.

B. and C. The flat tendon of the brachioradialis is sectioned at its insertion into the base of the styloid process of the radius. The tendons of the abductor pollicis longus and extensor pollicis brevis are divided at their musculotendinous junction and marked with 00 Tycron whip sutures as they traverse from the dorsal to the volar aspect on the brachioradialis tendon. Injury to neurovascular structures should be avoided. The radial artery lies on the volar margin of the brachioradialis tendon, and on the ulnar side of the radial vessels is the flexor carpi radialis tendon. The radial nerve runs along the lateral aspect of the forearm deep to the brachioradialis muscle. In the upper third of the forearm, the nerve is radial to the radial artery; in the middle of the forearm, it is immediately lateral to the artery; in the lower third of the forearm, the superficial branch of the nerve curves dorsally underneath the brachioradialis tendon to divide into the medial or lateral branches after penetrating the deep fascia on the dorsum of the wrist.

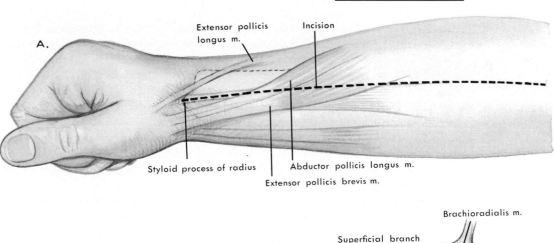

A.

Extensor pollicis longus m.

Incision

Styloid process of radius

Abductor pollicis longus m.

Extensor pollicis brevis m.

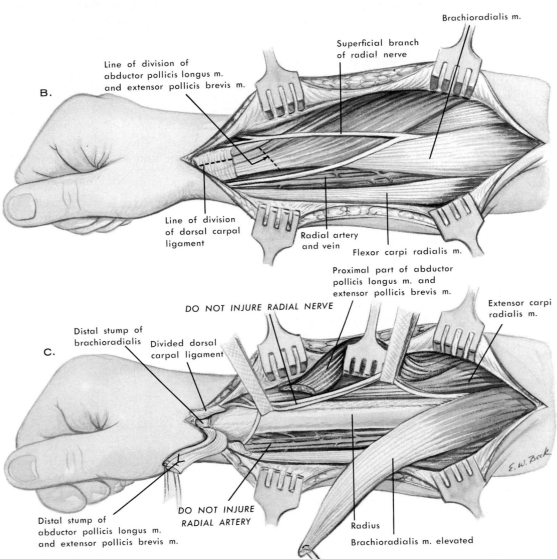

B.

Line of division of abductor pollicis longus m. and extensor pollicis brevis m.

Superficial branch of radial nerve

Brachioradialis m.

Line of division of dorsal carpal ligament

Radial artery and vein

Flexor carpi radialis m.

C.

Proximal part of abductor pollicis longus m. and extensor pollicis brevis m.

DO NOT INJURE RADIAL NERVE

Extensor carpi radialis m.

Distal stump of brachioradialis

Divided dorsal carpal ligament

Distal stump of abductor pollicis longus m. and extensor pollicis brevis m.

DO NOT INJURE RADIAL ARTERY

Radius

Brachioradialis m. elevated

E. W. Beck

Plate 62. **A.–E.,** Brachioradialis transfer to restore thumb abduction and extension.

D. By sharp and dull dissection, the brachioradialis muscle is freed from the antebrachial fascia and the adjacent muscles (extensor carpi radialis dorsally and flexor carpi ulnaris anteriorly). It is imperative to mobilize the brachioradialis as proximally as possible (preferably immediately distal to the elbow joint) to gain maximal excursion of the muscle action and to have a straight line of muscle pull.

E. The extensor pollicis longus and abductor pollicis brevis tendons are sutured to the brachioradialis tendon by interrupted 00 Tycron sutures, and the tendon ends interwoven. The tension on the transferred tendon should be moderate so that the first metacarpal can be passively adducted 1.5 cm. from the palm with the wrist in neutral position and passive pulp pinch is possible between the thumb and index finger.

The wound is closed in layers, and an above-elbow cast is applied with the elbow in 90 degrees of flexion, the wrist in neutral position, the first metacarpal in maximal abduction, and the thumb in neutral extension.

Postoperative Care. Three to four weeks following surgery, the cast is removed and active exercises are performed to develop function of the transferred brachioradialis muscle as an abductor and extensor of the thumb. Passive exercises are performed to maintain full range of motion of the joint. In the beginning, a below-elbow splint is worn to maintain the thumb metacarpal in maximum abduction. Functional therapy is very important, involving such exercises as holding water glasses of various sizes for thumb abduction and holding a pencil for thumb adduction.

REFERENCE

Henderson, E. D.: Transfer of wrist extensors and brachioradialis to restore opposition of the thumb. J. Bone Joint Surg., 44–A:513, 1962.

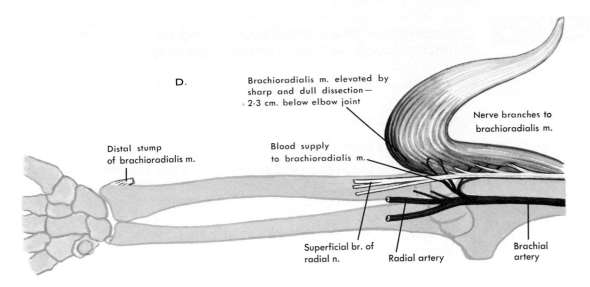

D.

Brachioradialis m. elevated by sharp and dull dissection— 2-3 cm. below elbow joint

Nerve branches to brachioradialis m.

Distal stump of brachioradialis m.

Blood supply to brachioradialis m.

Superficial br. of radial n.

Radial artery

Brachial artery

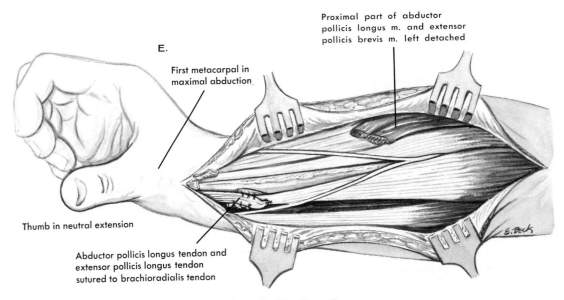

Proximal part of abductor pollicis longus m. and extensor pollicis brevis m. left detached

E.

First metacarpal in maximal abduction.

Thumb in neutral extension

Abductor pollicis longus tendon and extensor pollicis longus tendon sutured to brachioradialis tendon

Plate 62. (Continued)

PLATE 63   Capsulodesis of the Metacarpophalangeal Joint of the Thumb to Correct Hyperextension Deformity

Indications. Hyperextension deformity of the metacarpophalangeal joint of the thumb with dorsal subluxation.

Patient Position. Supine.

Operative Technique

A. Make a transverse incision parallel to the proximal flexor crease of the thumb. Divide subcutaneous tissue in line with the incision.

B. Identify the neurovascular bundles medially and laterally, and retract them out of harm's way. Expose the flexor pollicis longus tendon, and excise a part of its sheath over the metacarpophalangeal joint, including the thickened fibrous pulley between the two sesamoid bones.

C. Retract the flexor pollicis longus tendon, and expose the capsule and the volar plate of the metacarpophalangeal joint of the thumb. The growth plate of the proximal phalanx of the thumb is proximal; this should not be disturbed. With the help of a scalpel, incise the volar plate and the capsule at their proximal attachments and along each side, leaving their strong distal attachment intact.

Make the longitudinal incisions on either side of the plate outside the sesamoid bones. This technique divides the fibers of the intrinsic muscles, which insert to the volar plate, and leaves the fibers, which insert into the extensor wing and base of the proximal phalanx of the thumb, intact.

D.–F. Pass 00 or 000 Tycron (or other nonabsorbable) sutures through the volar plate and capsule. Make a slot in the metacarpal neck, then make two small holes through the neck of the metacarpal from its palmar to dorsal aspect.

Pass each end of the sutures through one of the drill holes, exiting on the skin on the dorsum of the thumb, and pull the proximal edge of the volar plate into the slot in the metacarpal neck. Flex the metacarpophalangeal joint 30 degrees, and firmly anchor the volar plate in the trap door. Pass the sutures through a piece of sterile felt and button, and tie them firmly. The flexed position of the joint is maintained by two small smooth Kirschner wires across the joint.

Close the wound in the usual fashion, and apply a below-elbow cast.

Postoperative Care. Four weeks postoperatively, remove the cast, the pins, and the pull-out sutures. Use a splint to hold the metacarpophalangeal joint in flexion for an additional two months.

REFERENCES

Filler, B. C., Stark, H. H., and Boyes, J. H.: Capsulodesis of the metacarpophalangeal joint of the thumb in children with cerebral palsy. J. Bone Joint Surg., 58–A:667, 1976.
Zancolli, E. A.: Structural and Dynamic Bases of Hand Surgery. 2nd ed. Philadelphia, J. B. Lippincott Co., 1979, pp. 212–213.

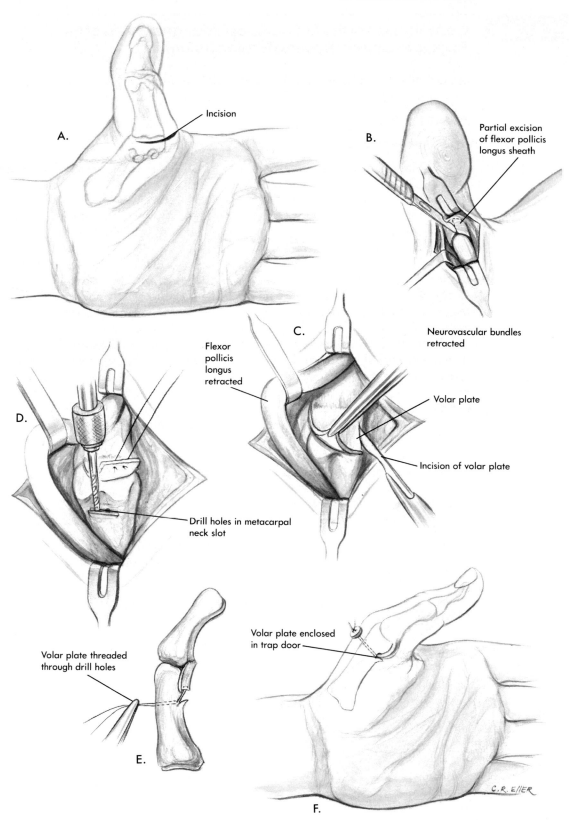

A. Incision

B. Partial excision of flexor pollicis longus sheath

Neurovascular bundles retracted

C. Volar plate

Incision of volar plate

D. Flexor pollicis longus retracted

Drill holes in metacarpal neck slot

E. Volar plate threaded through drill holes

F. Volar plate enclosed in trap door

C.R. Eller

Plate 63. A.–F., Capsulodesis of the metacarpophalangeal joint of the thumb to correct hyperextension deformity.

PLATE 64	Capsulodesis of the Metacarpophalangeal Joints of the Fingers to Correct Hyperextension Deformity

Indications. Hyperextension deformity with subluxation of the metacarpophalangeal joints of the fingers.

Patient Position. Supine.

Operative Technique

A. Make a transverse incision across the distal palm crease. Divide subcutaneous tissue in line with the skin incision.

B. Make longitudinal incisions in the peritendinous fascia and tendon sheaths, and expose the tendons of the flexor digitorum profundus and flexor digitorum superficialis. Retract the flexor tendon, and expose the volar plate of the metacarpophalangeal joints.

C.–E. The base of the proximal phalanx is dorsally displaced and hyperextended. Palmarflex the metacarpophalangeal joint, and resect an elliptical segment of the volar fibrocartilaginous plate. With the metacarpophalangeal joint in 20 degrees of flexion, repair the volar plate with two or three nonabsorbable sutures such as Tycron.

F. Insert a Kirschner wire transarticularly from the dorsum of the metacarpal into the proximal two thirds of the proximal phalanx with the metacarpophalangeal joint in 20 degrees of flexion. In the proximal phalanx, the tip of the Kirschner wire should just protrude from the dorsal cortex. Proximally it is left protruding across the dorsum of the metacarpal.

An alternate method of repair of the volar plate is by fixation to bone.

G. With a small drill bit, make two holes in the neck of the metacarpals proximal to the physis. Do not injure the growth plate.

H. Pass nonabsorbable sutures through the holes and into the distal part of the volar plate. Flex the metacarpophalangeal joint 30 degrees, and tie the sutures tightly. Insert a Kirschner wire transarticularly, as described in **F.**

Close the wound in the usual fashion, and apply a below-elbow cast.

Postoperative Care. Four weeks postoperatively, remove the cast, the pins, and the pull-out sutures. Use a splint to hold the metacarpophalangeal joints in flexion for an additional two months.

REFERENCE

Zancolli, E. A.: Structural and Dynamic Bases of Hand Surgery. 2nd ed. Philadelphia, J. B. Lippincott Co., 1979, p. 191.

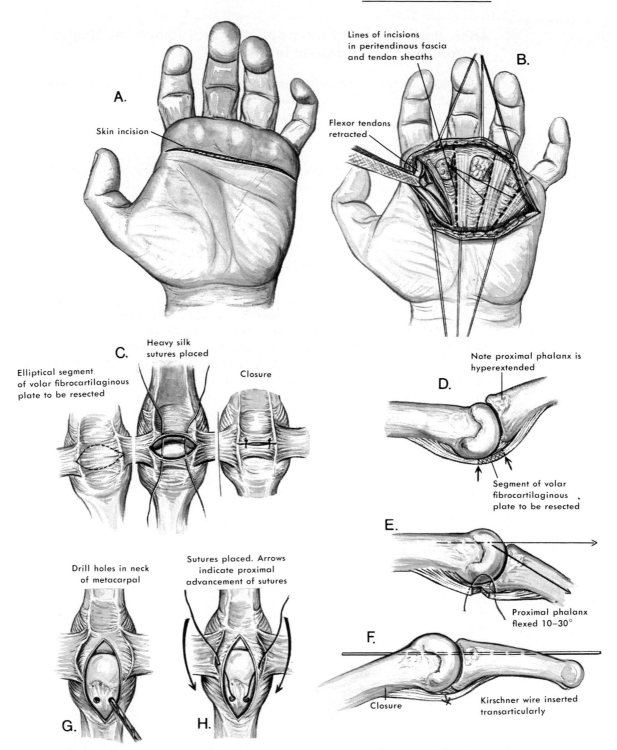

A.

Skin incision

Lines of incisions
in peritendinous fascia
and tendon sheaths

B.

Flexor tendons
retracted

C.

Elliptical segment
of volar fibrocartilaginous
plate to be resected

Heavy silk
sutures placed

Closure

D.

Note proximal phalanx is
hyperextended

Segment of volar
fibrocartilaginous
plate to be resected

E.

Proximal phalanx
flexed 10–30°

Drill holes in neck
of metacarpal

Sutures placed. Arrows
indicate proximal
advancement of sutures

F.

Closure

Kirschner wire inserted
transarticularly

G.

H.

Plate 64. A.–H., Capsulodesis of the metacarpophalangeal joints of the fingers to correct hyperextension deformity.

PLATE 65 **Arthrodesis of the Metacarpophalangeal Joint of the Thumb (Carroll-Hill Cup and Cone Technique)**

Indications. Marked instability and subluxation of the metacarpophalangeal joint of the thumb in the skeletally mature patient.

Patient Position. Supine.

Operative Technique

A. Make a dorsal incision to expose the metacarpophalangeal joint of the thumb. Incise the joint capsule, and resect the collateral ligaments. Expose the base of the proximal phalanx and the head of the first metacarpal.

B. By acute flexion and radial deviation of the thumb, expose the ends of the bones.

C. Hold the shaft of the first metacarpal steady with a small, bone-holding forceps. With a rongeur, shape the condyles into a tapered, rounded cone. Remove all articular cartilage.

D. Make multiple drill holes in the osteocartilaginous juncture of the base of the proximal phalanx. With an osteotome, connect the holes.

E. Remove a cone of bone from the diaphysis of the base of the proximal phalanx. With a curet, enlarge the cup to receive the end of the metacarpal.

F. Drill a Kirschner wire from the center of the cup distally to exit at the tip of the thumb. The metacarpal head is firmly anchored into the cup at the base of the proximal phalanx, and the metacarpophalangeal joint is fixed in 20 to 25 degrees of flexion with the thumb opposing the index finger by drilling the Kirschner wire into the metacarpal.

Insert a second Kirschner wire obliquely to control rotation. Apply a below-elbow cast.

Postoperative Care. Remove the cast and wires in 6 to 8 weeks, when fusion has taken place.

REFERENCE

Carroll, R. E., and Hill, N. A.: Small joint arthrodesis in hand reconstruction. J. Bone Joint Surg., 51–A:1219, 1969.

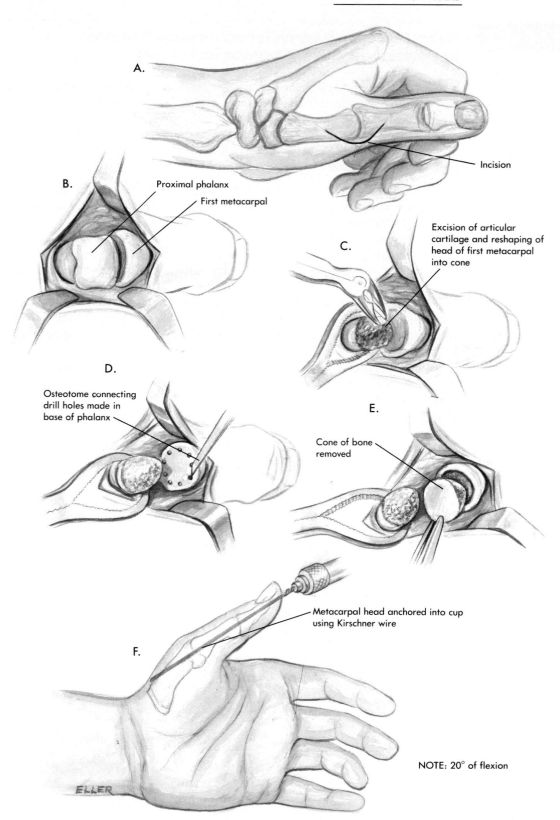

A.

Incision

B.

Proximal phalanx

First metacarpal

C.

Excision of articular
cartilage and reshaping of
head of first metacarpal
into cone

D.

Osteotome connecting
drill holes made in
base of phalanx

E.

Cone of bone
removed

F.

Metacarpal head anchored into cup
using Kirschner wire

NOTE: 20° of flexion

ELLER

Plate 65. A.–F., Arthrodesis of the metacarpophalangeal joint of the thumb (Carroll-Hill cup and cone technique).

| PLATE 66 | Flexor Digitorum Sublimis Tenodesis of the Proximal Interphalangeal Joint (Swanson Technique) |

Indications. Swan-neck deformity caused by chronic overpull on the middle extensor band by the spastic intrinsic muscles and by the tenodesis effect of the extensor digitorum longus when the wrist is in flexion.

Patient Position. Supine.

Operative Technique

A. Make a midlateral incision immediately dorsal to the flexion crease, beginning at the distal end of the middle phalanx and extending to the base of the proximal phalanx.

B. Divide subcutaneous tissue in line with the skin incision. Retract the wound edges with skin hooks. The digital vessels and nerves are dissected free with blunt scissors and retracted out of harm's way. Incise the flexor sheath longitudinally, and expose the flexor sublimis and profundus tendons.

C. Retract the flexor tendons palmarward and laterally. The distal half of the volar surface of the proximal phalanx is exposed subperiosteally by resection of the periosteum. Partially resect the proximal portion of the volar plate so that it will not interfere with the tenodesis.

With an electric drill, make two small drill holes through the neck of the proximal phalanx approximately 0.5 cm. apart. Drill in a palmar to dorsal direction. With a small curet, connect the two drill holes on the palmar aspect to form a bed of raw bone for firm attachment of the sublimis tendon.

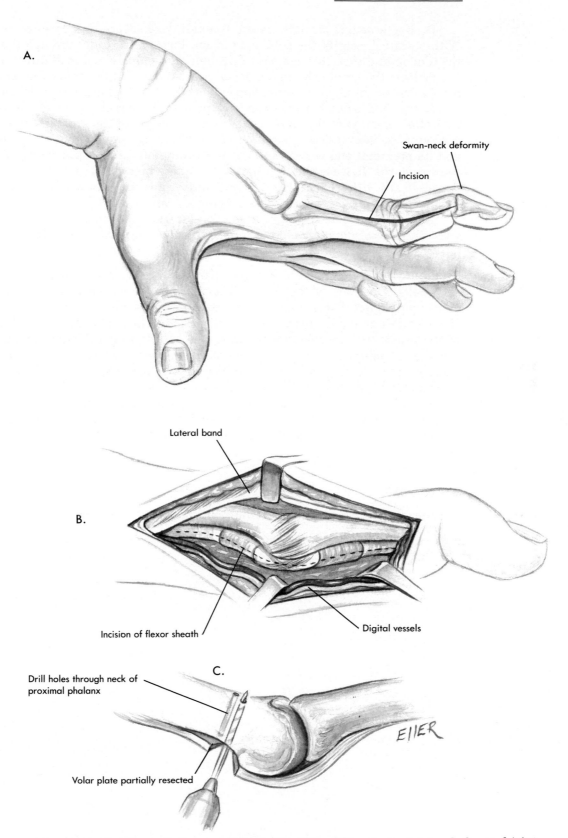

A.

Swan-neck deformity

Incision

Lateral band

B.

Incision of flexor sheath

Digital vessels

C.

Drill holes through neck of
proximal phalanx

Volar plate partially resected

ELLER

Plate 66. A.–F., Flexor digitorum sublimis tenodesis of the proximal interphalangeal joint
(Swanson technique).

D. Use a double straight needle Bunnell wire suture to secure the tenodesis. With a scalpel, scarify the sublimis tendon. Pass each needle through the edge of the tendon and then through each drill hole in a palmar to dorsal direction.

E. Pass the suture through a dorsal button, and firmly anchor the tendon into bone with the proximal interphalangeal joint in 20 to 30 degrees of flexion.

F. Insert a smooth Kirschner wire across the dorsal aspect of the proximal interphalangeal joint for more secure immobilization of the proximal interphalangeal joint in flexion. The distal end of the Kirschner wire is cut subcutaneously, and its proximal end is bent and left protruding out of the skin for facilitation of later removal. Release the tourniquet. Complete hemostasis is secured. Close the flexor sheath with 0000 or 00000 Vicryl sutures and the skin with 000 subcuticular nylon. Insert small silicone drains subcutaneously.

Apply an above-elbow cast; it should extend to the tip of the fingers with the wrist in neutral dorsiflexion, the forearm in full supination, and the elbow in 90 degrees of flexion.

Postoperative Care. Remove the cast, Kirschner wire, and suture wire in four to six weeks. One side of the wire is cut short under the button, and the wire is gently pulled out. Passive and active exercises are performed under supervision of the therapist and the parents to develop functional range of motion. Avoid extension of the proximal interphalangeal joints. Use splints that hold the proximal interphalangeal joints in flexion. These splints are worn during the day except for exercise periods for four to six weeks; then they are applied only at night, maintaining the patient's fingers in flexion for another two to three months.

In rare cases, dorsal dermadesis of the distal interphalangeal joint can be useful to improve flexion deformity of the joint. Fusion of the distal interphalangeal or proximal interphalangeal joint is not recommended in the child with cerebral palsy.

REFERENCES

Swanson, A. B.: Treatment of swan-neck deformity in cerebral palsied hand. Clin. Orthop., 48:167, 1966.
Swanson, A. B.: Surgery of the hand in cerebral palsy and muscle release procedures. Surg. Clin. North Am., 48:1129, 1968.

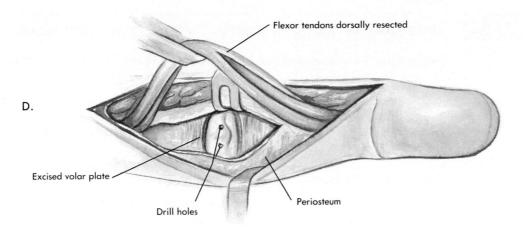

D.

Flexor tendons dorsally resected

Excised volar plate

Drill holes

Periosteum

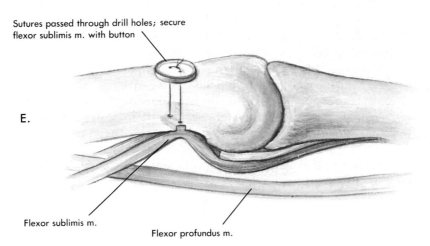

Sutures passed through drill holes; secure
flexor sublimis m. with button

E.

Flexor sublimis m.

Flexor profundus m.

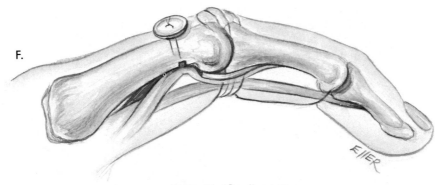

F.

Plate 66. (Continued)

PLATE 67 ## Restoration of Thumb Opposition by the Riordan Technique

Indications. Loss of opposition of the thumb caused by paralysis of the oppenens pollicis.

Requisites. Normal motor strength of the flexor sublimis of the ring finger.

Caution! Following transfer of the sublimis of the ring finger, there may be a varying degree of flexion contracture of the proximal interphalangeal joint.

Patient Position. Supine.

Operative Technique

A. A midlateral incision is made on the ulnar aspect of the ring finger centered over the proximal interphalangeal joint. The skin incision begins immediately dorsal to the flexor skin crease and extends distally and proximally for a distance of 3 cm. The volar and dorsal skin flaps are developed, with great care taken not to injure the neurovascular bundle.

B. and **C.** The sublimis tendon of the ring finger is isolated, and its two slips are sectioned at the level of the joint.

D. Next, an L-shaped skin incision is made over the flexor carpi ulnaris tendon. Subcutaneous tissue is divided in line with the skin incision, and the flexor carpi ulnaris tendon is identified. Do not injure the ulnar nerve and vessels.

E. The flexor carpi ulnaris tendon is split into two longitudinal halves from its insertion to the pisiform bone and extending proximally for a distance of 3 to 4 cm. Then the radial part of the split tendon is divided proximally and sutured to the remaining half at its distal insertion, creating a loop. The loop should be large enough for the sublimis tendon to glide through easily.

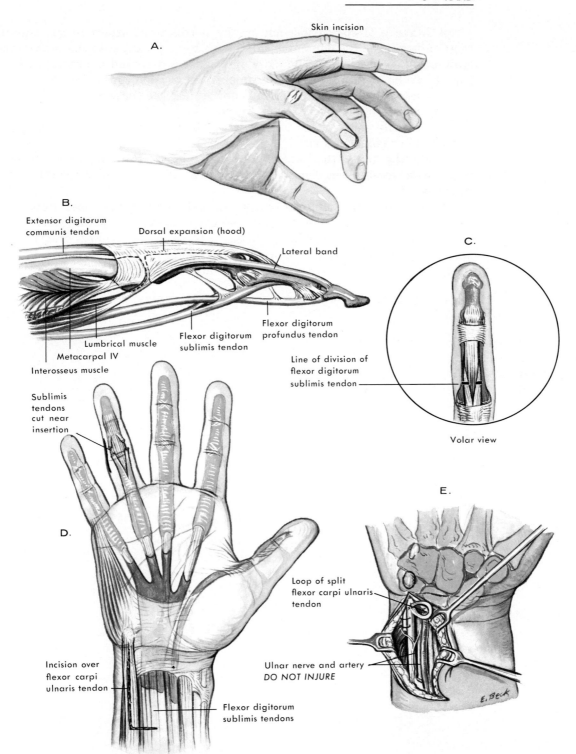

A.

Skin incision

B.

Extensor digitorum communis tendon

Dorsal expansion (hood)

Lateral band

Flexor digitorum profundus tendon

Flexor digitorum sublimis tendon

Lumbrical muscle

Metacarpal IV

Interosseus muscle

C.

Line of division of flexor digitorum sublimis tendon

Volar view

Sublimis tendons cut near insertion

D.

E.

Loop of split flexor carpi ulnaris tendon

Ulnar nerve and artery
DO NOT INJURE

E. BECK

Incision over flexor carpi ulnaris tendon

Flexor digitorum sublimis tendons

Plate 67. A.–N., Restoration of thumb opposition by the Riordan technique.

F. Make a C-shaped incision on the dorsolateral aspect of the thumb. The incision begins on the dorsum of the thumb 1 cm. proximal to the interphalangeal joint and then it extends proximally and volarward around the radial aspect of the thumb; at the metacarpal phalangeal joint the incision curves distally in line with the creases of the thenar eminence. Do not injure the sensory nerve branches from the superficial branch of the radial nerve.

G. Identify the tendons of extensor pollicis longus, extensor pollicis brevis, and abductor pollicis brevis.

H. At the wrist, the flexor sublimis tendon to the ring finger is identified through the forearm incision and the tendon is pulled and delivered into the wound in the wrist.

I. Next, pass the sublimis tendon through the loop fashioned from the flexor carpi ulnaris and, with a tendon passer, pass the tendon subcutaneously across the thenar eminence in line with the fibers of the abductor pollicis brevis. Fashion a small tunnel by making two parallel incisions in the abductor pollicis brevis tendon. Next, split the distal part of the sublimis tendon for approximately 3 cm.

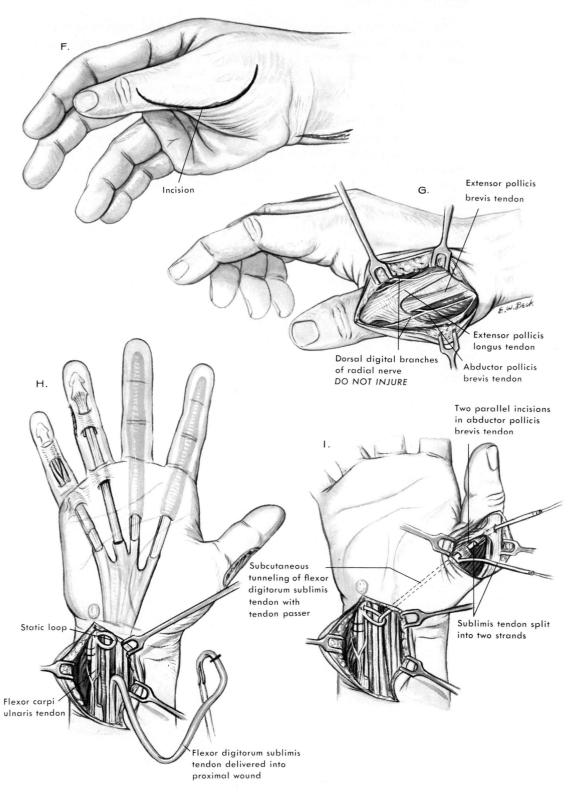

F.

Incision

G.

Extensor pollicis
brevis tendon

E.W.Beck

Extensor pollicis
longus tendon

Dorsal digital branches
of radial nerve
DO NOT INJURE

Abductor pollicis
brevis tendon

Two parallel incisions
in abductor pollicis
brevis tendon

H.

I.

Subcutaneous
tunneling of flexor
digitorum sublimis
tendon with
tendon passer

Static loop

Sublimis tendon split
into two strands

Flexor carpi
ulnaris tendon

Flexor digitorum sublimis
tendon delivered into
proximal wound

Plate 67. (Continued)

J. Separate the extensor aponeurosis from the periosteum of the proximal phalanx of the thumb; make a small incision through the aponeurosis and pass one half of the split sublimis tendon through it.

K.–N. Next, determine the proper tension for the transferred sublimis tendon. The two slips of the tendon are held together with a hemostat. With the wrist passively flexed, releasing the thumb should completely relax the transfer (**K.**). Dorsiflexion of the wrist to 45 degrees should apply enough traction on the transfer to bring the thumb into complete opposition and the interphalangeal joint into complete extension. Readjust the tension of the tendon if insufficient. When appropriate tension has been determined, suture the two slips of the sublimis tendon together. The transferred tendon should pass in the middle of the metacarpal head. If necessary, apply a single nonabsorbable suture fixing the tendon to the abductor pollicis brevis and the joint capsule.

Close the wounds in the usual fashion, and apply an above-elbow or below-elbow cast, holding the patient's wrist in 30 degrees of flexion and the fingers in functional position. The thumb should be in full opposition with the interphalangeal joint in complete extension.

Postoperative Care. Remove the cast in three to four weeks, and prescribe physical therapy to train the transferred tendon. Use a removable opponens splint during the night and part of the day for an additional two to three months.

REFERENCES

Riordan, D. C.: Tendon transplantations in median-nerve and ulnar-nerve paralysis. J. Bone Joint Surg., 35–A:312, 1953.

Riordan, D. C.: Surgery of the paralytic hand. In: Instructional Course Lectures, A.A.O.S., 16:79, 1959. St. Louis, C.V. Mosby.

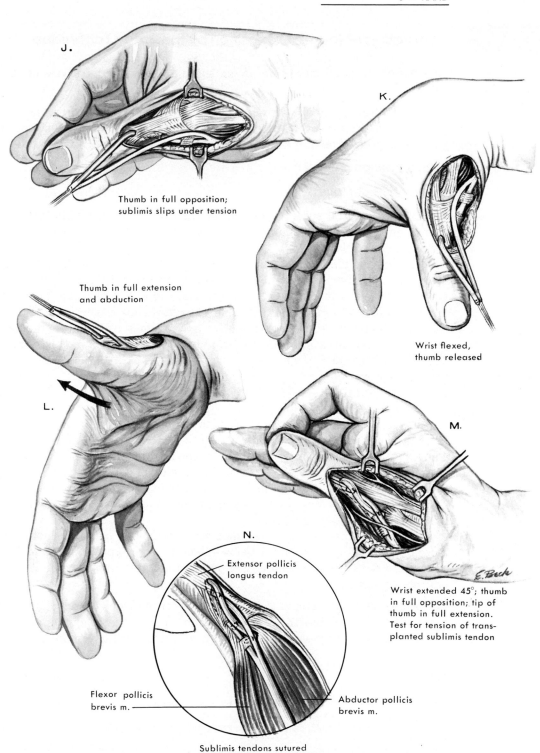

J. Thumb in full opposition; sublimis slips under tension

K. Wrist flexed, thumb released

Thumb in full extension and abduction

L.

M. Wrist extended 45°; thumb in full opposition; tip of thumb in full extension. Test for tension of transplanted sublimis tendon

N.

Extensor pollicis longus tendon

Flexor pollicis brevis m.

Abductor pollicis brevis m.

Sublimis tendons sutured

Plate 67. (Continued)

PLATE 68 — Restoration of Thumb Opposition by the Brand Technique

Indications. Loss of opposition of the thumb caused by paralysis of the oppenens pollicis.

Requisites. Normal motor strength of the flexor sublimis of the ring finger.

Caution! Following transfer of the sublimis of the ring finger, there may be a varying degree of flexion contracture of the proximal interphalangeal joint.

Patient Position. Supine.

Operative Technique

Division of the sublimis tendon of the ring finger and the incision over the thenar eminence of the thumb are similar to procedures described in the Riordan technique (see Plate 67).

A. Make a small incision on the volar surface of the forearm about 6 cm. proximal to the wrist, and the sublimis tendon from the ring finger is transferred into the forearm wound. Next, a 2-cm. longitudinal incision is made immediately distal and lateral to the pisiform bone. Subcutaneous tissue is divided in line with the skin incision, and the dissection is deepened until loose fat-like tissue is exposed. Do not injure a branch of the ulnar nerve that is in this fibrofatty tissue. Through the incision near the pisiform bone, insert a tendon passer that exits in the forearm wound.

B. The sublimis tendon to the ring finger is pulled into the palmar wound with the help of the tendon passer.

C. and D. Pass the sublimis tendon subcutaneously to the metacarpophalangeal joint of the thumb. The fibrous septa in the fat of the palm act as a pulley. The distal end of the sublimis tendon is split into two halves. The proximal slip of the sublimis tendon is sutured to the ulnar side of the metacarpophalangeal joint, and the distal slip is sutured to the tendons of abductor pollicis brevis and extensor pollicis longus; this step prevents shifting in the position of the tendon as it crosses the metacarpophalangeal joint.

The tourniquet is released, and after complete hemostasis the wounds are closed in the usual fashion; a below-elbow cast is applied, holding the thumb in opposition with the interphalangeal joint completely extended and the wrist in 30 degrees of flexion.

Postoperative Care. The cast is removed in three weeks, and physical therapy is performed to train the transferred tendon. A removable opponens splint is used during the night and part of the day for an additional two months.

REFERENCES

Brand, P. W.: Tendon grafting: Illustrated by a new operation for intrinsic paralysis of the fingers. J. Bone Joint Surg., 43–B:444, 1961.

Brand, P. W.: Tendon transfers for median and ulnar nerve paralysis. Orthop. Clin. North Am., 2:447, 1970.

Brand, P. W.: Rehabilitation of the hand with motor and sensory impairment. Orthop. Clin. North Am., 4:1135, 1973.

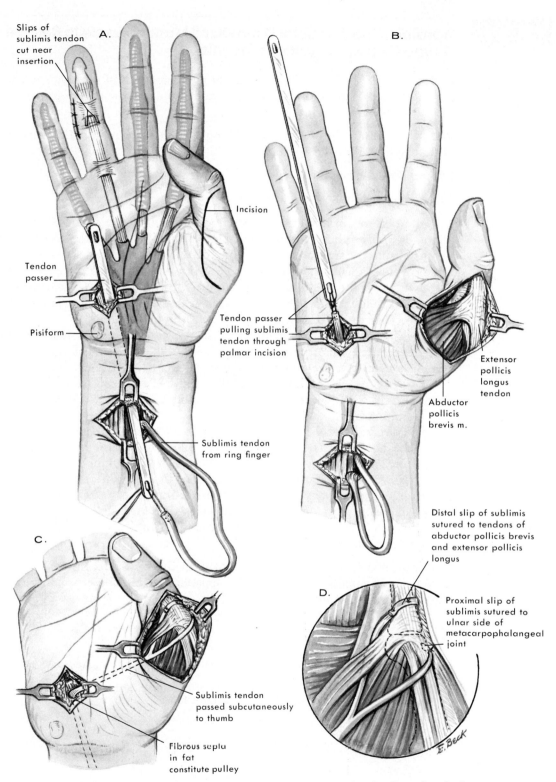

Slips of sublimis tendon cut near insertion

A.

B.

Incision

Tendon passer

Tendon passer pulling sublimis tendon through palmar incision

Pisiform

Extensor pollicis longus tendon

Abductor pollicis brevis m.

Sublimis tendon from ring finger

Distal slip of sublimis sutured to tendons of abductor pollicis brevis and extensor pollicis longus

Proximal slip of sublimis sutured to ulnar side of metacarpophalangeal joint

C.

D.

Sublimis tendon passed subcutaneously to thumb

Fibrous septa in fat constitute pulley

E. Beck

Plate 68. A.–D., Restoration of thumb opposition by the Brand technique.

PLATE 69   Transfer of the Abductor Digiti Quinti Manus Muscle to Restore Thumb Opposition (Littler's Technique)

Indications. Loss of opposition of the thumb as a result of paralysis of the oppenens pollicis when flexor sublimis is weak and the abductor digiti quinti is of normal motor strength.

Requisites. Stability of the metacarpophalangeal joint and the carpometacarpo-phalangeal joint of the thumb.

Patient Position. Supine.

Operative Technique

A. Make a curvilinear incision in the palm along the radial border of the abductor digiti quinti muscle belly. The incision begins from the radial side of the pisiform and terminates on the ulnar border of the middle phalanx of the little finger. Subcutaneous tissue is divided in line with the skin incision.

B. Expose the abductor digiti quinti distally until its two tendon slips of insertion are identified and divided. One of the tendinous insertions inserts to bone and the other to the extensor apparatus of the little finger.

C. The abductor digiti quinti muscle is lifted from its fascial compartment and elevated proximally until its neurovascular pedicle is identified and isolated. Avoid tension on muscle and neurovascular pedicle while freeing.

D. Proximally, the abductor digiti quinti is released from the pisiform bone, but its origin from flexor carpi ulnaris tendon is left intact. Do not injure the ulnar nerve and artery.

E. The abductor digiti quinti muscle is folded over about 170 degrees like the page of a book and is passed subcutaneously to its new position on the thumb. Avoid tension and angulation of the neurovascular bundle.

F. Next, the tendons of the abductor digiti quinti muscle are sutured to abductor pollicis brevis tendon at its insertion. The tourniquet is released, and after complete hemostasis the wound is closed in the usual manner. A below-elbow cast is applied, supporting the wrist in neutral position and the thumb in relaxed palmar abduction.

Postoperative Care. The cast is removed in three weeks, and active exercises are performed to oppose the thumb. An opponens splint is worn at night and part of the day for several months.

REFERENCES

Littler, J. W.: Tendon transfers and arthrodeses in combined median and ulnar nerve paralysis. J. Bone Joint Surg., 31–A:225, 1949.

Littler, J. W., and Cooley, S. G. E.: Opposition of the thumb and its restoration by abductor digiti quinti transfer. J. Bone Joint Surg., 45–A:1389, 1963.

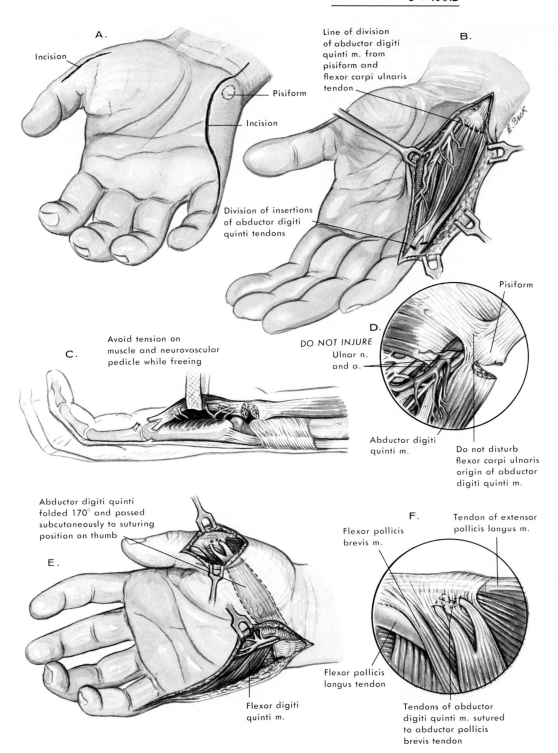

A.
Incision

Pisiform

Incision

Line of division
of abductor digiti
quinti m. from
pisiform and
flexor carpi ulnaris
tendon

B.

E. Beck

Division of insertions
of abductor digiti
quinti tendons

C.
Avoid tension on
muscle and neurovascular
pedicle while freeing

Pisiform

D.

DO NOT INJURE
Ulnar n.
and a.

Abductor digiti
quinti m.

Do not disturb
flexor carpi ulnaris
origin of abductor
digiti quinti m.

Abductor digiti quinti
folded 170° and passed
subcutaneously to suturing
position on thumb

E.

Flexor pollicis
brevis m.

F.

Tendon of extensor
pollicis longus m.

Flexor pollicis
longus tendon

Flexor digiti
quinti m.

Tendons of abductor
digiti quinti m. sutured
to abductor pollicis
brevis tendon

Plate 69. A.–F., Transfer of the abductor digiti quinti manus muscle to restore thumb
opposition (Littler's technique).

| PLATE 70 | Boyes Technique to Restore Thumb Opposition |

Indications. Paralysis of the thumb adductors.

Requisites

1. Normal motor strength of the brachioradialis.
2. Normal passive range of thumb adduction.

Patient Position. Supine.

Operative Technique

A. Make a longitudinal incision beginning at the radial styloid process and extending proximally for a distance of 7 to 10 cm. Subcutaneous tissue is divided in line with the skin incision; the wound flaps are undermined, mobilized, and retracted. The flat tendon of the brachioradialis is identified at its insertion and sectioned. The tendon is dissected, and its muscle is freed and mobilized proximally as far as its nerve supply permits.

Next, on the dorsum of the hand, two incisions are made: a 3-cm. longitudinal incision between the third and fourth metacarpals, and a curvilinear 2.5-cm. incision between the first and second metacarpals. An alternative surgical approach to expose the adductor tubercle of the thumb is by a 2.5-cm. incision in the palm in line with the skin crease of the metacarpophalangeal joint of the thumb.

B. A free tendon graft is taken either from the palmaris longus in the forearm or from the plantaris in the leg. First, the tendon graft is sutured to the adductor tubercle of the thumb and the insertion of adductor pollicis; next, with an Ober tendon passer the tendon graft is passed along the adductor muscle belly in the palm to exit through the third interosseous space on the dorsum of the hand in the incision between the third and fourth metacarpals.

C. A tendon passer is inserted deep to the extensor digitorum communis tendons, and the free tendon graft is delivered from the incision on the dorsum of the hand to the radial incision on the forearm.

D. The proximal end of the tendon graft is sutured to the brachioradialis tendon.

The tourniquet is released, and after complete hemostasis is obtained, the wounds are closed in routine fashion. A below-elbow cast is applied, holding the wrist in 45 degrees of dorsiflexion and the thumb in adduction.

Postoperative Care. The cast is removed in four to six weeks following surgery. Active exercises are performed to develop thumb adduction.

REFERENCES

Boyes, J. H.: Tendon transfers for radial palsy. Bull. Hosp. Joint Dis., 21:97, 1960.
Boyes, J. H.: Selection of a donor muscle for tendon transfer. Bull. Hosp. Joint Dis., 23:1, 1962.
Boyes, J. H.: Bunnell's Surgery of the Hand. 4th ed. Philadelphia, J. B. Lippincott Co., 1964.

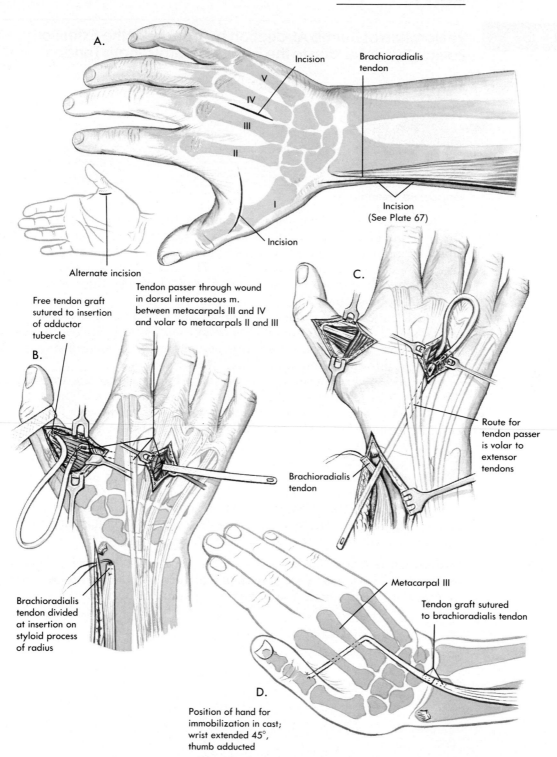

A.

Incision

Brachioradialis tendon

V

IV

III

II

I

Incision (See Plate 67)

Alternate incision

Incision

Free tendon graft sutured to insertion of adductor tubercle

Tendon passer through wound in dorsal interosseous m. between metacarpals III and IV and volar to metacarpals II and III

B.

C.

Brachioradialis tendon

Route for tendon passer is volar to extensor tendons

Brachioradialis tendon divided at insertion on styloid process of radius

Metacarpal III

Tendon graft sutured to brachioradialis tendon

D.

Position of hand for immobilization in cast; wrist extended 45°, thumb adducted

Plate 70. A.–D., Boyes technique to restore thumb opposition.

PLATE 71 — Restoration of Thumb Abduction by Transfer of the Extensor Pollicis Brevis Tendon to the Extensor Carpi Ulnaris Tendon

Indications. Paralysis of the thumb abductors.

Requisites

1. Normal motor strength of extensor pollicis brevis.
2. Normal range of passive abduction and adduction of thumb.

Patient Position. Supine.

Operative Technique

A. Make a 3-cm. transverse incision on the dorsoradial aspect of the distal forearm immediately proximal to the extensor retinaculum of the wrist over the musculotendinous junction of extensor pollicis tendon. The subcutaneous tissue is divided in line with the skin incision. The fasciae are divided by longitudinal incision, and the extensor pollicis brevis tendon is identified and divided at its musculotendinous junction.

Next, a 3-cm.-long incision is made on the dorsolateral aspect of the metacarpophalangeal joint of the thumb. Subcutaneous tissue is divided in line with the skin incision. The tendon of extensor pollicis brevis is identified at its insertion and pulled into the thumb wound from the wrist wound.

B. Make a curvilinear incision on the ulnar aspect of the wrist. It begins at the base of the fourth metacarpal and extends ulnarward and palmarward immediately distal to the ulnar styloid and then extends proximally for a distance of 3 cm. along the volar surface of the wrist. The extensor carpi ulnaris tendon is identified and divided at its insertion and freed proximally.

C. The extensor pollicis brevis tendon is passed subcutaneously toward the palmar surface of the hand and sutured to extensor carpi ulnaris tendon with the thumb in maximal abduction.

The tourniquet is released, and after complete hemostasis the wound is closed in the usual fashion. A below-elbow cast is applied, holding the wrist in neutral position and the thumb in maximal abduction.

Postoperative Care. The cast is removed four weeks following surgery. Active exercises are performed for active thumb abduction. A plastic splint, worn at night and part of the day, holds the thumb in maximal abduction.

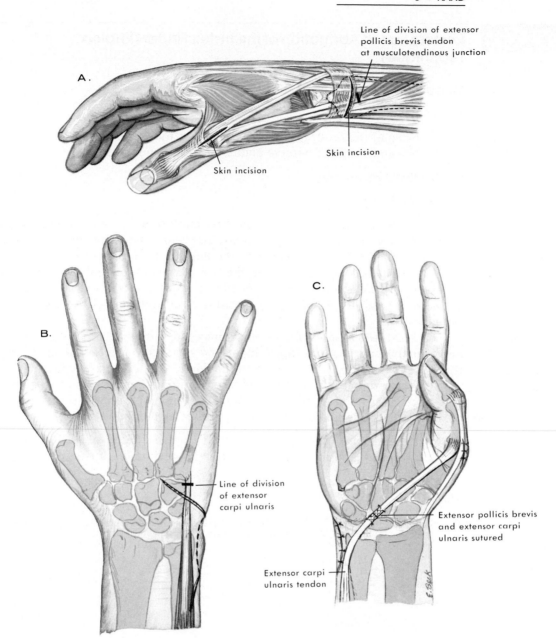

A.

Line of division of extensor
pollicis brevis tendon
at musculotendinous junction

Skin incision

Skin incision

B.

C.

Line of division
of extensor
carpi ulnaris

Extensor pollicis brevis
and extensor carpi
ulnaris sutured

Extensor carpi
ulnaris tendon

Plate 71. A.–C., Restoration of thumb abduction by transfer of the extensor pollicis brevis tendon to the extensor carpi ulnaris tendon.

PLATE 72   Restoration of Abduction of the Index Finger (Phalen Technique)

Indications. Paralysis of the abductor of the index finger.

Requisites

1. Normal motor strength of the extensor indicis proprius.
2. Normal range of passive abduction of the index finger.

Patient Position. Supine.

Operative Technique

A. Make a curved incision on the midlateral aspect of the index finger extending from the proximal phalanx to the radial aspect of the metacarpophalangeal joint; then extend it dorsally to the middle third of the index metacarpal.

B. The dorsal expansion over the metacarpophalangeal joint is incised. The extensor indicis proprius muscle is identified and sectioned at its insertion and pulled proximally. Do not injure dorsal digital branches of the radial artery and nerve.

C. Next, the tendon of extensor indicis proprius is passed distally to the radial and palmar aspects of the index finger and sutured to the tendon of the first dorsal interosseous muscle. The incision in the dorsal expansion is closed.

The tourniquet is released, and after complete hemostasis the wound is closed in the usual fashion. A below-elbow cast is applied, holding the wrist in neutral position and the index finger in 10 degrees of abduction.

Postoperative Care. The cast is removed three to four weeks following surgery, and active exercises are performed to provide abduction of the index finger.

REFERENCE

Phalen, G. S., and Miller, R. C.: The transfer of wrist extensor muscles to restore or reinforce flexion power of the fingers and opposition of the thumb. J. Bone Joint Surg., 39:993, 1947.

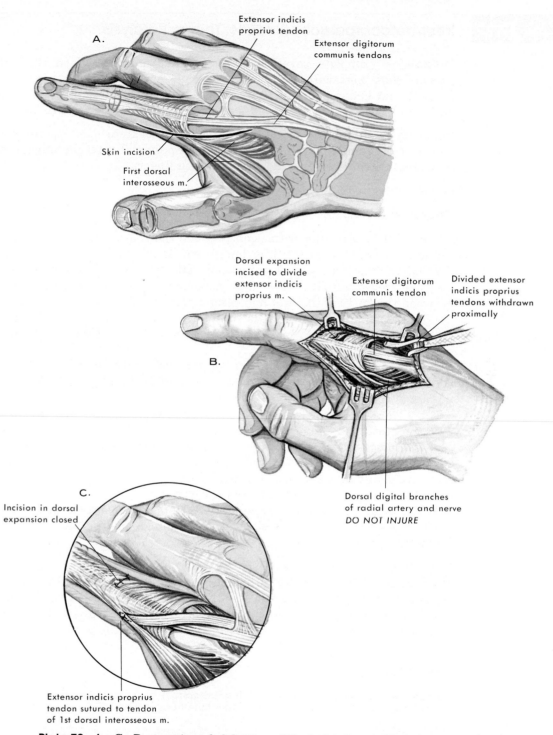

A.

Extensor indicis
proprius tendon

Extensor digitorum
communis tendons

Skin incision

First dorsal
interosseous m.

Dorsal expansion
incised to divide
extensor indicis
proprius m.

Extensor digitorum
communis tendon

Divided extensor
indicis proprius
tendons withdrawn
proximally

B.

Dorsal digital branches
of radial artery and nerve
DO NOT INJURE

C.

Incision in dorsal
expansion closed

Extensor indicis proprius
tendon sutured to tendon
of 1st dorsal interosseous m.

Plate 72. A.–C., Restoration of abduction of the index finger (Phalen technique).

PLATE 73   Intermetacarpal Bone Block for Thenar Paralysis

Indications. Complete paralysis of the thenar muscles. Warn the patient and parents that there will be difficulty with glove wear. If the carpometacarpophalangeal joint is unstable, the thumb and first metacarpal may drift into adduction and stabilization of the trapezoid-metacarpal joint may be required.

Requisites. Voluntary motor control of flexion and extension of the interphalangeal joint of the thumb and the interphalangeal, proximal interphalangeal, and metacarpophalangeal joints of the index and long fingers.

Patient Position. Supine.

Operative Technique

A. Make a curvilinear incision between the index and thumb metacarpals at the juncture of their distal third and proximal two thirds. Subcutaneous tissue is divided in line with the skin incision. The first dorsal interosseous muscle is elevated from the index and thumb metacarpals. Do not injure the radial artery between the bases of the first and second metacarpals.

B. The thumb metacarpal is rotated into full opposition, and the interspace between the thumb and index metacarpals is measured for length of iliac bone graft.

C. The interosseous muscle is split on the volar surface of the index and thumb metacarpals; a slot is made with a hand drill and gouges. Do not injure the physes of the index and thumb metacarpals.

D. The iliac bone graft is taken and shaped so that its ends are tapered to fit into the previously prepared slots.

E. The thumb metacarpal is fully abducted and rotated into neutral opposition, and the bone graft is inserted into the previously prepared slots. Chips of cancellous bone are placed at each end. A threaded Steinmann pin is used for internal fixation, transfixing the iliac graft to the metacarpals.

The tourniquet is released, and after complete hemostasis the wound is closed in the usual fashion; a below-elbow cast is applied, holding the thumb in maximal abduction and opposition.

Postoperative Care. The cast is changed in one month, and radiograms are made. If there is adequate healing, remove the pin; if not, leave the pin for another month. Usually, the graft heals within two to three months. When there are problems with bone healing, the Steinmann pin is left in as an internal fixator until bony union takes place. *Do not hurry to remove the pin!*

REFERENCE

Schnute, W. J., and Tachdjian, M. O.: Intermetacarpal bone block for thenar paralysis following poliomyelitis. An end result study. J. Bone Joint Surg., 45–A:1663, 1963.

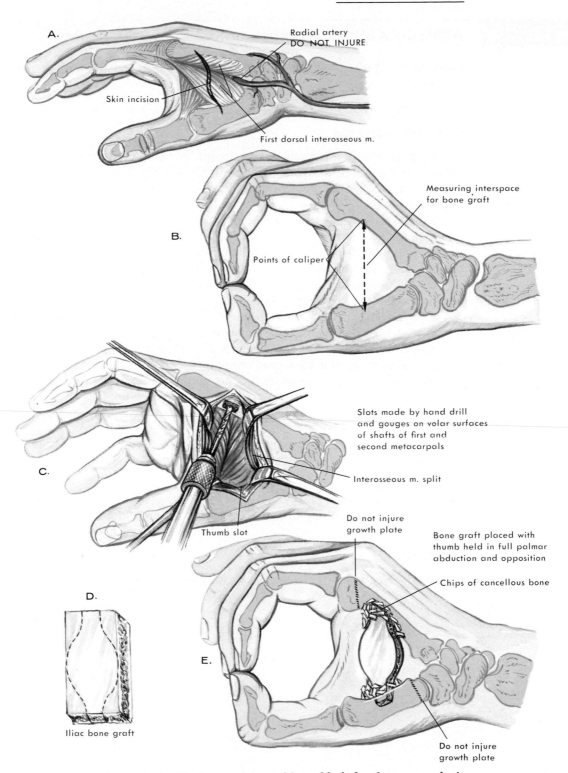

A.

Radial artery
DO NOT INJURE

Skin incision

First dorsal interosseous m.

B.

Measuring interspace
for bone graft

Points of caliper

C.

Slots made by hand drill
and gouges on volar surfaces
of shafts of first and
second metacarpals

Interosseous m. split

Thumb slot

D.

Iliac bone graft

E.

Do not injure
growth plate

Bone graft placed with
thumb held in full palmar
abduction and opposition

Chips of cancellous bone

Do not injure
growth plate

Plate 73. **A.–E.,** Intermetacarpal bone block for thenar paralysis.

| PLATE 74 | **Arthrodesis of the Carpometacarpal Joint of the Thumb** |

Indications. Marked instability and subluxation of the trapeziometacarpal joint of the thumb.

Patient Position. Supine.

Operative Technique

A. Expose the trapeziometacarpal joint by a curving incision on its dorsoradial aspect. Divide subcutaneous tissue in line with the skin incision. By blunt Metzenbaum scissors, expose and protect the sensory branches of the radial nerve and radial artery.

B. Make a longitudinal incision in the capsule of the carpometacarpal joint, and expose the opposing ends of the trapezoid and first metacarpal bones.

C. Denude the articular cartilage of the base of the first metacarpal, and with the help of rongeurs, shape it into a rounded, bullet-like contour.

D. Make small drill holes at the osteocartilaginous juncture of the trapezium and connect them with an osteotome.

E. Excise the articular cartilage. With the help of a curet and rongeur, create a cavity at the distal end of the trapezium.

F. Drive the proximal end of the first metacarpal into the trapezium with the thumb metacarpal in a 45-degree angle in both palmar and radial abduction from the plane of the index metacarpal. The thumb pulp should face that of the index and long fingers. Transfix the trapeziometacarpal joint with a single, strong Steinmann pin introduced in a retrograde fashion. To control rotation, introduce a second oblique wire.

Close the wound in the usual fashion. Make radiograms to check the position of the pins and angle of the fused joint.

Postoperative Care. Immobilize the hand, wrist, and forearm in a cast for eight to ten weeks. Remove the cast and pins, and prescribe active assisted and passive range of motion exercises to restore mobility of the digits.

REFERENCE

Carroll, R. E., and Hill, N. A.: Arthrodesis of the carpo-metacarpal joint of the thumb—a clinical and cineroentgenographic study. J. Bone Joint Surg., 55–B:292, 1973.

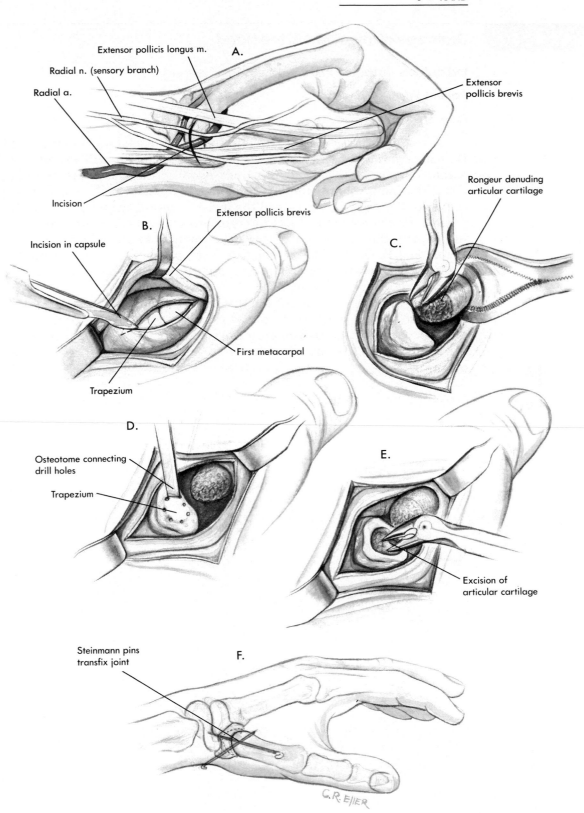

Extensor pollicis longus m.

Radial n. (sensory branch)

Radial a.

A.

Extensor pollicis brevis

Incision

Extensor pollicis brevis

B.

Incision in capsule

First metacarpal

Trapezium

C.

Rongeur denuding articular cartilage

D.

Osteotome connecting drill holes

Trapezium

E.

Excision of articular cartilage

Steinmann pins transfix joint

F.

C. R. Eller

Plate 74. A.–F., Arthrodesis of the carpometacarpal joint of the thumb.

PLATE 75 Drainage of Infections of the Hand

Indications. Infection and the presence of abscess.

Patient Position. Supine.

Operative Technique

A. and **B.** Drain the pulp space infection through a lateral longitudinal incision. Do not perform a "fishmouth" incision because the scar will retract and become painful. Begin the incision 0.5 to 1 cm. distal to the distal interphalangeal joint and 2 to 3 mm. volar to the lateral border of the nail wall, extending distally to the tip of the digit. Do not extend the incision toward the pulp, as the scar may be painful. Do not enter the distal interphalangeal joint. Divide subcutaneous tissue in line with the skin incision; retract the wound margins with hooks.

C. and **D.** Spread the wound flaps with a sharp, pointed tenotomy scissors. Identify the digital vessels and nerves, and retract them out of harm's way. Do not open the flexor tendon sheath.

With a scalpel, divide all fibrous septa across the pulp, and with a sharp, pointed scissors, spread the abscessed cavity and thoroughly irrigate the wound. A small catheter is inserted for drainage, and depending on the severity of infection, the wound edges may be left open for secondary closure or they may be sutured primarily.

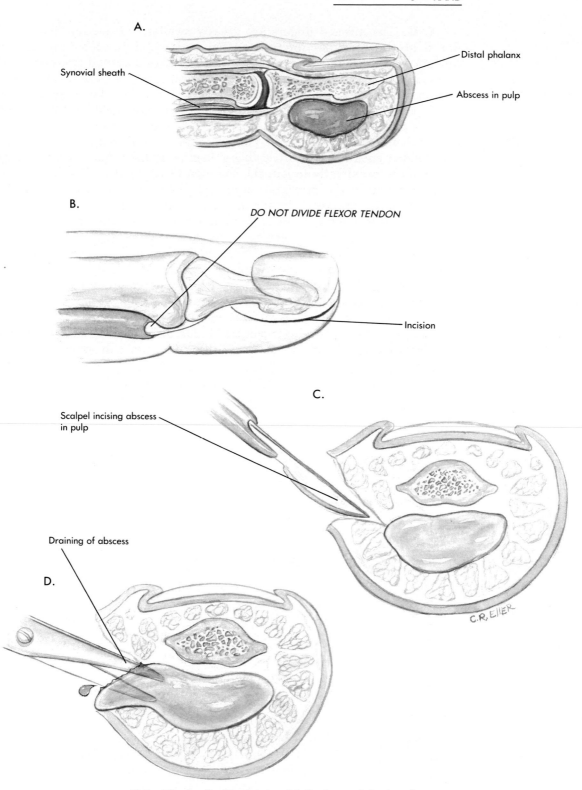

A.

Synovial sheath

Distal phalanx

Abscess in pulp

B.

DO NOT DIVIDE FLEXOR TENDON

Incision

C.

Scalpel incising abscess
in pulp

C.R. Eiler

Draining of abscess

D.

Plate 75. A.–L., Drainage of infections of the hand.

E.–G. The affected fingers are grossly swollen and tender. They are slightly flexed at the proximal interphalangeal and distal interphalangeal joints. The tendon sheaths of the index, long, and ring fingers extend from the neck of the metacarpals to the distal interphalangeal joints; these tendon sheaths are separate and do not communicate with the ulnar or radial bursa. The tendon sheath of the flexor pollicis longus begins distally at the interphalangeal joint of the thumb and extends proximally to the carpal tunnel. In the thenar eminence and at the wrist, the tendon sheath of the flexor pollicis longus is referred to as the *radial bursa*. The tendon sheath of the little finger begins at the distal interphalangeal joint and extends proximally to join the common flexor tendon sheath of all the finger flexor tendons in the proximal palm and distal forearm. The part of the flexor tendon sheath of the little finger in the hypothenar eminence and at the wrist is referred to as the *ulnar bursa*. Inflammatory processes can spread from the radial bursa to the ulnar bursa, creating a "horseshoe" abscess.

The space of Parona begins in the mid forearm proximally and extends distally to the superior margin of the carpal tunnel. The boundaries of Parona's space are the following: (1) the floor, formed by the pronator quadratus and interosseous membrane; (2) the roof, formed by the tendons of the flexor digitorum profundus distally and by the flexor digitorum sublimis muscle proximally; (3) the radial boundary, formed by the flexor pollicis longus; and (4) the medial boundary, formed by the flexor carpi ulnaris. Infections in the palm can extend to the space of Parona.

INFECTIONS OF THE FLEXOR TENDON SHEATHS

E.

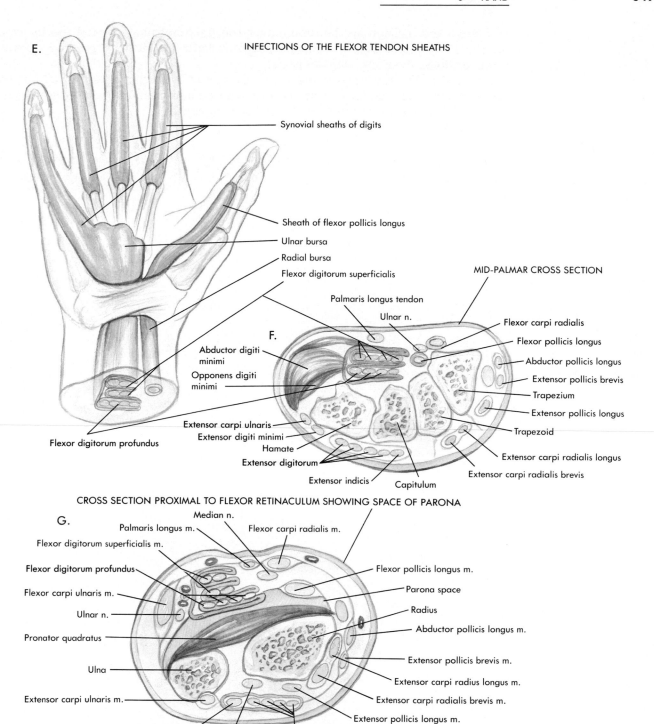

Synovial sheaths of digits

Sheath of flexor pollicis longus
Ulnar bursa
Radial bursa
Flexor digitorum superficialis

MID-PALMAR CROSS SECTION

Palmaris longus tendon
Ulnar n.

F.

Abductor digiti minimi
Opponens digiti minimi

Flexor carpi radialis
Flexor pollicis longus
Abductor pollicis longus
Extensor pollicis brevis
Trapezium
Extensor pollicis longus
Trapezoid
Extensor carpi radialis longus
Extensor carpi radialis brevis

Extensor carpi ulnaris
Extensor digiti minimi
Hamate
Extensor digitorum
Extensor indicis
Capitulum

Flexor digitorum profundus

CROSS SECTION PROXIMAL TO FLEXOR RETINACULUM SHOWING SPACE OF PARONA

G.
Median n.
Palmaris longus m.
Flexor carpi radialis m.
Flexor digitorum superficialis m.
Flexor digitorum profundus
Flexor carpi ulnaris m.
Ulnar n.
Pronator quadratus
Ulna
Extensor carpi ulnaris m.
Extensor digiti minimi
Extensor indicis
Extensor digitorum m.

Flexor pollicis longus m.
Parona space
Radius
Abductor pollicis longus m.
Extensor pollicis brevis m.
Extensor carpi radius longus m.
Extensor carpi radialis brevis m.
Extensor pollicis longus m.

Plate 75. (Continued)

Make the incision on the thumb over the proximal phalanx and the incision for the little finger over the middle phalanx; both the little finger and thumb, however, need incisions over the palm.

H. and **I.** The drainage of the index, long, and ring fingers is carried out by two incisions—one distally, centered over the middle phalanx, and a second one proximally, made over the distal end of the metacarpal.

INCISIONS

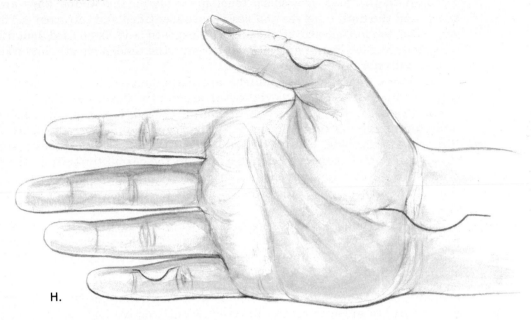

H.

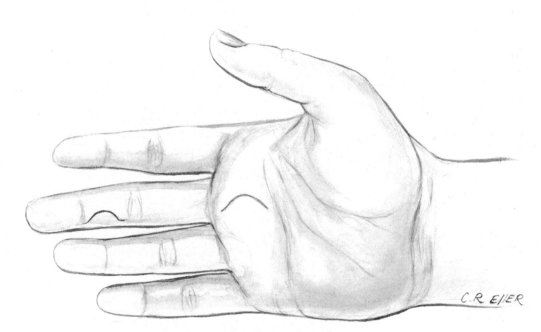

C.R. EIIER

Plate 75. (Continued)

J. With the help of a sharp tenotomy scissors, the wound flaps are spread apart, and the digital nerves and vessels are identified and retracted out of harm's way. The tendon sheath of the digit is exposed and is incised longitudinally, releasing the pus. Pass a fine catheter through the tendon sheath, and irrigate the wound with normal saline.

K. The ulnar and radial bursae are decompressed by an incision over the carpal tunnel. Excise the synovial tissue around the flexor tendons.

L. Drain the thenar infection through a curved, longitudinal incision in the mid palm overlying the index metacarpal; drain the mid palmar space infection through a transverse palmar incision. The thenar and mid palmar spaces are closed and do not connect proximally through the carpal tunnel into the forearm. This is in contrast to ulnar bursa and radial bursa infections, which are deep to the palmar aponeurosis and are freely connected to the carpal tunnel and with the forearm.

Obtain specimens for culture, and following thorough irrigation of the wounds, insert small Hemovac suction tubes. The wound is closed primarily, depending on the severity of infection and the delay of treatment; the wound may also be closed secondarily.

Postoperative Care. The hand is splinted in functional position, and appropriate antibiotics are given to control infection. Gentle active and passive exercises are performed to restore range of motion of the joints.

REFERENCES

Flynn, J. E.: Modern considerations of major hand infections. N. Engl. J. Med., 252:605, 1955.

Kanavel, A. B.: Infections of the Hand. A Guide to the Surgical Treatment of Acute and Chronic Suppurative Processes in the Fingers, Hand, and Forearm. 7th ed. Philadelphia, Lea & Febiger, 1943.

Milford, L. W.: The hand. Pyogenic infections. In: Crenshaw, A. H. (ed.): Campbell's Operative Orthopaedics. 5th ed. St. Louis, C. V. Mosby, 1971, pp. 390–397.

Neviaser, R. J.: Infections. In: Green, D. P. (ed.): Operative Hand Surgery. 2nd ed. New York, Churchill Livingstone, 1988, pp. 1027–1046.

Tubiana, R., McCullough, C. J., and Masquelet, A. C.: An Atlas of Surgical Exposures of the Upper Extremity. Philadelphia, J. B. Lippincott Co., 1990, pp. 317–324.

INCISIONS FOR MIDDLE OR LONG FINGER

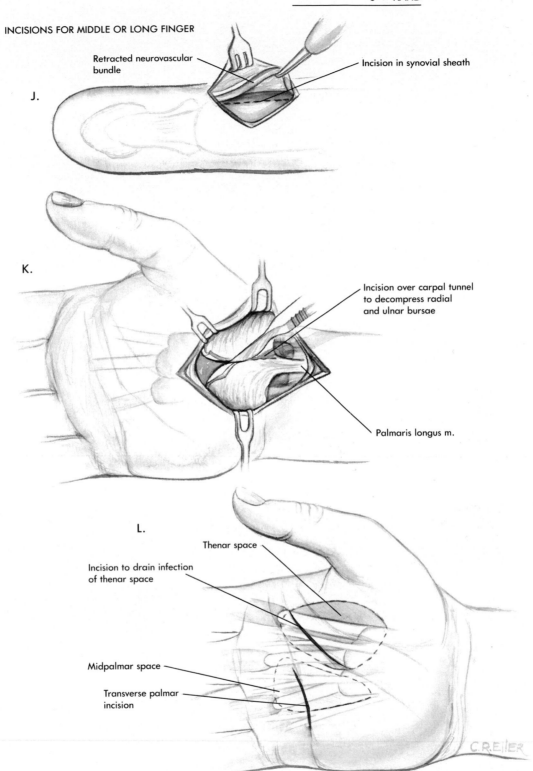

Retracted neurovascular bundle

Incision in synovial sheath

J.

K.

Incision over carpal tunnel to decompress radial and ulnar bursae

Palmaris longus m.

L.

Thenar space

Incision to drain infection of thenar space

Midpalmar space

Transverse palmar incision

C.R.Ejler

Plate 75. (Continued)

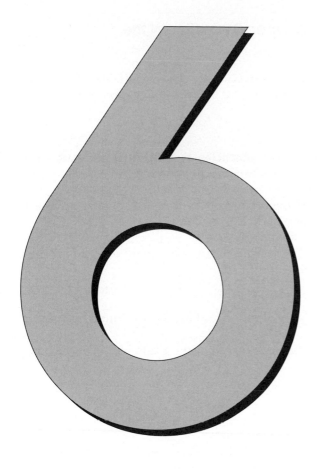

Pelvis–Hip–Proximal Femur

PLATE 76 ## Medial (Adductor) Approach for Open Reduction of the Congenitally Dislocated Hip

Indications. Inability to obtain concentric reduction by closed methods in a typical perinatal dislocation of the hip in a child under 12 months of age, preferably before standing and weight-bearing.

Requisites

1. The medial approach is used if the obstacles to concentric reduction are only medial and inferior, such as the psoas tendon constricting the capsule and a taut transverse acetabular ligament.

2. The capsule should not be redundant because through a medial approach it is difficult to perform capsulorrhaphy and tauten the capsule.

3. Patient should be younger than walking age.

4. Preliminary traction and an attempt at closed reduction have failed when the patient has been under general anesthesia.

Contraindications

1. Prenatal dislocation with a high-riding femoral head that cannot be brought down.

2. Capsular adhesions between the lateral wall of the ilium and femoral head.

3. Teratologic dislocations.

4. Redislocation of hips previously operated.

Blood for Transfusion. Yes.

Radiographic Control. Image intensifier.

Patient Position. The patient is placed in supine position, and the ipsilateral hip, hemipelvis, and entire lower limb are prepared and draped in the usual fashion, allowing free mobility of the limb during surgery.

Choice of Procedure. There are two alternative skin incisions, longitudinal and transverse. I prefer the transverse incision because of its better cosmesis. The iliopsoas tendon and hip joint capsule may be reached by an approach posterior to the adductor brevis, anterior to the adductor brevis and posterior to the pectineus, or anterior to the pectineus.

Operative Technique

Longitudinal Skin Incision with Surgical Approach Posterior to the Adductor Brevis

A. With the hip flexed 70 to 80 degrees, abducted, and laterally rotated, the adductor longus muscle tendon is palpated, and a straight longitudinal incision is made immediately behind the adductor longus muscle for a distance of 6 to 8 cm. It begins at the adductor tubercle and extends distally along the course of the muscle.

B. and C. The subcutaneous tissue is divided in line with the incision. The deep fascia is divided. The anterior and posterior margins of the adductor longus muscle are delineated, and the muscle is sectioned over a blunt elevator at its origin and retracted distally. The adductor brevis muscle is retracted anteriorly, and the anterior branches of the obturator nerve and vessels are visualized but not disturbed. By blunt digital dissection the interval posterior to the adductor brevis is developed; the lesser trochanter is easily palpated in the intermuscular interval. The iliopsoas tendon is exposed, and the fatty tissue and the bursa over the tendon are elevated. A curved hemostat is inserted beneath the iliopsoas tendon; the tendon is divided by a transverse incision and allowed to retract proximally.

D. Dissection is carried proximally until the femoral head is palpated. Two

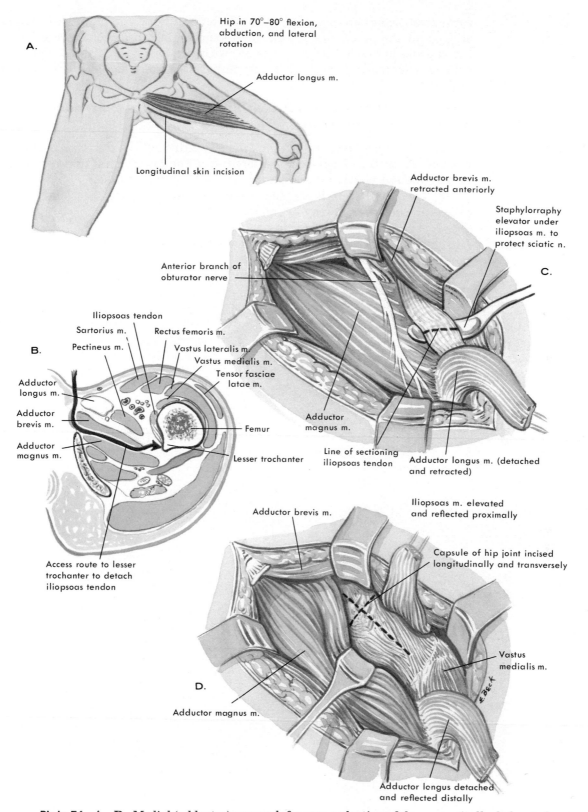

A.

Hip in 70°–80° flexion, abduction, and lateral rotation

Adductor longus m.

Longitudinal skin incision

Adductor brevis m. retracted anteriorly

Staphylorraphy elevator under iliopsoas m. to protect sciatic n.

C.

Anterior branch of obturator nerve

Iliopsoas tendon

Sartorius m.

Pectineus m.

Rectus femoris m.

Vastus lateralis m.

Vastus medialis m.

Tensor fasciae latae m.

B.

Adductor longus m.

Adductor brevis m.

Adductor magnus m.

Femur

Lesser trochanter

Adductor magnus m.

Line of sectioning iliopsoas tendon

Adductor longus m. (detached and retracted)

Access route to lesser trochanter to detach iliopsoas tendon

Iliopsoas m. elevated and reflected proximally

Adductor brevis m.

Capsule of hip joint incised longitudinally and transversely

Vastus medialis m.

D.

Adductor magnus m.

Adductor longus detached and reflected distally

Plate 76. A.–R., Medial (adductor) approach for open reduction of the congenitally dislocated hip.

curved retractors are placed around the femoral neck and capsule, one superolaterally and the other inferomedially to expose the capsule of the hip joint. Next, the capsule is divided by a T incision, with the longitudinal limb along the long axis of the femoral neck and the transverse limb along the margin of the acetabulum.

Transverse Skin Incision with Surgical Approach Anterior to the Adductor Brevis and Medial to the Pectineus

E. An alternative surgical approach is through a transverse oblique skin incision about 5 to 7 cm. long centered over the anterior margin of the adductor longus about 1 cm. distal and parallel to the inguinal crease.

F. The deep fascia is divided. Take care not to injure the saphenous vein; if necessary, however, it may be ligated and sectioned.

G. The adductor longus muscle is sectioned at its origin and reflected distally. At the anterior margin of the adductor longus, the fibers of the pectineus muscle are identified.

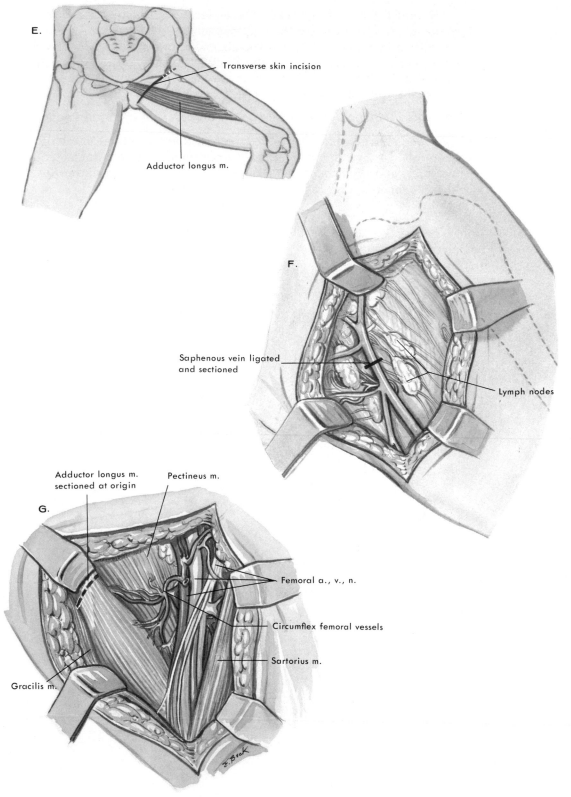

E.

Transverse skin incision

Adductor longus m.

F.

Saphenous vein ligated
and sectioned

Lymph nodes

G.

Adductor longus m.
sectioned at origin

Pectineus m.

Femoral a., v., n.

Circumflex femoral vessels

Sartorius m.

Gracilis m.

Plate 76. (Continued)

H. and **I.** One can approach the lesser trochanter by a route medial to the pectineus muscle to release the iliopsoas tendon. The pectineus muscle is retracted laterally, protecting the femoral vessels and nerve, and the adductor brevis muscle is retracted medially, bringing the iliopsoas tendon into view at its insertion to the lesser trochanter. A Kelly clamp is passed under the iliopsoas tendon and opened slightly, and the tendon is sectioned.

Transverse Skin Incision with Surgical Approach Lateral to the Pectineus

J. and **K.** Another route to the lesser trochanter to release the iliopsoas tendon is lateral to the pectineus muscle. The pectineus muscle is retracted medially and inferiorly, and the femoral vessels and nerve are retracted laterally, exposing the iliopsoas tendon at its insertion to the lesser trochanter.

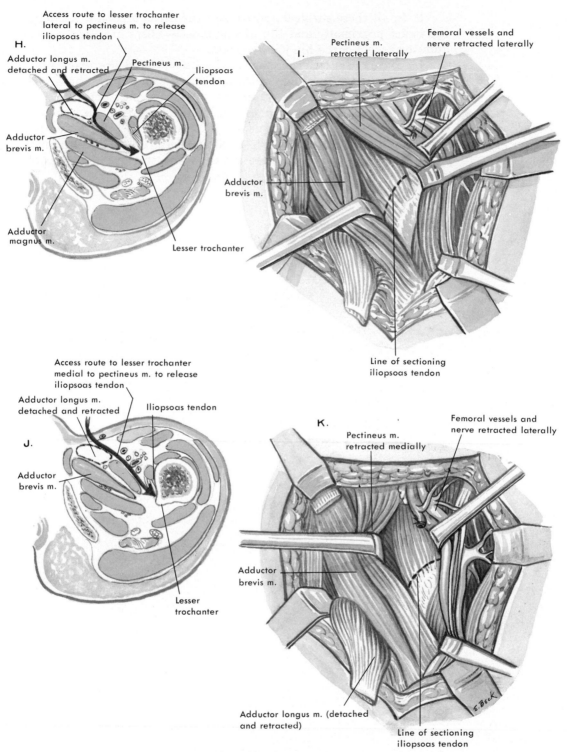

H.

Access route to lesser trochanter lateral to pectineus m. to release iliopsoas tendon

Adductor longus m. detached and retracted

Pectineus m.

Iliopsoas tendon

Adductor brevis m.

Adductor magnus m.

Lesser trochanter

I.

Pectineus m. retracted laterally

Femoral vessels and nerve retracted laterally

Adductor brevis m.

Line of sectioning iliopsoas tendon

J.

Access route to lesser trochanter medial to pectineus m. to release iliopsoas tendon

Adductor longus m. detached and retracted

Iliopsoas tendon

Adductor brevis m.

Lesser trochanter

K.

Pectineus m. retracted medially

Femoral vessels and nerve retracted laterally

Adductor brevis m.

Adductor longus m. (detached and retracted)

Line of sectioning iliopsoas tendon

E. Beck

Plate 76. (Continued)

L. In all these surgical approaches, the psoas tendon is sectioned and allowed to retract proximally and the iliacus muscle fibers are gently elevated from the anterior aspect of the hip joint capsule.

M. and **N.** The inferior part of the capsule and the transverse ligament are pulled upward with the femoral head. The capsule may adhere to the floor of the acetabulum, and the ligamentum teres may be hypertrophic.

O. The capsule is opened with a longitudinal incision along the long axis of the femoral neck and a transverse cut near the acetabular margin. Incisions in the capsule should be thorough, obtaining joint fluid and visualizing the femoral head. In the drawing, a cruciate cut is shown; this author, however, recommends a T-shaped cut, as illustrated in Plate 77.

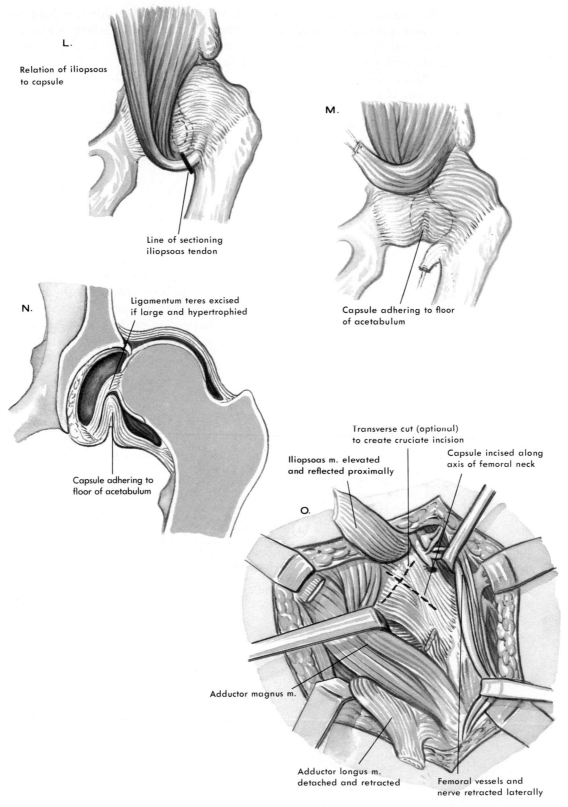

L.

Relation of iliopsoas
to capsule

Line of sectioning
iliopsoas tendon

M.

Capsule adhering to floor
of acetabulum

N.

Ligamentum teres excised
if large and hypertrophied

Capsule adhering to
floor of acetabulum

Transverse cut (optional)
to create cruciate incision

Iliopsoas m. elevated
and reflected proximally

Capsule incised along
axis of femoral neck

O.

Adductor magnus m.

Adductor longus m.
detached and retracted

Femoral vessels and
nerve retracted laterally

Plate 76. (Continued)

P. The transverse acetabular ligament is sectioned, and the ligamentum teres is excised if large and obstructive. The hypertrophied pulvinar is also removed.

Q. Following this, the femoral head can be easily reduced underneath the limbus, and reduction can be maintained by holding the hip in 30 degrees of abduction, 15 degrees of flexion, and 20 degrees of medial rotation. According to Ferguson, it is not necessary to repair the capsule. I strongly recommend its repair by plication as illustrated in Steps L and M of Plate 77. I also recommend reattaching the adductor longus tendon to its origin because it is esthetically more pleasing, preventing an ugly depression on the upper medial aspect of the thigh. Tubes are inserted for closed Hemovac suction, and the wound is closed in the usual fashion.

R. A one-and-one-half hip spica cast is applied with the hip in 30 degrees of flexion, 30 degrees of abduction, and 10 to 25 degrees of medial rotation. During application and setting of the cast, medially directed pressure is applied over the greater trochanter with the palm.

Postoperative Care. Ferguson recommends that the cast be changed at six-week to two-month intervals, with total duration of cast immobilization of about four months. I believe, however, that with repair of the capsule such prolonged immobilization in cast is unnecessary, and in about six to eight weeks the cast is removed. After removal of the cast, the patient is gradually mobilized. Initially, a hip containment splint (such as Denis-Browne) is used to maintain the hip abduction and flexion.

REFERENCES

Chiari, K.: Die operative Behandlung am Huftgelenk bei der angeborenen Huftgelenksverrenkung. Wien. Med. Wochenschr., 107:1020, 1957.

Dorr, W. M.: Zur offenen Reposition nach Ludloff. Verh. Dtsch. Orthop. Ges., 54:370, 1968.

Ferguson, A. B., Jr.: Primary open reduction of congenital dislocation of the hip using a median adductor approach. J. Bone Joint Surg., 55–A:671, 1973.

Ludloff, K.: Zur Pathogenese und Therapie der angeborenen Huftverrenkung. Klin. Jahrb., 10:1902.

Ludloff, K.: The open reduction of the congenital hip dislocation by an anterior incision. Am. J. Orthop. Surg., 10:438, 1913.

Ludloff, K.: Die Erfahrungen bei der blutigen Reposition der angeborenen Huftluxation mit seinem vorderen Schnitt. Zentralbl. Chir., 41:156, 1914.

Mau, H., Dorr, W. M., Henkel, L., and Lutsche, J.: Open reduction of congenital dislocation of the hip by Ludloff's method. J. Bone Joint Surg., 53–A:1281, 1971.

Salzer, M., and Zuckriegl, H.: Die Operationstechnik der offenen Huftgelenkreposition nach Ludloff. Z. Orthop., 103:409, 1967.

Staheli, L. T.: Medial approach open reduction for congenitally dislocated hips: A critical analysis of forty cases. In: Tachdjian, M. O. (ed.): Congenital Dislocation of the Hip. New York, Churchill Livingstone, 1982, pp. 295–303.

Tsuchiya, K., and Yamada, K.: Open reduction of congenital dislocation of the hip in infancy using Ludloff's approach. Int. Orthop., 1:337, 1978.

Weinstein, S. L., and Ponseti, I. V.: Congenital dislocation of the hip. J. Bone Joint Surg., 61–A:119, 1979.

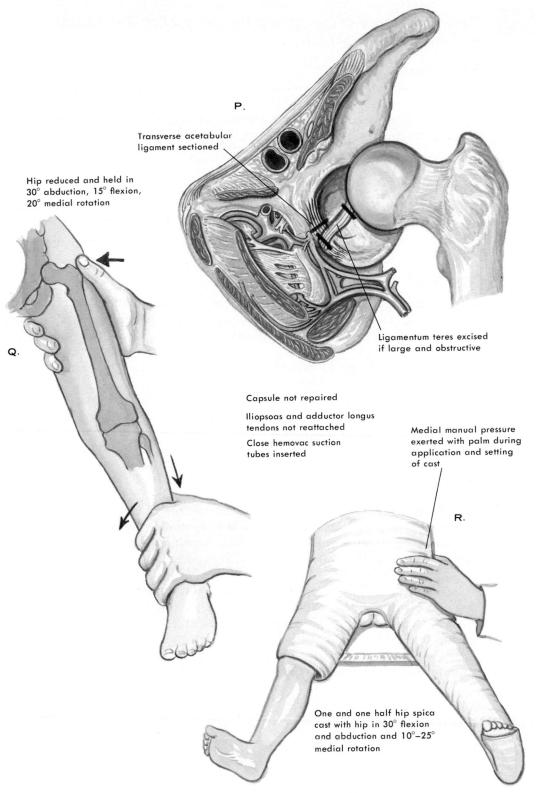

P.

Transverse acetabular ligament sectioned

Hip reduced and held in 30° abduction, 15° flexion, 20° medial rotation

Q.

Ligamentum teres excised if large and obstructive

Capsule not repaired

Iliopsoas and adductor longus tendons not reattached

Close hemovac suction tubes inserted

Medial manual pressure exerted with palm during application and setting of cast

R.

One and one half hip spica cast with hip in 30° flexion and abduction and 10°–25° medial rotation

Plate 76. (Continued)

PLATE 7 7 ## Open Reduction of Congenital Hip Dislocation Through the Anterolateral Approach

Indications

1. Inability to achieve concentric reduction of the hip, especially after walking age.

2. High dislocation that cannot be brought down with traction or that requires femoral shortening.

Blood for Transfusion. Yes.

Radiographic Control. Image intensifier.

Patient Position. The patient is placed in lateral position. The entire lower limb, affected half of the pelvis, and lower part of the chest are prepared and draped to allow free motion of the hip. Then the patient is turned to lie in completely supine position.

Operative Technique

A. The skin incision extends from the junction of the posterior and middle thirds of the iliac crest to the anterior superior iliac spine and then distally for about 7 to 10 cm. in the groove between the tensor fasciae latae and the sartorius muscles.

B. The deep fascia is incised over the iliac crest, and the fascia lata is opened in line with the skin incision.

The lateral femoral cutaneous nerve is identified; it crosses the sartorius muscle 2.5 cm. distal to the anterior superior iliac spine and lies close to the muscle's lateral border. A longitudinal incision is made over the medial part of the fascia covering the tensor fasciae latae; this 1 cm.-wide strip of fascia is mobilized by sharp dissection and used to protect the lateral femoral cutaneous nerve while the nerve is retracted medially with silicone (Silastic) tubing.

C. Blunt dissection is used to open the groove between the tensor fasciae latae muscle laterally and the sartorius and rectus femoris muscles medially; the fatty layer of tissue that covers the front of the capsule of the hip joint is exposed. The ascending branches of the lateral femoral circumflex vessels cross the midportion of the wound. If they are in the way, they must be isolated, clamped, cut, and ligated.

D. With a scalpel, the cartilaginous iliac apophysis is split through the middle down to bone from the junction of its posterior and middle thirds to the anterior superior iliac spine. With a broad periosteal elevator, the lateral part of the apophysis and the tensor fasciae latae and the gluteus medius and minimus muscles are subperiosteally stripped and reflected as a continuous sheet to the superior rim of the acetabulum anteriorly and the greater sciatic notch posteriorly.

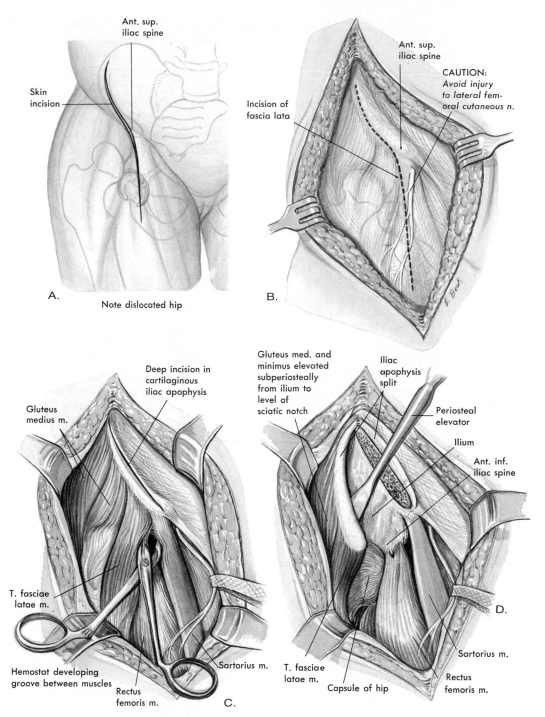

A.

Ant. sup.
iliac spine

Skin
incision

Note dislocated hip

B.

Ant. sup.
iliac spine

CAUTION:
*Avoid injury
to lateral fem-
oral cutaneous n.*

Incision of
fascia lata

E. Beck

C.

Gluteus
medius m.

Deep incision in
cartilaginous
iliac apophysis

T. fasciae
latae m.

Hemostat developing
groove between muscles

Rectus
femoris m.

Sartorius m.

D.

Gluteus med. and
minimus elevated
subperiosteally
from ilium to
level of
sciatic notch

Iliac
apophysis
split

Periosteal
elevator

Ilium

Ant. inf.
iliac spine

T. fasciae
latae m.

Capsule of hip

Sartorius m.

Rectus
femoris m.

Plate 77. A.–O., Open reduction of congenital hip dislocation through the anterolateral approach.

E. Next, the origin of the sartorius muscle is detached from the anterior superior iliac spine, and its free end is marked with 00 Tycron whip sutures for later reattachment. The sartorius muscle is reflected distally and medially. The two heads of the rectus femoris—the direct one from the anterior inferior iliac spine and the reflected one from the superior margin of the acetabulum—are divided at their origin, marked with 00 Tycron whip sutures, and reflected distally.

F. The hip is then flexed, abducted, and laterally rotated, exposing the iliacus muscle fibers, iliopsoas tendon, and lesser trochanter. A moist hernia tape is passed around the femoral nerve and gently retracted medially with the femoral vessels. With a moist sponge and a periosteal elevator, the iliacus muscle fibers are elevated and dissected free of the capsule, which is thus exposed superiorly, anteriorly, and inferiorly.

The iliopsoas muscle is usually short; it is lengthened by two transverse incisions of its tendinous fibers only. Take care not to injure the medial circumflex artery. When the hip is hyperextended, the tendinous fibers will slide and separate on the muscle, lengthening the iliopsoas. The iliacus and iliopsoas muscles are elevated medially, exposing the superolateral part of the superior ramus of the pubis.

G. At this point, an attempt is made to reduce the dislocated hip in order to determine the factors obstructing closed reduction. Manipulation should not be forcible. If reduction is not possible, either there are intracapsular factors in the obstruction or all obstructing extracapsular factors have not been relieved, or both.

H. The capsule and synovium are incised parallel to the superior and anterior margins of the acetabulum. Leave enough of a brim (usually 1 cm.) of the capsule medially and tag it with 0 or 00 Tycron sutures for later capsuloplasty. Anteroinferiorly, make a longitudinal incision parallel with the neck of the femur, converting the capsular incision into a T. The free edges of the capsule are marked with 0 or 00 Tycron sutures for traction and later plication.

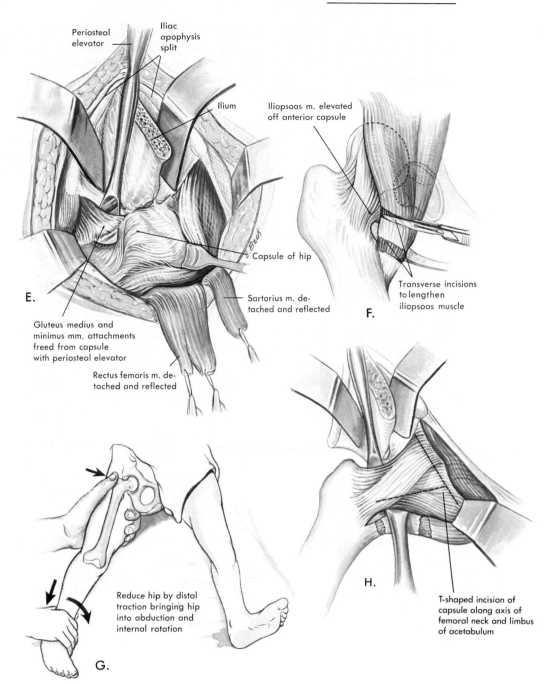

E. Periosteal elevator / Iliac apophysis split / Ilium / Capsule of hip / Sartorius m. detached and reflected / Gluteus medius and minimus mm. attachments freed from capsule with periosteal elevator / Rectus femoris m. detached and reflected

F. Iliopsoas m. elevated off anterior capsule / Transverse incisions to lengthen iliopsoas muscle

G. Reduce hip by distal traction bringing hip into abduction and internal rotation

H. T-shaped incision of capsule along axis of femoral neck and limbus of acetabulum

Plate 77. (Continued)

I. Inspect the hip joint for intra-articular factors obstructing reduction. The ligamentum teres is usually elongated and enlarged, preventing anatomic concentric reduction of the hip; it should be excised. First, the femoral head end of the ligamentum teres is divided, and the opposite end is traced to the acetabular notch at the lower part of the true acetabulum, where it is divided by two cuts—one anterior and the other posterior. In this way, injury to the acetabular branch of the obturator vessels is avoided and one can easily release the transverse acetabular ligament, which is displaced superiorly with the inferior part of the capsule.

J. Next, inspect the acetabulum. It may be filled with fibrofatty tissue, which may interfere with optimal seating of the femoral head within the socket; if so, it is excised with a sharp scalpel and curet.

Caution! Do not remove articular cartilage with it.

K. The limbus may be hypertrophic and inverted into the acetabulum. If the femoral head cannot be placed down and under the limbus and concentric reduction obtained, the free edge is everted with a blunt hook. If unable to evert the limbus, make two radiate incisions: one anteriorly and the other posteriorly; then evert it.

L. If the limbus is large and adherent to the acetabular rim, it may be impossible to evert it. In such an instance, it is grasped with a hemostat and its base is freed with either the tip of the hook or scalpel, and it is excised with strong curved scissors. *Do not injure the growth zones of the rim of the acetabulum.*

Next, inspect and determine (1) the depth of the acetabulum and the inclination of its roof, (2) the shape of the femoral head and the smoothness and condition of the articular hyaline cartilage covering it, (3) the degree of antetorsion of the femoral neck, and (4) the stability of the hip after reduction. Place the femoral head in the acetabulum under direct vision by flexing, abducting, and medially rotating the hip while applying traction and gentle pressure against the greater trochanter. This maneuver is reversed to redislocate the hip. When the femoral head comes out of the acetabulum, the position of the hip is determined and noted in the operative record. If necessary, a radiopaque dye is introduced into the hip for intraoperative arthrography or sterile fine-mesh tantalum gauze is wrapped around the cartilaginous femoral head to delineate it, the hip is reduced, and radiograms are made.

Remove the tantalum gauze. If the hip joint is unstable or if, upon reduction under direct vision, the femoral head is insufficiently covered superiorly and anteriorly, decide whether to perform an acetabuloplasty, Salter's innominate osteotomy, or a derotation osteotomy of the proximal femur at this time.

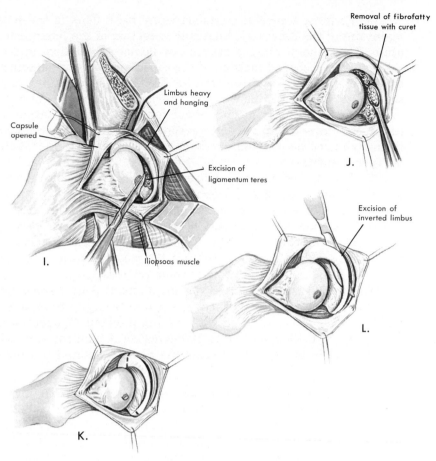

Removal of fibrofatty
tissue with curet

Limbus heavy
and hanging

Capsule
opened

Excision of
ligamentum teres

Iliopsoas muscle

I.

J.

Excision of
inverted limbus

L.

K.

Plate 77. (Continued)

M. Perform a careful capsulorrhaphy next. This is the most crucial step in maintaining the concentric anatomic reduction of the femoral head in the acetabulum. The femoral head is reduced by flexion, abduction, and medial rotation of the hip. The T-shaped incision of the capsule leaves a redundant proximal part of the superolateral flap of the capsule. Excise this triangular part of the flap with scissors or scalpel. In this way the T-incision is converted to a V.

N. With the hip in flexion, abduction, and medial rotation, bring the superior part of the lateral flap medially beyond the anteroinferior iliac spine; and suture it tautly to the periosteum and bone of the superior ramus of the pubis with 0 or 00 Tycron sutures.

O. The divided edges of the resected area of the capsule are brought together and firmly sutured with 00 Tycron interrupted sutures.

Skeletal fixation (e.g., a Steinmann pin to fix the proximal femur to the innominate bone) is unnecessary because the hip joint will be very stable following capsuloplasty, as just described. The two halves of the iliac apophysis are sutured together over the iliac crest; be sure the closure is taut. The rectus femoris and sartorius muscles are resutured to their origins.

The wound is closed in the routine manner. An anteroposterior radiograph of the hips is taken to double check the concentricity of reduction before a one-and-one-half spica cast is applied with the hip in about 45 degrees of abduction, 60 to 70 degrees of flexion, and 20 to 30 degrees of medial rotation. The knee is always flexed at 45 to 60 degrees to relax the hamstrings and to control rotation in the cast.

Postoperative Care. Immobilization in a hip spica cast following open reduction and capsuloplasty is for four to six weeks. When a simultaneous derotation femoral osteotomy or Salter's innominate osteotomy is also performed, the cast is kept on for six weeks. Following these periods, the cast is bivalved and radiographs of the hips are taken with the cast off. The child is allowed to move the lower limbs actively. Passive exercises should be avoided, as they stretch the shortened retinacular vessels. A bivalved hip spica cast, such as a hip abduction splint, is used at night.

As soon as functional range of motion of the hips is obtained, partial weight-bearing with a three-point crutch gait is begun. It may be difficult to teach this to the young child. Full weight-bearing is started in four to six weeks, following removal of the solid cast. The bivalved hip spica cast or a hip abduction splint is used at night for 6 to 12 months, depending on the age of the patient, the degree of femoral antetorsion, and the adequacy of the acetabular roof.

REFERENCES

Coleman, S. S.: Congenital Dysplasia and Dislocation of the Hip. St. Louis, C. V. Mosby, 1978.

Salter, R. B.: Innominate osteotomy in the treatment of congenital dislocation and subluxation of the hip. J. Bone Joint Surg., 43–B:518, 1961.

Scaglietti, O., and Calandriello, B.: Open reduction of congenital dislocation of the hip. J. Bone Joint Surg., 44–B:257, 1962.

Tönnis, D.: Congenital Dysplasia and Dislocation of the Hip in Children and Adults. With collaboration of Helmut Legal and Reinhard Graf. Berlin, Springer-Verlag, 1984.

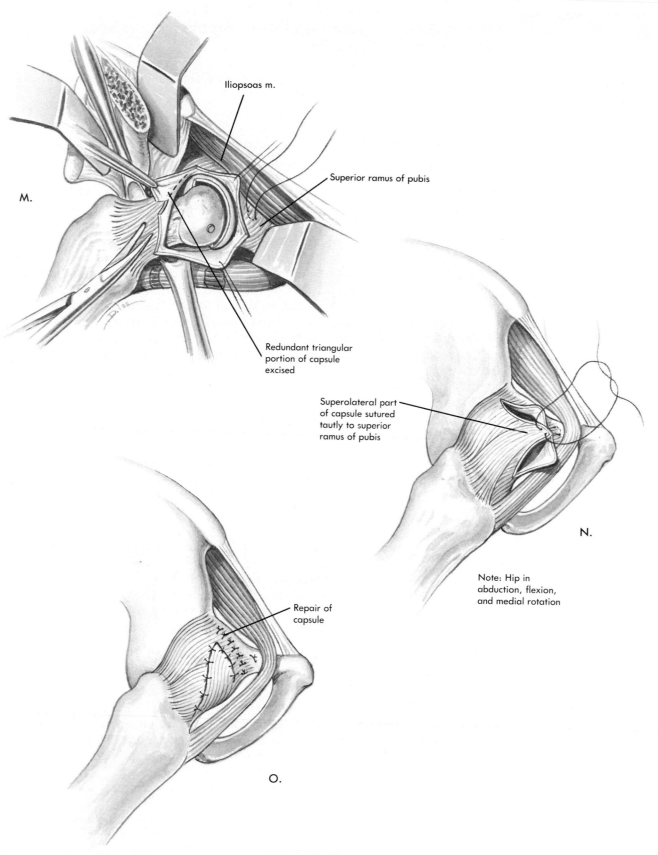

M.

Iliopsoas m.

Superior ramus of pubis

Redundant triangular
portion of capsule
excised

Superolateral part
of capsule sutured
tautly to superior
ramus of pubis

N.

Note: Hip in
abduction, flexion,
and medial rotation

Repair of
capsule

O.

Plate 77. (Continued)

PLATE 78 **Femoral Shortening and Derotation Osteotomy Combined with Open Reduction of the Hip**

Indications. High dislocation and a moderately displaced femoral head that cannot be reduced after preliminary traction.

Radiographic Control. Image intensifier.

Patient Position. Supine.

Blood for Transfusion. Yes.

Principle. This author performs femoral shortening and derotation osteotomy through a separate lateral longitudinal incision (See Plate 79, Steps **A.** and **B.**). (Coleman employs the iliofemoral approach and a large skin incision that begins at the mid part of the iliac crest, extends forward to the anterior superior iliac spine, then distally for 5 to 7 cm. over the upper thigh, paralleling the interval between the tensor fasciae latae and the sartorius muscles, and then curves posteriorly over the lateral aspect of the upper thigh, ending at the midlateral part of the upper femur. It is deepened, the tensor fasciae latae muscle is cut transversely, and the underlying vastus lateralis muscle is exposed by reflecting the divided tensor fasciae latae laterally. The tendinous insertion of the gluteus maximus, identified posteriorly, is left intact. The vastus lateralis muscle is detached at its origin, elevated, and reflected distally to expose the anterior and lateral surfaces of the intertrochanteric region and upper femoral shaft.)

Exposure of the upper femoral shaft through a separate longitudinal incision of the upper thigh is technically simpler, bleeding is less, and the scars esthetically more attractive. It is vital to expose a sufficient length of the upper femoral shaft subperiosteally.

In irreducible dislocation, femoral shortening facilitates reduction and, when reduction is difficult because of increasing pressure on the femoral head, decompresses the hip.

Operative Technique

A. The amount of shortening is determined preoperatively by measuring the distance between the inferior margin of the femoral head and the floor of the acetabulum. The roof of the true acetabulum may be oblique and deficient, and measuring from it to the top of the femoral head may pose problems. Avoid insufficient femoral shortening. If inadequate, it will not permit positioning of the femoral head in the true acetabulum, and postoperatively, pressure on the femoral head leads to cartilage necrosis and a stiff hip joint.

Another method of determining the amount of femoral shortening desired is to reduce the femoral head in the acetabulum and measure the overlap of the osteotomized segments.

Next, a "score" of adequate length is made on the anterior aspect of the femur parallel to its longitudinal axis to serve as an orientation mark to determine the degree of rotation after osteotomy and resection. As an added safety measure, I recommend insertion of threaded Steinmann pins of appropriate diameter, one in the upper femoral segment and another in the distal segment.

B. Next, the femur is shortened by two parallel transverse osteotomies; the first immediately distal to the inferior pole of the lesser trochanter and the second distal to it. The osteotomies are performed with an oscillating power saw. This author prefers to make a four-fifths osteotomy first at each of the two levels. Then the four-hole or five-hole plate of appropriate size is applied on the lateral aspect of the upper femoral shaft and firmly fixed with two screws to the upper segment. The osteotomies are completed, the segment of femur is resected, the distal segment is rotated laterally, and the bone surfaces are apposed.

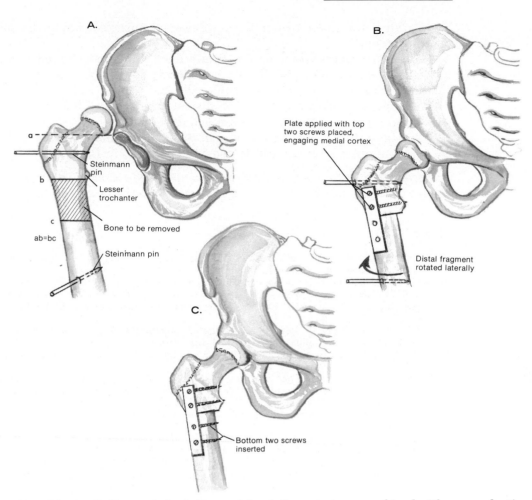

A.

a

Steinmann pin

b

Lesser trochanter

c

Bone to be removed

ab=bc

Steinmann pin

B.

Plate applied with top two screws placed, engaging medial cortex

Distal fragment rotated laterally

C.

Bottom two screws inserted

Plate 78. **A.–C.,** Femoral shortening and derotation osteotomy combined with open reduction of the hip.

C. Then the lower two or three screws are inserted, fixing the plate to the distal segment.

After the femoral osteotomy is firmly fixed, the femoral head is repositioned in the acetabulum. The stability of reduction is determined, and the adequacy of "decompression" of the hip is double checked. As a rule, the degree of hip decompression is adequate if one can distract the reduced femoral head from the socket for about 3 to 4 mm. without much tension.

The lateral thigh wound is closed in the usual manner. Repair of the hip joint capsule and other steps are illustrated and described in Plate 77.

Postoperative Care. Care is like that for open reduction of the hip. The plate is removed three to six months postoperatively when the osteotomy is solidly healed.

REFERENCES

Ashley, R. K., Larsen, L. T., and James, P. M.: Reduction of dislocation of the hip in older children. J. Bone Joint Surg., 54–A:545, 1972.

Coleman, S. S.: Congenital Dysplasia and Dislocation of the Hip. St. Louis: C. V. Mosby, 1978.

Galpin, R. D., Roach, J. W., Wenger, D. R., Herring, J. A., and Birch, J. G.: One-stage treatment of congenital dislocation of the hip in older children including femoral shortening. J. Bone Joint Surg., 71–A:734, 1989.

Herold, H. Z., and Daniel, D.: Reduction of neglected congenital dislocation of the hip in children over the age of six years. J. Bone Joint Surg., 61–B:1, 1979.

King, H. A., and Coleman, S. S.: Open reduction and femoral shortening in congenital dislocation of the hip. Orthop. Trans., 4:302, 1980.

Klisič, P., and Jankovic, L.: Combined procedure of open reduction and shortening of the femur in treatment of congenital dislocation of the hips in older children. Clin. Orthop., 119:60, 1976.

Schoenecker, P. L., and Strecker, W. B.: Congenital dislocation of the hip in children. Comparison of the effects of femoral shortening and of skeletal traction in treatment. J. Bone Joint Surg., 66–A:21, 1984.

Tönnis, D.: Congenital Dysplasia and Dislocation of the Hip in Children and Adults. With collaboration of Helmut Legal and Reinhard Graf. Berlin, Springer-Verlag, 1984.

Westin, G. W., Dallas, T. G., Watanabe, B. M., and Ilfeld, F. W.: Skeletal traction vs. femoral shortening in treatment of older children with congenital hip dislocation. Isr. J. Med. Sci., 16:318, 1980.

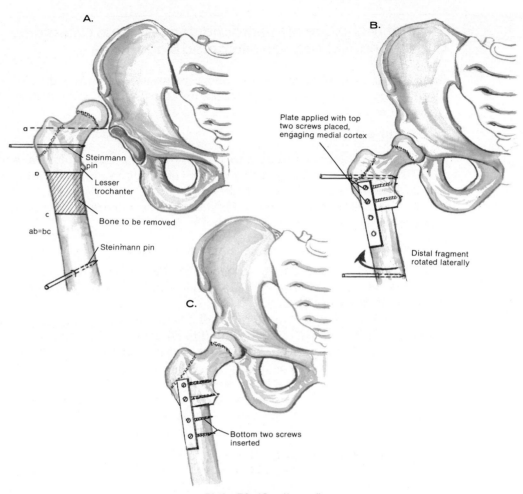

A.

a

Steinmann pin

b

Lesser trochanter

c

Bone to be removed

ab=bc

Steinmann pin

B.

Plate applied with top two screws placed, engaging medial cortex

Distal fragment rotated laterally

C.

Bottom two screws inserted

Plate 78. (Continued)

PLATE 79 **Wagner Technique of Intertrochanteric Oblique Osteotomy and Internal Fixation with Bifurcated Blade-Plate**

Indications. Instability of the hip and retardation of normal development of the acetabulum due to excessive femoral antetorsion and valgus deviation of the proximal femur.

Preoperative Assessment

1. Anteroposterior radiograms of hip, including upper femurs, with the hips in neutral rotation and in varying degrees of abduction and medial rotation.
2. True lateral projection of the hip.
3. Computed tomography (CT) to determine femoral and acetabular torsion and limb lengths.

Requisites

1. Concentric and stable reduction of the femoral head in the acetabulum when the hip is medially rotated (to neutralize antetorsion) and abduction (to compensate for coxa valga).
2. Functional or adequate range of hip motion (preferably an arc of 50 to 60 degrees of abduction–adduction, and 50 to 60 degrees of rotation).
Caution! Do not perform femoral osteotomy in the presence of restricted range of motion. It will cause a deformity in attitude.
3. Presence of deformation of the proximal femur.
4. When there is no femoral antetorsion, derotation osteotomy will cause retrotorsion and possible posterior subluxation. In the absence of coxa valga, varization osteotomy will cause deformation of the upper femur.

Contraindications. Presence of total necrosis of femoral head.
Caution! Osteotomy should be intertrochanteric. Do not create a deformity of the upper end of the femur. The tip of the greater trochanter should be in the center of the femoral head.

Radiographic Control. Image intensifier.

Blood for Transfusion. Yes.

Special Instrumentation. Wagner (Altdorf) bifurcated blade-plate, special holder and impacter.

Patient Position. The patient is in the supine position on a radiolucent operating table. Some surgeons prefer to operate on an older child on a fracture table because it is technically easier to make a lateral radiogram of the hip.

Operative Technique

A. A straight midlateral longitudinal incision is made, beginning at the tip of the greater trochanter and extending distally parallel with the femur for a distance of 10 to 12 cm. The subcutaneous tissue is divided in line with the skin incision.
B. The fascia lata is exposed by deepening the dissection and is first divided with a scalpel and then split longitudinally with scissors in the direction of its fibers. Division of the fascia lata should be posterior to the tensor fasciae latae in order to avoid splitting its muscle.
C. By retraction, visualize the vastus lateralis muscle. Next, expose the anterolateral region of the proximal femur and the trochanteric area. It is vital not to injure the greater trochanteric growth plate. The origin of the vastus lateralis muscle is divided transversely from the inferior border of the greater trochanter down to the posterolateral surface of the femur. Elevate the vastus lateralis muscle fibers from the lateral intramuscular septum and the tendinous insertion of the gluteus maximus.

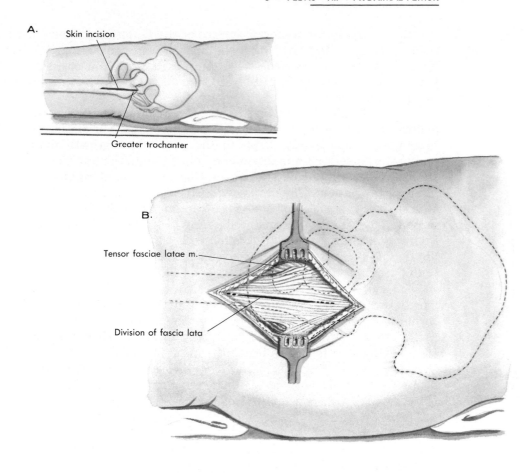

A.

Skin incision

Greater trochanter

B.

Tensor fasciae latae m.

Division of fascia lata

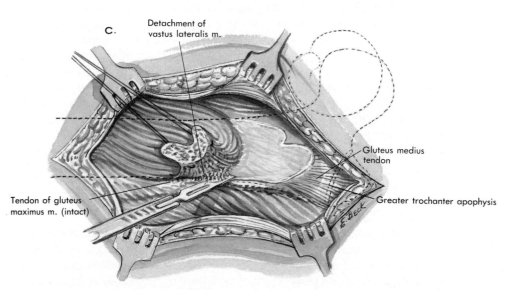

C.

Detachment of
vastus lateralis m.

Gluteus medius
tendon

Greater trochanter apophysis

E. Beck

Tendon of gluteus
maximus m. (intact)

Plate 79. A.–M., Wagner technique of intertrochanteric oblique osteotomy and internal fixation with bifurcated blade-plate.

D. To expose the posterior surface of the femur, use a curved wide osteotome to cut a thin cortical shell from the linea aspera. This technique avoids bleeding from the perforating vessels. The anterior, lateral, and posterior surfaces of the femur are exposed by insertion of Chandler or Cobra retractors anteromedially and posterolaterally.

E. and **F.** The femoral head is centered concentrically in the acetabulum by abduction and medial rotation of the hip; its position is checked by image intensifier. Immediately distal to the apophyseal growth plate of the greater trochanter, insert a 3-mm. Steinmann pin through the lateral cortex of the femoral shaft parallel to the floor of the operating room and at right angles to the median plane of the patient. The pin is drilled medially along the longitudinal axis of the femoral neck, stopping short of the capital femoral physis. This position of the proximal femur can be reproduced at any time during the operation by placing the Steinmann pin horizontally parallel to the floor and at 90 degrees to the longitudinal axis of the patient—a very dependable, simple method for proper orientation of the proximal femur.

G. With a slow oscillating saw, the intertrochanteric osteotomy is made parallel to the Steinmann pin and level with a point just below the inferomedial corner of the femoral neck. Avoid and do not enter the medial cortex of the femoral neck. The cut surfaces should be smooth to permit their accurate apposition and stable contact. It is best to be gentle and refrain from manipulating the proximal fragment by levering the Steinmann pin because the bone may be atrophic and easily cut through; instead the distal segment is manipulated. Insert a wide, flat osteotome into the osteotomy site, and open the osteotomy cleft by adducting and laterally rotating the lower limb into neutral position (with respect to adduction–abduction and medial-lateral rotation). Next, with an oscillating saw, remove a small wedge from the medial peak of the distal segment. Removal of a full wedge will sacrifice too much bone.

H. With the proximal fragment in the corrected position (i.e., the Steinmann pin parallel to the floor and at right angles to the median plane of the patient), the distal fragment is displaced medially about half the diameter of the shaft. The site of insertion of the bifurcated blade of the Altdorf hip clamp will determine the degree of medial displacement. More medial insertion of the blade will increase the amount of medial displacement of the distal fragment, which has a definite advantage. Varization osteotomy without medial displacement moves the greater trochanter and femoral shaft laterally away from the median line. This varus position of the limb axis subjects the proximal end of the femur to bending force, which interferes with bone healing. By displacing the distal fragment medially and bringing it closer to the center of hip rotation, the weight-bearing lever arm is shortened, bending force is decreased, and compression force is increased. Biomechanically, the medial displacement of the distal fragment stimulates bone healing and provides better bony support.

Next, choose the appropriate-sized blade-plate. The proximal end of the blade is bifurcated, and the blade itself is bent to make an angle of 130 degrees with the plate. The metal of the plate is flexible enough to allow bending with instruments to change the blade-plate angle if necessary. Immediately below the angulation of the blade and plate there is a round hole through which a screw is inserted into the proximal fragment. The plate has two oval screw holes, which provide leeway for compression. The blade is placed in the center of the femoral neck and should not protrude from its cortices, nor should the points of its bifurcated end penetrate and injure the capital femoral physis. The blade plate is held securely in a special holding instrument; by careful hammer blows, the bifurcated end is inserted into the osteotomy surface of the proximal fragment parallel to the longitudinal axis of the femoral neck. Check the position of the blade by image intensifier radiography.

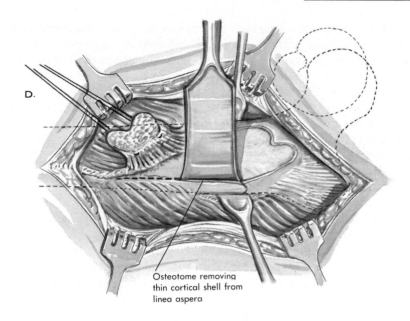

D.

Osteotome removing
thin cortical shell from
linea aspera

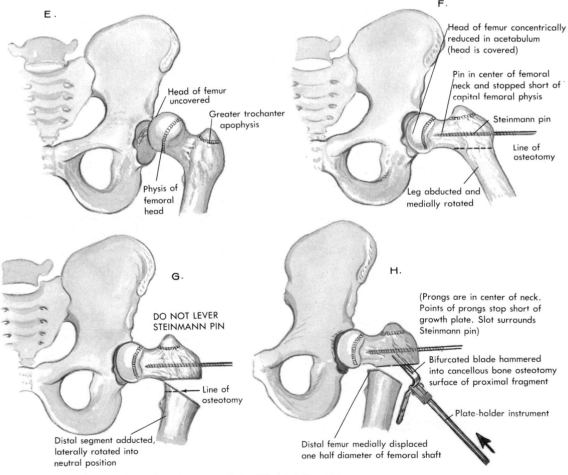

E.

Head of femur
uncovered

Greater trochanter
apophysis

Physis of
femoral
head

F.

Head of femur concentrically
reduced in acetabulum
(head is covered)

Pin in center of femoral
neck and stopped short of
capital femoral physis

Steinmann pin

Line of
osteotomy

Leg abducted and
medially rotated

G.

DO NOT LEVER
STEINMANN PIN

Line of
osteotomy

Distal segment adducted,
laterally rotated into
neutral position

H.

(Prongs are in center of neck.
Points of prongs stop short of
growth plate. Slot surrounds
Steinmann pin)

Bifurcated blade hammered
into cancellous bone osteotomy
surface of proximal fragment

Plate-holder instrument

Distal femur medially displaced
one half diameter of femoral shaft

Plate 79. (Continued)

I. and **J.** The blade is driven proximally into the osteotomy surface and buried almost to the angle with the plate. The holding instrument is removed, and the blade is impacted further with a punch. Next, a drill hole is made for the compression screw in the proximal fragment (small-fragment screws are used for the small and medium-sized blade plates and standard AO cortical screws are used for the large size). The screw is inserted into the proximal fragment, securely anchoring the bifurcated blade to the femoral neck. This type of fixation provides tremendous stability, which is essential in atrophic bone. (If the bone is not atrophic, some surgeons prefer to put the screw in the neck of the femur later.)

K. and **L.** Next, interfragmentary compression is achieved. First, fit the osteotomy surfaces together in the desired position, paying meticulous attention to keeping the Steinmann pin parallel to the floor and at right angles to the longitudinal axis of the patient and the distal fragment in neutral position as to abduction-adduction and medial-lateral rotation. Second, the osteotomized fragments are deliberately placed in slightly overcorrected position, the distal fragment brought into further medial displacement and the proximal fragment into further valgus displacement, so that only the distal tip of the plate touches the femoral shaft. This maneuver keeps a cleft 4 to 6 mm. wide at the osteotomy site, allowing impaction as the plate is anchored to bone. Insert a screw of appropriate size through the most distal hole of the plate first and then another screw through the next proximal hole. By tightening the second screw, one can pull the distal fragment laterally against the plate, which in turn lowers the proximal fragment into varus position. By this technique, the buttress point of the two fragments is compressed. If further compression is desired, the blade is impacted farther into the proximal fragment and the screws are tightened. The bone wedge removed earlier is placed between the two femoral fragments, and the previously inserted lag screw in the femoral neck is tightened, further compressing the fragments.

M. The vastus lateralis muscle is reattached to the tendinous insertion of the gluteus medius and minimus. Continuity of muscle structure of the gluteus medius and vastus lateralis takes much of the force on the lateral aspect of the upper femur and transforms bending force to compression force. One cannot overemphasize the importance of careful reattachment of the vastus lateralis to the gluteus medius insertion. A suction drainage tube is inserted underneath the free posterior margin of the vastus lateralis muscle. The fascia lata is sutured, and the subcutaneous tissues and skin are closed in the usual fashion. Skin closure should always be by a running subcuticular suture.

Postoperative Care. This type of osteosynthesis is so stable that it is safe not to apply a hip spica cast. Partial weight-bearing with crutches (three-point) is permitted on the fourth or fifth postoperative day when the child is comfortable. The osteotomy usually heals in about eight weeks, at which time crutch protection is discontinued. A hip spica cast is applied only when the femoral osteotomy is combined with open reduction of hip dislocation in which the cast is needed to maintain the stability of concentric reduction until the capsule and soft tissue heal.

REFERENCES

Alonso, J. E., Lowell, W. W., and Lovejoy, J. I.: The Altdorf hip clamp. J. Pediatr. Orthop., 6:399, 1986.
Wagner, H.: Femoral osteotomies for congenital hip dislocation. In: Weil, U. H. (ed.): Progress in Orthopedic Surgery. Vol. 2., Acetabular Dysplasia and Skeletal Dysplasia in Childhood. Heidelberg, Springer, 1978, p. 85.

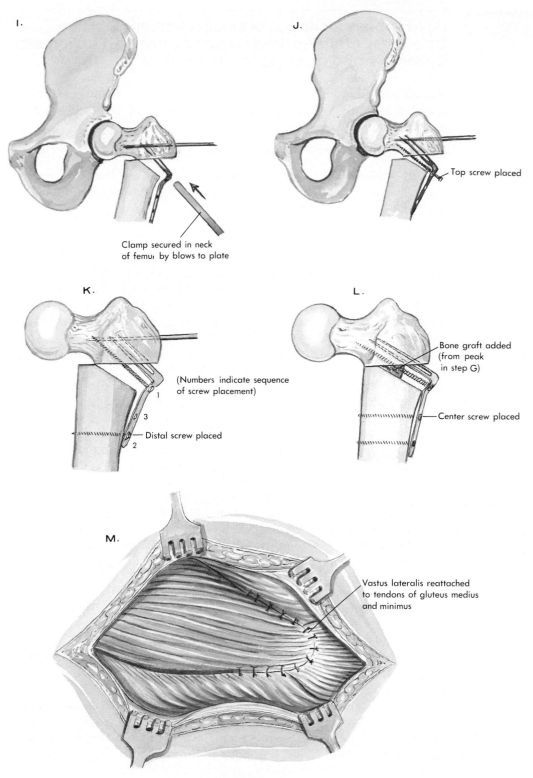

I.

Clamp secured in neck
of femur by blows to plate

J.

Top screw placed

K.

(Numbers indicate sequence
of screw placement)

1

3

Distal screw placed

2

L.

Bone graft added
(from peak
in step G)

Center screw placed

M.

Vastus lateralis reattached
to tendons of gluteus medius
and minimus

Plate 79. (Continued)

PLATE 80 **Lloyd Roberts Technique of Intertrochanteric Oblique Osteotomy of the Proximal Femur and Internal Fixation with Coventry Apparatus (Lag Screw and Plate)**

Indications. Instability of the hip and retardation of normal development of the acetabulum due to excessive femoral antetorsion and valgus deviation of the proximal femur.

Radiographic Control. Image intensifier.

Patient Position. The patient is placed supine on a radiolucent operating table. The iliac region, hip, and entire lower limb are prepared sterile and draped so that the limb can be manipulated freely.

Operative Technique

A. The incision begins 1 cm. posterior and inferior to the anterior superior iliac spine, curves across to the top of the greater trochanter, and continues distally along the femoral shaft for a distance of 6 to 8 cm. The subcutaneous tissue is divided in line with the skin incision. The deep fascia is incised, and the interval between the tensor fasciae latae anteriorly and the gluteus medius posteriorly is developed by blunt dissection. The vastus lateralis is divided longitudinally by an L-shaped or U-shaped incision, and the part of it that originates from the anterior aspect of the intertrochanteric area is detached.

With a periosteal elevator, expose the intertrochanteric region and the upper femoral shaft. At this time, the calcar femorale is visualized, and the femoral head can be palpated within the capsule. A sturdy stainless steel pin of appropriate diameter, usually 0.062 inch, is chosen; be sure that its diameter fits the hole in the lag screw. With the hip in full medial rotation, a 3-mm. hole is drilled through the center of the lateral cortex of the upper femoral shaft, 0.75 to 1.0 cm. below the growth plate of the greater trochanter. Avoid injury to the growth plate of the apophysis; verify its site with an image intensifier radiogram.

Insert the guide pin into the femoral neck parallel to the floor in a proximally inclined oblique plane parallel to the long axis of the femoral neck. The tip of the pin should stop immediately distal to the capital femoral physis. The proper placement of the guide pin is crucial; it is confirmed by anteroposterior and lateral image intensifier radiography.

B. A cannulated reamer (with a "stop" to prevent more than ½ inch penetration) is fitted over the guide pin; the lateral cortex of the upper femoral shaft is reamed to permit firm fixation of the lag screw in the cancellous bone.

C. Next, with the special lag screw inserter, a lag screw of appropriate length is inserted into the femoral neck. It should stop short of the capital physis. Avoid growth plate injury. Confirm the position of the screw by anteroposterior and lateral radiograms.

D. With an oscillating saw, the femoral osteotomy is performed at the intertrochanteric level parallel to the calcar; use the guide pin, which protrudes from the lag screw, to guide the direction of osteotomy and verify it by image intensifier radiography. (Drill holes may be used to mark the line of osteotomy.) Once the osteotomy is completed, gently strip the adjacent periosteum to mobilize the bone fragments and permit free rotation of the femoral shaft.

E. The side plate is bent to the appropriate angle. The guide pin is removed, and the top hole of the side plate is engaged to the protruding end of the lag screw. A cannulated lever with a handle is attached to the lag screw for firm control of the upper fragment. The distal fragment is adducted and rotated laterally to the desired degree. The oblique line of the osteotomy will often make a triangle of bone, at the upper end of the femoral shaft, that will protrude anteriorly; this is excised and used as a local bone graft. The osteotomized fragments are apposed

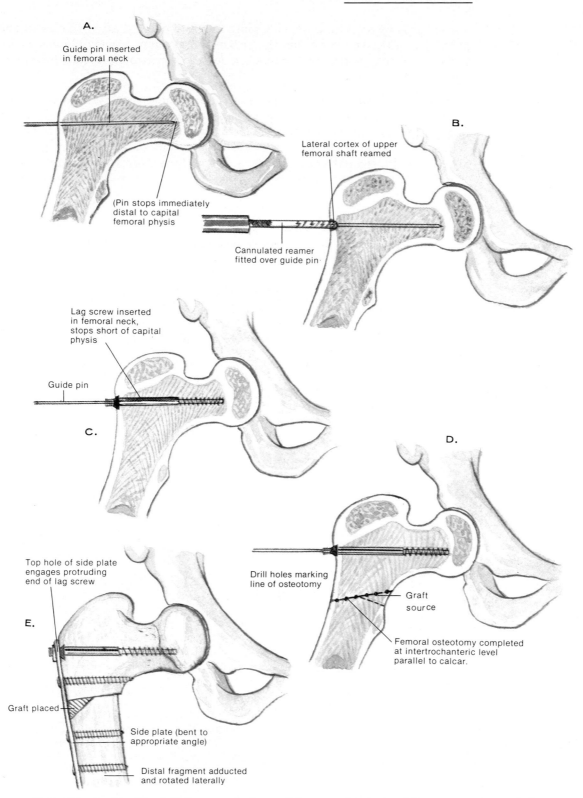

A.

Guide pin inserted
in femoral neck

(Pin stops immediately
distal to capital
femoral physis

B.

Lateral cortex of upper
femoral shaft reamed

Cannulated reamer
fitted over guide pin

Lag screw inserted
in femoral neck,
stops short of capital
physis

Guide pin

C.

D.

Drill holes marking
line of osteotomy

Graft
source

Femoral osteotomy completed
at intertrochanteric level
parallel to calcar.

Top hole of side plate
engages protruding
end of lag screw

E.

Graft placed

Side plate (bent to
appropriate angle)

Distal fragment adducted
and rotated laterally

Plate 80. A.–E., Lloyd Roberts technique of intertrochanteric oblique osteotomy of the proximal femur and internal fixation with Coventry apparatus (lag screw and plate).

and secured by attaching the side plate to the femoral shaft with screws and a nut at the top of the lag screw and the proximal fragment. Final radiograms are made to double check security of the fixation device. A one-and-one-half hip spica cast is applied.

Postoperative Care. The child is usually sent home three to four days postoperatively and readmitted to the hospital six weeks later. The plaster cast is removed, and the hip and knee are mobilized by active-assisted and gentle passive exercises. When able to ambulate with crutches (three-point partial weight-bearing on the affected limb), the patient is discharged, usually within two to four days.

The plate and screws are removed six to twelve months postoperatively.

REFERENCE

Canale, S. T., and Holand, R. W.: Coventry screw fixation of osteotomies about the pediatric hip. J. Pediatr. Orthop., 3:592, 1983.

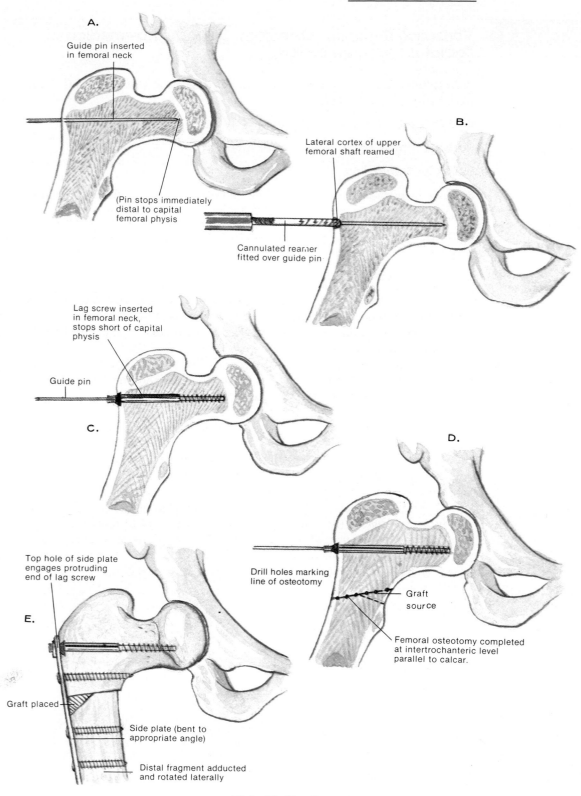

A.

Guide pin inserted
in femoral neck

(Pin stops immediately
distal to capital
femoral physis

B.

Lateral cortex of upper
femoral shaft reamed

Cannulated reamer
fitted over guide pin

Lag screw inserted
in femoral neck,
stops short of capital
physis

Guide pin

C.

D.

Drill holes marking
line of osteotomy

Graft
source

Femoral osteotomy completed
at intertrochanteric level
parallel to calcar.

Top hole of side plate
engages protruding
end of lag screw

E.

Graft placed

Side plate (bent to
appropriate angle)

Distal fragment adducted
and rotated laterally

Plate 80. (Continued)

PLATE 81 ## Varization Derotation Osteotomy Using the Howmedica Pediatric Hip Screw System

Indications. Valgus and antetorsion deformity of the proximal femur causing instability and subluxation of the hip joint.

Requisites. Concentricity of reduction of the hip joint.

Radiographic Control. Image intensifier.

Blood for Transfusion. Yes.

Special Instrumentation. Howmedica pediatric hip screw fixation system.

Patient Position. The patient is supine on a translucent operating table. Ensure that the heating pad is not obstructing the projection of the hip on the image intensifier.

Operative Technique

A. Make an incision beginning 1 cm. above the proximal tip of the greater trochanter extending distally on the lateral aspect of the thigh along the axis of the shaft of the femur. Subcutaneous tissue is divided in line with the skin incision. Superficial and deep fascia are incised.

B. Expose the vastus lateralis muscle. It is detached from its origin at the trochanteric ridge through an L-shaped incision, and the muscle is elevated and reflected anteriorly. The posterior aspect of the shaft of the femur is exposed only at the proposed site of the osteotomy.

Caution! Watch for the perforating vessels that can cause troublesome bleeding.

Make a longitudinal incision in the periosteum, and expose the upper shaft of the femur medially, anteriorly, and posterolaterally. Do not disturb the greater trochanteric apophyseal growth plate.

C. and **D.** Under image intensifier radiographic control, drill a 0.064 guide pin into the neck of the femur. Stop short of the capital femoral physis. Check its position in the anteroposterior and lateral projections to ensure that it is in the center of the femoral neck. The site of entry of the pin should be straight lateral, above the lesser trochanter in the intertrochanteric region.

A.

Incision

B.

Vastus lateralis reflected anteriorly

D.

LATERAL VIEW

ANTERIOR VIEW

C.

Guide pin

Caution: Stop short of
capital femoral epiphysis

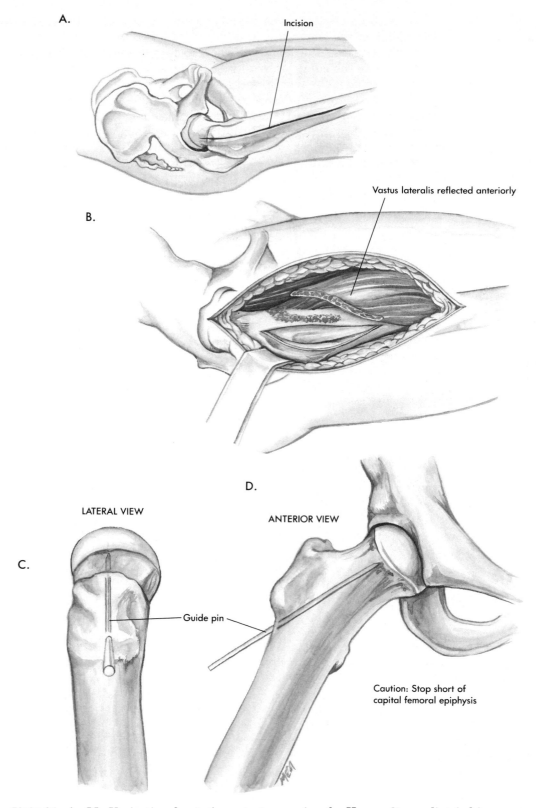

Plate 81. A.–M., Varization derotation osteotomy using the Howmedica pediatric hip screw
system.

E. With an electric power reamer, ream the lateral cortex of the intertrochanteric region of the femur.

F. To measure the length of the hip screw, place another pin of the same length next to the guide pin with its tip on the lateral cortex. The difference of the two pin lengths is the length of the screw.

G. Insert the cannulated tap over the guide pin; under image intensifier radiographic control, slowly tap the neck of the femur manually. Make anteroposterior and lateral radiograms with the image intensifier to be sure that the tap is in the center of the neck and stops short of the capital physis.

H. Insert the cannulated hip screw over the guide pin. Its tip should be 5 mm. short of the capital physis; laterally, several threads of the screw should protrude lateral to the cortex.

E.

Lateral cortex of intertrochanteric region is power reamed

F.

Length of hip screw

G.

Hand reamer

H.

5 mm.

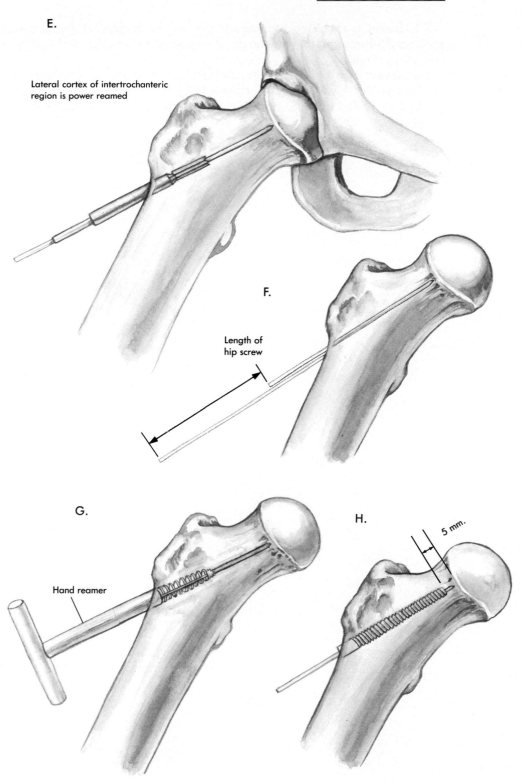

Plate 81. (Continued)

I. Insert a threaded Steinmann pin in the middle of the femoral shaft and another Steinmann pin over the greater trochanter to control the degree of rotation following osteotomy.

J. Insert two guide pins at the calculated angle of correction of the valgus deformity. The base of wedge of bone to be excised is medial. The position of the guide pins in the intertrochanteric area is determined by image intensifier radiographic control.

I.

ANTEROLATERAL VIEW

Threaded
Steinmann pin

Threaded
Steinmann pin

ANTERIOR VIEW

J.

Guide pins

Lines marking medially
based wedge osteotomy

Note: It includes upper
half of lesser trochanter

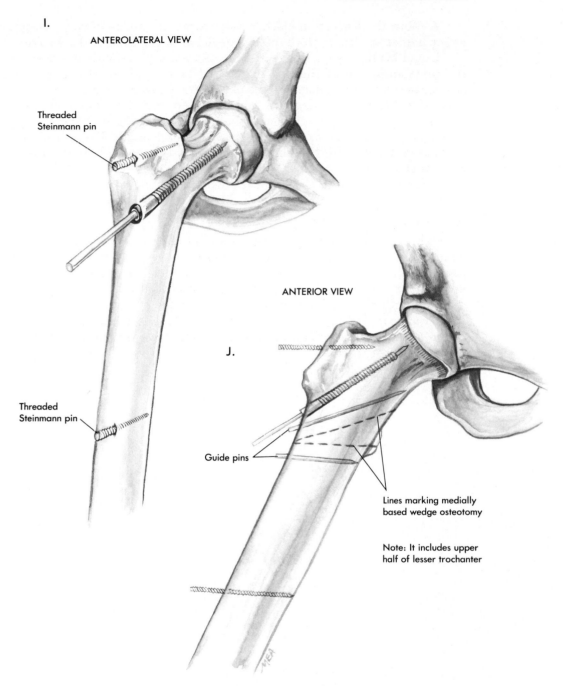

Plate 81. (Continued)

K. With the help of an electric saw, excise the wedge of bone. Ordinarily, the upper half of the lesser trochanter is included in the base of the wedge.

L. and **M.** Remove a wedge of bone. Secure a plate with the desired angle to the protruding end of the hip screw, and lock in place with a nut. The metal surface of the nut should appose the plate. The plates come in 20-degree increments (e.g., 100, 120 and 140 degrees) and have two, three, or four holes. The plate is anchored into the upper femoral shaft with the help of bone-holding forceps. Radiograms are made to measure the neck-shaft angle. If the desired degree of varization is achieved, the plate is screwed to the femoral shaft with the help of cortical screws.

Close the wound in the usual fashion, and apply a one-and-one-half hip spica cast.

Postoperative Care. Two to three weeks after surgery, radiograms are made through the cast. Remove the cast six weeks after surgery. Radiograms are made when the patient is out of the cast to ensure that the screws and plates are in good position. Ordinarily, the osteotomy is healed and the patient is admitted to the hospital for a few days for restoration of joint motion and muscle function and gait training with crutches or a walker protecting the operated lower limb. Crutch or walker support is discontinued when the bone is solidly healed and motor strength of the lower limb musculature is adequate. Remove the plate and screws 6 to 12 months after surgery.

K.

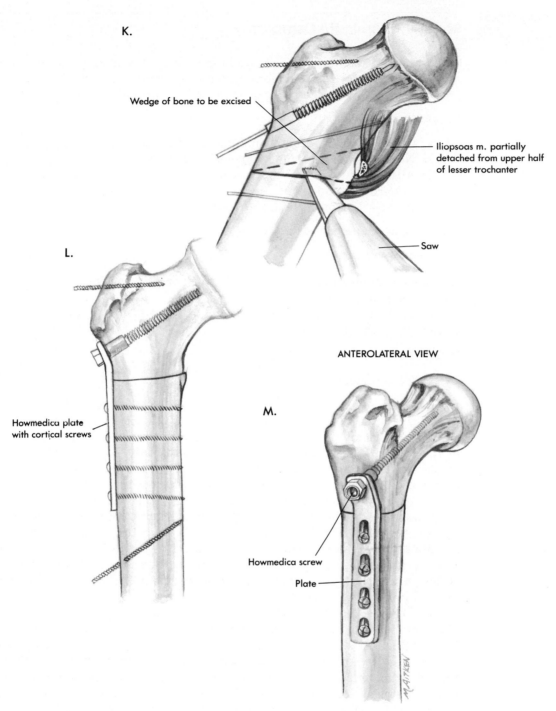

Wedge of bone to be excised

Iliopsoas m. partially
detached from upper half
of lesser trochanter

Saw

L.

Howmedica plate
with cortical screws

ANTEROLATERAL VIEW

M.

Howmedica screw

Plate

Plate 81. (Continued)

PLATE 82   Salter's Innominate Osteotomy

Indications. Instability of the reduced hip in weight-bearing position as a result of excessive acetabular antetorsion. Salter's innominate osteotomy is a derotation osteotomy—it does not decrease or increase the capacity of the acetabulum.

Requisites

1. Complete and concentric reduction of the hip.
2. Normal or near-normal range of hip motion.
3. Absence of myostatic contracture of iliopsoas and hip adductors.
4. Congruous hip joint.
5. Patient 18 months of age or older.

Blood for Transfusion. Yes.

Radiographic Control. Image intensifier.

Special Instrumentation. Rang retractors for ease of passing a Gigli saw through the sciatic notch.

Caution! Stay subperiosteal. Sciatic nerve palsy can occur. Be gentle during retraction in the sciatic notch.

Patient Position. Supine.

Operative Technique

A.–D. The Salter innominate osteotomy is based on redirection of the acetabulum as a unit by hinging and rotation through the symphysis pubis, which is mobile in children. It is performed by a transverse linear cut above the acetabulum at the level of the greater sciatic notch and the anterior inferior iliac spine. The whole acetabulum with the distal fragment of the innominate bone is tilted downward and laterally by rotating it. The new position of the distal fragment is maintained by a triangular bone graft taken from the proximal portion of the ilium and inserted in the open-wedge osteotomy site. Internal fixation is provided by two threaded Kirschner wires. Through the rotation and redirection of the acetabulum, the femoral head is covered adequately with the hip in normal weight-bearing position, i.e., the reduced dislocation or subluxation that was previously stable in the position of flexion and abduction is now stable in the extended and neutral position of weight-bearing.

E. Prepare the skin with the patient in the side-lying position so that the abdomen, lower part of the chest, and affected half of the pelvis can be draped to the midline anteriorly and posteriorly; the entire lower limb is also prepared and draped to allow free motion of the hip during the operation. Then the patient is turned on his or her back to lie completely supine. The range of abduction of the hip is tested. Maximum normal abduction must be present; if it is limited by contracted hip adductors, an adductor myotomy is performed first.

The skin incision is oblique, extending from the junction of the posterior and middle thirds of the iliac crest to a point 1 cm. below the anterior superior iliac spine, and then is extended medially to just below the midpoint of the inguinal ligament. The subcutaneous tissue is divided in line with the skin incision. The deep fascia is incised over the iliac crest. The wound edges are undermined, and pressure is applied with large sponges to minimize bleeding. Next, the fascia lata is opened over the medial border of the tensor fasciae latae and lateral to the groove between it and the sartorius muscles—this 1-cm. strip of fascia protects the lateral femoral cutaneous nerve from inadvertent injury.

F. With a scalpel, split the cartilaginous iliac apophysis in the middle down to bone from the junction of its posterior and middle thirds to the anterior superior iliac spine. By blunt dissection, the groove between the tensor fasciae latae and the sartorius and rectus femoris muscles is opened and developed. With a broad,

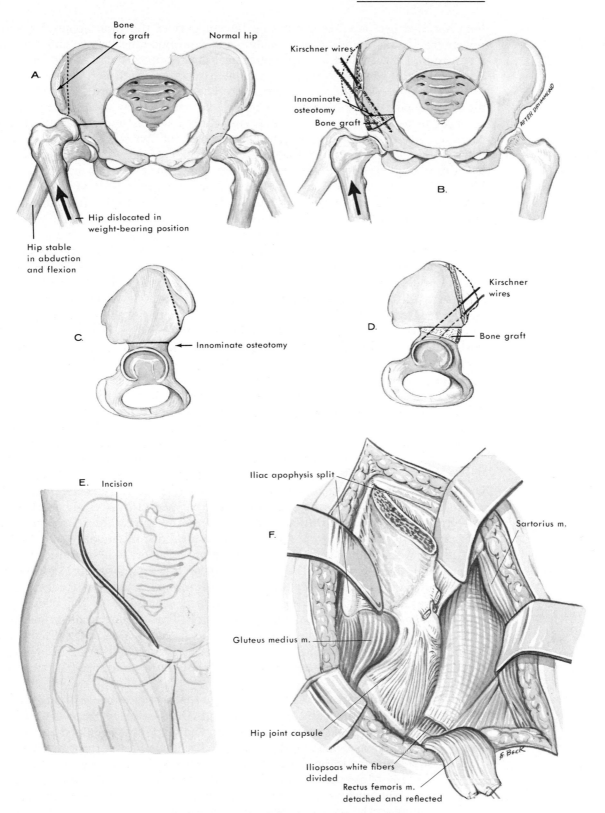

A. Bone for graft — Normal hip

Hip dislocated in weight-bearing position

Hip stable in abduction and flexion

B. Kirschner wires — Innominate osteotomy — Bone graft

AFTER DRUMMOND

C. Innominate osteotomy

D. Kirschner wires — Bone graft

E. Incision

F. Iliac apophysis split — Sartorius m. — Gluteus medius m. — Hip joint capsule — Iliopsoas white fibers divided — Rectus femoris m. detached and reflected

F. BECK

Plate 82. **A.–J., Salter's innominate osteotomy.**

long-handled periosteal elevator, the lateral part of the iliac apophysis and the tensor fasciae latae and gluteus medius and minimus muscles are subperiosteally stripped and reflected as a continuous sheet to the superior rim of the acetabulum anterolaterally and the greater sciatic notch posteromedially.

G. Next, elevate the periosteum from the medial and lateral walls of the ilium all the way posteriorly to the sciatic notch. It is vital to stay within the periosteum in order to prevent injury to the superior gluteal vessels and the sciatic nerve. A common pitfall is inadequate surgical exposure of the sciatic notch, making it difficult to pass the Gigli saw behind the notch. The space on the lateral wall of the ilium is packed with sponge to dilate the interval and to control oozing of blood. Next, the periosteum is elevated from the inner wall of the ilium in a continuous sheet, exposing the sciatic notch medially. Again, it is important to stay in the subperiosteal plane in order to avoid injury to vessels and nerves.

Pack the medial space with sponge. The sartorius muscle usually can be reflected medially with the medial half of the cartilaginous iliac apophysis. If it is difficult to do so or if more distal exposure is desired, the origin of the sartorius muscle is detached from the anterior superior iliac spine, its free end is marked with whip sutures for later reattachment and the muscle is reflected distally and medially. The two heads of origin of the rectus femoris, the direct one from the anterior inferior iliac spine and the reflected one from the superior margin of the acetabulum, are divided at their origin, marked with whip sutures, and reflected distally.

Next, on the deep surface of the iliopsoas muscle, expose the psoas tendon at the level of the pelvic rim. The iliopsoas muscle is rolled over so that its tendinous portion can be separated from the muscular portion. If identification is in doubt, use a nerve stimulator to distinguish the psoas tendon from the femoral nerve. A Freer elevator is passed between the tendinous and muscular portions of the iliopsoas muscle, and the psoas tendon is sectioned at one or two levels. The divided edges of the tendinous portion retract, and the muscle fibers separate; releasing contractures of the iliopsoas without disturbing the continuity of the muscle. Next, make two or three transverse incisions in the medial half of the cartilaginous apophysis of the ilium to allow lateral tilting and anterolateral rotation of the acetabulum; if necessary to provide greater lateral displacement.

Place two medium-sized Chandler elevator retractors, one introduced from the lateral and the other from the medial side of the ilium, subperiosteally in the sciatic notch. This step is crucial; besides keeping neurovascular structures out of harm's way, the Chandler retractors maintain continuity of the proximal and distal innominate segments at the sciatic notch. This author recommends the use of the Rang retractors,* which have a special groove inside and are larger than Chandler retractors. This facilitates the passing of the Gigli saw from the medial to the lateral side and maintains continuity of the osteotomized cortices at the sciatic notch.

A right-angled forceps (Mixter or Negus) is passed subperiosteally from the medial side of the ilium and guided through the sciatic notch to the outer side with the index finger of the opposite hand. The Gigli saw is introduced from the lateral side, the loop of one end is grasped by the blades of the right-angled forceps, and the saw is passed through the sciatic notch from the lateral to the medial side.

H. The line of osteotomy extends from the sciatic notch to the anterior inferior iliac spine, perpendicular to the sides of the ilium. It is vital to begin the osteotomy well inferiorly in the sciatic notch; the tendency is to start too high. Determine its exact site by image intensifier radiographic control. The handles of the Gigli saw are kept widely separated and at a continuous tension in order to keep the saw from binding in the soft cancellous bone. The osteotomy, which emerges anteriorly immediately above the anterior inferior iliac spine, is completed with the Gigli

---

*Rang retractors may be obtained through the manufacturer: Jantek Engineering Inc., 570 Trafford Crescent, Oakville, Ontario, Canada L6L 3T3.

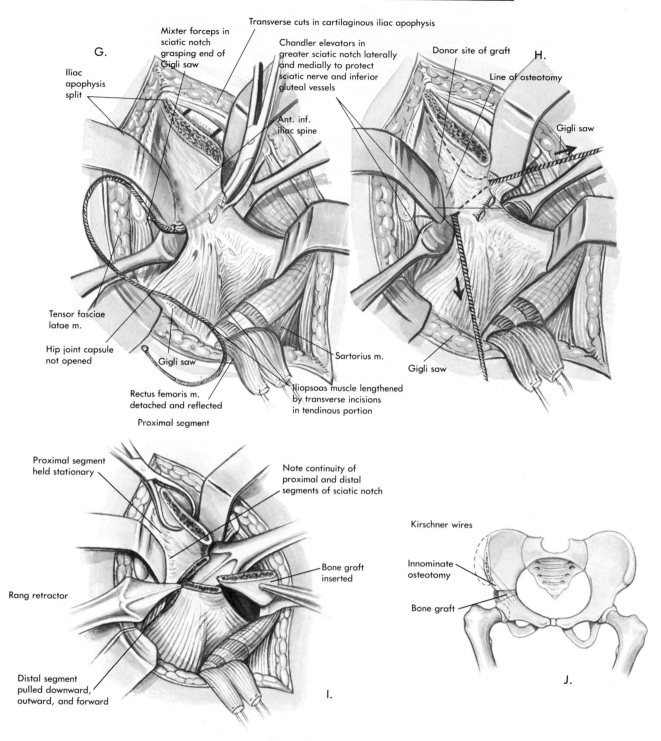

G.

Iliac apophysis split

Mixter forceps in sciatic notch grasping end of Gigli saw

Transverse cuts in cartilaginous iliac apophysis

Chandler elevators in greater sciatic notch laterally and medially to protect sciatic nerve and inferior gluteal vessels

Ant. inf. iliac spine

Tensor fasciae latae m.

Hip joint capsule not opened

Gigli saw

Rectus femoris m. detached and reflected

Proximal segment

Sartorius m.

Iliopsoas muscle lengthened by transverse incisions in tendinous portion

H.

Donor site of graft

Line of osteotomy

Gigli saw

Gigli saw

Proximal segment held stationary

Note continuity of proximal and distal segments of sciatic notch

Rang retractor

Bone graft inserted

Distal segment pulled downward, outward, and forward

I.

Kirschner wires

Innominate osteotomy

Bone graft

J.

Plate 82. (Continued)

saw. Use of an osteotome may subject the superior gluteal artery and sciatic nerve to iatrogenic damage. A Midas power saw may be used instead of a Gigli saw, particularly if a curvilinear cut is planned.

I. The two Chandler or Rang retractors are kept constantly at the sciatic notch by an assistant to prevent posterior or medial displacement of the distal segment and loss of bony continuity posteriorly. A triangular full-thickness bone graft is removed from the anterior part of the iliac crest with a large, straight, double-action bone cutter. The length of the base of the triangular wedge represents the distance between the anterior superior and the anterior inferior iliac spines. The portion of bone to be removed as bone graft is held firmly with a Kocher forceps; be sure that it does not fall on the floor or become contaminated.

The proximal fragment of the innominate bone is held steady with a large towel clip forceps, and the distal fragment is grasped with a second stout towel forceps. The affected hip is placed in 90 degrees of flexion, maximal abduction, and 90 degrees of lateral rotation; a second assistant applies distal and lateral traction on the thigh. With the second towel clip placed well posteriorly on the distal fragment, the surgeon rotates the distal fragment downward, outward, and forward, thus opening the osteotomy site anteriorly. The site must be kept closed posteriorly. Leaving it open posteriorly displaces the hip joint distally without adequate rotation and redirection of the acetabulum at the symphysis pubis; furthermore, it will lengthen the lower limb unnecessarily. A large Cobb periosteal elevator may be used for lateral rotation and downward and lateral tilting of the distal fragment. Another technical error to avoid is opening the osteotomy site with a mechanical spreader (such as a laminectomy spreader or a self-retaining retractor) because that will do nothing but move the proximal fragment upward and the distal fragment downward without rotating the distal fragment through the symphysis pubis. The acetabular maldirection will not be corrected unless such rotation of the distal fragment takes place. Avoid posterior and medial displacement of the distal fragment. When the periosteum on the median wall of the ilium is taut, the cartilaginous apophysis of the ilium is divided at two or three levels; this will help to rotate the acetabulum.

J. Next, the bone graft is shaped with bone cutters to the appropriate size to fit the open osteotomy site. Ordinarily, the graft is about the correct size for the size of the patient because the base of the triangular graft represents the distance between the anterior superior and anterior inferior iliac spines. Avoid using a large graft and hammering it in to fit snugly into the osteotomy site; this will open the site posteriorly. With the osteotomy site open anteriorly and the distal segment rotated, insert the bone graft into the opened-up osteotomy. Keep the distal fragment of the innominate bone slightly anterior to the proximal fragment. When traction is released, the graft is firmly locked by the two segments of the bone.

Drill a stout, threaded Kirschner wire from the proximal segment across the osteotomy site, through the graft, and into the distal segment posterior to the acetabulum, preventing any future displacement of the graft or the distal segment. The wire should never point in the direction of the hip joint. Radiographs are made to check the adequacy of correction of the acetabular maldirection and the position of the Kirschner wire. Then a second Kirschner wire is drilled parallel to the first to further stabilize internal fixation of the osteotomy. To ensure security of fixation in the older patient, this author uses two three-hole semitubular plates with the most distal hole in the plate cut so that it is converted into two prongs. The prongs are hammered into the distal segment of the ilium, and the two proximal holes are secured to the wall of the ilium. Inadequate penetration of the wires into the distal fragment will result in loss of alignment of the osteotomy. They may bend or break, or if excessively heavy, they may fracture the graft or the innominate bone; the importance of choosing the correct diameter of wire or cancellous screw cannot be overemphasized. Penetration of the wires into the hip joint may cause chondrolysis of the hip or cause the wire to break at the joint level. The wires

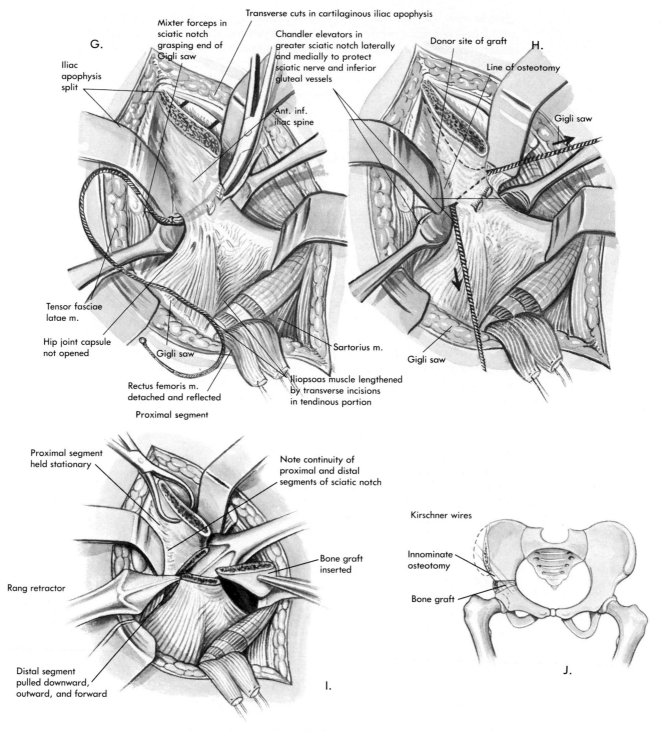

G.

Transverse cuts in cartilaginous iliac apophysis

Mixter forceps in sciatic notch grasping end of Gigli saw

Chandler elevators in greater sciatic notch laterally and medially to protect sciatic nerve and inferior gluteal vessels

Iliac apophysis split

Ant. inf. iliac spine

Tensor fasciae latae m.

Hip joint capsule not opened

Gigli saw

Sartorius m.

Rectus femoris m. detached and reflected

Iliopsoas muscle lengthened by transverse incisions in tendinous portion

Proximal segment

H.

Donor site of graft

Line of osteotomy

Gigli saw

Gigli saw

I.

Proximal segment held stationary

Note continuity of proximal and distal segments of sciatic notch

Rang retractor

Bone graft inserted

Distal segment pulled downward, outward, and forward

J.

Kirschner wires

Innominate osteotomy

Bone graft

Plate 82. (Continued)

should not be inserted upward from below, since they may pass medial to the proximal segment and injure retroperitoneal or intraperitoneal structures. An anteroposterior radiograph of the hips is taken to check the depth of the Kirschner wires and the degree of correction obtained.

The two halves of the cartilaginous iliac apophysis are sutured together over the iliac crest. The rectus femoris and sartorius muscles are reattached to their origins.

The wound is closed in the routine manner. Skin closure should be by continuous subcuticular 00 nylon. Cut the Kirschner wires so that their ends are in the subcutaneous fat and are easily palpable.

A one-and-one-half spica cast is applied with the hip in stable weight-bearing position. Avoid immobilization in a forced or extreme position because it will cause excessive and continuous compression of articular cartilage, osteonecrosis, permanent joint stiffness, and eventual degenerative arthritis. In the cast, the knee is bent to control the position of hip rotation. When there is excessive femoral antetorsion the hip is immobilized in slight medial rotation. A common pitfall is immobilization in marked medial rotation; this mistake will result in posterior subluxation or dislocation of the femoral head. In femoral retrotorsion, the hip should be immobilized in slight lateral rotation. It is obvious that prior to Salter's innominate osteotomy it is vital to determine the degree of femoral torsion accurately.

A radiograph of the hips through the cast is made before the child is discharged from the hospital. Another set of radiographs is made two to three weeks postoperatively to ensure that the graft has not collapsed, that the pins have not migrated, and that there is no medial displacement of the distal segments. In the older cooperative patient, when cancellous screws are used for internal fixation, a hip spica cast is not necessary.

Postoperative Care. The hips remain immobilized in the spica cast for a total of six weeks, following which the cast is bivalved and radiographs of the hip are made with the cast removed. It is best to readmit the child to the hospital, where bilateral split Russell's traction is applied, and gradual active exercises are performed to mobilize the lower limbs and develop muscle strength. An accidental fall during the first few weeks might result in collapse of the graft or stress fracture of the femur. When functional range of motion of the hips and knees is obtained, partial weight-bearing with a three-point crutch gait is begun. This may be difficult to teach to the two- or three-year-old child. Full weight-bearing is allowed four to six weeks following removal of the solid cast, or ten to 12 weeks postoperatively. This author recommends removal of the Kirschner wires when there is complete consolidation and revascularization of the graft (usually three to six months postoperatively). Ordinarily this is performed as an outpatient procedure using general anesthesia in the operating room.

REFERENCES

Gallien, R., Bertin, D., and Kirette, R.: Salter procedure in congenital dislocation of the hip. J. Pediatr. Orthop., 4:427, 1984.

Rab, G. T.: Biomechanical aspects of the Salter osteotomy. In: The Hip: Proceedings of the Fourth Meeting of the Hip Society, 1976. St. Louis, C. V. Mosby, 1976, pp. 67–74.

Rab, G. T.: Biomechanical aspects of Salter osteotomy. Clin. Orthop., 132:82, 1978.

Salter, R. B.: Innominate osteotomy in the treatment of congenital dislocation and subluxation of the hip. J. Bone Joint Surg., 43–B:518, 1961.

Salter, R. B.: The principle and technique of innominate osteotomy (motion picture with sound track). Chicago, Film Library, American Academy of Orthopedic Surgeons, 1966.

Tachdjian, M. O.: Salter's innominate osteotomy to derotate the maldirected acetabulum. In: Tachdjian, M. O. (ed.): Congenital Dislocation of the Hip. New York, Churchill Livingstone, 1982, pp. 525–541.

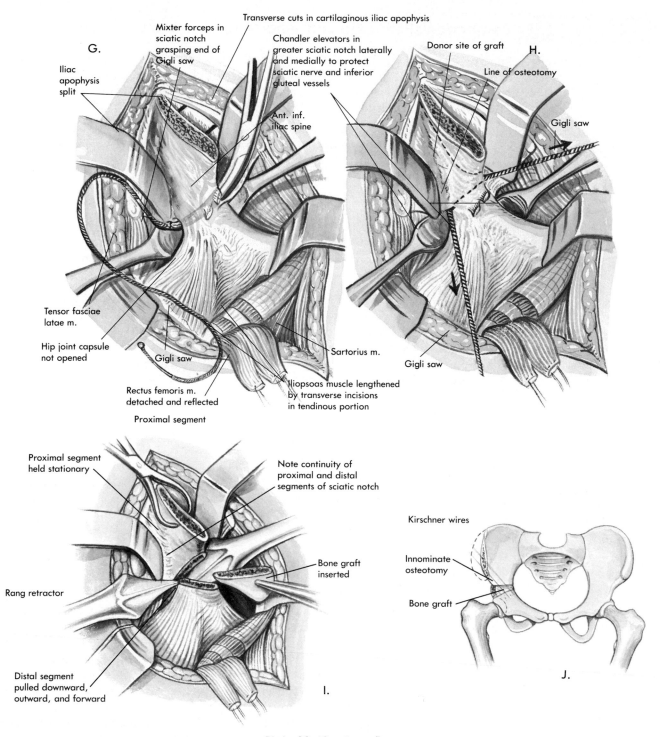

G.

Iliac apophysis split

Mixter forceps in sciatic notch grasping end of Gigli saw

Transverse cuts in cartilaginous iliac apophysis

Chandler elevators in greater sciatic notch laterally and medially to protect sciatic nerve and inferior gluteal vessels

Ant. inf. iliac spine

Tensor fasciae latae m.

Hip joint capsule not opened

Gigli saw

Rectus femoris m. detached and reflected

Proximal segment

Sartorius m.

Iliopsoas muscle lengthened by transverse incisions in tendinous portion

H.

Donor site of graft

Line of osteotomy

Gigli saw

Gigli saw

Proximal segment held stationary

Rang retractor

Distal segment pulled downward, outward, and forward

Note continuity of proximal and distal segments of sciatic notch

Bone graft inserted

I.

Kirschner wires

Innominate osteotomy

Bone graft

J.

Plate 82. (Continued)

PLATE 83 **Pemberton's Periacetabular Innominate Osteotomy**

Principle. The cut in the ilium begins in the anterosuperior and anteroinferior iliac spines and extends posteriorly around the acetabulum to the posterior rim of the triradiate cartilage, where it terminates. The fulcrum of rotation and angulation takes place at the triradiate cartilage.

Indications. Marked deficiency of the anterior and superolateral walls of the acetabulum in a child between two and six years of age with marked laxity of the capsule and hypermobility of the hip joint.

Requisites

1. Open triradiate cartilage.
2. Full range of hip motion.
3. Congruous hip joint.
4. Absence of myostatic contracture of the iliopsoas hip adductors.
5. Patient two to six years of age.

Preoperative Assessment. Perform computed tomography (CT), preferably with three-dimensional visualization of the cartilaginous acetabulum to depict the pathology. Be sure that the deficiency of the acetabulum is anterior and superior and not posterior. Posterior deficiency of the acetabulum is a contraindication to Pemberton's osteotomy.

Caution! Pemberton's pericapsular osteotomy can cause growth arrest and closure of the triradiate cartilage.

Blood for Transfusion. Yes.

Radiographic Control. Image intensifier.

Patient Position. The skin of the affected side of the abdomen and pelvis and the entire lower limb is prepared with the patient lying on his or her side, and is draped to allow free hip motion during surgery. Then the patient is placed completely supine. The operation is performed on a radiolucent operating table. It is imperative to have image intensifier fluoroscopy and radiographic control.

Operative Technique

A. The medial and lateral walls of the ilium and the hip joint are exposed through an anterolateral iliofemoral approach. The cartilaginous apophysis of the ilium is split according to Salter's technique. The sartorius muscle is sectioned at its origin from the anterior superior iliac spine, tagged with 00 Tycron or nonabsorbable suture, and reflected distally. Both heads of the rectus femoris are divided at their origin and reflected. The iliopsoas tendon is lengthened by transverse incisions. Pemberton's iliac osteotomy lengthens the pelvis. Division of the psoas tendon (not the iliacus muscle) decreases the pressure over the femoral head.

B. The ilium is exposed subperiosteally all the way posteriorly. The interval between the greater sciatic notch and the hip joint capsule posteriorly is developed gently and cautiously. The periosteal elevator meets resistance at the posterior limb of the triradiate cartilage. Chandler elevator retractors are placed in the greater sciatic notch medially and laterally in order to protect the sciatic nerve and the gluteal vessels and nerves. On the inner wall of the pelvis, the periosteum and the cartilaginous apophysis may be divided anteriorly to posteriorly at the level of the anteroinferior iliac spine as far as the sciatic notch; this facilitates opening up of the osteotomy.

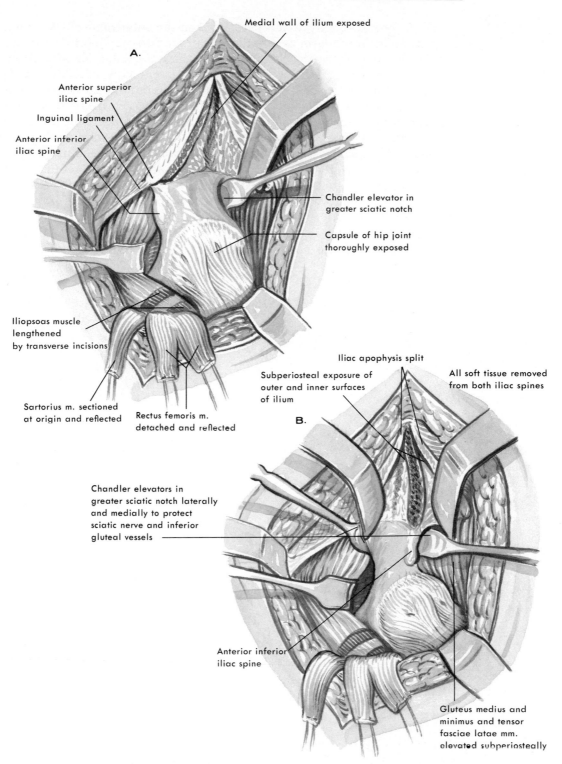

A.

Medial wall of ilium exposed

Anterior superior
iliac spine

Inguinal ligament

Anterior inferior
iliac spine

Chandler elevator in
greater sciatic notch

Capsule of hip joint
thoroughly exposed

Iliopsoas muscle
lengthened
by transverse incisions

Sartorius m. sectioned
at origin and reflected

Rectus femoris m.
detached and reflected

B.

Iliac apophysis split

Subperiosteal exposure of
outer and inner surfaces
of ilium

All soft tissue removed
from both iliac spines

Chandler elevators in
greater sciatic notch laterally
and medially to protect
sciatic nerve and inferior
gluteal vessels

Anterior inferior
iliac spine

Gluteus medius and
minimus and tensor
fasciae latae mm.
elevated subperiosteally

Plate 83. A.–I., Pemberton's periacetabular innominate osteotomy.

C.–E. The osteotomy is first performed on the outer table of the ilium. The cut is curvilinear, in the form of a semicircle around the hip joint on the lateral side at a level 1 cm. above the joint, between the anterosuperior and anteroinferior iliac spines. It is best to mark the line of osteotomy with indelible ink. The sharp edge of a thin osteotome is used to make the cut. The osteotomy ends at the posterior arm of the triradiate cartilage. This is most difficult to visualize if the exposure is inadequate. Image intensifier fluoroscopy with television control helps to determine the terminal point of the cut at the triradiate cartilage, which is anterior to the greater sciatic notch and posterior to the hip joint margin.

The next cut is made on the inner wall of the ilium and should be inferior to the level of the outer cut. The more distal the level of the inferior cut, the greater the extent of lateral coverage. If more anterior than superior coverage is required, the medial and lateral cuts in the ilium are parallel. The importance of sectioning the ilium as far posterior and inferior to the triradiate cartilage as possible cannot be overemphasized. Do not violate the articular cartilage of the acetabulum or enter the hip joint.

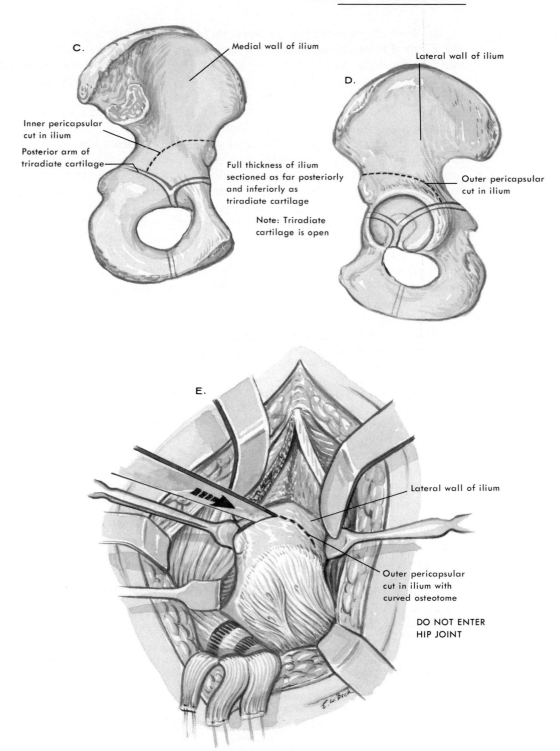

C.

Medial wall of ilium

Inner pericapsular
cut in ilium

Posterior arm of
triradiate cartilage

Full thickness of ilium
sectioned as far posteriorly
and inferiorly as
triradiate cartilage

Note: Triradiate
cartilage is open

D.

Lateral wall of ilium

Outer pericapsular
cut in ilium

E.

Lateral wall of ilium

Outer pericapsular
cut in ilium with
curved osteotome

DO NOT ENTER
HIP JOINT

Plate 83. (Continued)

F. With sharp curved osteotomes, join the cuts of the inner and outer table of the ilium. Periosteal elevators are used to mobilize the osteotomized fragments, and the inferior segment of the ilium is leveled laterally, anteriorly, and distally.

G. If necessary, a laminar spreader may be utilized to separate the iliac fragments. Be very gentle, however, and steady the upper segment of the ilium and push it distally. Take care not to fracture the acetabular segment by forceful manipulation or crushing with the laminar spreader.

H. and I. Next, resect a triangular wedge of bone from the anterior part of the iliac wing. In the young child, this author removes the wedge of bone more posteriorly and avoids the anterosuperior iliac spine. This gives greater stability to the iliac fragments. The wedge of bone graft may be shaped into a curve to fit the graft site. Pemberton and Coleman recommend that grooves be made on the opposing cancellous surfaces of the osteotomy. The graft is impacted into the grooves, and the osteotomized fragment is sufficiently stable to obviate the need for internal fixation. This author does not recommend cutting grooves because of problems with splintering and weakening of the acetabulum. The fragments are fixed internally with two threaded Kirschner pins or cancellous screws. The internal fixation allows one to remove the cast sooner, mobilize the hip, and prevent joint stiffness.

The sartorius muscle is reattached to its origin, the split iliac apophysis is sutured, and the wound closed in the usual fashion. A one-and-one-half hip spica cast is applied.

Postoperative Care. The cast is removed in four to six weeks, and the healing of the osteotomy is assessed by anteroposterior and oblique-lateral radiograms. The child is placed in bilateral split Russell's traction to mobilize the hip gradually. When joint motion and motor strength of the hip extensors, quadriceps, and triceps surae muscles are good, the child is allowed to ambulate. In the older patient, three-point crutch gait with toe touch on the limb that was operated on is used to protect the hip until the Trendelenburg test is negative.

REFERENCES

Coleman, S. S.: The incomplete pericapsular (Pemberton) and innominate (Salter) osteotomies. A complete analysis. Clin. Orthop., 98:116, 1974.

Faciszewski, T., Kiefer, G. N., and Coleman, S. S.: Pemberton osteotomy for residual acetabular dysplasia in children who have congenital dislocation of the hip. J. Bone Joint Surg., 75-A:650, 1993.

McKay, D. W.: Pemberton's innominate osteotomy: Indications, technique, results, pitfalls and complications: In: Tachdjian, M. O. (ed.): Congenital Dislocation of the Hip. New York: Churchill Livingstone, 1982, pp. 543–554.

McKay, D. W., Rising, E., and Keblisch, P.: Comparison of the innominate osteotomy (Salter) with the pericapsular osteotomy (Pemberton). Proc. Am. Acad. Orthop. Surg., 50–A:832, 1968.

Pemberton, P. A.: Osteotomy of the ilium with rotation of the acetabular roof for congenital dislocation of the hip. J. Bone Joint Surg, 40–A:724, 1958.

Pemberton, P. A.: Pericapsular osteotomy of the ilium for congenital subluxation and dislocation of the hip. J. Bone Joint Surg., 47–A:65, 1965.

Pemberton, P. A.: Pericapsular osteotomy of the ilium for the treatment of congenitally dislocated hips. Clin. Orthop., 98:41, 1974.

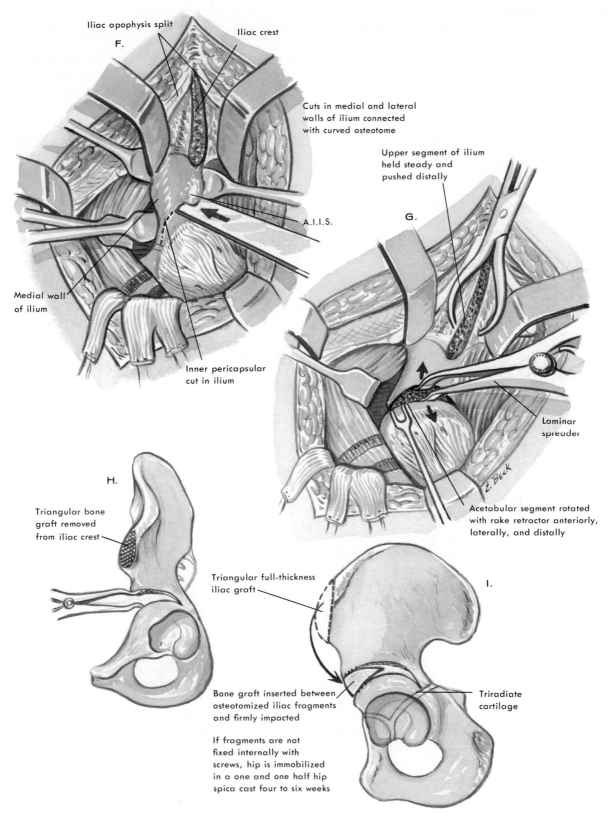

F.

Iliac apophysis split

Iliac crest

Cuts in medial and lateral
walls of ilium connected
with curved osteotome

Upper segment of ilium
held steady and
pushed distally

A.I.I.S.

G.

Medial wall
of ilium

Inner pericapsular
cut in ilium

Laminar
spreader

H.

Triangular bone
graft removed
from iliac crest

Triangular full-thickness
iliac graft

I.

Acetabular segment rotated
with rake retractor anteriorly,
laterally, and distally

Bone graft inserted between
osteotomized iliac fragments
and firmly impacted

Triradiate
cartilage

If fragments are not
fixed internally with
screws, hip is immobilized
in a one and one half hip
spica cast four to six weeks

E. Beck

Plate 83. (Continued)

PLATE 84   Pericapsular Acetabuloplasty

Principle. The acetabular roof is mobilized by a pericapsular covered dome osteotomy of the acetabulum. The procedure is extra-articular. Acetabuloplasty allows anterior, superior, and posterior coverage, whereas the Salter and Pemberton osteotomies provide only anterolateral coverage of the femoral head.

Salter's innominate osteotomy is a derotation procedure and does not change the capacity of the acetabulum, whereas acetabuloplasty does decrease the capacity of the acetabulum. Acetabuloplasty differs from Pemberton's pericapsular innominate osteotomy in the following way: In acetabuloplasty the acetabulum is mobilized through the cancellous bone of its roof; the growth of triradiate cartilage is not violated, and the inner cortex of the medial wall of the acetabulum is left intact.

Indications. Deficient and shallow acetabulum in a child under four years of age.

Requisites

1. Concentrically reduced hip.
2. Functional range of hip motion.
3. Absence of myostatic contracture of iliopsoas and hip adductors.
4. Congruous hip joint.
5. Patient 18 months of age or older.

Blood for Transfusion. Yes.

Radiographic Control. Image intensifier.

Patient Position. The patient is placed supine on a radiolucent operating table. The entire lower limb, the affected half of the pelvis, and the lower chest are washed with povidone-iodine (Betadine) soap, painted with Betadine solution, and draped to allow free motion of the hip and knee. The procedure can be performed during open reduction of a dislocated hip or staged at a later date.

Operative Technique

A. Expose the hip joint and lateral wall of the ilium through the anterolateral surgical approach, as described and illustrated in Plate 77.

B. If the hip joint is not concentrically reduced, perform open reduction of the hip first (Steps **H.–K.**, Plate 77).

The indication for acetabuloplasty is the deficient-shallow acetabulum. When the femoral head is placed deeply in the acetabulum, there will be a space between the femoral head and acetabular margin superoanteriorly and sometimes posteriorly.

C. Mark the line of osteotomy with the help of drill holes made with an electric drill. The osteotomy extends from the lateral wall of the ilium to its medial cortex; leave the cortex of the medial wall of the ilium intact. The line of osteotomy is curved parallel to the acetabular roof. It begins 7.5 to 10 mm. superior to the margin of the acetabulum and extends from the iliopectineal prominence anteriorly to the posterior limb of the triradiate cartilage posteriorly. It stops short of the growth plate of the Y-cartilage.

Avoid physeal damage! Do not cause growth arrest of the Y-cartilage and cartilaginous growth cells ("the umba zone") of the lateral rim of the acetabulum. It is best to make the drill holes and perform the osteotomy under image intensifier radiographic control.

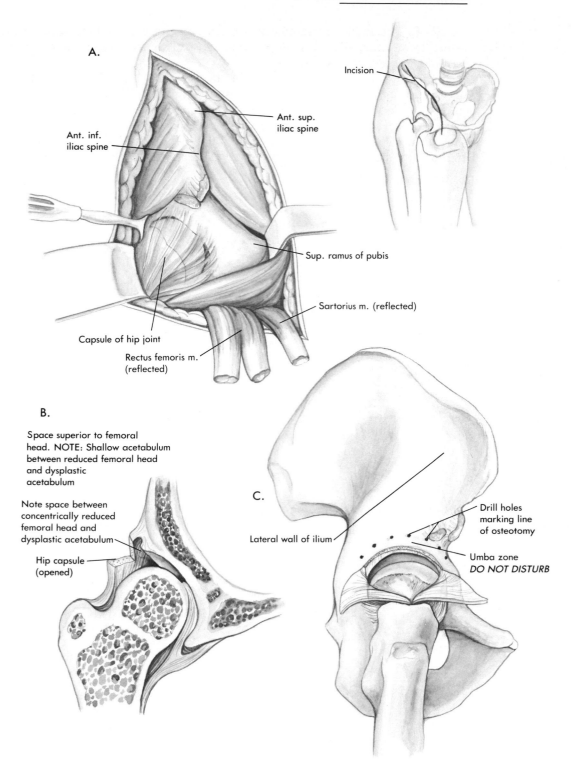

A.

Ant. inf.
iliac spine

Ant. sup.
iliac spine

Incision

Sup. ramus of pubis

Sartorius m. (reflected)

Capsule of hip joint

Rectus femoris m.
(reflected)

B.

Space superior to femoral
head. NOTE: Shallow acetabulum
between reduced femoral head
and dysplastic
acetabulum

Note space between
concentrically reduced
femoral head and
dysplastic acetabulum

Hip capsule
(opened)

C.

Lateral wall of ilium

Drill holes
marking line
of osteotomy

Umba zone
DO NOT DISTURB

Plate 84. A.–J., Pericapsular acetabuloplasty.

D.–F. The plane of osteotomy is curved in three directions: anteroposteriorly, laterally to medially, and superoinferiorly. The osteotomy is performed with straight and curved osteotomes.

With the help of broad periosteal elevators mobilize the acetabulum through its cancellous roof. The cartilaginous and bony roof of the acetabulum are turned inferiorly, laterally and anteriorly, covering the concentrically reduced femoral head anteriorly, superiorly, and posteriorly.

Caution! Leave the medial cortex of the ilium and the posterior limb of the triradiate cartilage intact.

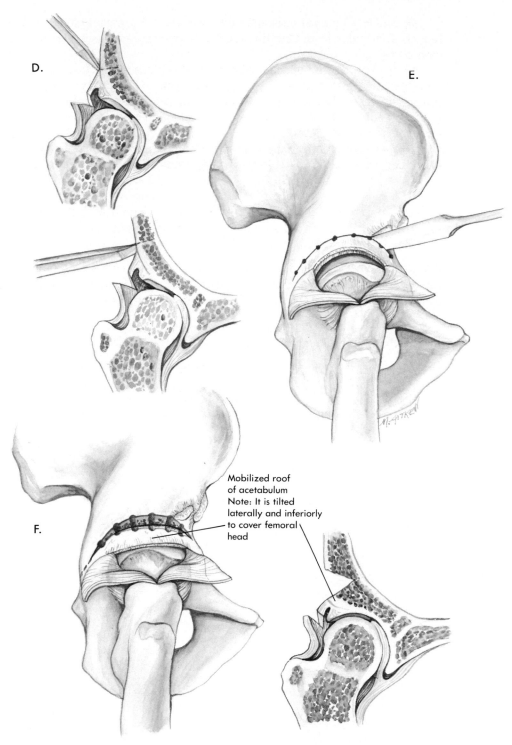

D.

E.

F.

Mobilized roof
of acetabulum
Note: It is tilted
laterally and inferiorly
to cover femoral
head

Plate 84. (Continued)

G. and **H.** Next, take three or four wedges of bicortical bone graft of appropriate length and width from the iliac crest and insert them securely into the cleft of the osteotomy.

I and **J.** Pack the spaces between the wedges of cortical bone with cancellous bone graft from the lateral wall of the ilium. Ordinarily, internal fixation with pins and screws is not required. Following adequate acetabuloplasty, the concentrically reduced femoral head will be fully covered, with no space between the femoral head and acetabulum.

If open reduction of the hip is performed, a capsulorrhaphy is performed, as described in Plate 77. The split cartilaginous iliac apophysis is tautly closed. The rectus femoris and sartorius muscles are reattached at their origin.

The wound is closed in the usual manner. The skin closure should be subcuticular with 00 nylon. Apply a one-and-one-half hip spica cast, with the patient's hip immobilized in a stable position. Avoid extreme positions of the hip in order to prevent compression of articular cartilage and osteonecrosis.

Postoperative Care. The cast is removed in six weeks. Radiograms of the hip are made with the cast off. The hip is gradually mobilized. Full weight-bearing is not allowed until four to six weeks after removal of the solid cast.

REFERENCES

Dega, W.: Transiliac osteotomy in the treatment of congenital hip dysplasia. Chir. Narzadow Ruchu Orthop. Pol., 39:601, 1974.

Hughes, J. R.: The surgical treatment of the dysplastic acetabulum in childhood. Proceedings 12th Congress International Society of Orthopedic Surgery, Traumatology. Tel Aviv, Oct. 9–12, 1972.

Hughes, J. R.: Acetabular dysplasia in congenital dislocation of the hip. Proc. R. Soc. Med., 67:1178, 1974.

Hughes, J. R.: Acetabular dysplasia and acetabuloplasty. In: Tachdjian, M. O. (ed.): Congenital Dislocation of the Hip. New York: Churchill Livingstone, 1982, pp. 665–693.

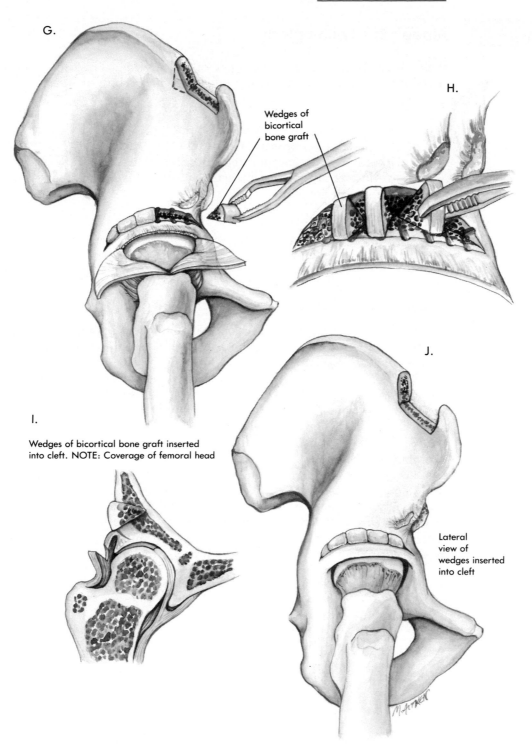

G.

H.

Wedges of
bicortical
bone graft

I.

Wedges of bicortical bone graft inserted
into cleft. NOTE: Coverage of femoral head

J.

Lateral
view of
wedges inserted
into cleft

Plate 84. (Continued)

PLATE 85   ## Albee's Shelf Arthroplasty

Indications. Dysplasia and deficiency of the acetabulum with uncoverage of the femoral head in which acetabular enlargement is required.

Requisites

1. Infant or child up to six years of age.
2. Complete and concentric reduction of the hip.
3. Normal or near-normal range of hip motion.
4. Absence of myostatic contracture of iliopsoas and hip adductors.
5. Congruous hip joint.

Blood for Transfusion. Yes.

Radiographic Control. Image intensifier.

Patient Position. The patient is placed supine on a radiolucent operating table with the ipsilateral pelvis raised 15 to 20 degrees on a pad.

Operative Technique

A. The hip is exposed in a routine iliofemoral approach through a "bikini" incision (see Plate 82). Often, the Albee shelf is performed simultaneously with open reduction of the hip.

B. The tendon of the reflected head is detached and reflected anteriorly. The capsule of the hip joint is exposed anteriorly, superiorly, and posteriorly. Identify the joint line by image intensifier radiography by inserting a small Kirschner wire into the capsule. The reflected head of rectus femoris is anterior.

C. The level of osteotomy is immediately above the cartilaginous roof of the acetabulum. Make drill holes parallel to the roof of the acetabulum. The line of osteotomy is curvilinear, extending more anteriorly if there is excessive acetabular and femoral antetorsion and more posteriorly if the acetabulum is deficient posteriorly. It extends from the iliopectineal eminence to the posterior limb of the triradiate cartilage. The cut stops short of the growth plate of the Y cartilage. The osteotomy extends from the lateral wall of the ilium to its medial cortex, but the medial cortex is not divided. Also, the line of osteotomy is directed superoinferiorly.

A.

Incision

B.

Tensor fasciae latae m.

Kirschner wire

Iliopsoas m.

Sartorius m. (reflected)

Rectus femoris m. (reflected)

Hip capsule

Labrum

Kirschner wire

Capsule

NOTE: Dysplastic acetabulum and marked uncoverage of femoral head

C.

Rectus femoris m. (reflected)

Greater sciatic notch

Drill holes making curvilinear line of osteotomy

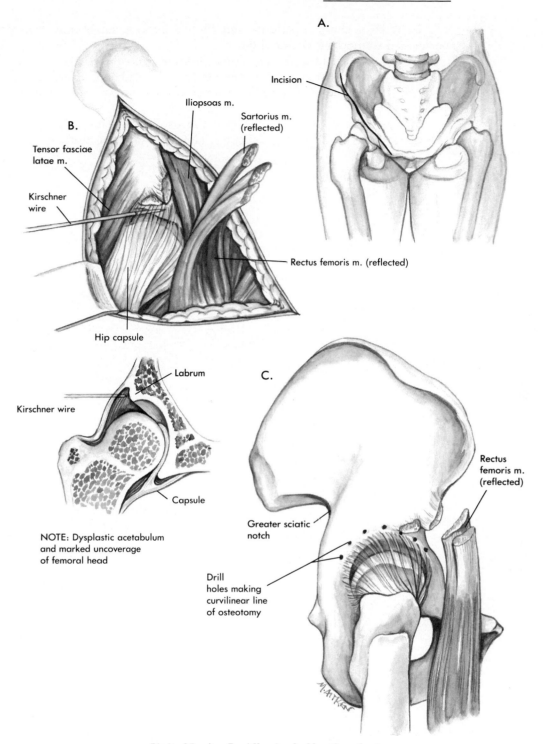

Plate 85. A.–J., Albee's shelf arthroplasty.

D. With a sharp, straight, and then a curved osteotome, the osteotomy is performed connecting the drill holes.

E. The acetabulum is mobilized through cancellous bone of its roof. The cartilage and bony roof of the acetabulum are turned inferiorly and laterally covering the concentrically reduced femoral head anteriorly, superiorly, and posteriorly.

F. Place a curved osteotome into the osteotomy site, with the concave side facing superiorly, and make a superior slot deep into the cleft.

D.

Straight osteotome

E.

Acetabular roof
turned inferiorly
and laterally

F.

Curved osteotome
making a notch
superomedially

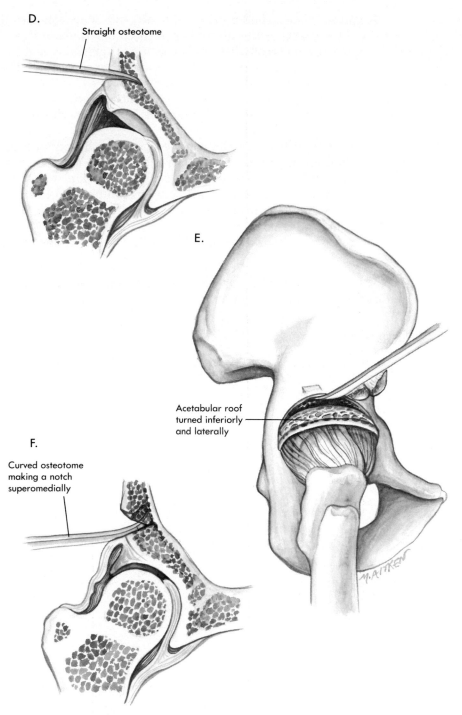

Plate 85. (Continued)

G. and **H.** Take a solid unicortical bone graft of appropriate size from the crest and the lateral wall of the ilium. Leave the inner table of the ilium intact. Turn down the acetabular roof with a large periosteal elevator, and insert the graft into the cleft. The lateral margin of the graft extends beyond the acetabular rim covering the femoral head.

I. Then triangular wedges of cortical and cancellous bone of appropriate size are taken from the crest of the ilium and inserted superior to the graft in the cleft and firmly impacted into place.

J. Any spaces between the bone wedges are packed with strips of cancellous bone taken from the lateral wall of the ilium, which should extend laterally to the edge of the solid plate of bone graft. Internal fixation with pins or screws is not required. There should be no space between the femoral head and the acetabular roof. The gap should be firmly closed. Radiograms are made to check the adequacy of coverage of the femoral head.

Close the wound in the usual fashion, and apply a one-and-one-half hip spica cast.

Postoperative Care. The cast is removed when there is adequate bone healing, ordinarily in about six weeks.

REFERENCE

Albee, F. H.: The bone graft wedge. Its use in the treatment of relapsing, acquired and congenital dislocation of hip. N. Y. Med. J., 102:433, 1915.

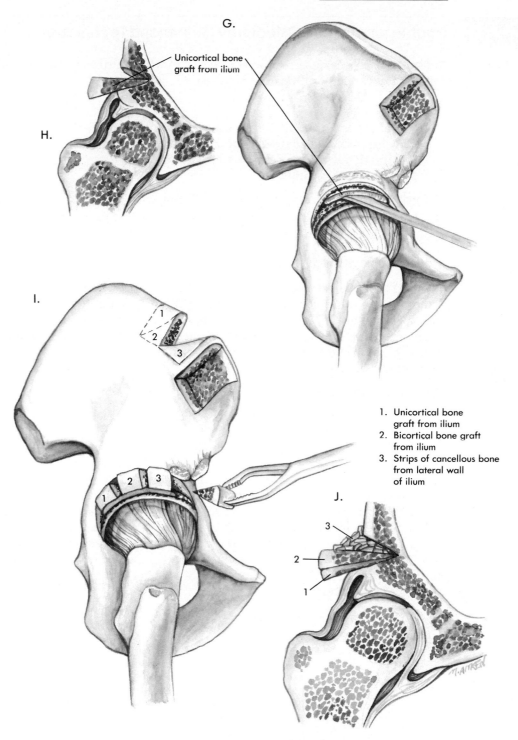

G.

H.

Unicortical bone
graft from ilium

I.

1. Unicortical bone
   graft from ilium
2. Bicortical bone graft
   from ilium
3. Strips of cancellous bone
   from lateral wall
   of ilium

J.

Plate 85. (Continued)

PLATE 86   Double Innominate Osteotomy (Sutherland Technique)

Indications. Hip dysplasia in an adolescent in whom anterior, lateral, and posterior coverage of the femoral head is required.

Requisites

1. Congruous hip that can be concentrically reduced.
2. A hip with adequate articular cartilage space.
3. Functional range of hip motion.
4. No upper age limit.

Contraindications. Incongruous and stiff hip with loss of its articular cartilage space and degenerative arthritis.

Blood for Transfusion. Yes.

Radiographic Control. Image intensifier.

Patient Position. The operation is performed with the patient in supine position on a radiolucent table. It is vital that image intensifier fluoroscopy and radiographic control be utilized. The bladder is emptied at the time of surgery by inserting a Foley catheter, which will remain in place for two days. Skin preparation and draping, which should include the contralateral hip, is carried out. Salter's innominate osteotomy is performed first, as illustrated in Plate 82.

Operative Technique

A. A transverse suprapubic incision 7 to 10 cm. long is centered over the symphysis pubis.

B. The subcutaneous tissue and suprapubic fat are divided in line with the skin incision, and the wound edges are retracted. The spermatic cords in the male or the round ligaments in the female are retracted laterally. The aponeurosis of the external abdominal oblique muscle is identified.

C. By dull dissection, the attachments of the rectus abdominus and pyramidalis muscles are identified and sharply sectioned from their attachment on the upper border of the pubis. Do not injure the spermatic cords or the round ligaments.

D. Next, the tendons of the adductor longus and gracilis muscles are identified at their origin, freed, and elevated with a periosteal elevator from the anterior surface of the pubis.

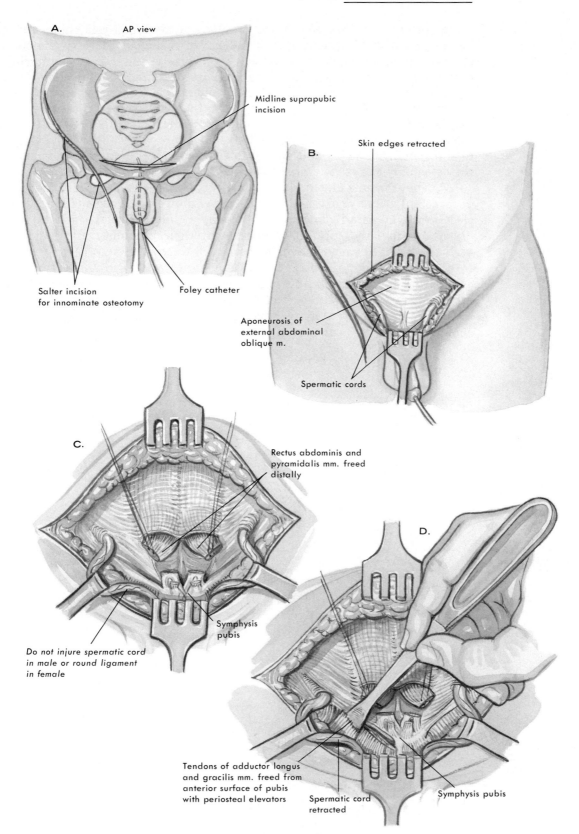

A. AP view

Midline suprapubic incision

Salter incision for innominate osteotomy

Foley catheter

B. Skin edges retracted

Aponeurosis of external abdominal oblique m.

Spermatic cords

C.

Rectus abdominis and pyramidalis mm. freed distally

Symphysis pubis

Do not injure spermatic cord in male or round ligament in female

D.

Tendons of adductor longus and gracilis mm. freed from anterior surface of pubis with periosteal elevators

Spermatic cord retracted

Symphysis pubis

Plate 86. A.–M., Double innominate osteotomy (Sutherland technique).

E. Insert a Keith needle in the cartilage of the symphysis pubis, and confirm its position with an anteroposterior radiogram of the pelvis. Next, the periosteum of the symphysis pubis is sectioned transversely and elevated anteriorly and posteriorly, and Chandler retractors are passed around the pubic bone to protect soft tissues during surgery. The internal pudendal artery curves around the medial margin of the inferior ramus of the pubis; the subperiosteal dissection should be gentle and cautious to prevent inadvertent injury to this vessel. The level of osteotomy is marked by drilling a Kirschner wire vertically immediately lateral to the symphysis pubis and medial to the obturator foramen. Again, location of the osteotomy site is visualized by image intensifier radiography.

F. The urogenic diaphragm attaches at the inferior margin of the pubis. The deep dorsal nerve and vessels of the penis pierce the urogenic diaphragm very close to the arcuate ligaments of the penis in the midline. These vital structures are away from the surgical approach, but their proximity and position in the midline should be remembered. With a small rongeur, remove a wedge of bone 0.7 to 1.3 cm. wide from the pubic bone. Do not enter the obturator foramen.

G. and **H.** The lateral pubic segment is elevated with a towel clip, and the attachments of the lower part of the periosteum of the urogenic diaphragm are freed from the inferior margin of the pubis. The stripping of the urogenic diaphragm should extend 2 to 3 cm. laterally.

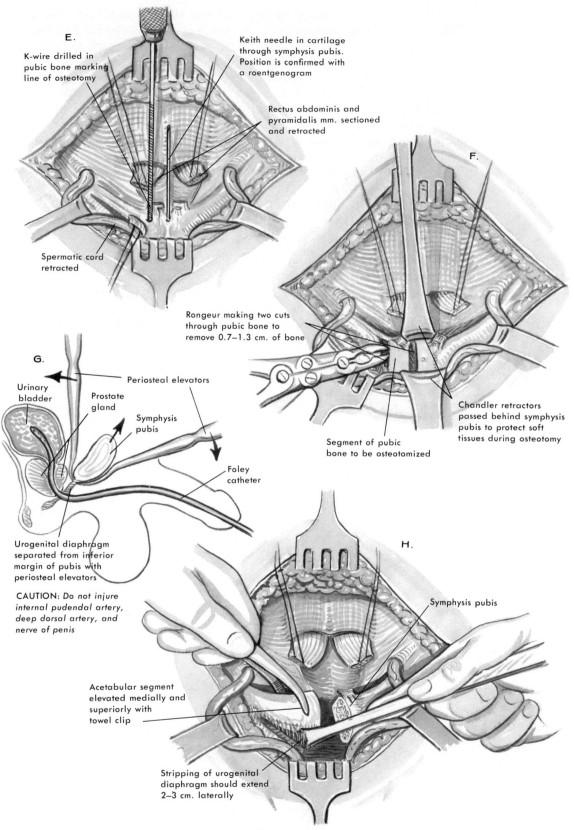

E.

K-wire drilled in pubic bone marking line of osteotomy

Keith needle in cartilage through symphysis pubis. Position is confirmed with a roentgenogram

Rectus abdominis and pyramidalis mm. sectioned and retracted

Spermatic cord retracted

F.

Rongeur making two cuts through pubic bone to remove 0.7–1.3 cm. of bone

Chandler retractors passed behind symphysis pubis to protect soft tissues during osteotomy

Segment of pubic bone to be osteotomized

G.

Periosteal elevators

Urinary bladder

Prostate gland

Symphysis pubis

Foley catheter

Urogenital diaphragm separated from inferior margin of pubis with periosteal elevators

CAUTION: *Do not injure internal pudendal artery, deep dorsal artery, and nerve of penis*

H.

Symphysis pubis

Acetabular segment elevated medially and superiorly with towel clip

Stripping of urogenital diaphragm should extend 2–3 cm. laterally

Plate 86. (Continued)

I. and **J.** Use a laminar spreader at the site of the Salter iliac osteotomy to mobilize the lateral segment. (Do not use a laminar spreader to effect acetabular rotation.) With a towel clip, the lateral acetabular segment is pulled downward and forward and the medial end of the acetabular segment is pulled upward and medially. The acetabular segment should be displaced superiorly at the site of the pubic osteotomy. By this maneuver, the acetabulum is rotated anteriorly and laterally and the hip joint is displaced medially.

K. One or two medium-sized threaded Steinmann pins are used to transfix the pubic osteotomy. Do not direct the Steinmann pins in a posterior or inferior direction.

L. and **M.** The osteotomized iliac segments of the Salter osteotomy are fixed with two heavy threaded Kirschner wires transfixing the graft; in the distal fragment, they should be posterior and medial to the acetabulum. Closed-suction drainage tubes are inserted, and the wound is closed. A one-and-one-half hip spica cast is applied.

Postoperative Care. In children and adolescents, the cast is removed at six weeks and radiograms are made to determine the healing of the osteotomy. The pubic pin is removed, and gradually the hip is mobilized. The iliac pins are not removed for six months or more. The hip that was operated on is protected with a three-point crutch gait until its functional strength is restored and the Trendelenburg test is negative.

REFERENCES

Sutherland, D. H.: Double innominate osteotomy in congenital hip dislocation or dysplasia. In: Tachdjian, M. O. (ed.): Congenital Dislocation of the Hip. New York: Churchill Livingstone, 1982, pp. 595–608.

Sutherland, D. H., and Greenfield, R.: Medial pubic osteotomy in difficult Salter procedures. (Proc. West. Orthop. Assoc.) J. Bone Joint Surg., 57–A:135, 1975.

Sutherland, D. H., and Greenfield, R.: Double innominate osteotomy. J. Bone Joint Surg., 59–A:1082, 1977.

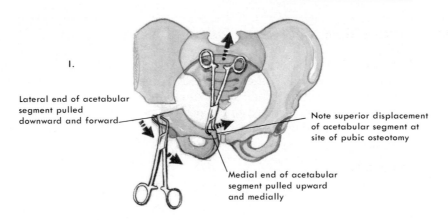

I.

Lateral end of acetabular segment pulled downward and forward

Note superior displacement of acetabular segment at site of pubic osteotomy

Medial end of acetabular segment pulled upward and medially

Arrows show directions of pull to produce anterior and lateral rotation of acetabulum and medial shift of hip joint

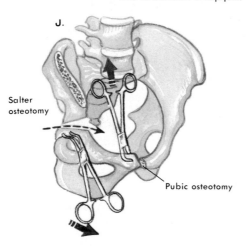

J.

Salter osteotomy

Pubic osteotomy

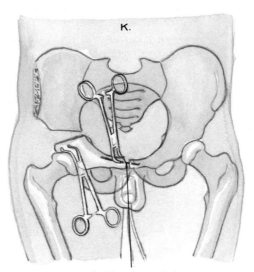

K.

Position of acetabular segment maintained while pubic osteotomy is secured with one or two medium-sized Steinmann pins

L.

Two heavy threaded Kirschner wires transfixing graft

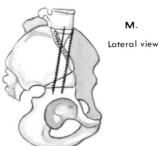

M.

Lateral view

Note anterior displacement of acetabulum and anterior rotation of acetabular segment at site of Salter osteotomy

Plate 86. (Continued)

PLATE 87   Steel's Triple Innominate Osteotomy

Principle. Three cuts are made: the first, through the ilium similar to Salter's innominate osteotomy; the second, through the ramus of the pubis; and the third, through the ischium. The three osteotomies allow free mobility of the acetabular segment, which is directed to the desired position, fully covering the femoral head by normal articular cartilage and providing stability of the hip in weight-bearing position.

Indications

1. Dysplastic hip in an adolescent that requires more than 25 degrees of abduction to contain the femoral head concentrically in the acetabulum.

2. Bilateral dysplasia of the hip in an adolescent in whom less than 25 degrees of abduction is required to concentrically contain the hip. In the adolescent in whom the symphysis pubis is not flexible, the bilateral Salter technique is contraindicated because if it is performed on one side, it increases the uncoverage of the femoral head on the opposite side.

3. Hip joint instability and pain.

Requisites

1. A congruous hip that can be concentrically reduced.
2. A hip with adequate articular cartilage space.
3. Functional range of hip motion.
4. No upper age limit.

Contraindications

1. Incongruous and stiff hip with loss of its articular cartilage space and degenerative arthritis.

2. A femoral head that is enlarged, flattened, and uncovered. Triple innominate osteotomy does not enlarge the capacity of the hip joint. Rotating the acetabulum to cover the anterior and lateral parts of the femoral head uncovers its posterior part and results in posterior instability of the hip joint—a biomechanically undesirable problem in the adult when total joint replacement is performed.

3. Paralytic hip subluxation–dysplasia (such as in cerebral palsy or myelomeningocele). The results of shelf acetabular augmentation are more effective.

Blood for Transfusion. Yes.

Radiographic Control. Image intensifier.

Special Instrumentation. Rang retractors, Gigli saw, nerve stimulator.
Note. Ask the anesthesiologist not to paralyze the patient until ischial osteotomy is performed.

Patient Position. The patient is placed supine on a radiolucent operating table, and the affected hemipelvis, abdomen, lower part of the chest, and entire lower limb are prepared sterile and draped. Preparation of the buttock inferiorly and appropriate shielding of the perineum are important. The draping should allow free motion of the hip and knee during the operation. A nerve stimulator should be available.

Operative Technique

A. and B. The acetabulum is freed and mobilized by osteotomies of the ischium, superior ramus of the pubis, and ilium from the greater sciatic notch posteriorly to an area between the anterior superior and anterior inferior iliac spines anteriorly. The acetabular segment is rotated to cover the femoral head anteriorly and laterally; the iliac osteotomy is stabilized by a wedge of iliac bone and internal fixation with threaded Steinmann pins or screws.

A.

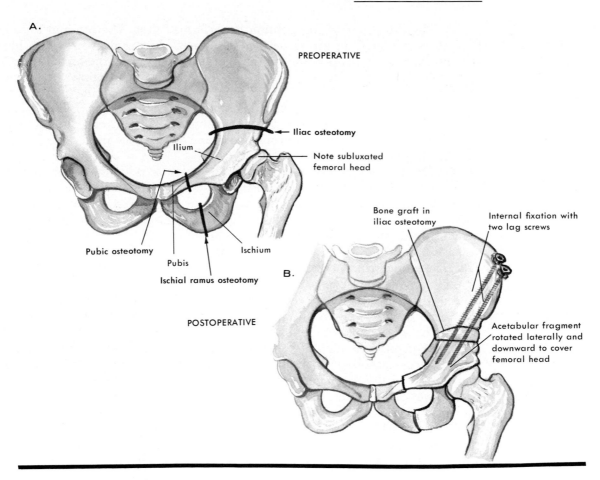

PREOPERATIVE

Iliac osteotomy

Ilium

Note subluxated femoral head

Pubic osteotomy

Pubis

Ischial ramus osteotomy

Ischium

Bone graft in iliac osteotomy

Internal fixation with two lag screws

B.

POSTOPERATIVE

Acetabular fragment rotated laterally and downward to cover femoral head

C.

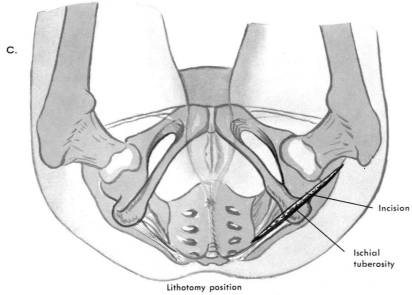

Incision

Ischial tuberosity

Lithotomy position

Plate 87. A.–N., Steel's triple innominate osteotomy.

C. The osteotomy of the ischium is performed first. The hip and knee of the limb to be operated on are flexed at 90 degrees. (In the drawing, both hips are shown in the lithotomy position; on the operating table, only the hip on the affected side is flexed.) An assistant holds the limb with the hip in neutral position with respect to rotation and adduction–abduction. The ischial tuberosity, which is readily palpated, is marked with indelible ink. A 7- to 9-cm. long transverse incision is made 1 cm. proximal to the subnatal crease and centered over the ischial tuberosity. The subcutaneous tissue and deep fascia are incised in line with the skin incision.

D. The inferior border of the gluteus maximus is delineated and retracted laterally. The sciatic nerve lies immediately deep to the medial and inferior fibers of the gluteus maximus. Watch for the sciatic nerve and be cautious. It is not necessary to expose the nerve, but its visualization helps to protect it from inadvertent injury during surgery.

The ischial bursa, which is superficial to the ischial tuberosity, is identified. The three hamstring muscles take origin from the ischial tuberosity: the biceps femoris is the most superficial, the semitendinosus (which is membranous at its origin) is lateral to the biceps femoris, and the semimembranosus (which is tendinous near its origin) is immediately proximal and lateral to the semitendinosus. The sciatic nerve and semimembranosus muscle look alike; they should not be mistaken for each other. After its exit from the greater sciatic notch, the sciatic nerve courses posterior to the ramus of the ischium and down the limb parallel and lateral to the semimembranosus. It lies far enough laterally to stay out of harm's way. If in doubt, use a nerve stimulator. (The leg will jump! Be sure that the patient's foot does not hit the assistant's head, contaminating the field.)

E. and **F.** The origins of the biceps femoris, the semitendinosus, and the semimembranosus may be detached and tagged with sutures for later reattachment. The periosteum over the ischial ramus and tuberosity is incised.

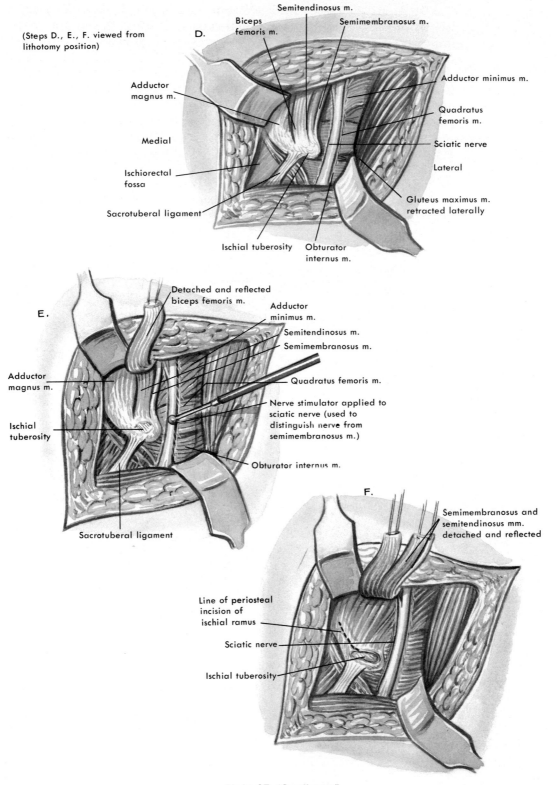

(Steps D., E., F. viewed from lithotomy position)

D.

Semitendinosus m.

Biceps femoris m.

Semimembranosus m.

Adductor magnus m.

Adductor minimus m.

Quadratus femoris m.

Medial

Sciatic nerve

Lateral

Ischiorectal fossa

Gluteus maximus m. retracted laterally

Sacrotuberal ligament

Ischial tuberosity

Obturator internus m.

E.

Detached and reflected biceps femoris m.

Adductor minimus m.

Semitendinosus m.

Semimembranosus m.

Adductor magnus m.

Quadratus femoris m.

Nerve stimulator applied to sciatic nerve (used to distinguish nerve from semimembranosus m.)

Ischial tuberosity

Obturator internus m.

Sacrotuberal ligament

F.

Semimembranosus and semitendinosus mm. detached and reflected

Line of periosteal incision of ischial ramus

Sciatic nerve

Ischial tuberosity

Plate 87. (Continued)

G. A curved kidney pedicle forceps is passed subperiosteally superior to the ischial tuberosity, around the ischial ramus, and into the obturator foramen. The importance of staying beneath the periosteum cannot be overemphasized. The internal pudendal vessels and nerves should be protected; they run in Alcock's canal, enclosed in the obturator internus fascia, and emerge from the pelvis to innervate and supply blood to the external genitalia. *The site and level of osteotomy are verified by image intensifier fluoroscopy.* The lower part of the ischial ramus is sectioned obliquely with an osteotome directed lateromedially.

H. The detached hamstring muscles are resutured to their origin. Hemostasis is obtained; blood loss is usually minimal. Catheters are inserted for closed suction.

I. The edge of the gluteus maximus is sutured to the fascial envelope, and the wound is closed in the usual fashion. Because this phase of the operation is performed in close proximity to the perineum, it is advisable to change instruments, gown, and gloves. Appropriate redraping is recommended for the anterior approach.

Patient in lithotomy position

G.

Kidney pedicle forceps passed
behind ischium subperiosteally
elevating origin of obturator mm.

Note: Kidney pedicle forceps
exteriorized at inferior margin
of ischium, kept in contact
with bone to protect internal
pudendal vessels and nerves

Sciatic nerve

Osteotome sectioning
ischial ramus obliquely

H.

Hamstrings resutured
to ischial tuberosity

I.

Gluteus maximus m. resutured
to fascial envelope

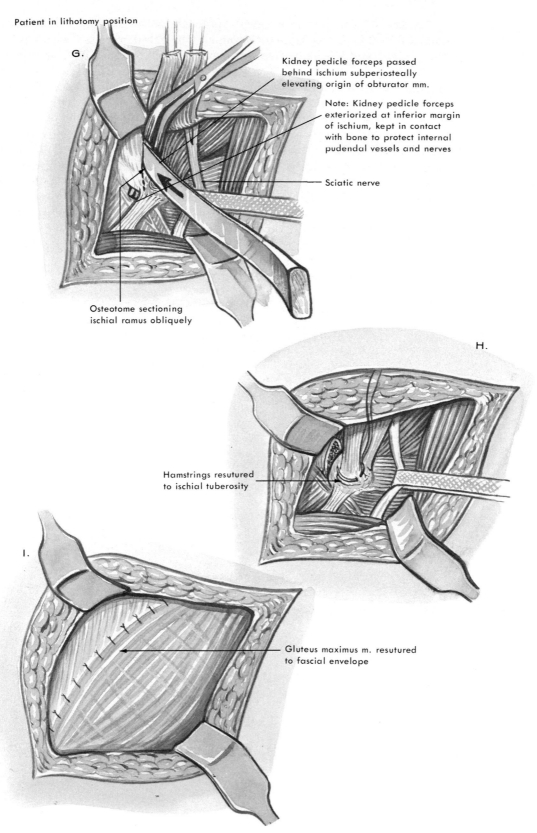

Plate 87. (Continued)

J. and **K.** The second surgical approach is the standard iliofemoral one employed for other innominate osteotomies. The cartilaginous iliac apophysis is split; the gluteal and iliac muscles are elevated subperiosteally from the lateral and medial walls of the ilium. The sartorius is sectioned at its origin and reflected distally, and the lateral attachments of the inguinal ligament are detached and reflected medially. Both heads of the rectus femoris are divided, elevated, and reflected distally. Keeping the dissection subperiosteal and deep to the iliacus and psoas muscles protects the femoral nerve and vessels. Exposure of the superior ramus of the pubis is facilitated by flexing the hip. The ramus is subperiosteally exposed circumferentially 1 cm. medial to the iliopectineal prominence. There is a tendency to perform the osteotomy too far laterally—in the medial wall of the acetabulum; verify the site radiographically. A curved kidney pedicle forceps is introduced subperiosteally from the upper border of the ramus into the obturator foramen. Avoid injury to the obturator vessels and nerves. If the pubic bone is very thick, a second forceps may be introduced subperiosteally below and pushed superiorly to meet the upper forceps. The pubic bone is osteotomized with a sharp osteotome directed posteromedially—15 degrees medial from the perpendicular.

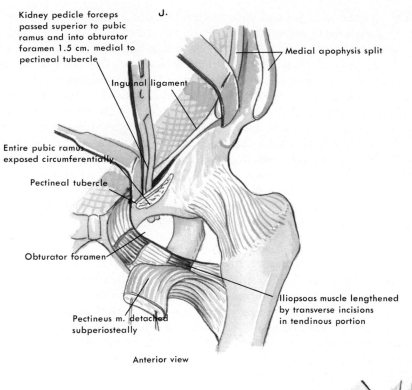

J.

Kidney pedicle forceps passed superior to pubic ramus and into obturator foramen 1.5 cm. medial to pectineal tubercle

Medial apophysis split

Inguinal ligament

Entire pubic ramus exposed circumferentially

Pectineal tubercle

Obturator foramen

Iliopsoas muscle lengthened by transverse incisions in tendinous portion

Pectineus m. detached subperiosteally

Anterior view

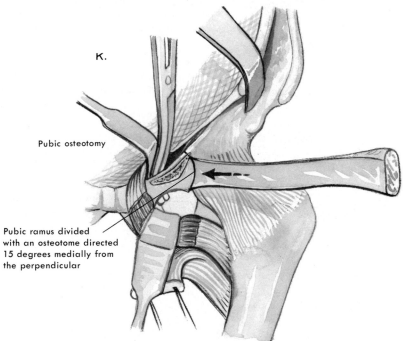

K.

Pubic osteotomy

Pubic ramus divided with an osteotome directed 15 degrees medially from the perpendicular

Plate 87. (Continued)

L. The iliac bone is divided with a Gigli saw, utilizing the technique described for Salter's innominate osteotomy.

M. After sectioning the iliac bone, mobilize the acetabular segment with a laminar spreader and periosteal elevator. When free, the acetabular segment is manipulated into the desired position to cover the femoral head. Avoid lateralization of the acetabulum; the medially directed oblique cuts of the ischium and pubis will facilitate its medial shift. With the acetabulum in the proper position, remove a triangular fragment of bone from the superior margin of the ilium.

N. The iliac segments and the graft are transfixed with two threaded Steinmann pins. The pins may be introduced from below and directed superiorly into the upper iliac segment, or from superior to inferior. They should not penetrate the hip joint. This author prefers fixation with two cancellous screws or two pronged tubular plates as in the Wagner technique. Immobilization of the hip in a hip spica cast is unnecessary. (Steel and Coleman apply a one-and-one-half hip spica cast.)

Postoperative Care. I recommend placing the patient in bilateral split Russell's traction. Gluteus medius and minimus, gluteus maximus, quadriceps femoris, and triceps surae exercises are begun as soon as possible. The patient is allowed to be up and around, walking with three-point, toe-touch crutch gait for 10 to 12 weeks.

Steel and Coleman retain the hip spica cast for eight to ten weeks. When the triple osteotomies show healing, partial weight-bearing with crutches is allowed. Full weight-bearing is allowed six months postoperatively, at which time the internal fixation device is removed.

REFERENCES

Guille, J. T., Forlin, E., Kumar, S. J., and MacEwen, G. D.: Triple osteotomy of the innominate bone in treatment of developmental dysplasia of the hip. J. Pediatr. Orthop., 12:718, 1992.

LeCoeur, P.: Correction des défauts d'orientation de l'articulation coxofémorale par ostéotomie de l'isthme iliaque. Rev. Chir. Orthop., 51:211, 1965.

LeCoeur, P.: Osteotomie isthmique de bascule. In: Chapchal, G. (ed.): Beckenosteotomie—Pfannendachplastik. Stuttgart, Thieme, 1965.

Steel, H. H.: Triple osteotomy of the innominate bone. J. Bone Joint Surg., 55–A:343, 1973.

Steel, H. H.: Triple ostotomy of the innominate bone. A procedure to accomplish coverage of the dislocated or subluxated femoral head in the older patient. Orthop. Clin., 122:16, 1977.

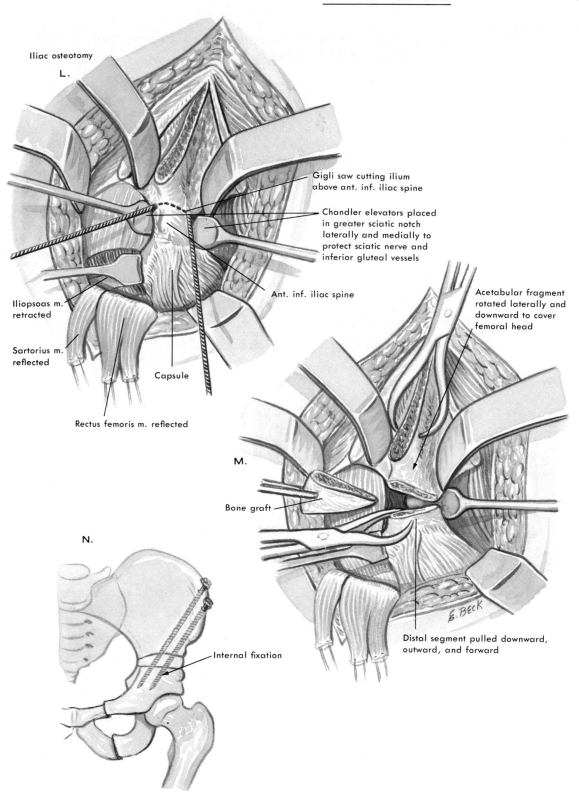

Iliac osteotomy

L.

Gigli saw cutting ilium above ant. inf. iliac spine

Chandler elevators placed in greater sciatic notch laterally and medially to protect sciatic nerve and inferior gluteal vessels

Ant. inf. iliac spine

Iliopsoas m. retracted

Sartorius m. reflected

Capsule

Rectus femoris m. reflected

Acetabular fragment rotated laterally and downward to cover femoral head

M.

Bone graft

E. BECK

Distal segment pulled downward, outward, and forward

N.

Internal fixation

Plate 87. (Continued)

PLATE 88 ## Periacetabular Triple Innominate Osteotomy Through the Subinguinal Adductor Approach

Indications

1. Dysplastic hip in an adolescent that requires more than 25 degrees of abduction to contain the femoral head concentrically in the acetabulum.

2. Bilateral dysplasia of the hip in an adolescent in whom less than 25 degrees of abduction is required to concentrically contain the hip.

Requisites

1. A congruous hip that can be concentrically reduced.
2. A hip with adequate articular cartilage space.
3. Functional range of hip motion.
4. No upper age limit.

Contraindications. Incongruous and stiff hip with loss of its articular cartilage space and degenerative arthritis.

Blood for Transfusion. Yes.

Radiographic Control. Image intensifier.

Special Instrumentation. Rang retractors, Gigli saw, nerve stimulator.

Note. Ask the anesthesiologist not to paralyze the patient until ischial osteotomy is performed.

Principle. This approach allows performance of a triple innominate osteotomy close to the hip joint and avoids turning the patient from prone to supine and repreparing and redraping (as in the Tönnis gluteal approach).

Patient Position. The patient is placed in completely supine position on a radiolucent operating table so that a C-arm image intensifier can be used. The abdomen, affected side of the pelvis, perineal area, and entire lower limb are prepared and draped to allow free motion of the hip. Adequate shielding, preparing, and draping of the perineum is crucial.

Operative Technique

A. Two separate skin incisions are used: first, an oblique iliac incision for the usual Salter innominate osteotomy; and second, a transverse adductor incision, such as is used for routine adductor myotomy.

B.–D. The subcutaneous tissue and fascia are divided. The adductor longus, gracilis, and adductor brevis muscles are detached at their origins, tagged, and retracted distally. Avoid injury to the obturator nerves and vessels.

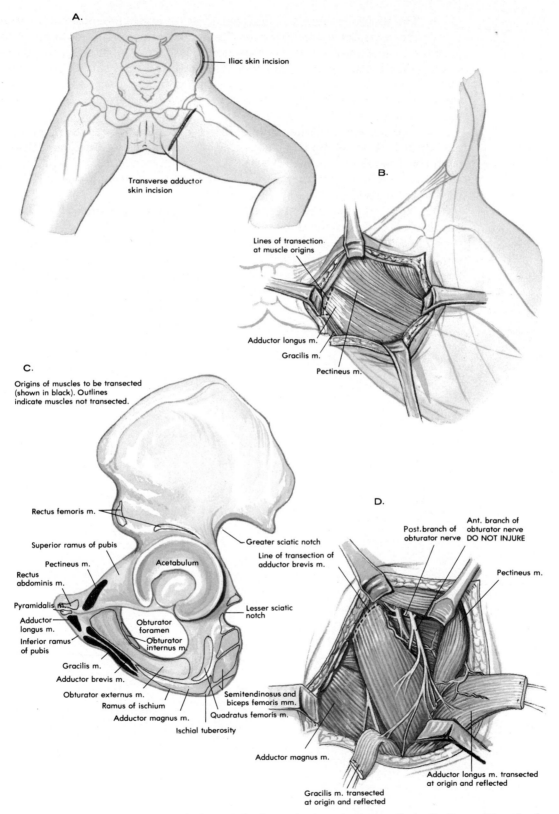

A.

Iliac skin incision

Transverse adductor
skin incision

B.

Lines of transection
at muscle origins

Adductor longus m.

Gracilis m.

Pectineus m.

C.

Origins of muscles to be transected
(shown in black). Outlines
indicate muscles not transected.

Rectus femoris m.

Superior ramus of pubis

Pectineus m.

Rectus
abdominis m.

Pyramidalis m.

Adductor
longus m.

Inferior ramus
of pubis

Gracilis m.

Adductor brevis m.

Obturator externus m.

Ramus of ischium

Adductor magnus m.

Ischial tuberosity

Greater sciatic notch

Line of transection of
adductor brevis m.

Acetabulum

Lesser sciatic
notch

Obturator
foramen

Obturator
internus m.

Semitendinosus and
biceps femoris mm.

Quadratus femoris m.

D.

Post. branch of
obturator nerve

Ant. branch of
obturator nerve
DO NOT INJURE

Pectineus m.

Adductor magnus m.

Gracilis m. transected
at origin and reflected

Adductor longus m. transected
at origin and reflected

Plate 88. A.–O., Periacetabular triple innominate osteotomy through the subinguinal
adductor approach.

E. The iliopsoas muscle is lengthened at its musculotendinous junction.

F. The avascular plane between the abductor magnus and obturator externus muscles is developed by blunt dissection. The ramus of the ischium is identified and verified by the image intensifier. Tissue in the interval between the adductor magnus and obturator externus is divided with electrocautery, and the ischial ramus is exposed subperiosteally. Place two Chandler elevator retractors completely around the ischial ramus.

G. Use a broad flat osteotome to resect a wedge of the ischium, based laterally and anteriorly, about 1.5 to 2.0 cm. inferior to the acetabulum. Direct the osteotome from the lateral to the medial side. The osteotomy should be complete. Taking a wedge of bone prevents lateral displacement of the acetabular segment and allows rotation and medialization of the acetabulum.

H. Next, the superior ramus of the pubis is identified by palpation and verification under image intensifier; it is relatively subcutaneous at this level. The iliopsoas muscle is retracted laterally and the pectineus muscle is elevated. The site of osteotomy of the superior ramus of the pubis is 1.5 cm. medial to the acetabulum, which is verified by image intensifier radiography. The pubic bone is subperiosteally exposed, and two Chandler elevator retractors are inserted behind the pubic ramus.

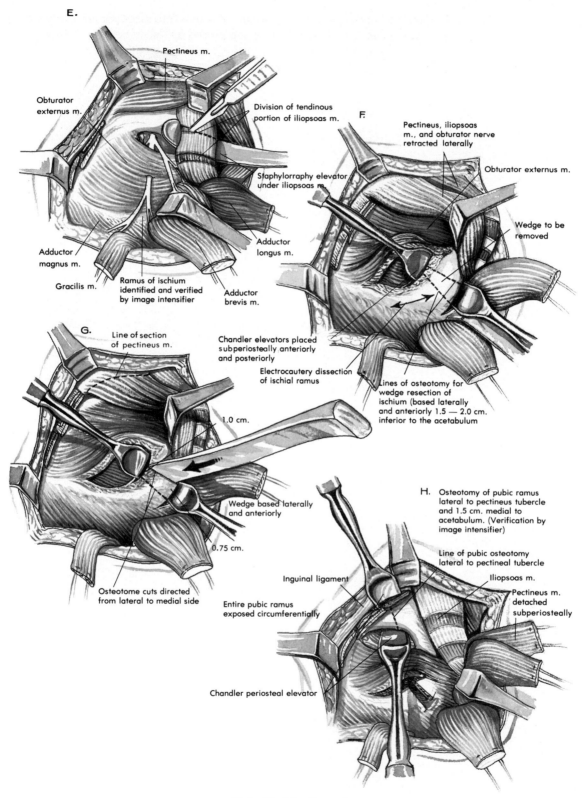

E.

Pectineus m.

Obturator externus m.

Division of tendinous portion of iliopsoas m.

Staphylorraphy elevator under iliopsoas m.

Adductor longus m.

Adductor magnus m.

Gracilis m.

Ramus of ischium identified and verified by image intensifier

Adductor brevis m.

F.

Pectineus, iliopsoas m., and obturator nerve retracted laterally

Obturator externus m.

Wedge to be removed

Chandler elevators placed subperiosteally anteriorly and posteriorly

Electrocautery dissection of ischial ramus

Lines of osteotomy for wedge resection of ischium (based laterally and anteriorly 1.5 — 2.0 cm. inferior to the acetabulum

G. Line of section of pectineus m.

1.0 cm.

Wedge based laterally and anteriorly

0.75 cm.

Osteotome cuts directed from lateral to medial side

H. Osteotomy of pubic ramus lateral to pectineus tubercle and 1.5 cm. medial to acetabulum. (Verification by image intensifier)

Line of pubic osteotomy lateral to pectineal tubercle

Iliopsoas m.

Pectineus m. detached subperiosteally

Inguinal ligament

Entire pubic ramus exposed circumferentially

Chandler periosteal elevator

Plate 88. (Continued)

I. Perform a pubic osteotomy with the osteotome directed medially and upward.

J. and **K.** The iliac osteotomy is completed as described by Salter.

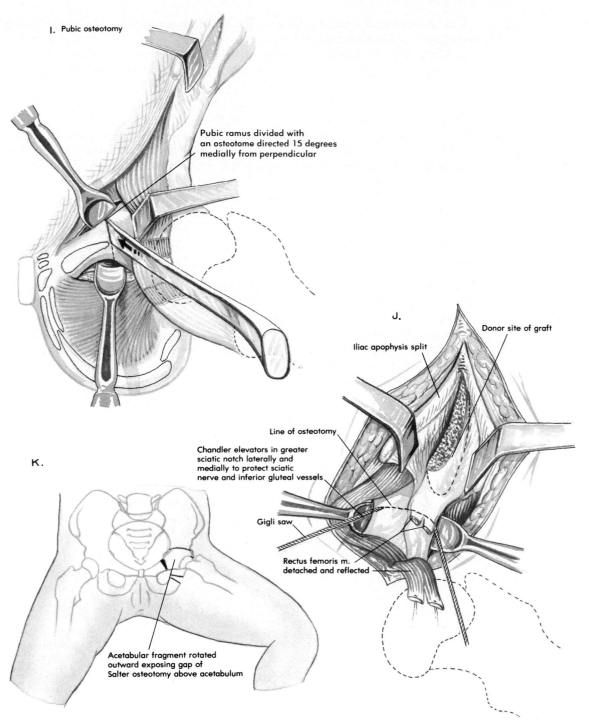

I. Pubic osteotomy

Pubic ramus divided with an osteotome directed 15 degrees medially from perpendicular

J.

Iliac apophysis split

Donor site of graft

Line of osteotomy

Chandler elevators in greater sciatic notch laterally and medially to protect sciatic nerve and inferior gluteal vessels

Gigli saw

Rectus femoris m. detached and reflected

K.

Acetabular fragment rotated outward exposing gap of Salter osteotomy above acetabulum

Plate 88. (Continued)

L. Rotating the acetabular fragment and manipulating the lower limb provide excellent anterior and lateral coverage.

M. and **N.** A wedge of bone taken from the ilium is inserted at the iliac osteotomy site and fixed by two threaded Steinmann pins, which may be inserted either superoinferiorly and medially or retrograde inferosuperiorly.

O. Additional fixation by one semitubular plate is recommended. Cut the inferior holes of the semitubular plates with a large pin cutter to create prongs. The sharp prongs are impacted into the rotated acetabulum; cortical screws are inserted from the lateral to the medial surface of the ilium, transfixing the plates. The pubic and ischial osteotomies do not require fixation, but the former may be grafted with a wedge of bone taken from the ischium or ilium.

Final radiograms are made for a permanent record. The tendons of the adductor longus, adductor brevis, and gracilis are resutured to their origins. Closed suction tubes are used for 48 hours.

The wound is closed in routine fashion. A hip spica cast is not needed unless a concurrent varus femoral osteotomy is performed.

Postoperative Care. The patient is placed in bilateral split Russell's traction. Active assisted and gentle passive exercises are commenced the second day postoperatively. In about seven to ten days postoperatively, the patient is allowed to be up and around, with a three-point crutch gait protecting the limb that was operated on. Full weight-bearing is delayed until the osteotomies are solidly healed, about two to three months. Internal fixation devices are removed four to six months postoperatively.

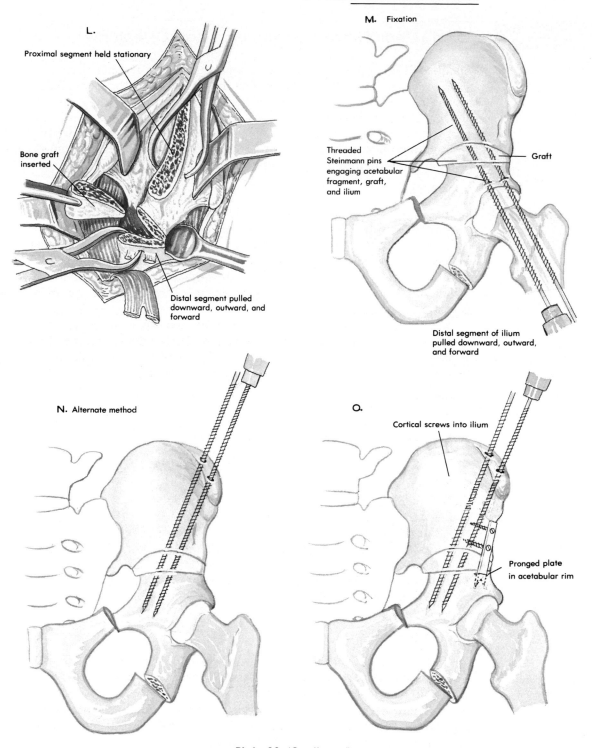

L.

Proximal segment held stationary

Bone graft inserted

Distal segment pulled downward, outward, and forward

M. Fixation

Threaded Steinmann pins engaging acetabular fragment, graft, and ilium

Graft

Distal segment of ilium pulled downward, outward, and forward

N. Alternate method

O.

Cortical screws into ilium

Pronged plate in acetabular rim

Plate 88. (Continued)

PLATE 89 ## Chiari's Medial Displacement Innominate Osteotomy

Principle. Chiari's pelvic osteotomy is a salvage, not a reconstructive procedure. It is a form of capsular arthroplasty. The innominate bone is osteotomized between the anterior inferior iliac spine and the greater sciatic notch, immediately above the origin of the capsule of the hip joint. The cut extends upward and medially, and the inferior segment of the innominate bone is displaced medially. The upper fragment becomes the shelf. The interposed capsule between the femoral head and the shelf converts into fibrocartilage.

Indications

1. An irreducible lateral subluxation of the hip with moderate incongruity of the joint in an adolescent or young adult.

2. Pain. The pain is alleviated by Chiari's innominate osteotomy. Medial displacement of the fulcrum of the hip joint shortens the medial arm of the hip abductor lever system, improves the hip mechanics, and diminishes the load on the femoral head. It also relieves abnormal joint pressure by increasing the acetabular capacity.

3. Progressive instability of the hip in an adolescent with moderate or severe incongruity of the hip joint and coxa magna. The enlarged femoral head requires an acetabular enlargement operation. Stability of the hip is determined by the Trendelenburg test and standing radiograms of the hips.

Requisites

1. Adequate articular cartilage space. A hip with severe osteoarthritis and marked destruction of articular cartilage cannot be salvaged by Chiari's innominate osteotomy; for such a hip, total joint replacement is required.

2. Functional range of hip motion. Chiari's innominate osteotomy is contraindicated in a stiff hip.

3. Moderate incongruity of the hip. A congruous hip is best treated by triple innominate osteotomy, if there is no coxa magna, or by shelf arthroplasty by slotted acetabular augmentation (Staheli), if there is coxa magna.

4. In the subluxated hip, the femoral head should be low enough so that the osteotomy will not extend into the sacroiliac joint. Chiari's innominate osteotomy is contraindicated when the femoral head is high.

5. Preferably, no surgical scarring around the sciatic notch and nerve from previous pelvic osteotomies.

Disadvantages

1. Coverage of the femoral head is provided by fibrocartilage and not by hyaline cartilage. Fibrocartilage is less durable than hyaline cartilage under the stresses of weight-bearing and loading.

2. There may be postoperative narrowing of the pelvis. Forewarn the patient and parents that a narrowed pelvic outlet may obstruct full-term vaginal delivery and that cesarean section may be necessary.

3. There may be shortening of the lower limb as a result of medial and upward displacement of the acetabulum.

4. Sciatic nerve paresis may result in angulation of the nerve at the osteotomy site or direct injury by bone splintering at the sciatic notch. Use a Gigli saw or very sharp, thin AO osteotomes. Keep subperiosteal in your exposure of the ilium.

5. If the osteotomy level is too low (close to the femoral head), it may enter the hip joint and damage articular hyaline cartilage. Determine the proper level of osteotomy by image intensifier radiographic control. Provide sufficient interval between the femoral head and the ilium to accommodate the capsule.

6. If the osteotomy level is too high (a problem when the acetabulum is shallow and in high subluxation), the osteotomy line may extend into the sacroiliac joint and cause painful sacroiliac arthritis.

7. Posterior slipping of the distal fragment may cause an ugly prominence of the anterior superior iliac spine and a flexion deformity of the hip. Prevent it by curving the osteotomy line into a dome shape, keeping a retractor posterior to the distal segment before the osteotomy is completed and using secure internal fixation.

8. Limitation of hip flexion due to bony block of the proximal segment. Forewarn the patient.

9. Penetration of screws or threaded Steinmann pins into the hip joint. Avoid by appropriate radiographic control.

10. Non-union may occur. If the degree of displacement is more than 50 per cent, fill the osteotomy site with autogenous bone graft from the ilium, especially in the skeletally mature child.

11. When dictating the operative note, accurately record and map the position of the screws or pins. This facilitates their removal and obviates the necessity of extensive stripping of the glutei from the lateral wall of the ilium; the latter may cause persisting gluteus medius lurch.

Radiographic Control. Image intensifier.

Blood for Transfusion. Yes.

Special Instrumentation. Rang retractors; Gigli saw; sharp, thin AO osteotomes; AO instrumentation.

Patient Position. The patient is placed supine on a radiolucent operating table. Image intensifier fluoroscopy and radiographic control are vital to control the level, direction, and degree of medial displacement of the osteotomy accurately. Some surgeons prefer to perform the operation on a fracture table with the patient's feet secured to the traction plate; this facilitates the application of a hip spica cast. This author fixes the iliac osteotomy internally with cancellous screws and does not apply a spica cast; therefore, the fracture table, which is cumbersome (especially the perineal post), is unnecessary.

The skin of the affected side of the lower part of the chest, abdomen, pelvis, and entire lower limb is prepared and draped to allow free motion of the hip as it is being operated.

Operative Technique

A. and **B.** The medial and lateral walls of the ilium are exposed by an anterolateral approach similar to that described for Salter's innominate osteotomy (Plate 82). Adequate posterior exposure to visualize the sciatic notch is vital. Also it is imperative to stay in the subperiosteal plane in order to avoid injury to the sciatic nerve and gluteal vessels and nerves. Distal exposure is important. The sartorius muscle must be detached from the anterior superior iliac spine, its free end marked with non-absorbable suture (such as 00 Tycron) for later reattachment, and reflected inferiorly and medially.

C. In adolescent hip dysplasia, the capsule is thickened and often adherent to the lateral wall of the ilium; the capsule is dissected and elevated off the ilium to the rim of the acetabulum. If the capsule is very thick, it is best to thin it by partial excision of its superior part. Occasionally, one may have to make a small opening in the hip joint capsule anterosuperiorly to ascertain the correct level of osteotomy. Expose the capsule from anterior to posterior for adequate visualization of the superior aspect of the hip.

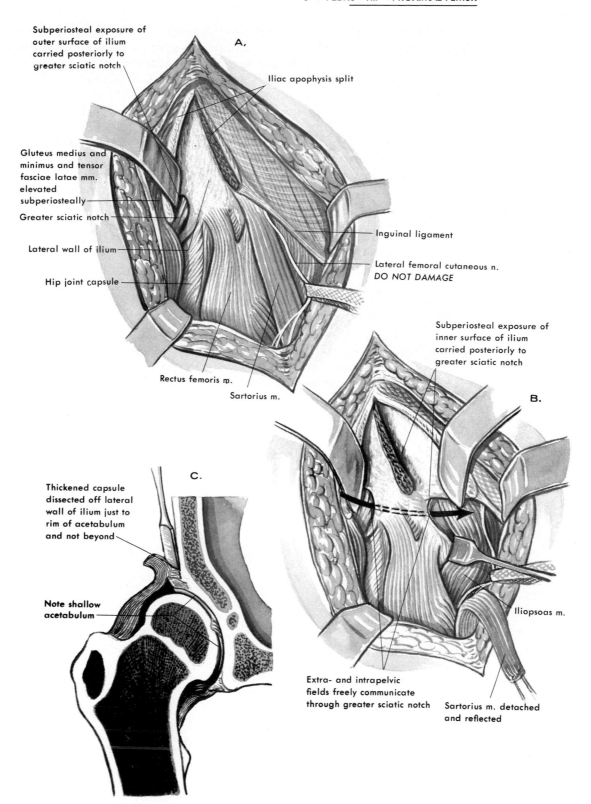

Subperiosteal exposure of
outer surface of ilium
carried posteriorly to
greater sciatic notch

A.

Iliac apophysis split

Gluteus medius and
minimus and tensor
fasciae latae mm.
elevated
subperiosteally

Greater sciatic notch

Lateral wall of ilium

Hip joint capsule

Inguinal ligament

Lateral femoral cutaneous n.
DO NOT DAMAGE

Rectus femoris m.

Sartorius m.

Subperiosteal exposure of
inner surface of ilium
carried posteriorly to
greater sciatic notch

B.

Thickened capsule
dissected off lateral
wall of ilium just to
rim of acetabulum
and not beyond

C.

**Note shallow
acetabulum**

Iliopsoas m.

Extra- and intrapelvic
fields freely communicate
through greater sciatic notch

Sartorius m. detached
and reflected

Plate 89. A.–Q., Chiari's medial displacement innominate osteotomy.

D. Next, the reflected head of the rectus femoris is elevated and detached from the superior margin of the acetabulum. In the older patient, the capsule and the reflected head of the rectus femoris may not be separately identifiable. The direct head of the rectus femoris is detached from its origin at the anterior inferior iliac spine; both heads are reflected distally. Do not damage the hip joint capsule. The taut iliopsoas muscle is lengthened by two transverse incisions of its tendinous fibers only; the underlying muscle fibers are left intact. If there is no hip flexion deformity, routine iliopsoas lengthening is not recommended because, postoperatively, temporary weakness of hip flexion is a problem.

E.–G. The ideal level of osteotomy is just above the capsular attachment between the capsule and the reflected head of the rectus femoris. Too low a level will damage the interposed capsule, and too high a level will not provide adequate coverage. The ilium is cut at an angle directed 10 to 15 degrees upward and medially. The osteotomy angle is the angle between the plane of the pelvic osteotomy and the horizontal. If it is directed more than 15 to 20 degrees superiorly, the osteotomy may violate the sacroiliac joint. The danger of entering the joint is great if the acetabulum is shallow. The roof angle is the angle formed between the horizontal and a line joining the original outer acetabular lip to the new acetabular lip. With remodeling of the osteotomy, the "step" region fills in and the roof angle represents the increased acetabular overhang. The center edge (CE) angle of Wiberg does not accurately express the adequacy of femoral head coverage, because innominate osteotomies at different levels and angles can give the same CE angle but widely varying degrees of acetabular improvement.

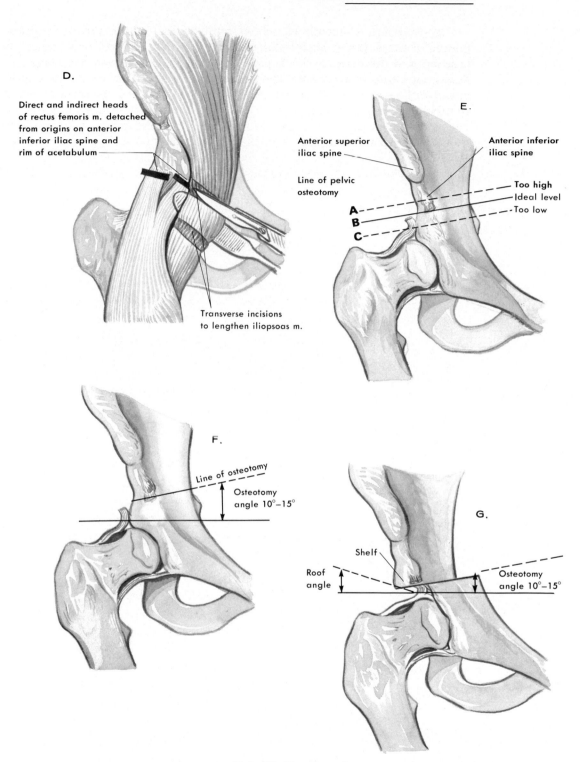

D.

Direct and indirect heads of rectus femoris m. detached from origins on anterior inferior iliac spine and rim of acetabulum

Transverse incisions to lengthen iliopsoas m.

E.

Anterior superior iliac spine

Anterior inferior iliac spine

Line of pelvic osteotomy

Too high
Ideal level
Too low

A
B
C

F.

Line of osteotomy

Osteotomy angle 10°–15°

G.

Shelf

Roof angle

Osteotomy angle 10°–15°

Plate 89. (Continued)

H.–J. Insert a smooth Kirschner wire or Steinmann pin as a guide at the middle of the superior acetabular rim at the proposed level and angle. The exact position and direction of the angle of the pin is determined by image intensifier fluoroscopy and radiograms. The angle should be 10 to 15 degrees medial and upward. The line of osteotomy, which may be marked by multiple drill holes, should be curved, terminating inferior to the anterior inferior iliac spine anteriorly and to the lower part of the greater sciatic notch posteriorly. The curved osteotomy should correspond to the shape of the femoral head.

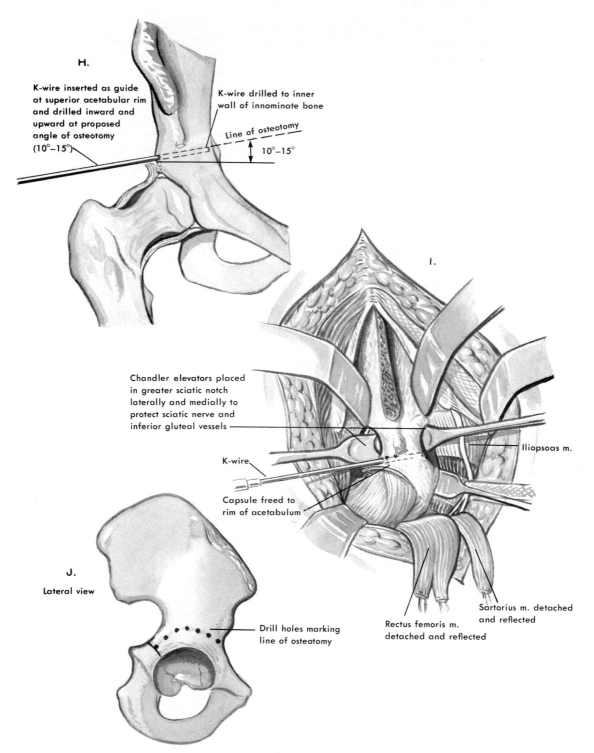

H.

K-wire inserted as guide at superior acetabular rim and drilled inward and upward at proposed angle of osteotomy (10°–15°)

K-wire drilled to inner wall of innominate bone

Line of osteotomy

10°–15°

I.

Chandler elevators placed in greater sciatic notch laterally and medially to protect sciatic nerve and inferior gluteal vessels

K-wire

Capsule freed to rim of acetabulum

Iliopsoas m.

Sartorius m. detached and reflected

Rectus femoris m. detached and reflected

J.

Lateral view

Drill holes marking line of osteotomy

Plate 89. (Continued)

K. *Caution!* Straight-line osteotomy may cause posterior displacement of the distal segment that will produce an ugly prominence of the anterior superior iliac spine and a flexion deformity of the hip. Curve the osteotomy line!

L. Posterior displacement of the distal segment may also cause angulation and kinking of the sciatic nerve and neurapraxia.

M. The osteotomy is performed with ½- or ⅜-inch-wide osteotomes, which should be thin and sharp. Avoid splintering and greenstick fracture of the inner wall of the ilium. The position and the direction of the angle of the osteotomes should be double checked by image intensifier fluoroscopy. Cut the lateral cortex first, and then osteotomize the medial cortex. Several osteotomes are used side by side and advanced together. Osteotomy cuts are first made anteriorly around the capsule and then posteriorly. Narrower osteotomes ensure an adequate curve. An assistant will indicate when the osteotomes penetrate the medial wall of the ilium.

Do not use osteotomes to cut the cortex of the sciatic notch; the bone will splinter and cause sciatic nerve damage.

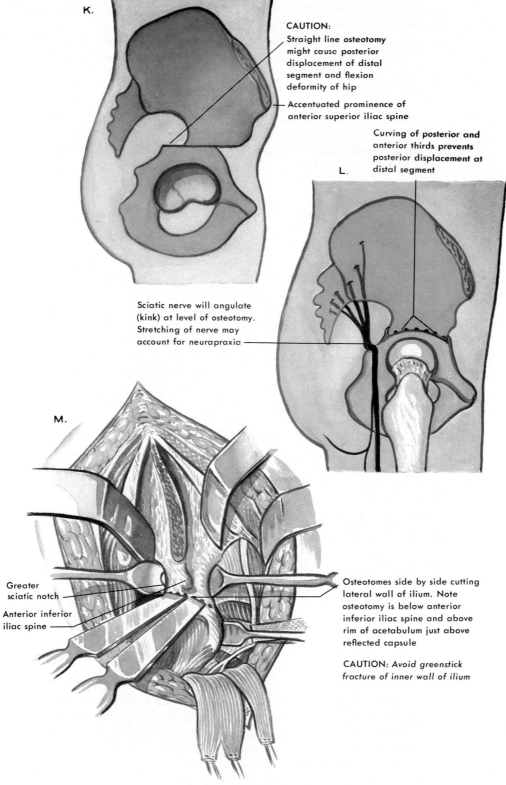

K.

CAUTION:
Straight line osteotomy
might cause posterior
displacement of distal
segment and flexion
deformity of hip

Accentuated prominence of
anterior superior iliac spine

Curving of posterior and
anterior thirds prevents
posterior displacement at
distal segment

L.

Sciatic nerve will angulate
(kink) at level of osteotomy.
Stretching of nerve may
account for neurapraxia

M.

Greater
sciatic notch

Anterior inferior
iliac spine

Osteotomes side by side cutting
lateral wall of ilium. Note
osteotomy is below anterior
inferior iliac spine and above
rim of acetabulum just above
reflected capsule

CAUTION: *Avoid greenstick
fracture of inner wall of ilium*

Plate 89. (Continued)

N. Using Rang retractors in the sciatic notch, cut the last posterior 1 or 2 cm. of the ilium with a Gigli saw.*

O. and **P.** Upon completion of the osteotomy, the cut is opened first by wide osteotomes, periosteal elevators, and then gently by a laminar spreader. The iliac fragments should be fully mobilized. The hip is widely abducted, and the femoral head is displaced medially by the surgeon as an assistant holds the anterior iliac crest firmly. The Rang or Chandler retractors should be kept in the greater sciatic notch to prevent posterior displacement and sciatic nerve injury. The hip joint capsule should disappear under the new roof of cancellous bone of the inferior surface of the proximal iliac fragment. The medial displacement or shift is expressed as a percentage of the thickness of the ilium at the level of osteotomy. Remember, the ilium cross section is thin anteriorly and wide posteriorly. A common pitfall is hinging at the greater sciatic notch when the distal iliac fragment is rotated medially. Complete the osteotomy by connecting the cuts of the lateral and medial cortices. The distal pelvic segment has rotated inward. The "hinged" osteotomy may give the pseudoappearance of excellent head coverage. Oblique radiograms, however, will show the curve at the greater sciatic notch to be unbroken. The medial wall of the iliac wing is a reliable benchmark to assess the degree of medial displacement. With 50 per cent medial displacement, approximately 1.5 cm. of femoral head coverage is provided. Complete separation of the iliac fragments is not desirable and must be avoided. If greater coverage and cupping of the femoral head is required, the Chiari osteotomy is combined with a shelf procedure. Corticocancellous strips of bone ½ inch wide are taken from the ilium and wedged into a slot in the distal iliac segment. The bone grafts are angled a few degrees cephalad and interposed between the capsule and the proximal iliac segment. This is most important anteriorly when the ilium is thin.

Q. Two threaded Steinmann pins are used to transfix the iliac fragments obliquely under image intensifier radiographic control. An anteroposterior radiogram is made to determine the degree of femoral head coverage provided. Then, two cannulated, cancellous screws with washers are used to transfix the iliac fragments obliquely. It is best to drill from the superior wall of the proximal iliac segment into the distal ilium, directing the guide pins and then the screws obliquely, medially, and distally and posteriorly. Cancellous screws should not penetrate the hip joint.

Remove the guide pins and the threaded Steinmann pins. The split iliac apophysis is sutured, the sartorius muscle reattached to its origin, and the wound closed in routine fashion. A hip spica cast is not necessary.

Postoperative Care. The patient is placed in bilateral split Russell's traction. Active assisted and gentle passive exercises are begun as soon as the patient is comfortable. On the second to the third postoperative day he is allowed to be up and around with a three-point crutch gait protecting the limb by toe-touch. When the patient is not walking, counterpoised traction is replaced until painless functional range of motion of the hip is achieved and maintained. Crutch protection is continued until complete bony healing has taken place, usually in about six to eight weeks. The screws are removed four to six months postoperatively.

When the patient is comfortable, side-lying hip abduction exercises are performed to increase motor strength of the gluteus medius and minimus. When bony healing has taken place, standing Trendelenburg exercises are performed until gluteus medius lurch has disappeared. This may take as long as six months.

REFERENCES

Bailey, T. E., and Hall, J. E.: Chiari medial displacement osteotomy. J. Pediatr. Orthop., 5:635, 1985.
Benson, M. K. D., and Jameson Evans, D. C.: The pelvic osteotomy of Chiari: An anatomical study of the hazards and misleading radiographic appearances. J. Bone Joint Surg., 58–B:164, 1976.

*Rang retractors are available from the manufacturer: Jantek Engineering Inc., 570 Trafford Crescent, Oakville, Ontario, Canada L6L 3T3.

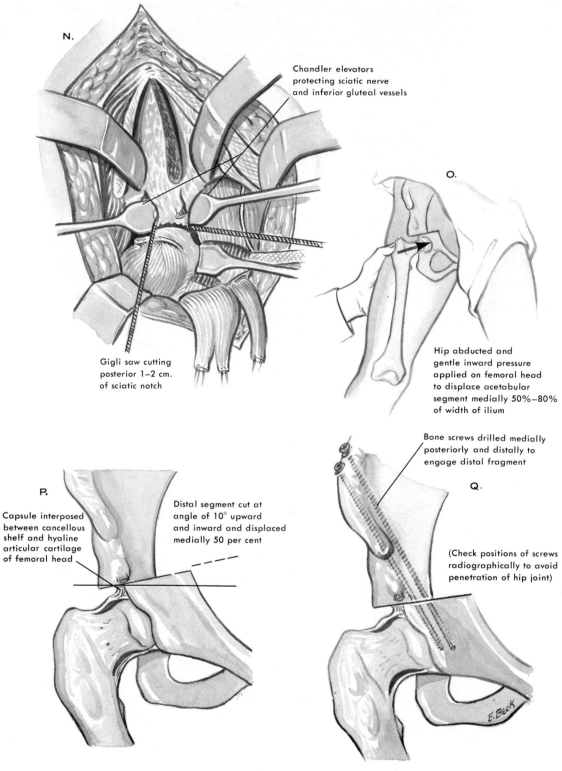

N.

Chandler elevators
protecting sciatic nerve
and inferior gluteal vessels

Gigli saw cutting
posterior 1–2 cm.
of sciatic notch

O.

Hip abducted and
gentle inward pressure
applied on femoral head
to displace acetabular
segment medially 50%–80%
of width of ilium

P.

Capsule interposed
between cancellous
shelf and hyaline
articular cartilage
of femoral head

Distal segment cut at
angle of 10° upward
and inward and displaced
medially 50 per cent

Bone screws drilled medially
posteriorly and distally to
engage distal fragment

Q.

(Check positions of screws
radiographically to avoid
penetration of hip joint)

E. Beck

Plate 89. (Continued)

Betz, R. R., Kumar, S. J., Palmer, C. T., and MacEwen, G. D.: Chiari pelvic osteotomy in children and young adults. J. Bone Joint Surg., 70–A:182, 1988.

Chiari, K.: Ergebnisse mit der Beckenosteotomie als Pfannendachplastik. Z. Orthop., 87:14, 1955.

Chiari, K.: Die operative Behandlung am Huftgelenk bei der angeborenen Huftgelenksverrenkung. Wien. Med. Wochenschr., 107:1020, 1957.

Chiari, K.: In: Proceedings of Société Internationale de Chirurgie Orthopédique et de Traumatologie. Neuvième congrès, Vienna, September 1–7, 1964.

Chiari, K.: Die Beckenosteotomie in der Coxarthrose. Beitr. Orthop., 15:163, 1968.

Chiari, K.: Pelvic osteotomy for hip subluxation. J. Bone Joint Surg., 52–B:174, 1970.

Chiari, K.: Spatergebnisse nach Beckenosteotomie—Verhutung der Praarthrose. Z. Orthop., 112:603, 1974.

Chiari, K.: Medial displacement osteotomy of the pelvis. Clin. Orthop., 98:55, 1974.

Chiari, K.: Bericht uber die Beckenosteotomie als Pfannendachplastik nach eigener Methode. In: Chapchal, G. (ed.): Beckenosteotomie—Pfannendachplastik. Stuttgart, Thieme, 1975, pp. 70–75.

Colton, C. L.: Chiari osteotomy for acetabular dysplasia in young subjects. J. Bone Joint Surg., 54–B:578, 1972.

Fernandez, D. L., Isler, B., and Muller, M.: Chiari's osteotomy: A note on technique. Clin. Orthop., 185:53, 1984.

Hogh, J., and Macnicol, M. F.: The Chiari pelvic osteotomy. A long-term review of clinical and radiographic results. J. Bone Joint Surg., 69–B:365, 1987.

Renoirte, P. and Saussez, M.: L'ostéotomie de Chiari dans les dysplasies coxofémorales acquisés de la second enfance. Acta Orthop. Belg., 36:209, 1970.

Salvati, E. A., and Wilson, P. D.: Treatment of irreducible hip subluxation by Chiari. Clin. Orthop., 98:151, 1974.

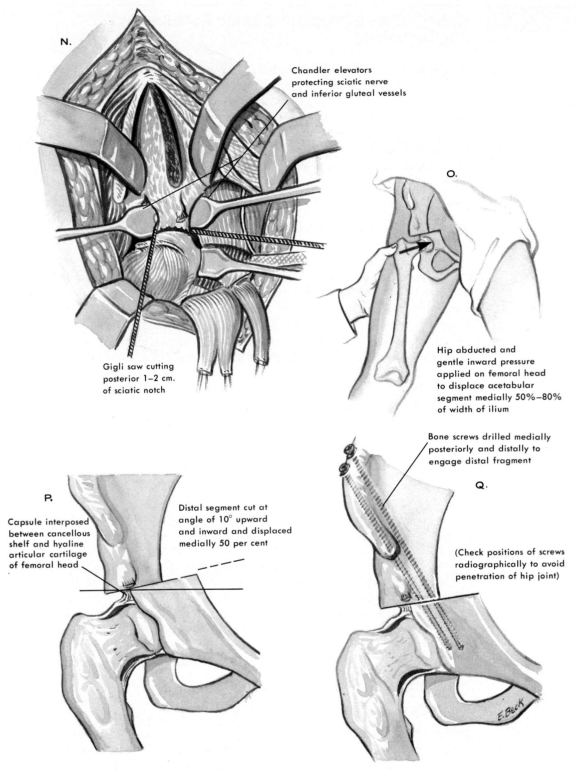

N.

Chandler elevators
protecting sciatic nerve
and inferior gluteal vessels

Gigli saw cutting
posterior 1–2 cm.
of sciatic notch

O.

Hip abducted and
gentle inward pressure
applied on femoral head
to displace acetabular
segment medially 50%–80%
of width of ilium

P.

Capsule interposed
between cancellous
shelf and hyaline
articular cartilage
of femoral head

Distal segment cut at
angle of 10° upward
and inward and displaced
medially 50 per cent

Bone screws drilled medially
posteriorly and distally to
engage distal fragment

Q.

(Check positions of screws
radiographically to avoid
penetration of hip joint)

E.Beck

Plate 89. (Continued)

PLATE 90 ### Staheli's Shelf Arthroplasty (Slotted Acetabular Augmentation)

Principle. The roof of the acetabulum is extended outward (laterally, posteriorly, and anteriorly) by the addition of autogenous corticocancellous bone taken from the adjacent ilium. The grafts are inserted into a deep slot at the acetabular margin and added in layers directly over the capsule of the uncovered femoral head. The procedure (1) increases the capacity of the deficient acetabulum, (2) stabilizes the hip by preventing superolateral migration of the femoral head, and (3) increases the weight-bearing area of the hip and decreases pressure forces across the joint.

Indications

1. A dysplastic and deficient acetabulum and a large femoral head requiring an acetabular enlargement in a child or an adolescent with a hip that has aspherical congruity.

2. A dysplastic hip with spherical congruity that requires more than 25 degrees of hip abduction for concentric containment of the femoral head. In such patients, acetabular redirection anteriorly and laterally will not cover the femoral head posteriorly.

3. Pain and instability of the hip and a very shallow acetabulum. In such an instance, Chiari's medial displacement innominate osteotomy may violate the sacroiliac joint.

4. Pain and instability in a dysplastic hip that had multiple pelvic operations with scarring around the sciatic notch or that was associated with congenital anomalies of the lumbosacral spine; in such an instance, there is increased risk of injury to the sciatic nerve.

Advantages

1. The procedure is extra-articular. There is no danger of progressive stiffness of the hip joint.

2. The viability of the articular cartilage and circulation of the femoral head are not damaged.

3. The pelvic ring anatomy and integrity are not disturbed.

4. Danger of injury to the sciatic nerve is nil or minimal.

5. The procedure provides a congruous extension of the acetabulum and dome-shaped coverage of the femoral head.

6. The operation does not cause shortening of the lower limb.

7. The operation does not aggravate or cause gluteus medius limp.

8. There is no danger of injury to sacroiliac joint.

9. Technically, the procedure is simple and safe.

Radiographic Control. Image intensifier.

Blood for transfusion. Yes.

Patient Position. The patient is placed on a radiolucent operating table, with the involved side raised and tilted about 15 degrees on a pad. Heavy patients are best placed on a fracture table, with the affected lower limb draped free.

Operative Technique

A. Expose the lateral wall of the ilium and hip joint via an iliofemoral approach through a bikini incision made 2 to 3 cm. below and parallel to the iliac crest.

B. The tendon of the reflected head of rectus femoris is sectioned in its anterior part and elevated and reflected posteriorly (later this tendon will be reattached to stabilize the graft). Expose the capsule of the hip joint anteriorly, superiorly, and posteriorly.

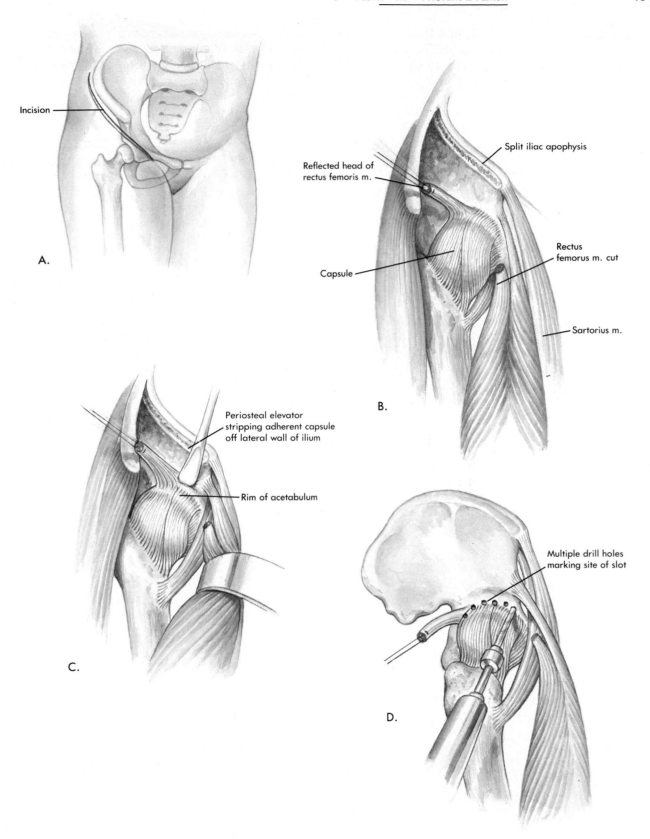

Incision

Reflected head of
rectus femoris m.

Split iliac apophysis

Capsule

Rectus
femorus m. cut

Sartorius m.

A.

B.

Periosteal elevator
stripping adherent capsule
off lateral wall of ilium

Rim of acetabulum

Multiple drill holes
marking site of slot

C.

D.

Plate 90. A.–L., Staheli's shelf arthroplasty (slotted acetabular augmentation).

C. and **D.** Note the thickened capsule, which is adherent to the lateral wall of the ilium. With a periosteal elevator, elevate the capsule from the ilium and reflect it distally to the acetabular rim (see p. 431). With image intensifier radiographic control, identify the joint line. Some surgeons prefer to make a small aperture in the capsule to determine the level of the femoral head.

The next step is to make a slot *exactly* at the margin of the acetabulum. Insert a smooth Kirschner wire at the proposed site of the slot, and confirm its exact location by an anteroposterior radiogram. The slot should be 10 mm. deep and 5 mm. wide; its floor is the subchondral bony plate and articular cartilage of the acetabulum. Its roof is cancellous bone. Drill holes with a 5/32-inch bit; the depth of the holes should be at least 1 cm. The extent of coverage required determines the length of the slot. When there is excessive femoral antetorsion, the slot extends more anteriorly. When the acetabulum is deficient posteriorly, it is extended backward.

E. With a narrow rongeur, join the drill holes producing the slot. An alternate method to make the slot is by the use of a Hall air drill.

F. Next, determine the width of the augmentation and the total length of the graft. This is done on a preoperative standing anteroposterior radiogram of the hips. The actual CE angle and the desired normal CE angle of 35 degrees are drawn on the film. The extra width necessary to extend the existing socket to obtain the normal CE angle is measured; this is the width of augmentation (WA). The graft length (GL) is the sum of the width of augmentation and the slot depth (SD).

G. Strips of cortical and cancellous bone are harvested from the lateral wall of the ilium. Leave the inner table of the ilium intact. The bone graft strips extend from the iliac crest to the upper border of the slot. This shallow decortication ensures rapid fusion of the graft to the ilium.

H. Carry out acetabular augmentation in the following layers. *The first layer* consists of thin strips of cancellous bone 1 mm. thick and 1 cm. wide and of appropriate length, as determined on the anteroposterior radiogram. These strips of bone graft are inserted into the slot in a radial fashion with the concave side down, thereby providing congruous coverage on the femoral head.

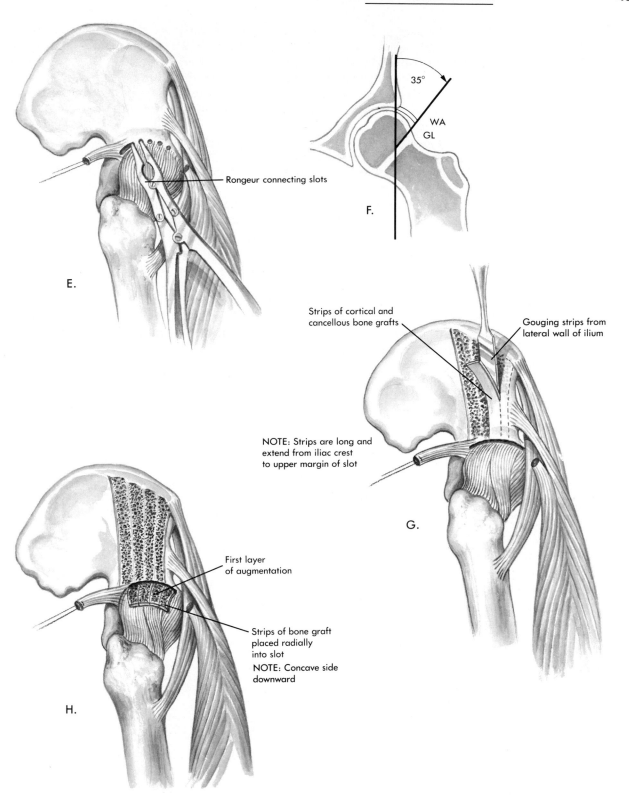

Rongeur connecting slots

E.

F.

35°

WA
GL

Strips of cortical and
cancellous bone grafts

Gouging strips from
lateral wall of ilium

NOTE: Strips are long and
extend from iliac crest
to upper margin of slot

G.

First layer
of augmentation

Strips of bone graft
placed radially
into slot

NOTE: Concave side
downward

H.

Plate 90. (Continued)

I. The *second layer* consists of thicker bone graft strips (about 2 mm.) with their length equal to the length of extension. They are placed parallel to the acetabulum at right angles to the first layer of extension. Do not extend the augmentation too far anteriorly because it will limit hip flexion.

J. The detached reflected head of rectus femoris is pulled forward over the grafts and sutured to its original site. This measure ensures that the grafts are held in place.

K. If necessary, make a capsular flap by slicing the thickened capsule and suturing it over the grafts securing them to the ilium.

L. The *third layer* consists of small pieces of bone that are packed above the first two layers and above the reattached reflected head of rectus femoris. The third layer of augmentation should not protrude beyond the initial two layers. The hip abductors are reattached to the iliac crest, holding the third layer in place.

In paralytic hip dysplasia (such as in cerebral palsy or myelomeningocele), when the ilium is atrophic and thin, bank bone is used for acetabular augmentation. It is imperative not to disrupt the integrity of the slot by harvesting bone grafts from the lateral wall of the iluim.

The position and width of the augmentation are verified by an anteroposterior radiogram of the hip. The wound is closed in the routine fashion, and a single hip spica cast is applied, with the hip in 15 degrees of abduction and 20 degrees of flexion and internal rotation.

Postoperative Care. Immobilization in the cast is for six weeks. The cast is then removed, and three-point, crutch-walking gait is permitted with partial weight-bearing on the affected limb until the graft is radiographically shown to be incorporated, usually about three to four months.

REFERENCES

Staheli, L. T.: Slotted acetabular augmentation. J. Pediatr. Orthop., 1:321, 1981.
Staheli, L. T., and Chew, D. E.: Slotted acetabular augmentation in childhood and adolescence. J. Pediatr. Orthop., 12:569, 1992.

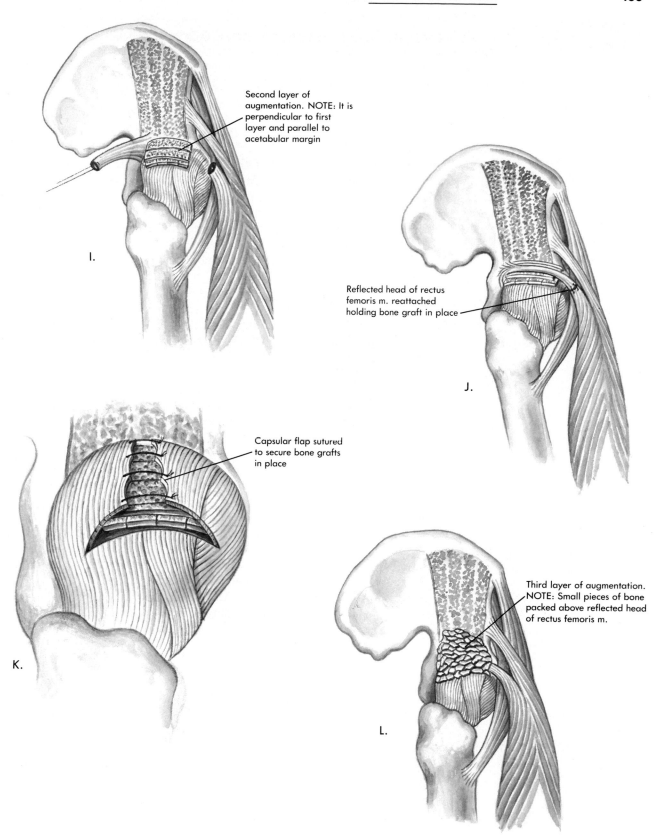

Second layer of augmentation. NOTE: It is perpendicular to first layer and parallel to acetabular margin

I.

Reflected head of rectus femoris m. reattached holding bone graft in place

J.

Capsular flap sutured to secure bone grafts in place

K.

Third layer of augmentation. NOTE: Small pieces of bone packed above reflected head of rectus femoris m.

L.

Plate 90. (Continued)

PLATE 91 ## Greater Trochanteric Apophyseodesis (Langenskiöld Technique)

Indications. Arrest of growth of the capital femoral physis in a child six years of age or under.

Caution!

1. Be unequivocally sure that there is no further growth from the physis of the femoral head.

2. Fifty per cent of the growth of the greater trochanter can be stopped by apophyseodesis; 50 per cent of the growth of the greater trochanter occurs by appositional bone growth at its cephalic cartilaginous portion on which the hip abductors insert.

3. Greater trochanteric apophyseodesis does not lateralize the greater trochanter or functionally lengthen the femoral neck.

4. The procedure does not restore neck-shaft angle, and correction of coxa vara does not occur.

Radiographic Control. Image intensifier.

Patient Position. The patient is placed supine with a sandbag under the ipsilateral hip. The entire lower limb, hip, and pelvis are prepared and draped to permit free passive motion of the hip.

Operative Technique

A. A 5- to 7-cm. long transverse incision is centered over the apophysis of the greater trochanter. If so desired, a longitudinal incision may be made, especially if distal transfer of the greater trochanter is anticipated in the future.

B. The site of origin of the vastus lateralis from the upper part of the intertrochanteric line, the anteroinferior border of the greater trochanter, the lateral tip of the gluteal tuberosity, and the upper part of the lateral tip of the linea aspera is shown.

C. Subcutaneous tissue is divided in line with the skin incision. The wound edges are retracted. A longitudinal incision is made in the fascia of the tensor fasciae latae muscle.

D. The tensor fasciae latae muscle is retracted anteriorly, and the origin of the vastus lateralis is detached and elevated extraperiosteally.

E. A Keith needle is inserted into the soft growth plate of the greater trochanteric apophysis. Anteroposterior radiograms are made to verify the position of the Keith needle and the growth plate.

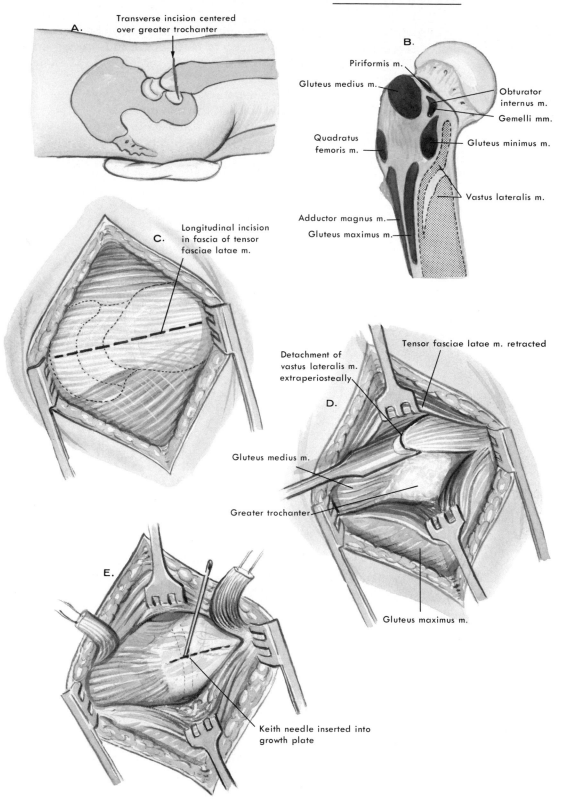

A. Transverse incision centered over greater trochanter

B.
Piriformis m.
Gluteus medius m.
Obturator internus m.
Gemelli mm.
Quadratus femoris m.
Gluteus minimus m.
Vastus lateralis m.
Adductor magnus m.
Gluteus maximus m.

C. Longitudinal incision in fascia of tensor fasciae latae m.

D.
Detachment of vastus lateralis m. extraperiosteally
Tensor fasciae latae m. retracted
Gluteus medius m.
Greater trochanter
Gluteus maximus m.

E.
Keith needle inserted into growth plate

Plate 91. A.–M., Greater trochanteric apophyseodesis (Langenskiöld technique).

F. Divide the periosteum by one longitudinal and two horizontal incisions. The dotted rectangle marks the bone plug to be removed and turned around. *Note.* It is 2 cm. long and 1.25 cm. wide. In the smaller child, the rectangle is ⅜ inch (1 cm.) long and ¼ inch (0.6 cm.) wide.

G. and **H.** With straight osteotomes, remove the bone plug. Note that the growth plate is in the proximal third of the rectangle.

I. A diamond-shaped drill and curets are used to destroy the growth plate. Be careful not to enter the trochanteric fossa and injure circulation to the femoral head.

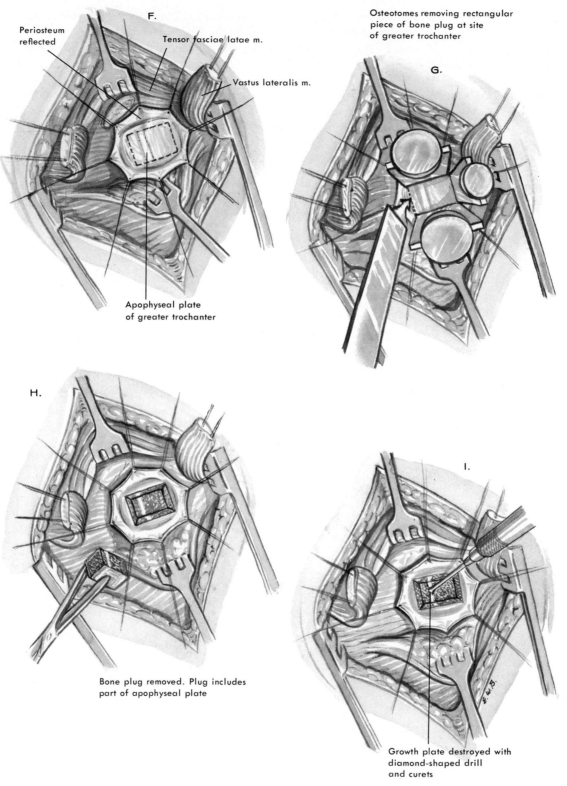

F.

Periosteum
reflected

Tensor fasciae latae m.

Vastus lateralis m.

Apophyseal plate
of greater trochanter

Osteotomes removing rectangular
piece of bone plug at site
of greater trochanter

G.

H.

Bone plug removed. Plug includes
part of apophyseal plate

I.

Growth plate destroyed with
diamond-shaped drill
and curets

Plate 91. (Continued)

J. With a curved osteotome, remove cancellous bone from the proximal femoral shaft and pack into the defect at the site of the growth plate.

K. and **L.** The bone plug is rotated 180 degrees, replaced in the defect in the greater trochanter, and with an impactor and mallet, is securely seated.

M. The muscles are resutured to their insertion sites, and the vastus lateralis is attached to gluteus medius–minimus tendons at their insertion after closure of the periosteum. The fascia lata is closed with interrupted sutures, and the wound is closed with interrupted and subcuticular skin sutures. It is not necessary to immobilize the hip in any cast.

Postoperative Care. The patient is allowed to be up and around the first day postoperatively, as soon as he or she is comfortable, and is discharged home within a few days. The limb that was operated on is protected with a three-point crutch gait for three to four weeks.

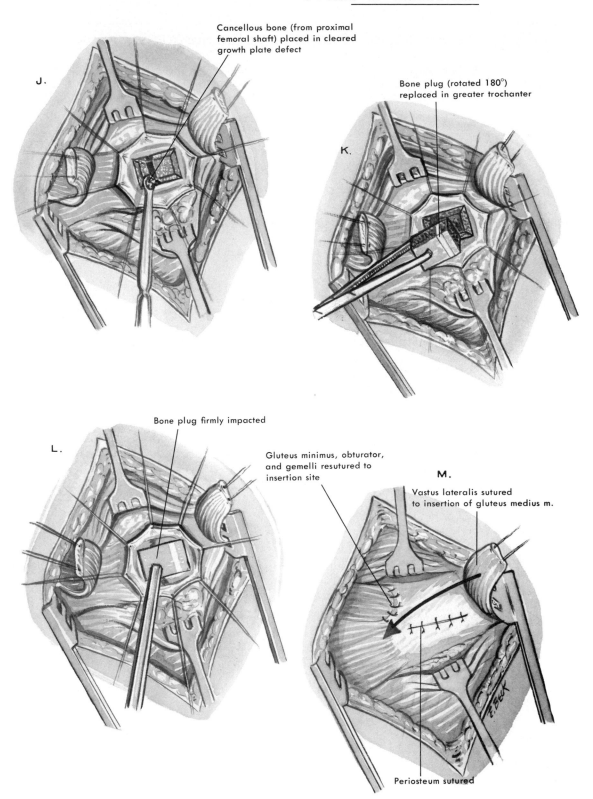

Cancellous bone (from proximal femoral shaft) placed in cleared growth plate defect

J.

Bone plug (rotated 180°) replaced in greater trochanter

K.

Bone plug firmly impacted

L.

Gluteus minimus, obturator, and gemelli resutured to insertion site

M.

Vastus lateralis sutured to insertion of gluteus medius m.

Periosteum sutured

Plate 91. (Continued)

PLATE 92 ## Distal and Lateral Transfer of the Greater Trochanter

Indications

1. Relative overgrowth of the greater trochanter with its tip at the joint line.
2. A short femoral neck.
3. Positive Trendelenburg sign (immediate or delayed).
4. Lower age limit of eight years.

Requisites

1. Congruous and concentric reduction of hip joint.
2. A femoral neck–shaft angle of at least 110 degrees. (If it is less than 110 degrees, perform a lateral closing-wedge osteotomy of the proximal femur combined with greater trochanteric arrest.)
3. Functional range of hip motion with total arc of hip abduction–adduction of at least 45 degrees.
4. Preoperative hip abductor muscle strength of at least fair minus.
5. Femoral antetorsion of less than 40 degrees.
6. Lower age limit of eight years.

Blood for Transfusion. Yes. Type and cross-match for 1 unit of blood.

Radiographic Control. Image intensifier.

Patient Position. The patient is placed on the fracture table with the affected hip in neutral position as to adduction–abduction and in 20 to 30 degrees of medial rotation to bring the greater trochanter forward to facilitate exposure. The opposite hip is placed in 40 degrees of abduction. Image intensifier anteroposterior fluoroscopy is used to show the femoral head and neck, the greater trochanter, and the upper femoral shaft. Rotate the hip medially so that the greater trochanter is seen in profile and not superimposed over the femoral neck. It is crucial to visualize the trochanteric fossa. Prepare and drape the affected hip and upper two thirds of the thigh in the usual manner.

Operative Technique

A. and **B.** A straight lateral longitudinal incision is made from the tip of the greater trochanter and extending distally for 10 cm. The subcutaneous tissue is divided in line with the skin incision.

C. The fascia lata is split longitudinally in the direction of its fibers.

D. and **E.** The vastus lateralis is detached proximally from the abductor tubercle by a proximally based, horseshoe-shaped incision and elevated subperiosteally from the femoral shaft for 5 to 7 cm. Be sure that the vastus lateralis is elevated in its entire width.

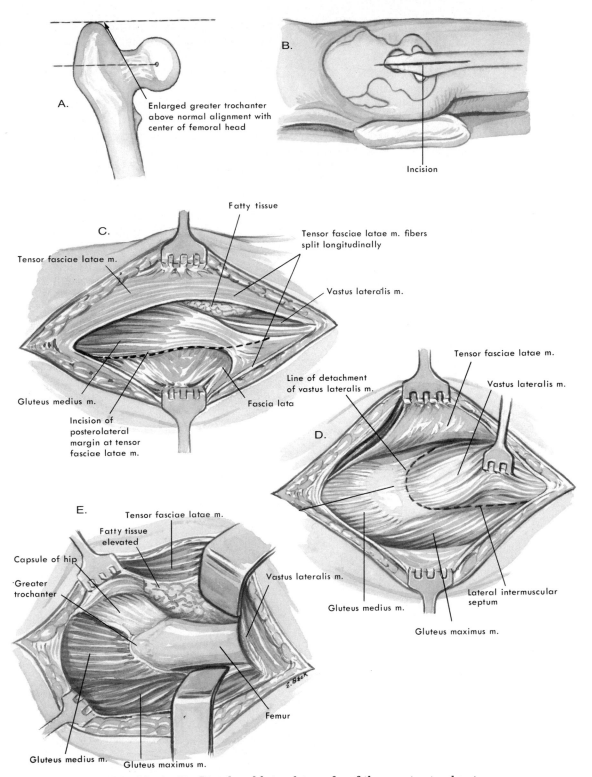

A. Enlarged greater trochanter above normal alignment with center of femoral head

B. Incision

C. Fatty tissue
Tensor fasciae latae m. fibers split longitudinally
Tensor fasciae latae m.
Vastus lateralis m.
Line of detachment of vastus lateralis m.
Gluteus medius m.
Incision of posterolateral margin at tensor fasciae latae m.
Fascia lata

D. Tensor fasciae latae m.
Vastus lateralis m.
Gluteus medius m.
Lateral intermuscular septum
Gluteus maximus m.

E. Tensor fasciae latae m.
Fatty tissue elevated
Capsule of hip
Greater trochanter
Vastus lateralis m.
Gluteus medius m.
Gluteus maximus m.
Femur

Plate 92. A.–P., Distal and lateral transfer of the greater trochanter.

F. Identify the anterior border of the gluteus medius, and introduce a blunt elevator-retractor beneath its deep surface, pointing in the direction of the trochanteric fossa.

G. At this time, to orient the plane of the trochanteric osteotomy properly, insert a smooth Kirschner wire at the level of the abductor tubercle, pointing to the trochanteric fossa along a line continuous with the upper cortex of the femoral neck. Radiography with image intensification will verify the proper level and depth of the guide wire. The point of the Kirschner wire must not protrude through the medial cortex into the trochanteric fossa.

H. Place a blunt flat retractor beneath the posterior border of the greater trochanter to protect the soft tissues. The previously applied anterior retractor protects the soft tissues ventrally. With a 2- to 3-cm.-wide reciprocating saw, divide the greater trochanter in the anteroposterior direction, following the proximal border of the Kirschner wire. Take care to stop the cut 3 cm. short of the medial cortex of the trochanteric fossa. Avoid injury to the vessels in the trochanteric fossa to prevent necrosis of the femoral head.

I. A 3-mm.-wide flat osteotome is driven through the osteotomy cleft, and the osteotomy site is wedged open by moving the handle of the osteotome craniad. By leverage with the osteotome in the cleft, a greenstick fracture of the medial cortex is produced.

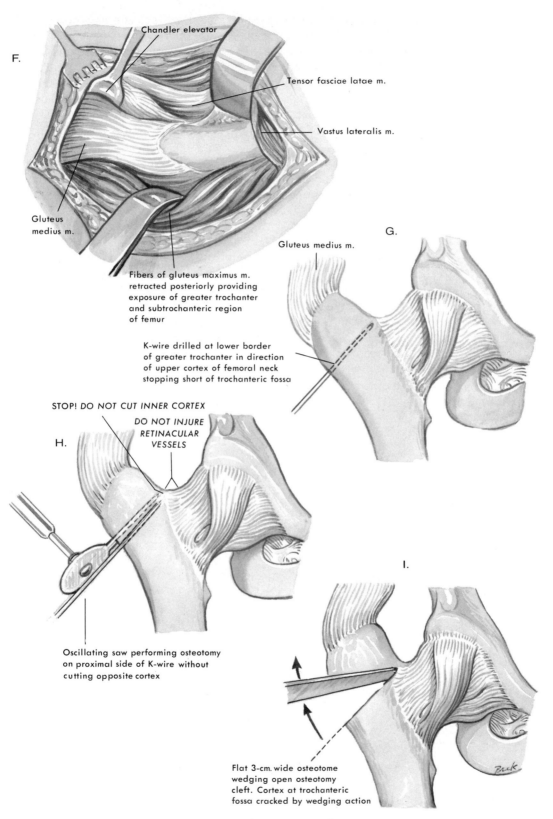

F.

Chandler elevator

Tensor fasciae latae m.

Vastus lateralis m.

Gluteus medius m.

Fibers of gluteus maximus m. retracted posteriorly providing exposure of greater trochanter and subtrochanteric region of femur

G.

Gluteus medius m.

K-wire drilled at lower border of greater trochanter in direction of upper cortex of femoral neck stopping short of trochanteric fossa

STOP! *DO NOT CUT INNER CORTEX*

DO NOT INJURE RETINACULAR VESSELS

H.

Oscillating saw performing osteotomy on proximal side of K-wire without cutting opposite cortex

I.

Flat 3-cm. wide osteotome wedging open osteotomy cleft. Cortex at trochanteric fossa cracked by wedging action

Plate 92. (Continued)

J. Place a large periosteal elevator deep into the osteotomy cleft, opening it up medially by gently levering the handle up and down. The trochanteric fragment is lifted superolaterally with a Lewin bone clamp, and adhesions between the joint capsule and the medial aspect of the greater trochanter are released. This must be done very carefully in order not to injure retinacular blood vessels in the capsule.

Do not fracture the greater trochanter! Mobilization is sufficient when, upon lateral and distal traction on the greater trochanter, the muscle response is elastic; if there is still muscle resistance, it means that further adhesions are present that must be freed.

K. After sufficient mobilization of the greater trochanter, the recipient site on the lateral surface of the upper femoral shaft is prepared with a curved osteotome to create a flattened surface. Do not remove too much bone laterally. Next, the greater trochanter is displaced distally and laterally; in excessive femoral antetorsion it may be moved slightly forward. If additional distal advancement is desired, the hip may be abducted on the fracture table.

L. and **M.** The trochanter is held in the desired position and temporarily fixed to the femur with two threaded Kirschner wires of adequate size that are drilled upward and medially. At this point, the accuracy of the position of the greater trochanter is verified by image intensifier radiography. As stated previously, the tip of the greater trochanter should be level with the center of the femoral head and at a distance from it of two to two and a half times the radius of the femoral head. If there are problems with proper visualization, place a long Kirschner wire horizontally and parallel to both anterior superior iliac spines, crossing the center of the femoral head; then check the position of the tip of the greater trochanter.

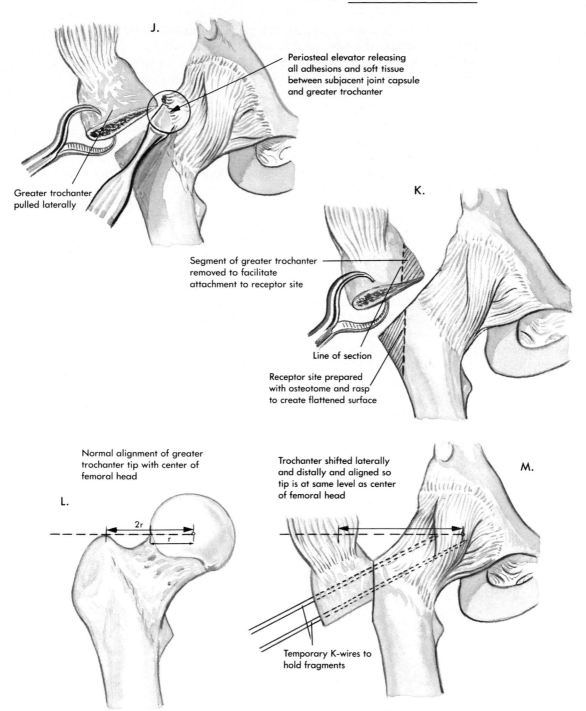

J.

Periosteal elevator releasing all adhesions and soft tissue between subjacent joint capsule and greater trochanter

Greater trochanter pulled laterally

K.

Segment of greater trochanter removed to facilitate attachment to receptor site

Line of section

Receptor site prepared with osteotome and rasp to create flattened surface

L.

Normal alignment of greater trochanter tip with center of femoral head

$2r$

r

M.

Trochanter shifted laterally and distally and aligned so tip is at same level as center of femoral head

Temporary K-wires to hold fragments

Plate 92. (Continued)

N. Prior to osteosynthesis, the gluteal muscle is split in the direction of the fibers to expose the bone and to avoid muscle necrosis. The greater trochanter is fixed to the lateral surface of the upper femur with two lag screws (each equipped with a washer), which are directed medially and distally at a 45-degree angle to counteract the pull of the hip abductors. For large trochanters, 6.5-mm. cancellous screws with drill bits of appropriate size are used; with smaller trochanters, 3.2-mm. screws are used. The outer cortex of the greater trochanter may be overdrilled. Tapping of the outer cortex is optional. The washers increase the surface area, avoid cutting through the cortex, ensure more secure fixation, and allow early motion. After both screws are inserted, the initial Kirschner wires are removed. At present, I use cannulated hip screws; they are simpler to insert.

O. An alternative method of fixation is the use of two heavy threaded Kirschner wires directed medially and upward. The resultant pull of the hip abductors through the direction of the wires provides force that will compress the greater trochanter against the lateral surface of the femur. This author does not recommend internal fixation by this method because screw fixation is more stable. However, in an obese or uncooperative patient, threaded Kirschner wires may be used in addition to screw fixation; or a tension wire band may be used as described in lateral advancement of the greater trochanter (see Plate 93).

P. Make final intraoperative radiograms to ensure that the trochanter has been advanced to the desired site. Next, the detached origin of the vastus lateralis is firmly sutured to the tendinous insertion of the gluteus medius and minimus muscles. This tension-band suture absorbs the pull of the hip abductors and reinforces the internal fixation of the greater trochanter. A suction drain is inserted, and the remainder of the wound is closed in routine fashion. The skin closure is subcuticular.

Postoperative Care. The patient is placed in split Russell's traction with each hip in 35 to 40 degrees of abduction. Active assisted exercises are begun as soon as the patient is comfortable, usually the third postoperative day. Adduction and excessive flexion of the hip should be avoided. Hip abduction exercises are performed supine, which eliminates the effect of gravity. Sitting is not permitted for three weeks because, with 60 to 90 degrees of hip flexion, the posterior fibers of the gluteus medius muscle exert a strong lateral rotatory force on the greater trochanter and may loosen its fixation.

The patient is allowed to be out of bed on crutches on the third postoperative day and instructed to walk; a three-point gait with partial weight-bearing protects the limb that was operated. The patient is discharged home as soon as he or she is independent and secure on crutches. Three weeks after surgery, side-lying hip abduction exercises are started, and the child is allowed to sit and to return to school. At six weeks bony consolidation is usually adequate to begin use of one crutch on the opposite side (to protect the hip that was operated) and to perform standing Trendelenburg exercises. One-crutch protection should be continued until hip abductor muscles are normal or good in motor strength and Trendelenburg's sign is negative.

The screws are removed three to six months postoperatively. During removal, be very cautious not to damage the gluteus medius and minimus muscle fibers. After removal of the screws, the hip is protected by three-point partial weight-bearing on crutches for two to three weeks, and exercises consisting of side-lying hip abduction and standing Trendelenburg exercises are performed to regain the motor strength of the hip abductor muscles.

REFERENCES

Kelikian, A. S., Tachdjian, M. O., Askew, M. J., and Jasty, M.: Greater trochanteric advancement of the proximal femur: A clinical and biomechanical study. In: Hungerford, D. S. (ed.): The Hip:

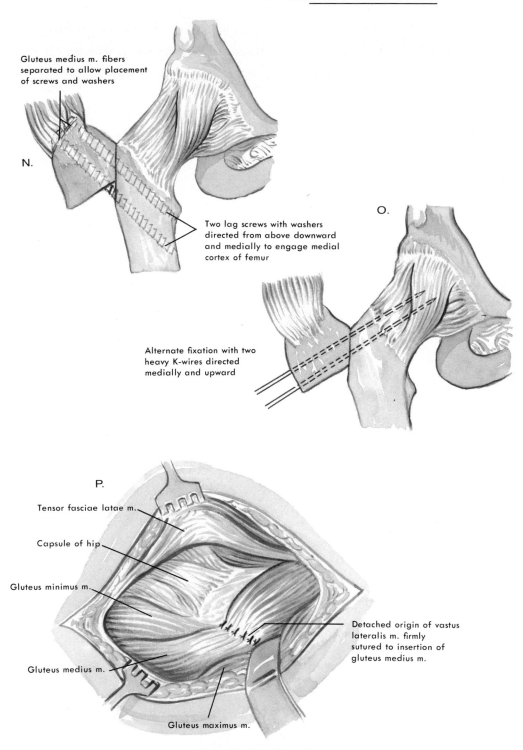

Gluteus medius m. fibers separated to allow placement of screws and washers

N.

O.

Two lag screws with washers directed from above downward and medially to engage medial cortex of femur

Alternate fixation with two heavy K-wires directed medially and upward

P.

Tensor fasciae latae m.

Capsule of hip

Gluteus minimus m.

Gluteus medius m.

Gluteus maximus m.

Detached origin of vastus lateralis m. firmly sutured to insertion of gluteus medius m.

Plate 92. (Continued)

Proceedings of the 11th Open Scientific Meeting of the Hip Society, 1983. St. Louis, C. V. Mosby, 1983, pp. 77–105.

Macnicol, M. F., and Makris, D.: Distal transfer of the greater trochanter. J. Bone Joint Surg., 73–B:838, 1991.

Tachdjian, M. O., and Kelikian, A. S.: Distal and lateral advancement of the greater trochanter. In: Tachdjian, M. O. (ed.): Congenital Dislocation of the Hip. New York, Churchill Livingstone, 1982, pp. 721–739.

Tauber, C., Ganel, A., Horoszowski, H., and Farine, I.: Distal transfer of the greater trochanter in coxa vara. Acta Orthop. Scand., 51:611, 1980.

Wagner, H.: Femoral osteotomies for congenital hip dislocation. In: Weil, U. H. (ed.): Progress in Orthopedic Surgery. Vol. 2. Acetabular Dysplasia and Skeletal Dysplasia in Childhood. Heidelberg, Springer, 1978. p. 85.

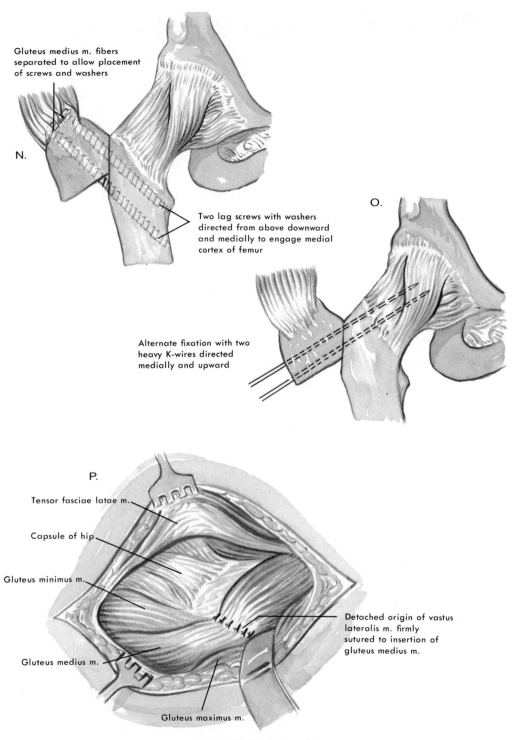

Gluteus medius m. fibers separated to allow placement of screws and washers

N.

Two lag screws with washers directed from above downward and medially to engage medial cortex of femur

O.

Alternate fixation with two heavy K-wires directed medially and upward

P.

Tensor fasciae latae m.

Capsule of hip

Gluteus minimus m.

Gluteus medius m.

Gluteus maximus m.

Detached origin of vastus lateralis m. firmly sutured to insertion of gluteus medius m.

Plate 92. (Continued)

PLATE 93   Lateral Advancement of the Greater Trochanter

Indications

1. Short femoral neck.
2. Tip of the greater trochanter level with the center of the femoral head (i.e., there is no relative overgrowth of the greater trochanter).

Requisites

1. Congruous and concentric reduction of hip joint.
2. A femoral neck–shaft angle of at least 110 degrees. (If it is less than 110 degrees, perform a lateral closing-wedge osteotomy of the proximal femur combined with greater trochanteric arrest.)
3. Functional range of hip motion, with total arc of hip abduction–adduction of at least 45 degrees.
4. Preoperative hip abductor muscle strength of at least fair minus.
5. Femoral antetorsion of less than 40 degrees.
6. Lower age limit of eight years.

Blood for Transfusion. Yes.

Radiographic Control. Image intensifier.

Patient Position. Supine on a fracture table.

Operative Technique

A. The surgical exposure of the greater trochanter and upper femoral shaft is similar to that for distal and lateral transfer of the greater trochanter (see Plate 92, Steps **A.** to **K.**).

B. The tip of the greater trochanter is at its normal level, so it is not necessary to advance it distally. It is kept horizontally level with the center of the femoral head, and its position is maintained by two wide-threaded, positional cancellous screws. Insert the screws horizontally perpendicular to the osteotomized lateral surface of the upper femur. The threads of these "positioning" screws grip the trochanter as well as the intertrochanteric region of the femur without compression. The cleft between the greater trochanter and femur is filled with autogenous cancellous iliac bone, taken through a separate incision over the iliac apophysis.

C. Internal fixation is augmented by a taut tension band of heavy wire suture that extends from the neck of each trochanteric screw to a small unicortical screw, anchored 6 cm. distally in the femur. This wire tension band counteracts the pull of the hip abductors.

D. Suture the detached vastus lateralis to the insertion of the gluteus medius. Close the subcutaneous tissue and the skin in the usual manner.

Postoperative Care. Care is similar to that following distal and lateral transfer of the greater trochanter (see Plate 92).

REFERENCES

Kelikian, A. S., Tachdjian, M. O., Askew, M. J., and Jasty, M.: Greater trochanteric advancement of the proximal femur: A clinical and biomechanical study. In: Hungerford, D. S. (ed.): The Hip: Proceedings of the 11th Open Scientific Meeting of the Hip Society, 1983. St. Louis, C. V. Mosby, 1983, pp. 77–105.

Tachdjian, M. O., and Edelstein, D.: Periacetabular osteotomy through the subinguinal medial adductor approach. Paper presented at the American Orthopedic Association Annual Meeting, 1985, San Diego. Orthop. Trans., 9: No. 2, Spring 1985.

Wagner, H.: Femoral osteotomies for congenital hip dislocation. In: Weil, U. H. (ed.): Progress in Orthopedic Surgery. Vol. 2. Acetabular Dysplasia and Skeletal Dysplasia in Childhood. Heidelberg, Springer, 1978, p. 85.

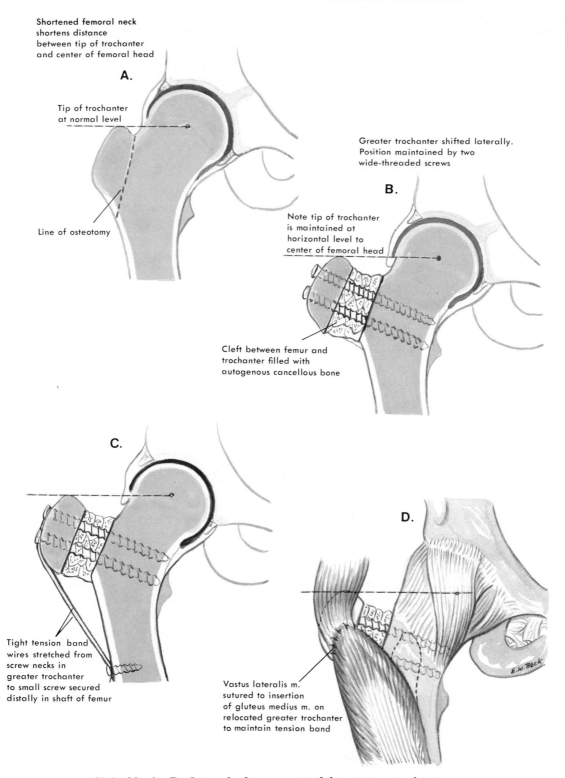

Shortened femoral neck
shortens distance
between tip of trochanter
and center of femoral head

A.

Tip of trochanter
at normal level

Line of osteotomy

Greater trochanter shifted laterally.
Position maintained by two
wide-threaded screws

B.

Note tip of trochanter
is maintained at
horizontal level to
center of femoral head

Cleft between femur and
trochanter filled with
autogenous cancellous bone

C.

Tight tension band
wires stretched from
screw necks in
greater trochanter
to small screw secured
distally in shaft of femur

D.

Vastus lateralis m.
sutured to insertion
of gluteus medius m. on
relocated greater trochanter
to maintain tension band

E.W. BECK

Plate 93. A.–D., Lateral advancement of the greater trochanter.

PLATE 94 ## Wagner's Intertrochanteric Double Femoral Osteotomy

Indications. Marked overgrowth of greater trochanter when its tip abuts the lateral wall of the ilium with a very short femoral neck and a femoral neck–shaft angle decreased from normal to 110 degrees.

Requisite. Relative congruity of the hip.

Blood for Transfusion. Yes.

Radiographic Control. Image intensifier.

Principle. The first step of the operation is a soft-tissue release of the hip adductors and iliopsoas muscle through a separate medial incision. Compressive forces between the femoral head and acetabulum should be relieved, since elongation of the femoral neck will increase intra-articular pressure. The objectives are to elongate the femoral neck, restore the neck-shaft angle to normal, and displace the greater trochanter laterally and distally.

The bony procedure consists of two horizontal osteotomies: the first at the base of the greater trochanter at the level of the upper border of the femoral neck; and the second through the upper end of the femoral shaft (above the lesser trochanter), level with the lower margin of the femoral neck. The double osteotomy creates three fragments that can be moved and redirected independently of each other.

Patient Position. Supine on a fracture table.

Operative Technique

A. The proximal part of the femur is exposed through a lateral longitudinal approach, as described for distal and lateral transfer (see Plate 92, Steps **A.** through **K.**).

First, insert a heavy threaded Steinmann pin in the center of the axis of the femoral head. The pin should stop short of the capital femoral physis. The level of the two horizontal osteotomies is determined under image intensifier. The first should be at the base of the greater trochanter and the second at the upper end of the femoral shaft immediately distal to the base of the femoral neck. These levels are marked by inserting smooth Kirschner wires into bone.

B. A heavy threaded Steinmann pin is inserted in the midportion of the greater trochanter, stopping short of its medial cortex. Next, perform the two horizontal osteotomies under image intensifier radiographic control. It is vital to avoid injury to the vessels in the trochanteric fossa and the retinacular vessels.

The deep ends of the osteotomies should stop short of the medial cortex, in which a greenstick fracture is made. First the greater trochanter is pulled cephalad to facilitate exposure. Next, the femoral neck fragment is pushed downward and medially into the desired position; then the distal femoral fragment is pulled laterally so that the medial cortex of the upper end of the femoral shaft serves as a buttress to the inferomedial corner of the femoral neck. This maneuver elongates the femoral neck.

C. When the femoral head and neck and the femoral shaft have been brought into the corrected position, three smooth Kirschner wires are used to transfix and temporarily hold the fragments. Next, the greater trochanter is transferred distally and laterally and fixed to the femoral neck with the threaded pin previously inserted in its midportion. Make radiograms to check the realignment of the three fragments and the correction achieved.

D. Perform osteosynthesis by a molded semitubular plate, which is prepared as follows. With a powerful wire cutter, a vertical slot is cut out from the plate's upper end to the first screw hole. The bifurcated limbs are trimmed at their tips to sharp points and bent inward to form hooks. The semitubular plate is reshaped to fit the superolateral surface of the upper femur. The hooks are inserted in the

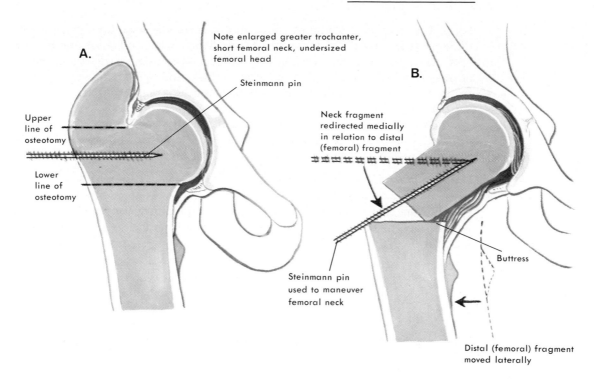

A.

Note enlarged greater trochanter, short femoral neck, undersized femoral head

Steinmann pin

Upper line of osteotomy

Lower line of osteotomy

B.

Neck fragment redirected medially in relation to distal (femoral) fragment

Buttress

Steinmann pin used to maneuver femoral neck

Distal (femoral) fragment moved laterally

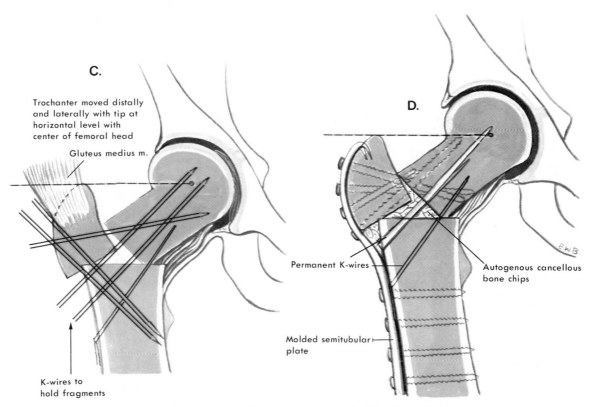

C.

Trochanter moved distally and laterally with tip at horizontal level with center of femoral head

Gluteus medius m.

K-wires to hold fragments

D.

Permanent K-wires

Autogenous cancellous bone chips

Molded semitubular plate

Plate 94. A.–D., Wagner's intertrochanteric double femoral osteotomy.

tip of the greater trochanter, deep into cancellous bone for firm anchorage. The diagonally inserted Kirschner wires transfix the neck and shaft and prevent medial shifting of the femoral neck on the buttress provided by the upper medial cortex of the femoral shaft. Insert all the screws and pack the spaces between the fragments with autogenous cancellous bone obtained from the ilium through a separate incision.

Some surgeons may prefer to use other methods of internal fixation, such as a 90- or 130-degree AO right-angle plate, and stabilization of the fragments with multiple screws.

Postoperative Care. Osteosynthesis is secure, permitting active assisted exercises three or four days postoperatively. The patient is kept in bilateral split Russell's traction for three weeks, until the hip develops functional range of motion. Then partial weight-bearing is permitted with three-point crutch gait protection. Bone healing is usually solid in three months, at which time full weight-bearing is allowed.

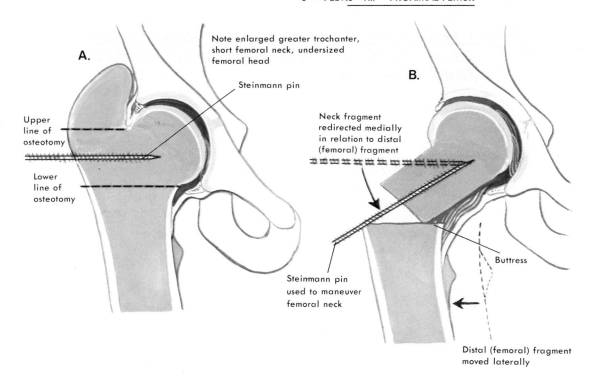

A.

Note enlarged greater trochanter, short femoral neck, undersized femoral head

Steinmann pin

Upper line of osteotomy

Lower line of osteotomy

B.

Neck fragment redirected medially in relation to distal (femoral) fragment

Buttress

Steinmann pin used to maneuver femoral neck

Distal (femoral) fragment moved laterally

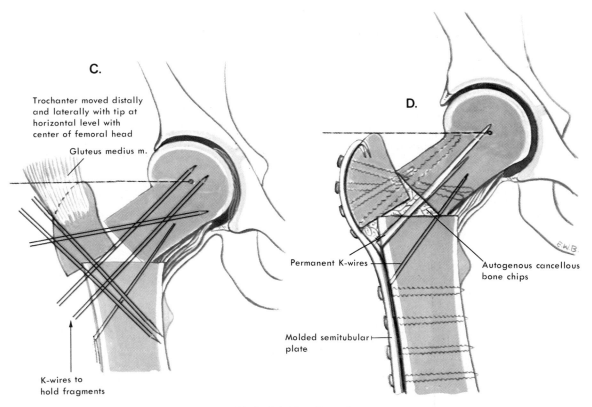

C.

Trochanter moved distally and laterally with tip at horizontal level with center of femoral head

Gluteus medius m.

K-wires to hold fragments

D.

Permanent K-wires

Autogenous cancellous bone chips

Molded semitubular plate

Plate 94. (Continued)

PLATE 95

Lateral-Based Closing-Wedge Valgization Osteotomy of the Proximal Femur with Distal-Lateral Advancement of the Greater Trochanter

Indications. Coxa vara deformity (femoral neck–shaft angle of less than 110 degrees) with relative overgrowth of the greater trochanter.

Requisites

1. Congruous and concentric reduction of hip joint.
2. Functional range of hip motion with total arc of hip abduction–adduction of at least 45 degrees.
3. Preoperative hip abductor muscle strength of at least fair minus.
4. Femoral antetorsion of less than 40 degrees.
5. Lower age limit of eight years.

Blood for Transfusion. Yes.

Radiographic Control. Image intensifier.

The greater trochanter and the upper femoral shaft are exposed according to the technique described in Plate 92, Steps **A.** through **K.** If the hip adductors are taut, they are released through a separate medial incision.

Patient Position. Supine on a fracture table.

Operative Technique

A. and **B.** The greater trochanter is osteotomized following the technique described for distal and lateral advancement. Then two threaded Steinmann pins are inserted to serve as guides for the level and angle of osteotomy. The apex of the osteotomy stops 1 cm. short of the medial cortex. The length of the base of the wedge depends on the degree of correction of coxa vara required. The wedge of bone is resected with an oscillating saw.

C. With a straight osteotome and the leverage of the pins anchored in the femur, a greenstick fracture is produced in the medial cortex, converting the osteotomy to a short-stemmed Y.

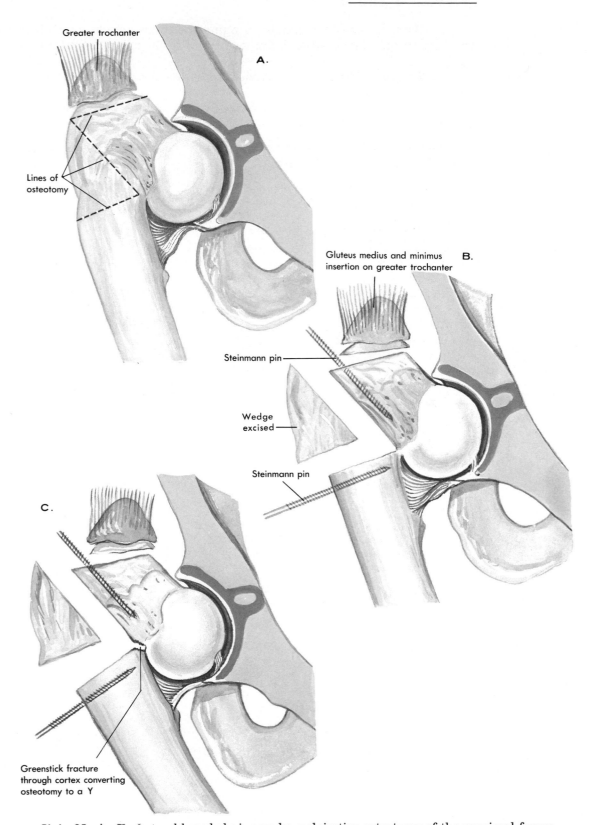

Greater trochanter

Lines of
osteotomy

A.

Gluteus medius and minimus
insertion on greater trochanter

B.

Steinmann pin

Wedge
excised

Steinmann pin

C.

Greenstick fracture
through cortex converting
osteotomy to a Y

Plate 95. A.–F., Lateral-based closing-wedge valgization osteotomy of the proximal femur
with distal-lateral advancement of the greater trochanter.

D. Close the osteotomy gap by bringing the two Steinmann pins together and by aligning the neck shaft and greater trochanter at a preoperatively determined angle.

E. The greater trochanter is transfixed with a threaded Steinmann pin driven into the neck of the femur.

F. The three fragments are then fixed with a pre-bent trochanteric hook plate and screws.

Postoperative Care. Care is similar to that after Wagner's intertrochanteric double femoral osteotomy (see Plate 94).

REFERENCE

Kelikian, A. S., Tachdjian, M. O., Askew, M. J., and Jasty, M.: Greater trochanteric advancement of the proximal femur: A clinical and biomechanical study. In: Hungerford, D. S. (ed.): The Hip: Proceedings of the 11th Open Scientific Meeting of the Hip Society, 1983. St. Louis: C. V. Mosby, 1983, pp. 77–105.

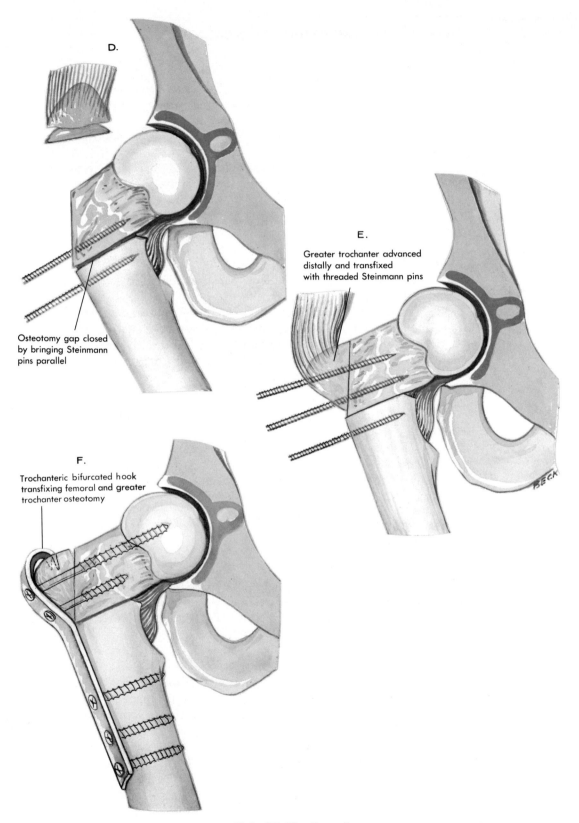

D.

Osteotomy gap closed
by bringing Steinmann
pins parallel

E.

Greater trochanter advanced
distally and transfixed
with threaded Steinmann pins

F.

Trochanteric bifurcated hook
transfixing femoral and greater
trochanter osteotomy

Plate 95. (Continued)

PLATE 96　## Pauwels' Intertrochanteric Y-Osteotomy

Objectives

1. Correction of the femoral neck–shaft angle to normal alignment.
2. Simultaneous correction of associated retrotorsion of the upper part of the femur.
3. Conversion of position of the capital femoral physis from nearly vertical to horizontal.
4. Stimulation of ossification and healing of the defective femoral neck.
5. Restoration of normal biomechanics of the hip and muscle physiology of gluteus medius–minimus.
6. Prevention of development of secondary dysplastic changes in the acetabulum.

Indications

1. Femoral neck–shaft angle of less than 105 degrees.
2. A defect in the femoral neck.
3. Hilgenreiner epiphyseal (HE) angle of greater than 60 degrees. The HE angle, measured on the anteroposterior radiogram of the hip, is the angle between the Hilgenreiner line on the horizontal axis and the line through the metaphyseal side of the defect on the femoral neck on the vertical axis.
4. Progression of varus deformity.

Age. The best age for this surgery is between one and two years.

Caution! Rule out associated dysplasia of the acetabulum. Perform CT scan with three-dimensional reconstruction or magnetic resonance imaging (MRI). If there is a deficient acetabulum (usually posterior because of femoral retrotorsion), correct it by acetabuloplasty or Albee shelf arthroplasty at the time of valgization osteotomy of the proximal femur. Provision of a stable hip joint is vital because the femur is short and will require lengthening in the future.

Radiographic Control. Image intensifier.

Blood for Transfusion. Yes.

Patient Position. The patient is placed supine on a radiolucent operating table. The hip and the upper end of the femur should be clearly visualized on the image intensifier. The entire hip and the whole lower limb are prepared and draped to permit free passive motion. The child older than six to eight years of age is best operated on while lying on a fracture table.

Operative Technique

A. The upper end of the femur and the trochanteric region are exposed through a direct lateral approach. On a transparent paper placed on the radiogram, draw the hip joint, physis, and axis of the shaft of the femur. First, draw a horizontal line "H," which transects the axis of the femoral shaft 4 to 6 cm. below the lesser trochanter. Second, draw an interrupted line "Ps" through the physis and extend it inferiorly until it intersects the horizontal line H. Third, from the point of intersection of the lines H and Ps, draw a line inclined upward 16 degrees from the horizontal and extend it laterally to intersect the axis of the femoral shaft (this line is approximately at right angles to the direction of the resultant compressive force R). The angle formed between the third line (inclined upward) and the interrupted line Ps is the angle of the wedge of bone based laterally to be resected (50 degrees in the drawing).

B. Next, draw the upper line of the intertrochanteric osteotomy. It should extend medially to transect the capital physis at the zone of resorption in the femoral neck. Then draw the wedge to be resected with its apex reaching the upper

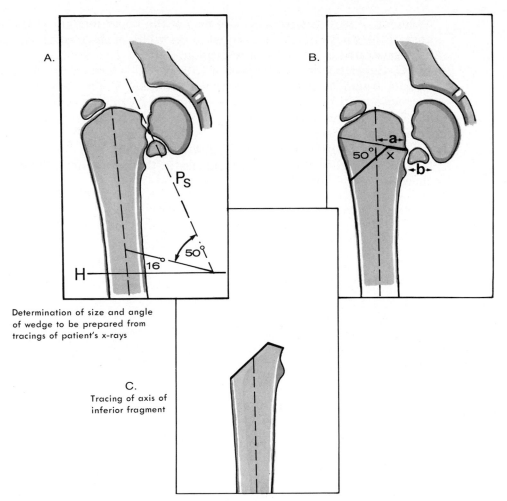

A.

P_S

50°

H   16°

Determination of size and angle
of wedge to be prepared from
tracings of patient's x-rays

B.

a

50°   x

b

C.
Tracing of axis of
inferior fragment

Plate 96. A.–L., Pauwels' intertrochanteric Y-osteotomy.

osteotomy line at the point X. The part of the upper femoral shaft vertical to the apex of the wedge (X) must be equal to the width of the medial part of the femoral neck separated by the zone of resorption.

C. Superimpose a new sheet of transparent paper on the first, and trace the inferior fragment of the osteotomy with its axis. Rotate the upper tracing sheet clockwise until the osteotomy lines of the two fragments coincide (see p. 463).

D. Trace the upper fragment. The two axes of the femoral shaft should form an angle of 50 degrees.

E. Rotate the upper tracing sheet back, sliding it upward parallel to the femoral axis until the femoral head lies in the acetabular socket of the original sheet; trace the acetabulum.

E.
Upper tracing sheet rotated back and slid upward parallel to axis of femur until femoral head lies in socket of original sheet. Socket is then traced

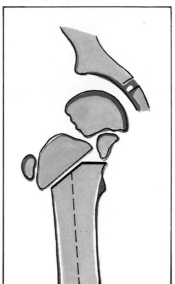

D.
Upper tracing sheet rotated clockwise until osteotomy lines of two fragments coincide. Two axes then form angle of 50°

50°

Plate 96. (Continued)

F. Resect the angle of the bone wedge as prepared from tracings of the radiogram.

G. Under image intensifier radiographic control, determine the lines of osteotomy by drilling Kirschner wires above and below the wedge resection lines. The upper Kirschner wire should stop short of the capital physis and the defect in the neck of the femur, and the tip of the lower Kirschner wire should be just below the upper osteotomy line and terminate medial to the point X, which marks the apex of the bone to be resected.

H. With an oscillating saw, perform the upper intertrochanteric osteotomy and resect the wedge of bone.

I. Remove the wedge of bone with flat osteotomes.

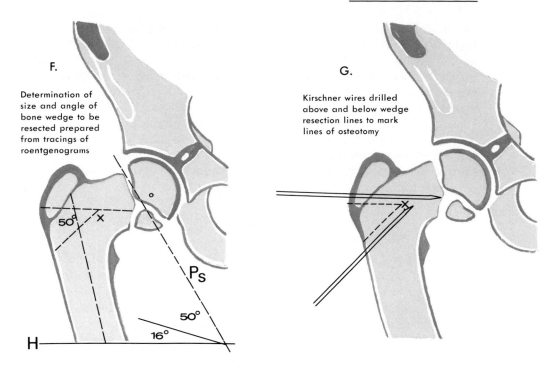

F.

Determination of size and angle of bone wedge to be resected prepared from tracings of roentgenograms

50°

X

Ps

50°

16°

H

G.

Kirschner wires drilled above and below wedge resection lines to mark lines of osteotomy

X

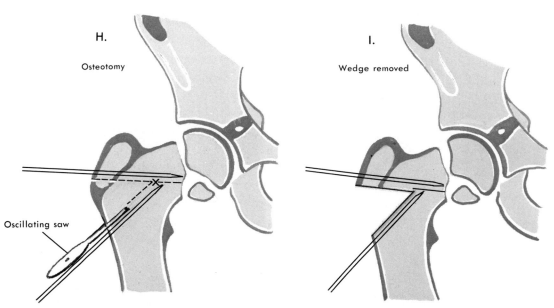

H.

Osteotomy

Oscillating saw

X

I.

Wedge removed

Plate 96. (Continued)

J. A hook over the greater trochanter is used to pull the upper segment distally, and the two Kirschner wires are made parallel to each other, closing the gap.

K. Pauwels recommends fixing the osteotomy fragments with a metal tension band. First, two holes are made with 2-mm. Kirschner wires parallel to the osteotomy surfaces, the first 1 cm. below and the second 1 cm. above the osteotomy line. These Kirschner wires are directed from the middle of the lateral surface of the shaft to the anterior aspect of the femoral neck. A wire is passed through the two holes and twisted on the lateral aspect of the femur. Pauwels finds that this method of fixation is adequate and maintains the osteotomized surfaces in compression, and he applies a plaster of Paris spica cast for six to eight weeks.

L. This author prefers internal fixation with screws and a band plate hooked over the greater trochanter. In the cooperative child over six years of age, hip spica cast immobilization is not necessary.

Postoperative Care. The hip spica cast is removed in six to eight weeks when the osteotomy is healed. Gentle passive and active exercises are performed to restore normal motor strength of muscles controlling the hip, knee, and ankle and normal range of motion of joints. Protect the hip by walker or crutches, depending on the age of the child. Prevent falls; stress fracture of the osteoporotic bone can occur.

Remove the internal fixation device six to twelve months postoperatively. Following hardware removal, protect the hip in a single spica cast until screw holes are filled in with bone.

REFERENCES

Pauwels, F.: Zur Therapie der kindlichen Coxa vara. Z. Orthop., 64:372, 1936.
Pauwels, F.: Uber die Coxa vara. Verh. Dtsch. Orthop. Ges., 24:8, 1930.
Pauwels, F.: Zur Therapie der Klinischen Coxa vara. Verh. Dtsch. Orthop. Ges., 30:372, 1935.
Pauwels, F.: Biomechanics of the Normal and Diseased Hip. New York, Springer, 1976.

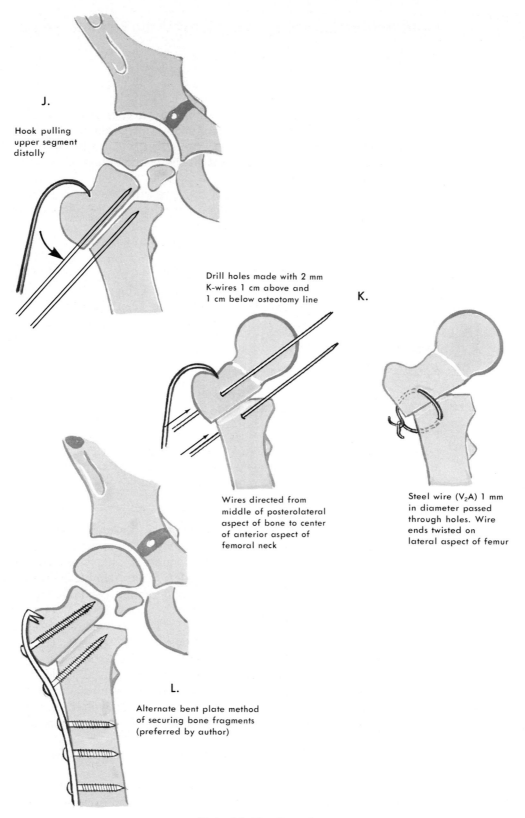

J.

Hook pulling upper segment distally

Drill holes made with 2 mm K-wires 1 cm above and 1 cm below osteotomy line

K.

Wires directed from middle of posterolateral aspect of bone to center of anterior aspect of femoral neck

Steel wire (V₂A) 1 mm in diameter passed through holes. Wire ends twisted on lateral aspect of femur

L.

Alternate bent plate method of securing bone fragments (preferred by author)

Plate 96. (Continued)

PLATE 97   ## Intertrochanteric Valgus Osteotomy of the Proximal Femur

Indications

1. Femoral neck–shaft angle of less than 105 degrees.
2. A defect in the femoral neck.
3. Hilgenreiner epiphyseal (HE) angle of greater than 60 degrees. The HE angle, measured on the anteroposterior radiogram of the hip, is the angle between the Hilgenreiner line on the horizontal axis and the line through the metaphyseal side of the defect on the femoral neck on the vertical axis.
4. Progression of varus deformity.
5. In the adolescent, with segmental avascular necrosis of the femoral head, when valgization and extension osteotomy will remove the avascular segment of the femoral head from the weight-bearing portion.
6. Hinged abduction of the hip in Legg-Calvé-Perthes disease; when the hip is congruent in adduction and some flexion and has a functional range of hip adduction beyond the point of congruity. The objective is to align the lower limb in the middle of the arc of movement, provide a congruent position of the femoral head with the acetabulum in weight-bearing position, relieve the hinging, and improve the remodeling process with rounding of the femoral head.

Blood for Transfusion. Yes.

Radiographic Control. Image intensifier.

Special Instrumentation. AO instrumentation. This author recommends the biologic plating using the limited-contact dynamic compression plate (LC-DCP).

Patient Position. With the patient supine on a radiolucent operating table, the entire hip and lower limb are prepared and draped to permit free passive motion without contaminating the operative field. The proximal femur and intertrochanteric region are exposed through a direct lateral surgical approach.

Operative Technique

A. The osteotomy is intertrochanteric with a wedge based laterally. The size of the wedge of bone to be resected is determined from drawings of the radiogram. Do not disturb the greater trochanteric apophysis. Determine the wedge resection lines by drilling Kirschner wires. The inferior wire should be immediately at the upper margin of the lesser trochanter and drilled cephalad and medially. The proximal wire is drilled perpendicular to the femoral shaft, more or less parallel to the inferior cortex of the femoral neck. The osteotomy lines converge at the medial cortex at the base of the neck of the femur.

B. With a power drill, insert two threaded Steinmann pins from the greater trochanter to the line of the upper osteotomy at a 50- to 70-degree angle. Do not cross the line of osteotomy. Insert a large threaded Steinmann pin penetrating the medial cortex of the femoral shaft. The upper and lower fragment pins should be at a predetermined rotational plane so that, with valgization, femoral retrotorsion can be corrected simultaneously.

C. With an oscillating saw and flat, sharp osteotomes, perform the osteotomy and resect the wedge of bone.

D. The distal femoral fragment is abducted and rotated and internally fixed with criss-cross threaded Steinmann pins. The wound is closed in the usual fashion. A one-and-one-half hip spica cast is applied.

Postoperative Care. Remove the pins in four weeks using general anesthesia. Apply another hip spica cast for an additional two to three weeks until there is adequate bone healing.

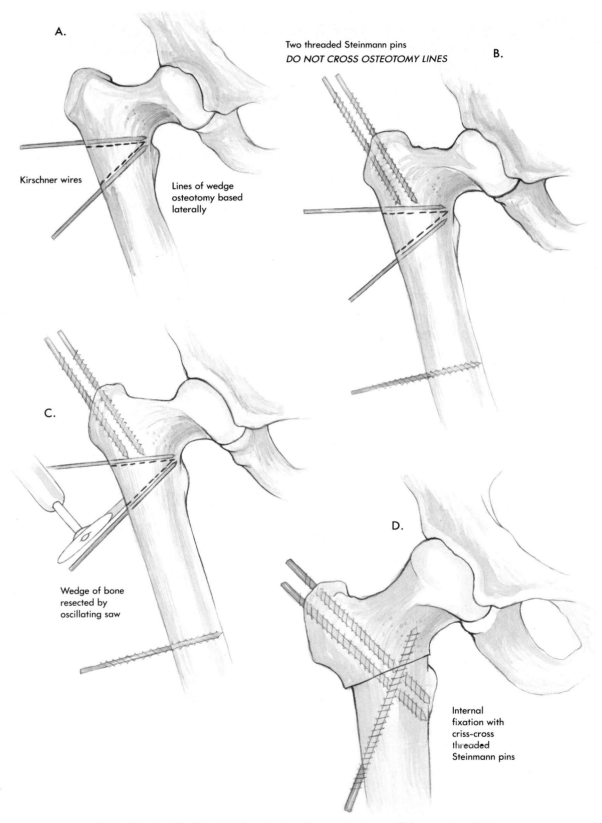

A.

Kirschner wires

Lines of wedge
osteotomy based
laterally

B.

Two threaded Steinmann pins
DO NOT CROSS OSTEOTOMY LINES

C.

Wedge of bone
resected by
oscillating saw

D.

Internal
fixation with
criss-cross
threaded
Steinmann pins

Plate 97. A.–D., Intertrochanteric valgus osteotomy of the proximal femur.

PLATE 98	**Rotation and Angulation (Valgization or Varization) Intertrochanteric Oblique Osteotomy (MacEwen and Shands Technique)**

Principle. An oblique cut through the bone in a single plane permits a change in both the angulation and rotation of the fragments if the osteotomized fragments are kept in contact. The direction and obliquity of the osteotomy determine the relative change in angulation and rotation. If an oblique osteotomy is made at the intertrochanteric level running from the anterior surface of the femur distally and posteriorly, *adduction* of the distal fragment will decrease *coxa valga* and *antetorsion* and *abduction* of the lower fragment will correct *coxa vara* and *retrotorsion*. The more oblique the cut, the less the correction of torsion and the greater the correction of angulation. The closer the plane of osteotomy to a right angle to the long axis of the femur, the greater the correction of torsion.

Indications. Excessive coxa valga with antetorsion or excessive coxa vara with retrotorsion. Proponents of this technique perform the procedure when both torsional and angular deformities necessitate simultaneous correction. They find the procedure relatively simple.

Preoperative Studies

A. Assess the degree of femoral torsion by CT scan, and determine the precise angle of the osteotomy in relation to the line of axis on the femur on the graph published by Merle d'Aubigne. The degree of change of rotation is plotted on the abscissa. The point of intersection of the two lines determines the angle of the cut in relation to the long axis of the femur.

Blood for Transfusion. Yes.

Radiographic Control. Image intensifier.

Patient Position. In the older child, the operation is preferably performed with the patient supine on a fracture table with both feet attached to the foot plate. The hip to undergo operation is rotated medially so that the femoral head and neck are parallel to the floor and aligned with the plane of osteotomy.

Expose the upper femoral shaft and the greater trochanter through a direct lateral approach (see Plate 92).

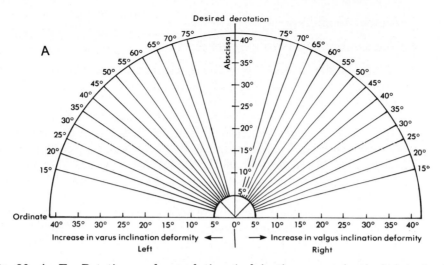

Plate 98. A.–F., Rotation and angulation (valgization or varization) intertrochanteric oblique osteotomy (MacEwen and Shands technique). (From MacEwen, G. D., and Shands, A. R.: Oblique trochanteric osteotomy. J. Bone Joint Surg., 49A:345, 1967.

Operative Technique

Correction of Coxa Vara and Retrotorsion

B.–D. Under image intensifier radiographic control, insert a heavy threaded Steinmann pin into the neck of the femur along its longitudinal axis. The tip should stop short of the capital femoral physis.

Insert a second heavy threaded Steinmann pin into the middle third of the femoral shaft at a predetermined angle of rotation and angulation so that when the lower fragment is abducted, the distal pin will be parallel to the proximal pin. Be sure that the deep end of the distal pin engages the medial cortex. (*Note.* MacEwen and Shands do not insert a distal pin, but this author finds that it ensures accuracy of the degree of correction obtained.)

Determine the level of the proposed osteotomy under image intensifier radiographic control. In the anteroposterior plane, the osteotomy is level with the lower margin of the lesser trochanter and is dome-shaped. In the lateral projection, the osteotomy line extends from anterosuperior to posteroinferior at a predetermined angle.

Next, with an electric drill, make holes along the line of osteotomy. Complete the osteotomy with an electric saw and sharp AO osteotomes.

E. For correction of coxa vara and femoral retrotorsion abduct the distal fragment, keeping the osteotomized fragments in close approximation.

Check the position of the fragments and degree of correction obtained by anteroposterior and lateral radiograms.

The osteotomized fragments are fixed by a five-hole or, preferably, a six-hole plate.

Correction of Coxa Valga with Femoral Antetorsion

F. The distal fragment is adducted, with the osteotomized fragments kept apposed. The wounds are closed in layers. The pins are removed, and a one-and-one-half hip spica cast is applied.

Check the position of the fragments and degree of correction obtained by anteroposterior and lateral radiograms.

The osteotomized fragments are fixed by a five-hole or, preferably, a six-hole plate.

Postoperative Care. Remove the cast six to eight weeks postoperatively when the osteotomy is healed. Exercises are performed to regain range of motion. Remove the plate and screws six to nine months later by a second open operation.

REFERENCES

MacEwen, G. D., and Shands, A. R.: Oblique trochanteric osteotomy. J. Bone Joint Surg., 49–A:345, 1967.

Merle D'Aubigné, R., and Descamps, L.: L'ostéotomie plane oblique dans la correction des déformations des mêmbres. Mem. Acad. Chir., 78:271, 1952.

Merle D'Aubigné, R., and Vaillant, J. M.: Correction simultanée des angles d'inclinaison et de torsion du col fémoral par l'ostéotomie plane oblique. Rev. Chir. Orthop., 47:94, 1961.

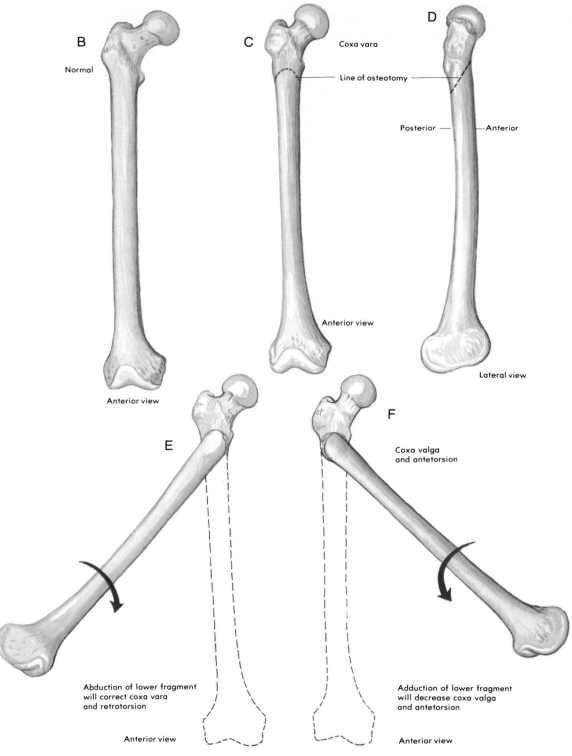

B

Normal

Anterior view

C

Coxa vara

Line of osteotomy

Anterior view

D

Posterior ——— Anterior

Lateral view

E

Abduction of lower fragment
will correct coxa vara
and retrotorsion

Anterior view

F

Coxa valga
and antetorsion

Adduction of lower fragment
will decrease coxa valga
and antetorsion

Anterior view

Plate 98. (Continued)

PLATE 99

Intertrochanteric Proximal Femoral Varus Osteotomy Using a 90-Degree AO Blade-Plate for Internal Fixation

Indications. Coxa valga deformity and instability of the hip in an obese, large adolescent in whom rigid, strong and secure fixation of the osteotomized fragments is required.

Requisites. In addition to those requisites listed for Plate 79, the technique warrants careful radiographic preoperative planning and a surgeon experienced with AO technique.

Radiographic Control. Image intensifier.

Blood for Transfusion. Yes.

Equipment. Fracture table.

Preoperative Assessment. The degree of femoral antetorsion is determined accurately by CT. Also, prior to surgery, anteroposterior radiograms are made with the hips in carefully measured degrees of medial rotation and abduction to position the femoral head concentrically in the acetabulum. The amount of medial rotation determines the degree of derotation angle required, and the amount of abduction determines the degree of varus angle necessary for concentricity of the hip in weight-bearing position. On the fracture table, medially rotate and abduct the hip in the amount determined preoperatively. Often apparent coxa valga is due to excessive femoral antetorsion. Don't be fooled. The degree of medial displacement is determined by preoperative planning on transparencies of the hip and lower limb in weight-bearing position.

Varization elevates the greater trochanter and decreases the torsion of the hip abductor muscles. Following varization osteotomy, the tip of the greater trochanter should be level with the center of the femoral head and the distance from the greater trochanter to the center of the femoral head is two to two-and-one-half times the radius of the femoral head. The purpose of femoral osteotomy is to correct valgus axial deformation of the proximal femur and not to create a varus deformity.

Changes in the femoral neck axis will alter congruity of the femoral head in relation to the acetabulum. Excessive varization of a congruous hip may result in inferior subluxation.

Intertrochanteric varus osteotomy will produce varus derotation of the entire lower limb with resultant genu varum deformity. Correct it by medial displacement of the distal fragments of the femur to restore normal biomechanical axis and alignment of the lower limb.

Patient Position. The patient is placed supine on a fracture table with the image intensifier introduced from the opposite side. To make the osteotomy at the correct level and place the AO blade-plate properly, it is vital to obtain adequate anteroposterior and lateral radiograms of the proximal femur and the hip during surgery.

The following biomechanical effects of varus intertrochanteric osteotomy should be considered.

Operative Technique.

A. and **B.** The anterior, lateral, and posterior surfaces of the proximal femoral shaft are subperiosteally exposed. Proximally the surgeon should be able to palpate the anterior surface of the base of the femoral neck and the lesser trochanter. In the growing child, do not disturb the greater trochanteric apophysis.

C. Next, introduce a smooth Kirschner wire superficially on the anterior aspect of the femoral neck until it touches the femoral head. This measure determines the degree of femoral antetorsion.

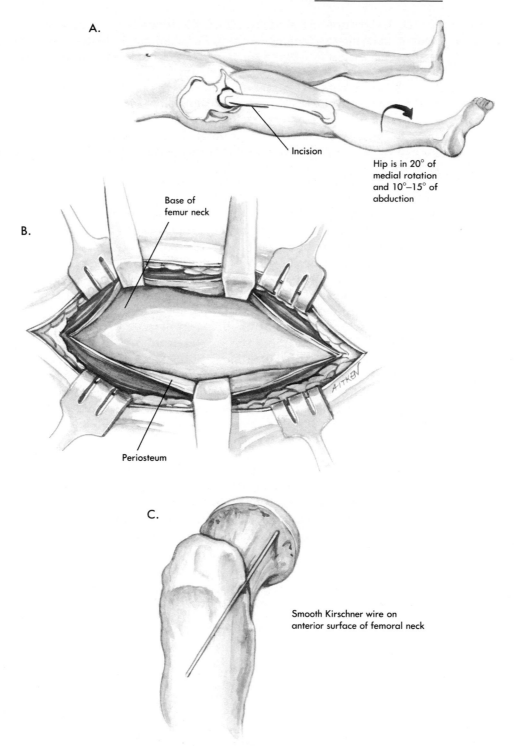

A.

Incision

Hip is in 20° of
medial rotation
and 10°–15° of
abduction

B.

Base of
femur neck

Periosteum

C.

Smooth Kirschner wire on
anterior surface of femoral neck

Plate 99. A.–I., Intertrochanteric proximal femoral varus osteotomy using a 90-degree AO
blade-plate for internal fixation.

D. Determine the angle at which the blade is to be inserted into the femoral neck in relation to the femoral shaft. For example, if 40 degrees of varus correction is planned with a 90-degree blade plate, the blade should enter the femoral neck at a 50-degree angle to the femoral shaft.

Choose a template of the appropriate angle (50 degrees in the illustration), and place it on the *lateral* surface of the femoral shaft.

Drill a second smooth Kirschner wire on the most superior part of the femoral neck parallel to the superior margin of the template. The degree of antetorsion is guided by the first K-wire on the anterior aspect of the femoral neck. Remove the first wire.

The second K-wire on the superior aspect of the femoral neck serves as a guide to the direction of the seating of the chisel and blade. The amount of correction of angular deformity will be corrected by the degree of the template.

E. Next, under image intensifier radiographic control, determine the level of osteotomy that should be at the superior border of the lesser trochanter. Mark it with an osteotome or indelible ink marker. Insert a smooth Kirschner wire into the lesser trochanter perpendicular to the femoral shaft, 0.5 to 1.0 cm. inferior to the intended level of osteotomy. Be sure that the Kirschner wire in the lesser trochanter is anteriorly placed, allowing insertion of the seating chisel.

F. Insert large Chandler (or Bennet) retractors subperiosteally to protect the soft tissues. Then determine the correct level and exact site of insertion of the chisel. The chisel is inserted in line with the femoral neck and somewhat anteriorly in the greater trochanter. Ignore the flat surface of the greater trochanter because it faces and lies 20 to 30 degrees posterior to the axis of the femoral neck.

Caution! If you start the chisel posteriorly on the flat surface of the greater trochanter, it will cut out of the posterior cortex of the femoral neck. Such an error has serious consequences!

The level of entry of the chisel is measured directly on the plate. Next, select the correct chisel corresponding to the size of the blade-plate to be used.

Place the chisel guide on the lateral surface of the femoral shaft. Following insertion of the blade into the femoral neck, the plate should be directly lateral on the femoral shaft, not anterior or posterior. Make appropriate adjustments for flexion or extension and rotation as planned preoperatively.

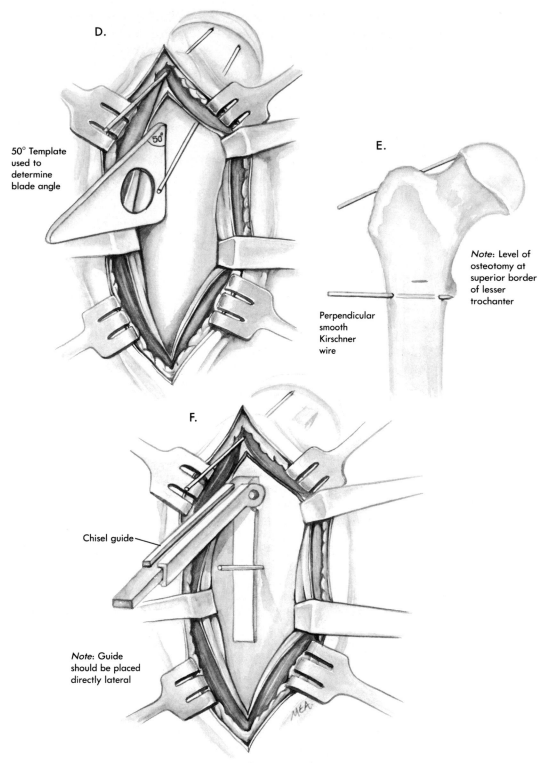

D.

50° Template used to determine blade angle

E.

Note: Level of osteotomy at superior border of lesser trochanter

Perpendicular smooth Kirschner wire

F.

Chisel guide

Note: Guide should be placed directly lateral

Plate 99. (Continued)

Under image intensifier radiographic control, hammer the chisel into the femoral neck using the superior Kirschner wire and chisel guide as guides. The depth of penetration of the chisel is assessed on the scale on its inferior surface and on the radiogram.

G. With the use of an oscillating saw and sharp AO osteotomes, perform a transverse osteotomy perpendicular to the femoral shaft.

H. After completion of the transverse osteotomy, use the seating chisel as a lever and tilt the proximal fragment into varus by elevating the tip of the greater trochanter.

With an oscillating saw, excise an appropriate wedge of bone from the medial half of the proximal segment of the femur as planned preoperatively.

I. Remove the seating chisel, and insert the blade-plate. Avoid making a false channel by inserting the blade by hand and controlling its site by image intensifier.

After complete seating of the blade into the femoral neck, the plate of the blade-plate is coapted to the femoral shaft with bone clamps.

Make appropriate adjustments for rotation and flexion–extension as necessary. The pins in the femoral neck and lesser trochanter will serve as a guide to double check rotation.

Under image intensification, check the position of the blade-plate and the degree of varization obtained. Make regular radiograms for a larger field of visualization if necessary.

Then fix the plate to the femoral shaft by screws.

The wound is copiously irrigated. The vastus lateralis is sutured to its origin and to the tendinous insertion of the gluteus medius–minimus. Hemovac suction drains are inserted, and the wound is closed in the usual fashion.

Postoperative Care. It is not necessary to immobilize the hip in a spica cast. As soon as the patient is comfortable, he or she is permitted to be up and around, with three-point crutch gait and partial weight-bearing on the operated lower limb. Active and passive exercises are performed to restore range of hip and knee motion and to increase motor strength of the muscles controlling the hip and lower limb. The osteotomy ordinarily takes eight weeks to heal. When there is bone union, crutches are discarded and full weight-bearing is permitted.

REFERENCES

Beauschesne, R., Miller, F., and Moseley, C.: Proximal femoral osteotomy using the AO fixed-angle blade plate. J. Pediatr. Orthop., 12:735, 1992.

Muller, M. E., Allgower, M., Schneider, R., and Willenegger, H.: Manual of Internal Fixation, 2nd ed. Berlin, Springer-Verlag, 1979.

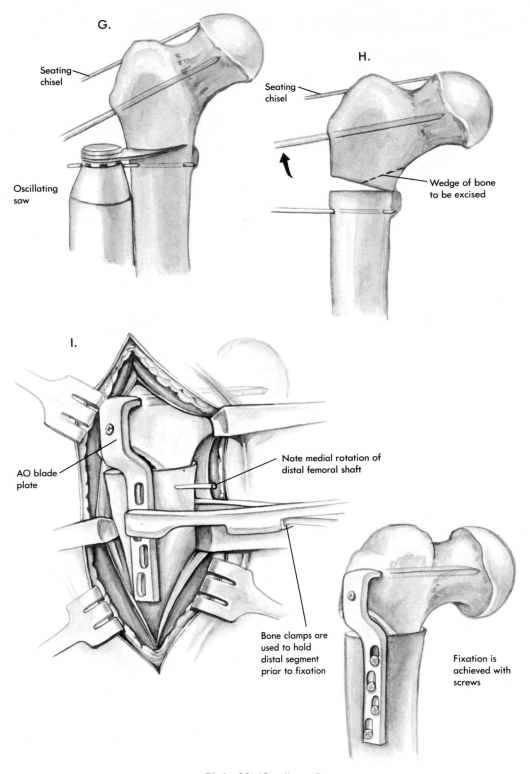

G.

Seating chisel

Oscillating saw

H.

Seating chisel

Wedge of bone to be excised

I.

AO blade plate

Note medial rotation of distal femoral shaft

Bone clamps are used to hold distal segment prior to fixation

Fixation is achieved with screws

Plate 99. (Continued)

PLATE 100   ## Derotation Osteotomy of the Proximal Femur

Indications

1. Excessive femoral antetorsion causing instability of the hip in developmental hip dysplasia.

2. Severe femoral antetorsion causing marked toeing-in and functional disability and unsightliness in a 10-year-old or older child, especially one who is uncoordinated or handicapped by a neuromuscular disorder.

Requisites

1. The degree of femoral antetorsion is more than 45 degrees as measured by CT scan or MRI.

2. The hip in extension cannot be rotated laterally to neutral and medial rotation is 90 degrees.

3. Lateral tibial torsion is less than 35 degrees.

Caution! Inform the parents and patient that the surgical procedure is major and carries a significant complication rate. Asymmetric growth stimulation and lower limb length disparity are potential problems. The extent of operative scars may be unsightly. There is no definite evidence that increased femoral antetorsion causes degenerative arthritis of the hip or knee that results in pain or functional disability in the adult. Do not perform derotation osteotomy when the hip joint is stable in a child eight years of age or under.

Blood for Transfusion. Yes.

Radiographic Control. Image intensifier.

Patient Position. Supine on a fracture table.

Operative Technique

A. With the hip held in internal rotation, a midlateral, longitudinal incision is made, beginning at the base of the greater trochanter and extending distally for 4 inches in line with the femoral shaft. The subcutaneous tissue is divided, and the skin margins are retracted.

B. The fascia lata and iliotibial band are divided in line with the skin incision.

C. With rake retractors, the posterior and anterior margins of the fascia lata are retracted. The vastus lateralis muscle is split in the direction of its fibers from the base of the greater trochanter to 2 inches below the lesser trochanter. Do not disturb the greater trochanteric epiphyseal plate. The periosteum is divided longitudinally in the anterior third of the lateral surface of the shaft of the femur.

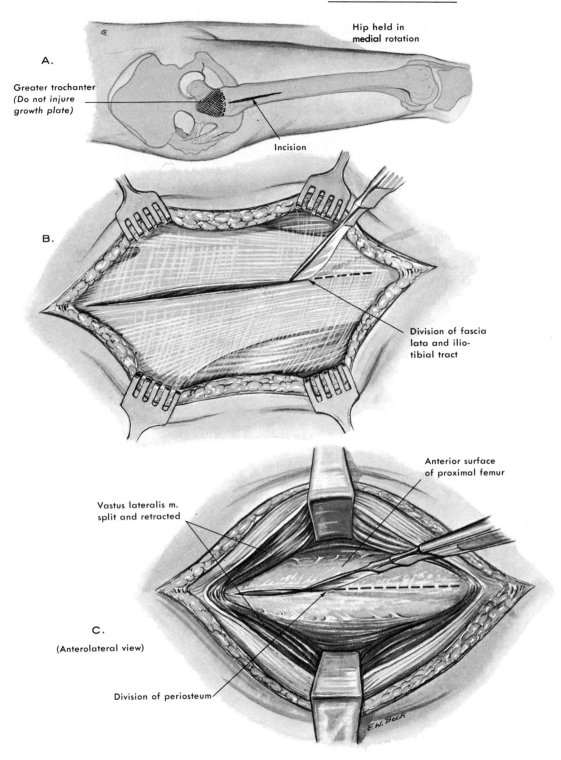

A.

Hip held in
medial rotation

Greater trochanter
*(Do not injure
growth plate)*

Incision

B.

Division of fascia
lata and ilio-
tibial tract

Anterior surface
of proximal femur

Vastus lateralis m.
split and retracted

C.

(Anterolateral view)

Division of periosteum

E.W. Beck

Plate 100. A.–H., Derotation osteotomy of the proximal femur.

D. and **E.** Anteversion is 60 degrees compared with the normal 12.

F. Expose the anterior and lateral surfaces of the proximal shaft of the femur by subperiosteal elevation of the vastus lateralis muscle. Next, hold the hip in maximal internal rotation and use Bennett retractors for retraction. With starter and drill, outline the line of a transverse osteotomy with drill holes through both anterior and posterior cortices ⅜ inch distal to the lesser trochanter.

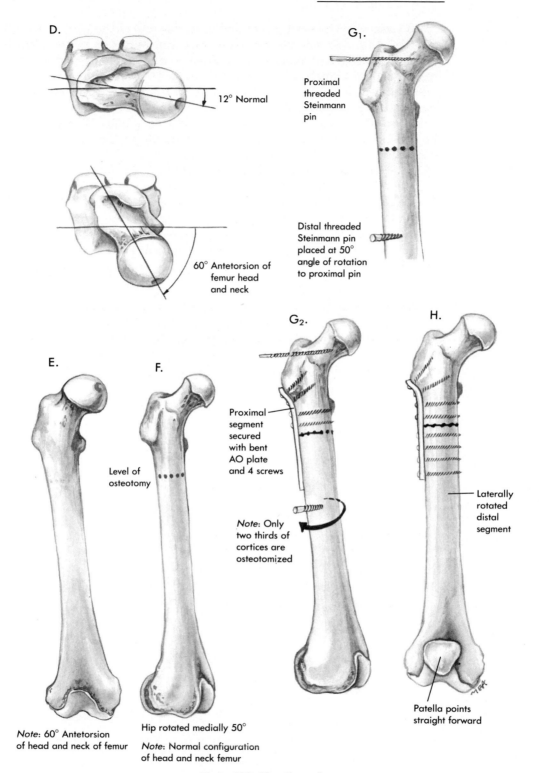

D.

12° Normal

60° Antetorsion of femur head and neck

G₁.

Proximal threaded Steinmann pin

Distal threaded Steinmann pin placed at 50° angle of rotation to proximal pin

E.

Note: 60° Antetorsion of head and neck of femur

F.

Level of osteotomy

Hip rotated medially 50°

Note: Normal configuration of head and neck femur

G₂.

Proximal segment secured with bent AO plate and 4 screws

Note: Only two thirds of cortices are osteotomized

H.

Laterally rotated distal segment

Patella points straight forward

Plate 100. (Continued)

G1 and **G2**. The periosteum and posterior flap of the wound are lifted forward, and, through stab wounds separate from and posterior to the skin incision, one large threaded Steinmann pin or Schanz screw is inserted into the proximal fragment, one aiming at the femoral neck. Then one large threaded Steinmann pin or Schanz screw is drilled in the distal fragment at a predetermined angle of rotation to the proximal ones, so that when the distal fragment is laterally rotated it will be parallel to the proximal pins. The deep ends of the pins should engage the medial cortex of the femur. The osteotomy is then carried out with a thin osteotome.

H. With the proximal fragment still held in internal rotation, the distal fragment is laterally rotated until the patella points straight anteriorly toward the ceiling. The degree of rotation of the distal femoral pins in relation to the proximal pins indicates the degree of derotation of the femur. Under direct vision and by palpation, the position of the osteotomized bone fragments is double-checked, and they are transfixed with a 7-hole or 8-hole AO plate and screws. The wound is closed in the usual fashion and a one-and-one-half hip spica cast is applied.

Postoperative Care. The cast is removed when the bone is healed (six to eight weeks), and active and passive exercises are performed to achieve functional range of motion of the hips and knees and increase motor strength of the muscles.

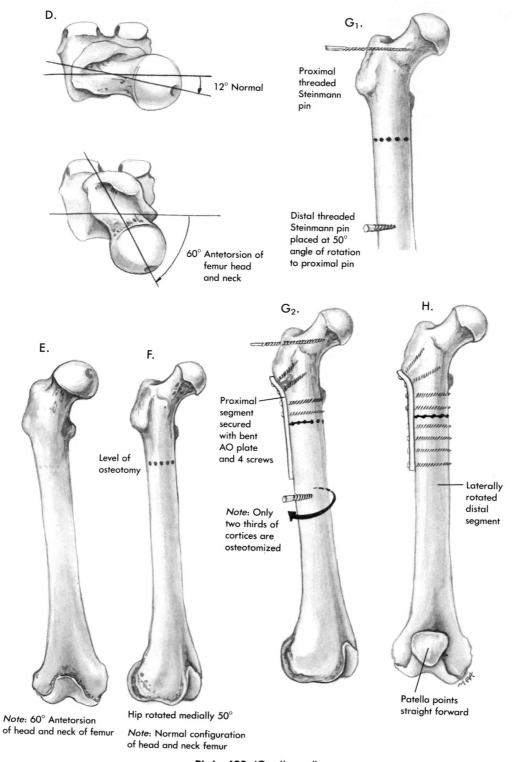

D.

12° Normal

60° Antetorsion of femur head and neck

G₁.

Proximal threaded Steinmann pin

Distal threaded Steinmann pin placed at 50° angle of rotation to proximal pin

E.

Note: 60° Antetorsion of head and neck of femur

F.

Level of osteotomy

Hip rotated medially 50°

Note: Normal configuration of head and neck femur

G₂.

Proximal segment secured with bent AO plate and 4 screws

Note: Only two thirds of cortices are osteotomized

H.

Laterally rotated distal segment

Patella points straight forward

Plate 100. (Continued)

PLATE 101

Percutaneous Hip Pinning with the Cannulated AO Screw for a Slipped Capital Femoral Epiphysis

Objective. To stabilize the capital femoral epiphysis and prevent further slipping until solid bony fusion has occurred.

Indications. Slipped capital femoral epiphysis less than 65 degrees (according to Southwick's method of mensuration) or less than two thirds of its diameter.

Note. The strong cannulated screws that have been developed are safe for in situ fixation. Use one screw for chronic slipped capital femoral epiphysis and two screws for acute slipped capital femoral epiphysis when the epiphysis is unstable after one screw fixation.

Radiographic Control. Image intensifier.

Chronic Slip. It is mandatory to have adequate radiographic control. Prior to anesthetizing the patient, a competent x-ray technician should be in the operating room and the image intensifier C-arm fluoroscopic machine should be in working order. Schedule ahead, and don't be caught short without a competent technician or without a functioning image intensifier.

Patient Position. The patient is positioned supine on a fracture table with the affected hip abducted 10 to 15 degrees and medially rotated (as far as it will rotate without force). Medial rotation of the hip will position the femoral neck parallel to the floor, thereby enabling one to obtain true anteroposterior and lateral projections of the hip.

Preoperative Assessment

A. and **B.** An image intensifier fluoroscopic C-arm is used for radiographic control. The opposite nonoperated lower limb is flexed and maximally abducted. The image intensifier is placed between the thighs so that by rotating the tube around the arc of the midline one can obtain both anteroposterior and lateral projections at right angles to each other without moving the lower limb or repositioning the patient.

The recording tube should be closest to the femoral head, i.e., along the lateral wall of the ilium in the lateral projection and under the hip for the anteroposterior view.

Prior to preparing and draping, obtain both anteroposterior and lateral images. Assess the quality of the pictures. In both the anteroposterior and lateral projections, the articular cartilage space of the hip, the subchondral bony plate of the femoral head, the capital femoral physis, and the femoral neck should be clearly depicted. In the very obese patient, when images of the hip are inadequate, use a portable x-ray machine for the lateral projection and the image intensifier for the anteroposterior view.

The hip, ilium, and thigh are prepared and draped in the usual fashion. The lateral and anterior surface of the hip and upper thigh should be sterile and freely accessible as far medially as the pubis in the inguinal area. The C-arm of the image intensifier should be rotated 90 degrees without contaminating the operating field.

Operative Technique

C. Determine the starting point; this should be precise. The objective of in situ fixation of chronic slipped capital femoral epiphysis with a single cannulated screw is to place the screw into the center of the capital femoral epiphysis perpendicular to its physis, and no closer than 5 mm. to the subchondral bone of the femoral head.

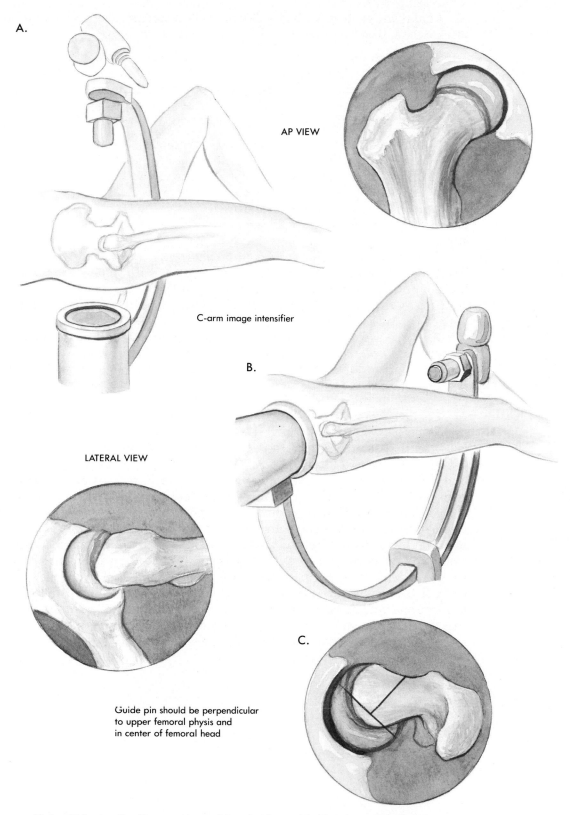

A.

AP VIEW

C-arm image intensifier

B.

LATERAL VIEW

Guide pin should be perpendicular
to upper femoral physis and
in center of femoral head

C.

Plate 101. A.–O., Percutaneous hip pinning with the cannulated AO screw for a slipped capital femoral epiphysis.

Lindaman et al described a fluoroscopic technique for determination of the incision site; it is based on the following geometric axioms:

1. Through any plane there is one and only one line that is perpendicular to any given point on that plane.

2. A plane and a line not part of that plane will intersect at one and only one point.

3. Two intersecting lines form a single line.

If there is any degree of slip, a lateral entry site will position the pin incorrectly in the femoral head. When the pin is inserted in the lateral cortex and positioned posteriorly to the slipped femoral epiphysis, the pin will exit posteriorly out of the femoral neck and then enter obliquely into the femoral head; in such an instance, internal fixation is inadequate and there is increased risk of unrecognized pin penetration. The entry site is moved anteriorly according to the degree of posterior slip.

The entry site of the pin should be above the level of the lesser trochanter. Fracture may occur at the pin entry site, especially if the pins are inserted at the level of or distal to the level of the lesser trochanter. Ten cases of subtrochanteric fracture were reported by Schmidt and Gregg as a complication for pinning of slipped capital femoral epiphysis.

D. Place a guide pin on the skin of the anterior aspect of the hip and upper thigh; in the anteroposterior image, this pin should be directed to the center of the displaced femoral head and in the appropriate varus-valgus position so that it is perpendicular to the capital femoral physis. With a sterile marking pen, draw the position of the guide pin on the anterior surface of the thigh (**C.** and **D.**).

E. Next, rotate the C-arm of the image intensifier so that a true lateral projection of the hip is obtained. Place the guide pin on the lateral aspect of the thigh so that it is in the correct anteroposterior plane on the image, i.e., in the center of the femoral head and perpendicular to its physis. As the femoral epiphysis is displaced posteriorly, the guide pin is directed anteroposteriorly, appearing to enter at the anterior part of the base of the femoral neck on the image.

F. The two skin lines are extended, and the site of intersection of these two lines is the correct starting point. Make a simple stab (puncture) wound or a skin incision 1 cm. long. The guide pin, drill, and screw are inserted through this wound. It behooves the surgeon to remember that the soft tissues of the upper thigh are mobile, the guide wires are flexible, and they may move along the cortical bone to an undesirable site. Therefore, by image intensifier fluoroscopy, confirm and monitor the starting point, proper alignment, position, and depth of insertion. The more severe the slip (i.e., the posterior displacement of the capital epiphysis), the more anterior the starting point.

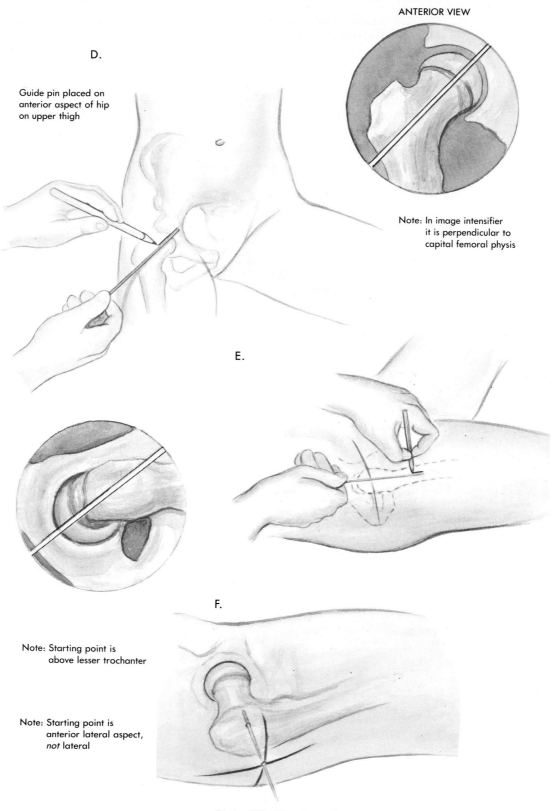

ANTERIOR VIEW

D.

Guide pin placed on
anterior aspect of hip
on upper thigh

Note: In image intensifier
it is perpendicular to
capital femoral physis

E.

Note: Starting point is
above lesser trochanter

Note: Starting point is
anterior lateral aspect,
not lateral

F.

Plate 101. (Continued)

G. The blood supply of the superior weight-bearing area of the femoral head is solely by branches of the lateral epiphyseal vessels that traverse the superoposterior quadrant of the femoral head. Pins or screws inserted into the posterior and superior quadrant of the femoral head will damage the blood supply to the weight-bearing position of the epiphysis and will result in avascular necrosis. During in situ pin fixation, this intricate vascular anatomy should be kept in mind. Do not place any fixation device in the superior quadrant of the femoral head.

H. and I. Internal fixation of a slipped capital femoral epiphysis is different from that of a subcapital fracture of the hip in an adult patient. The femoral head is displaced posteriorly, and the architecture of the upper end of the femur is distorted. When pins are inserted through the lateral femoral cortex, they may traverse outside the posterior or inferior cortex of the femoral neck before they re-enter the femoral head. In their journey posterior to the femoral neck, the posterior superior retinacular vessels may be injured, resulting in avascular necrosis of the femoral head. To prevent these complications, insert the pin anteriorly on the base of the femoral neck. Also, the part of the screw which is out of the cortical bone of the femoral neck is subject to marked stress. The segment of the screw that exits the femoral neck before it enters the femoral head may break.

Anterior protrusion of the guide pin or pins and screws may damage femoral vessels and result in pseudo-aneurysm.

J. The screws inserted distal to the level of the lesser trochanter may result in subtrochanteric fracture.

K. Avoid multiple drilling of the base of the femoral neck because it will weaken the bone and result in fracture.

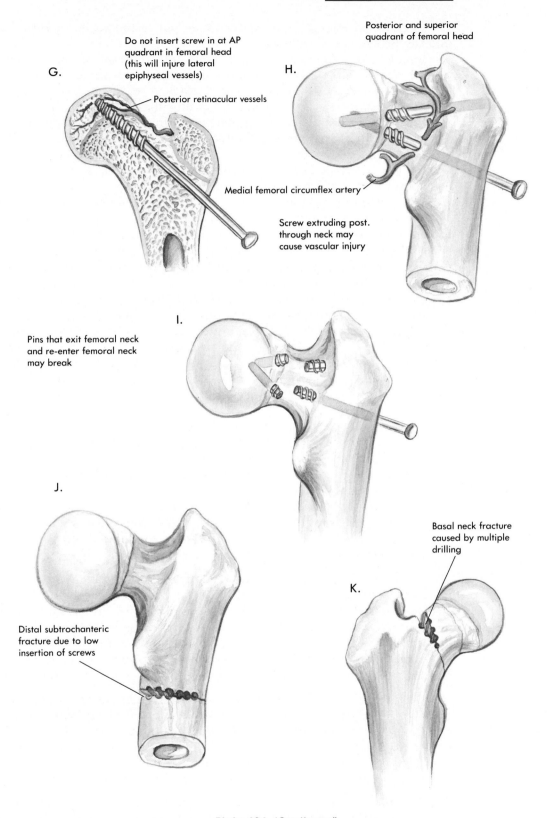

G. Do not insert screw in at AP quadrant in femoral head (this will injure lateral epiphyseal vessels)

Posterior retinacular vessels

H. Posterior and superior quadrant of femoral head

Medial femoral circumflex artery

Screw extruding post. through neck may cause vascular injury

I. Pins that exit femoral neck and re-enter femoral neck may break

J. Distal subtrochanteric fracture due to low insertion of screws

K. Basal neck fracture caused by multiple drilling

Plate 101. (Continued)

L. The next step is to insert the guide pin in the correct position and depth into the femoral neck and head.

Insert a Metzenbaum or dull scissors into the stab wound, spread the soft tissues, and push the scissor tips deep until they touch bone.

Use a special AO 2-mm. pin (with threads at its tip) as the guide pin. Prior to drilling the guide pin, check that it fits into the cannula of the AO cannulated screw. Using the skin lines as a guide and using image intensifier radiograms as a control (in the anteroposterior, lateral, and oblique projections), drill the guide pin, advancing slowly toward the center of the femoral head, perpendicular to the upper femoral physis. The tip of the pin should stop 5 mm. short of the subchondral bony plate of the capital femoral epiphysis.

When penetrating the cortex on the anterior femoral neck, advance the pin slowly with minimal force. Once the pin passes the cortex of the point of entry on the anterior femoral neck, further increased resistance to advancement indicates penetration of the posterior cortex. Check it on the image intensifier in multiple planes. Estimate the degree of the posterior slip and direct the guide pin toward the center of the femoral head.

Caution! Avoid making multiple drill holes at the base of the femoral neck; stress fracture may occur postoperatively.

Upon advancement of the pin to the capital physis, increased resistance will be met. Check the pin's position. Be sure that it is perpendicular to the growth plate. Then advance the guide pin slowly under repeated image intensifier radiographic control. The tip of the guide pin is placed in the center of the femoral head, stopping 5 mm. short of the subchondral bony plate in multiple planes.

Next, select a screw of the correct length. Insert a second guide pin of equal length down to bone through the stab incision alongside the guide pin drilled into the femoral head–neck. Under image intensifier, check the position of the tip of the measuring pin; it should be exactly at the point of entry of the first pin. Residual pin length of the second pin is measured; the difference between the pins represents the screw length.

M. and **N.** Utilizing a soft tissue protector, first advance the cannulated drill bit over the guide pin; remove the drill bit and then advance the cannulated tap over the guide pin into the femoral neck–head to the same depth. Two important technical details:

1. When advancing the drill, use image intensifier fluoroscopy repeatedly to ensure that the guide pin is not advanced deeper across the subchondral bone into the hip joint; this often is caused by impingement of the cannulated instrument on the guide pin, requiring cautious removal and readvancement.

2. When the cannulated drill bit and tap are being removed, the guide pin will sometimes retract with them; therefore, check under image intensifier fluoroscopy and advance it to its original depth if it comes out with the instruments.

O. Insert the correct length screw over the guide pin, monitoring its advancement in the lateral and anteroposterior projection of image intensifier fluoroscopy.

Check for penetration of the screw into the hip joint by liberating the lower limb from traction and by moving the hip in all planes and scrutinizing the hip joint through image intensifier radiograms.

Remove the guide pin, and close the skin with one or two absorbable sutures.

Postoperative Care. In chronic slip, the patient is placed in counterpoised split Russell's traction for comfort and is allowed to be ambulatory with the help of crutches (partial weight-bearing on the involved limb). Usually within a week to ten days, the crutches are discarded. In acute slip, crutch protection and partial weight-bearing are continued for a period of six to eight weeks.

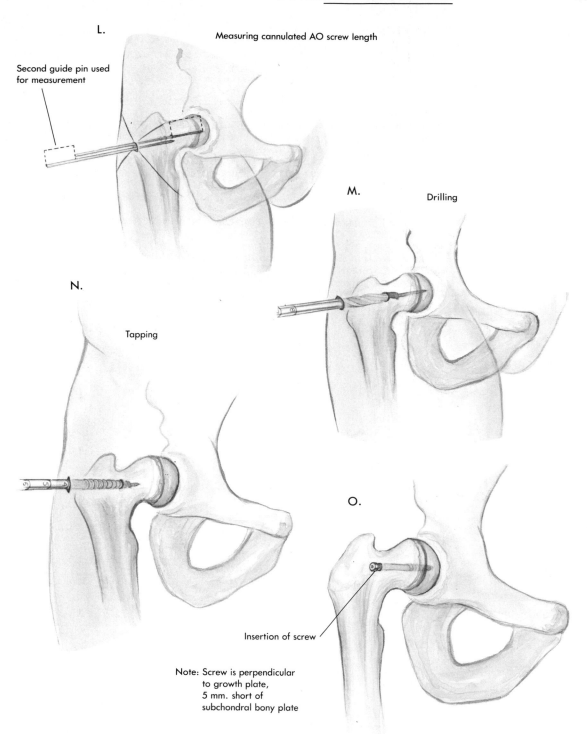

L.

Measuring cannulated AO screw length

Second guide pin used
for measurement

M.   Drilling

N.

Tapping

O.

Insertion of screw

Note: Screw is perpendicular
to growth plate,
5 mm. short of
subchondral bony plate

Plate 101. (Continued)

REFERENCES

Aronson, D. D., and Carlson, W. E.: Slipped capital femoral epiphysis. A prospective study of fixation with a single screw. J. Bone Joint Surg., 74–A:810, 1992.

Brodetti, A.: The blood supply of the femoral neck and head in relation to the damaging effects of nails and screws. J. Bone Joint Surg., 42–B:794, 1960.

Crock, H. V.: The Blood Supply of the Lower Limb Bones in Man. Edinburgh: E. & S. Livingstone, 1967, p. 11.

Lehman, W. B., Menche, D., Grant, A., Norman, A., and Pugh, J.: The problem of evaluating in situ pinning of slipped capital femoral epiphysis: An experimental model and a review of 63 consecutive cases. J. Pediatr. Orthop., 4:297, 1984.

Lindaman, L. M., Canale, S. T., Beaty, J. H., and Warner, W. C.: A fluoroscopic technique for determining the incision site for percutaneous fixation of slipped capital femoral epiphysis. J. Pediatr. Orthop., 11:397, 1991.

Morrissy, R. T.: In situ fixation of chronic slipped capital femoral epiphysis. A.A.O.S. Instructional Course Lectures, 3:319, 1984. St. Louis, C. V. Mosby.

Morrissy, R. T.: Slipped capital femoral epiphysis technique of percutaneous in situ fixation. J. Pediatr. Orthop., 10:347, 1990.

Nguyen, D., and Morrissy, R. T.: Slipped capital femoral epiphysis: Rationale for the technique of percutaneous in situ fixation. J. Pediatr. Orthop., 10:341, 1990.

Riley, P. M., Weiner, D. S., Gillespie, R., and Weiner, S. D.: Hazards of internal fixation in the treatment of slipped capital femoral epiphysis. J. Bone Joint Surg., 72–A:1500, 1990.

Ward, W. T., Stefko, J., Wood, K. B., and Stanitski, C. L.: Fixation with a single screw for slipped capital femoral epiphysis. J. Bone Joint Surg., 74–A:799, 1992.

L.

Measuring cannulated AO screw length

Second guide pin used
for measurement

M.   Drilling

N.

Tapping

O.

Insertion of screw

Note: Screw is perpendicular
to growth plate,
5 mm. short of
subchondral bony plate

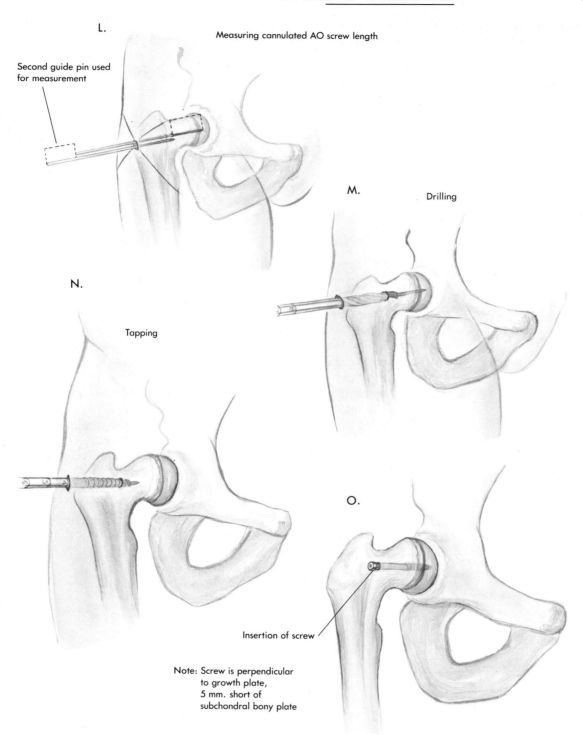

Plate 101. (Continued)

| PLATE 102 | Hip Pinning with the Asnis Guided Screw System |

Objective. To stabilize the capital femoral epiphysis and prevent further slipping until solid bony fusion has occurred.

Indications. A slipped capital femoral epiphysis less than 65 degrees (according to Southwick's method of mensuration) or less than two thirds of its diameter.

Patient Position. The patient is placed on the fracture table with the involved hip in 10 to 20 degrees of medial rotation. Biplane image intensifier fluoroscopy is set and tested to be certain that the hip (particularly the capital femoral epiphysis) can be adequately visualized. This can sometimes be a problem in the very obese patient.

Operative Technique

A. and **B.** Make a longitudinal incision in muscle on the lateral aspect of the upper thigh, beginning 3 to 4 cm. distal to the prominence of the greater trochanter and extending distally for about 3 to 7 cm. The fascia lata is incised, and the vastus lateralis muscle is split to expose the anterolateral aspect of the upper femoral shaft. A 9-inch long 5⁄32 inch drill is placed in the pin driver attached to a power drill. The more severe (i.e., the more posterior) the slip, the more anteriorly on the femoral cortex the hole must be drilled. The site of the drill hole should be above the lesser trochanter in the intertrochanteric region; it should not be subtrochanteric. Under image intensifier radiographic control, drill a hole through the lateral femoral cortex. The largest smooth Kirschner wire that will easily slide through the cannulated screw (usually 0.062 mm.) is then drilled through the hole in the lateral femoral cortex, up the center of the femoral neck, across the physis, and into the epiphysis so that it is centered in both the anteroposterior and lateral projections. The hip joint should not be penetrated. To confirm that the tip of the pin is not in the joint, the hip is carefully rotated under image intensifier fluoroscopy to check both anteroposterior and lateral projections.

C1.–C3. The "blind spot" is the space in the radiographic shadow of the femoral head in which the tip of the pin is projected within the boundaries of the femoral head in the radiogram; the tip of the pin appears to be in the femoral head, but it is not. With one x-ray beam, the space of the "blind spot" is large; with an increasing number of x-ray views, the volume of the "blind spot" becomes progressively smaller.

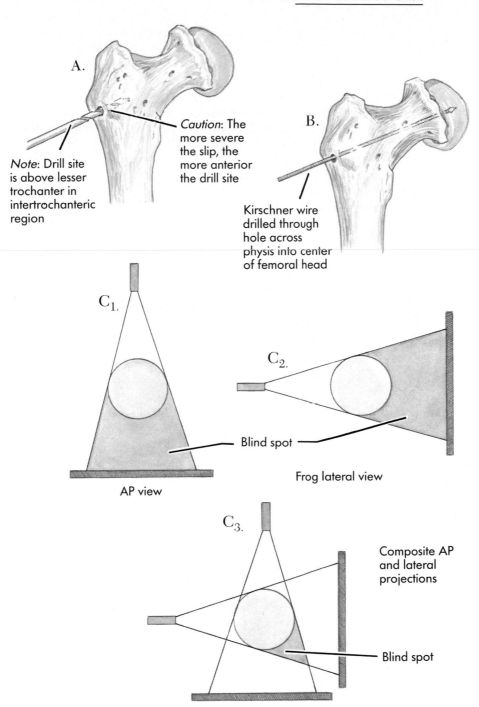

A.

Note: Drill site is above lesser trochanter in intertrochanteric region

Caution: The more severe the slip, the more anterior the drill site

B.

Kirschner wire drilled through hole across physis into center of femoral head

C₁.

Blind spot

AP view

C₂.

Frog lateral view

C₃.

Composite AP and lateral projections

Blind spot

Plate 102. A.–I., Hip pinning with the Asnis guided screw system.

D. The radiographic projection that shows the tip of the pin in its true position with respect to the articular surface and the subchondral bony plate of the femoral head is the *critical view*. This is visualized by the "tangential" x-ray beam. The "equator" around the femoral head is delineated by the points on its surface touched by the tangential x-ray beams. The tip of the pin should lie in the plane of this equator in the critical view.

E1.–E3. Next, elicit and detect the "approach-withdraw" phenomenon to identify the critical view, which shows the tip of the pin in its true relationship to the surface of the femoral head. The hip is rotated about the longitudinal axis, with the image intensifier in place, first to provide an anteroposterior projection of the hip and then a lateral view. Thereby, the femoral head should rotate around an axis perpendicular to the central beam of the image intensifier.

If the pin tip is moving toward the plane of the equator, it appears to move closer to the surface of the head in the two-dimensional projected view; conversely, if it is moving away from the equator, it appears to move away from the projected surface of the head. If it moves through the equatorial plane, its tip will appear to first approach and then withdraw from the surface of the head. The critical view can therefore be identified at the moment the pin tip appears to change the direction of its motion with respect to the surface of the head. If, on elicitation of the approach-withdraw phenomenon, the pin tip appears to be within the femoral head, it is in actuality within the head. If the pin appears to have penetrated the femoral head, with or without elicitation of the approach-withdraw phenomenon, the tip of the pin is in the joint. If one cannot elicit the approach-withdraw phenomenon or identify pin penetration into the joint, it indicates that the rotation of the hip has not included the critical view; this usually occurs when the pin is placed posteriorly. To visualize the posterior surface of the femoral head, an oblique view of the hip is obtained either by tilting the image intensifier or by elevating the contralateral hip. If the pin is placed superiorly, the hip is flexed and extended to elicit the approach-withdraw phenomenon.

D.

CRITICAL VIEW

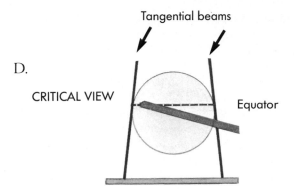

APPROACH-WITHDRAW PHENOMENON

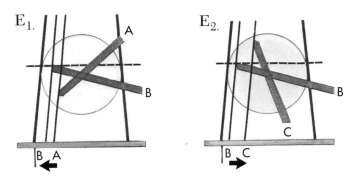

$E_1.$ $E_2.$

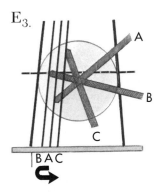

$E_3.$

Plate 102. (Continued)

F. Abduction-adduction views of the hip are of no assistance, as the hip movement takes place about an axis parallel to and not perpendicular to the x-ray beam. The reliability of the approach-withdraw phenomenon is dependent on the axis of hip rotation being roughly perpendicular to the central beam of the x-ray.

G. Once it is verified that the guide pin is in the center of the epiphysis, a ⁵⁄₃₂-inch drill bit is attached to a power drill and, with the pin as a guide, the drill bit is drilled through the lateral femoral cortex, up the center of the neck, across the physis, and into the center of the epiphysis. The tip of the drill bit should be within 0.5 mm. of the subchondral bony plate. In case of doubt, regular radiograms are made under image intensifier fluoroscopy, to double-check the exact position and depth of the drill. The drill bit is removed.

H1.–H2. At this time, the surgeon may choose to use either the tap directly or an optional guide pin assembly. Once a hole is drilled, the tap will follow the drill hole even without a guide pin. If the assembly is used, a guide pin (which fits in the hole of the cannulated screw) is driven up the predrilled channel, and its position is verified by image intensifier fluoroscopy. The inner pin is tapped with a mallet, and the outer component is removed. Next, the cannulated tap is placed over the guide wire and driven through the lateral cortex, the femoral neck, and across the physis into the epiphysis. The shank of the tap is calibrated by shiny and dull etchings. The holes in the tap show the guide pin in the distal hole when the tap is 25 mm. from the end of the pin. Stop when the guide pin is seen in the proximal hole; only 5 mm. is left.

I. The tap is removed, leaving the guide wire in place. A screw of the appropriate length and a washer are selected and placed over the wire, across the physis, and well into the femoral epiphysis.

The guide wire is removed, and if there is any question of joint penetration by the screw, renografin dye may be injected through the cannulated portion of the screw into the epiphysis. If the radiograph shows that any dye enters the hip joint, the screw must be backed out an appropriate distance. A second screw can be placed posterior and inferior to the first in cases of acute slips.

The wound is closed in layers in the usual manner.

Postoperative Care. Immediately after the patient leaves the operating room, the hip is protected by placing the patient in bilateral split Russell's traction, with medial rotation straps on the thigh. Active assisted and gentle passive exercises to develop motion in the affected hip are performed while the child is in bed. As soon as the patient is comfortable (usually in two to three days) he or she is allowed to be ambulatory, protecting the hip by three-point crutch gait, with a gradual increase of weight-bearing on the involved side. When muscle spasm has completely subsided and the hip has functional range of motion, crutch protection is gradually discontinued and full weight-bearing is allowed. In an *acute* slip, crutch protection is continued with toe-touch gait for a period of six weeks.

REFERENCES

Asnis, S. E.: The guided screw system in intracapsular fractures of the hip. Contemp. Orthop., 10:33, 1985.

Asnis, S. E.: The guided screw system in slipped capital femoral epiphysis. Contemp. Orthop., 11:27, 1985.

F.

Note: Axis of hip rotation is perpendicular to anterior beam of x-ray

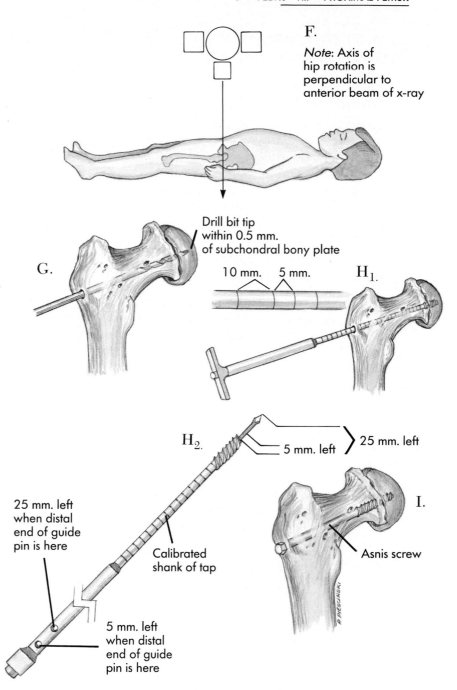

Drill bit tip within 0.5 mm. of subchondral bony plate

G.

10 mm.   5 mm.

H₁.

H₂.

5 mm. left

25 mm. left

25 mm. left when distal end of guide pin is here

Calibrated shank of tap

5 mm. left when distal end of guide pin is here

I.

Asnis screw

Plate 102. (Continued)

PLATE 103

Open Epiphyseodesis with an Autogenous Bone Graft in a Slipped Capital Femoral Epiphysis

Indications. This author recommends open epiphyseodesis of slipped capital femoral epiphysis only as follows:

1. When proper placement of the screw or screws is difficult because of technical reasons: (a) in the very obese child in whom adequate visualization of the site and depth of the screw in the epiphysis is difficult; (b) valgus slip; and (c) very severe slips that are difficult to pin.

2. In severe acute slip in patients in whom the femoral head is avascular (as demonstrated by technetium 99m bone scan and following decompression of the hip joint by aspiration) and when circulation does not return. Curettage of the growth plate and autogenous bone grafting will enhance vascularization of the femoral head.

Advantages

1. Pin penetration into the hip joint is not a problem, and the possibility of acute cartilage necrosis (chondrolysis) is extremely minimal.

2. The incidence of avascular necrosis as a postoperative complication is very low.

3. A second operation to remove the hardware is not necessary.

Disadvantages

1. There is a greater magnitude of surgical exposure and blood loss.

2. Curetting the growth plate and inserting a graft across the capital physis temporarily decreases the stability, converting a stable condition to an unstable one in which further slipping can occur, acutely or slowly. Stability, however, ceases to become a problem once the physis is closed and the bone graft bridges epiphyseal to metaphyseal bone. During the unstable period, the hip should be protected in a spica cast followed by protection with crutches.

3. The autogenous bone graft may fail to bridge the physis; it may absorb or undergo stress fracture.

Blood for Transfusion. Yes.

Radiographic Control. Image intensifier.

Special Instrumentation. Hollow mill.

Patient Position. The patient is placed in supine position on a radiolucent operating table.

Operative Technique

A. The anterior capsule of the hip joint is exposed through an anterolateral approach (see Plate 77). The joint is opened through an H-shaped incision into the anterosuperior part of the capsule. The proximal transverse incision is parallel to the acetabular margin and 1 cm. distal to it; the longitudinal incision is on the anterior aspect of the femoral neck; the distal transverse incision is at the base of the femoral neck.

B. With the help of a Freer elevator, the capsule and synovium are gently elevated from the femoral neck–head.

Caution! Do not disturb the retinacular blood supply.

Place two Cobra or Chandler elevators within the capsule to expose the femoral head–neck and the site of the slipped epiphysis. With a small Kirschner wire or drill point, a rectangular window is fashioned on the anterosuperior aspect of the femoral neck. Use radiographic control for proper placement of the window.

C. A large hollow mill is inserted through the window, and under image

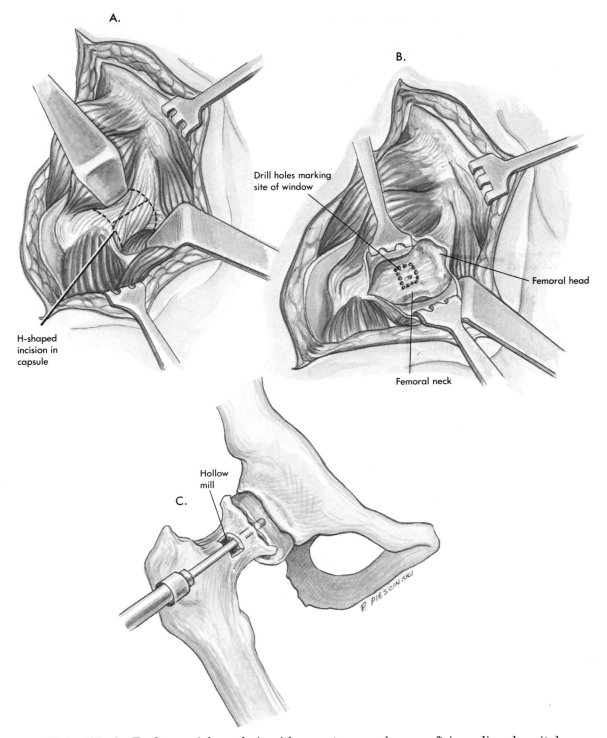

A.

H-shaped
incision in
capsule

B.

Drill holes marking
site of window

Femoral head

Femoral neck

C.

Hollow
mill

R. PIESCINSKI

Plate 103. A.–F., Open epiphyseodesis with an autogenous bone graft in a slipped capital femoral epiphysis.

intensifier control it is drilled across the physis into the capital femoral epiphysis. It is best initially to insert a guide wire for proper placement of the hollow mill into the center of the femoral head and avoid penetration of the joint. The cylindrical core of bone, containing the portions of capital epiphysis, physis, and metaphysis, is removed.

An alternative method is to insert progressively larger-sized drills through the window in the femoral neck and drill the metaphysis, physis, and epiphysis. The drill may be inserted through a separate small incision over the lateral intertrochanteric region.

D. Use a small curet to enlarge the cylindrical tunnel. The capital physis is curetted, with additional portions of the growth plate removed. Do not damage the articular cartilage or penetrate the hip joint.

E. and **F.** From the outer wall of the ilium, take corticocancellous strips of bone graft of appropriate size, apposed as a "sandwich," and drive as a composite bone peg across the capital physis into the femoral head. Make radiograms in the anteroposterior and lateral projections to verify bridging by the graft across the physis and into the epiphysis. Firmly replace the cortical bone removed from the femoral neck.

The capsule is closed, and the wound is closed in the usual fashion.

Postoperative Care. The patient is placed in counterpoised bilateral split Russell's traction. Within two to four days, as soon as the patient is comfortable, he or she is allowed to be ambulatory with a three-point, toe-touch crutch gait. In cases of acute slip, a bilateral hip spica cast is worn for six weeks, following which the patient is allowed to be ambulatory with a three-point crutch gait. In case of doubt of the stability of bone grafting across the physis, this author recommends a hip spica cast, even in chronic slip. Crutch protection is continued until the radiographic appearance of growth plate closure, which averages two-and-one-half months. Full weight-bearing is then allowed.

REFERENCES

Crawford, A. H.: Current concepts review. Slipped capital femoral epiphysis. J. Bone Joint Surg., 70–A:1422, 1988.

Heyman, C. H., and Herndon, C. H.: Epiphyseodesis for early slipping of the upper femoral epiphysis. J. Bone Joint Surg., 36–A:539, 1954.

Ward, W. T., and Wood, K.: Open bone graft epiphyseodesis for slipped capital femoral epiphysis. J. Pediatr. Orthop., 10:14, 1990.

Weiner, D. S., Weiner, S., Melby, A., and Hoyt, W. A.: A 30-year experience with bone graft epiphysiodesis in the treatment of slipped capital femoral epiphysis. J. Pediatr. Orthop., 4:145, 1984.

D.

Curet enlarging
cylindrical tunnel

E.

Corticocancellous
bone graft from
lateral wall of
ilium sandwiched and
driven as peg across
physis into femoral head

F.

Original bone plug
removed from femoral neck
and replaced in window

P. PIESCINSKI

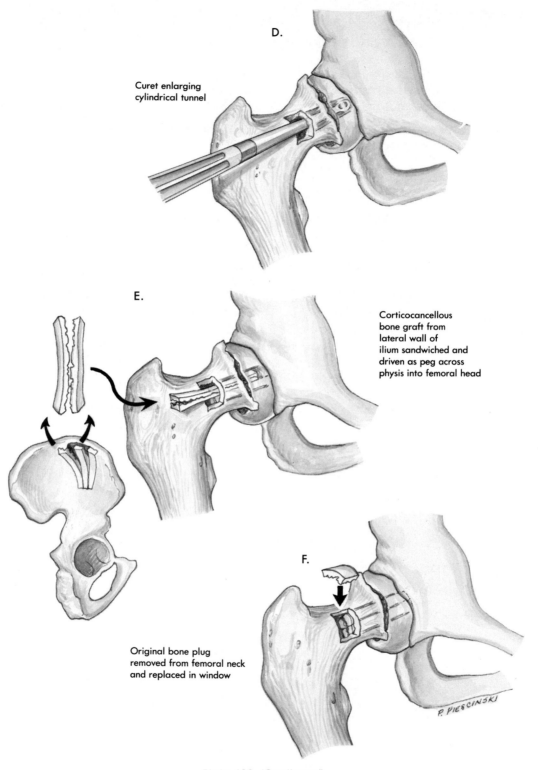

Plate 103. (Continued)

PLATE   104 **Dunn Procedure. Open Reduction of Displaced Femoral Head by Shortening the Femoral Neck**

Indications. Subacute slip (acute slip with more than three weeks elapsed since the acute episode) when more than three fourths (or more than 80 per cent) of the femoral head has slipped.

Requisites. Experienced pediatric orthopedic hip surgeon. Technically, the procedure is very demanding.

Blood for Transfusion. Yes.

Radiographic Control. Image intensifier.

Patient Position. The patient is supine on a fracture table.

Operative Technique

A. The incision begins 2 cm. inferior and lateral to the anterior superior iliac spine and extends toward the greater trochanter and distally along the shaft for a distance of about 10 cm. The subcutaneous tissue is divided in line with the skin incision. The deep fascia is incised. The gluteus maximus fibers are reflected posteriorly, and the tensor fasciae latae and rectus femoris are reflected anteriorly.

B. The vastus lateralis and intermedius muscles are detached from their origin and reflected distally. The anterior and posterior margins of the gluteus medius and minimus muscles are identified, incised, and mobilized. The base of the greater trochanter is exposed.

C. With the oscillating saw, the greater trochanter is detached, due care being taken not to injure the vessels in the intertrochanteric fossa. It is important that the superomedial cortex not be cut; rather, a greenstick fracture is produced. A Kirschner wire is used as a guide in making the osteotomy under image intensifier radiographic control.

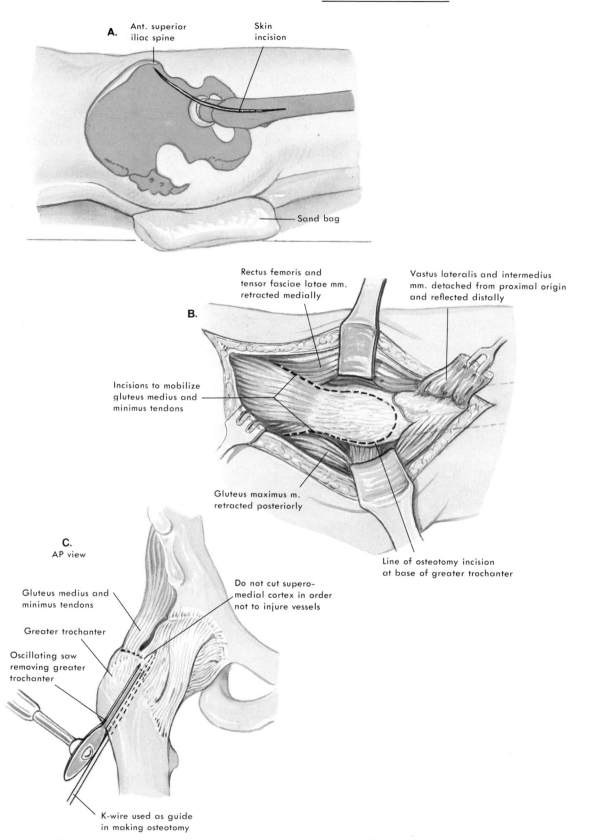

A.

Ant. superior iliac spine

Skin incision

Sand bag

B.

Rectus femoris and tensor fasciae latae mm. retracted medially

Vastus lateralis and intermedius mm. detached from proximal origin and reflected distally

Incisions to mobilize gluteus medius and minimus tendons

Gluteus maximus m. retracted posteriorly

Line of osteotomy incision at base of greater trochanter

C.
AP view

Gluteus medius and minimus tendons

Do not cut supero-medial cortex in order not to injure vessels

Greater trochanter

Oscillating saw removing greater trochanter

K-wire used as guide in making osteotomy

Plate 104. A.–Q., Dunn procedure. Open reduction of the displaced femoral head by shortening of the femoral neck.

D. Once the greater trochanter is detached and reflected proximally, a T-shaped incision is made in the capsule around the edge of the acetabulum, down the lateral aspect of the hip joint to the base of the greater trochanter.

E. When the hip joint is open, it is striking to see the dull white covering on the anterior aspect of the femoral neck and the highly vascularized, velvety membrane at the back. In an acute slip, there is no callus; in an acute and chronic slip, there will be callus extending from the upper end of the femoral neck from which the capital epiphysis has been displaced. Often it is difficult to determine where the white fibrocartilage ends and where the articular cartilage of the femoral head begins. A longitudinal incision is made on the anterolateral aspect of the femoral neck anterior to the vascular area of the edge and around the anterior margin of the femoral head. The posteroinferior retinacular vessels are shortened.

F. The synovium is gently elevated from the anterior and posterolateral surface of the femoral neck with a periosteal elevator. Do not injure the retinacular vessels.

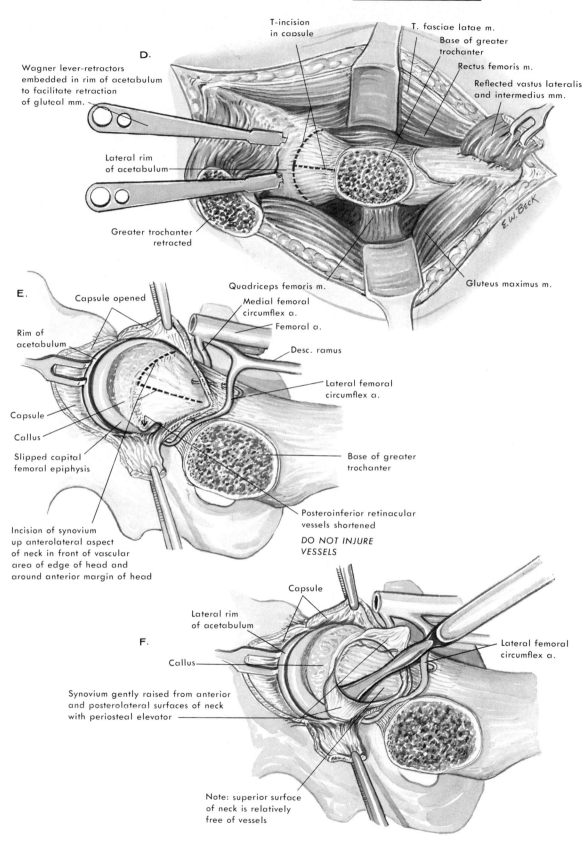

D.

Wagner lever-retractors
embedded in rim of acetabulum
to facilitate retraction
of gluteal mm.

Lateral rim
of acetabulum

Greater trochanter
retracted

T-incision
in capsule

T. fasciae latae m.

Base of greater
trochanter

Rectus femoris m.

Reflected vastus lateralis
and intermedius mm.

E.W. BECK

Quadriceps femoris m.

Gluteus maximus m.

E.

Rim of
acetabulum

Capsule

Callus

Slipped capital
femoral epiphysis

Incision of synovium
up anterolateral aspect
of neck in front of vascular
area of edge of head and
around anterior margin of head

Capsule opened

Medial femoral
circumflex a.

Femoral a.

Desc. ramus

Lateral femoral
circumflex a.

Base of greater
trochanter

Posteroinferior retinacular
vessels shortened

*DO NOT INJURE
VESSELS*

F.

Capsule

Lateral rim
of acetabulum

Callus

Synovium gently raised from anterior
and posterolateral surfaces of neck
with periosteal elevator

Lateral femoral
circumflex a.

Note: superior surface
of neck is relatively
free of vessels

Plate 104. (Continued)

G. With a gouge, the head is freed of all of the fibrocartilage and callus.

H. The osteotomy line on the upper end of the femoral neck is made for excision of the trapezoid bone segment. The purpose of bone shortening is to prevent stretching of the retinacular vessels when the femoral head is replaced on the femoral neck.

On the back of the femoral neck there will be an osseous beak, which is excised by rongeurs until it is level.

I. and **J.** Next, the head of the femur is replaced on the femoral neck, and three threaded Steinmann pins are used to transfix the shaft, neck, and head of the femur. Use two cancellous screws to fix the greater trochanter in its normal position.

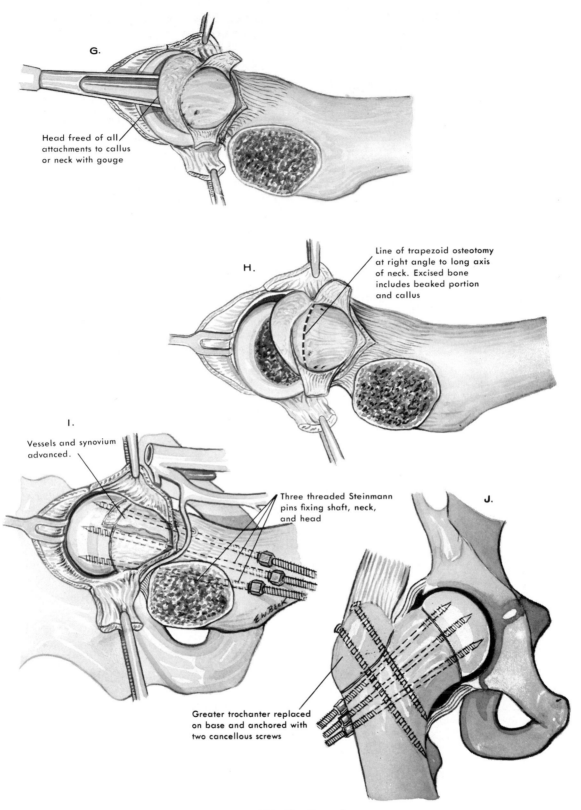

G.

Head freed of all attachments to callus or neck with gouge

H.

Line of trapezoid osteotomy at right angle to long axis of neck. Excised bone includes beaked portion and callus

I.

Vessels and synovium advanced.

Three threaded Steinmann pins fixing shaft, neck, and head

J.

Greater trochanter replaced on base and anchored with two cancellous screws

Plate 104. (Continued)

K.–Q. The importance of excision of a trapezoid segment of bone from the upper neck of the femur in order to prevent stretching of retinacular vessels is illustrated.

The wound is closed in layers.

Postoperative Care. The pins are removed when the osteotomy is healed and the growth plate is closed.

The patient is placed in split Russell's traction with a medial rotation strap on the thigh. When comfortable, the patient is allowed to stand and ambulate with a three-point crutch gait and toe-touch on the operated lower limb. Active assisted and passive exercises are performed to restore range of motion of the hip and increase motor strength of muscles controlling the hip and knee.

Caution! The hip is at risk for avascular necrosis and chondrolysis. If the hip joint becomes stiff, perform a bone scan with technetium 99m to rule out development of these complications.

REFERENCES

Dunn, D. M.: The treatment of adolescent slipping of the upper femoral epiphysis. J. Bone Joint Surg., 46–B:621, 1964.

Dunn, D. M., and Angel, J. C.: Replacement of the femoral head by open operation in severe adolescent slipping of the upper femoral epiphysis. J. Bone Joint Surg., 60–B:394, 1978.

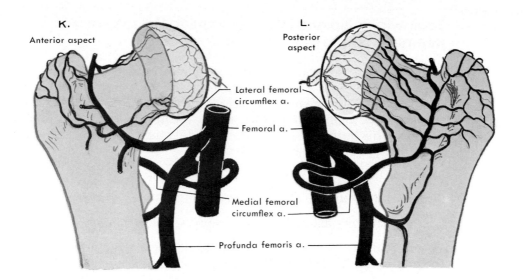

K.
Anterior aspect

L.
Posterior aspect

Lateral femoral circumflex a.

Femoral a.

Medial femoral circumflex a.

Profunda femoris a.

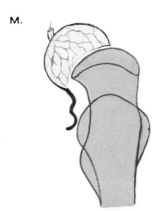

M.

Acute on chronic slip.
Retinacular vessels shorten
after few days

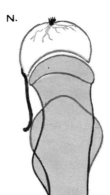

N.

Attempted closed reduction
will stretch blood vessels.
Only blood supply to head
is from artery of lig. teres

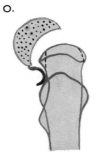

O.

Immediate injury

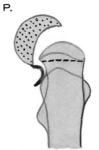

P.

Trapezoid osteotomy
of neck

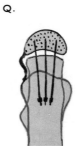

Q.

Neck shortened.
Retinacular
vessels relaxed

Plate 104. (Continued)

PLATE 105   ## Southwick's Biplane Intertrochanteric Osteotomy with Internal Compression Fixation

Indications. Lateral rotation and extension deformity of the hip as a residual from in situ fixation for a slipped capital femoral epiphysis.

Note. The proponents of this procedure regard this biplane intertrochanteric osteotomy as a primary method of treatment when the slip is greater than 30 degrees. This author does not recommend its use as a primary method of management because of the risk of chondrolysis.

Blood for Transfusion. Yes.

Radiographic Control. Image intensifier.

Special Instrumentation. Internal compression fixation device.

Patient Position. The patient is placed supine on a radiolucent operating table with the lower limb draped free. The anterior and lateral surfaces of the proximal femur are exposed subperiosteally at the level of the lesser trochanter. Dissection of the posterior surfaces of the femur is not necessary. The psoas tendon is detached at its insertion to the lesser trochanter (see steps **E.** and **F.**).

Operative Technique

A. The junction of the anterior and lateral surfaces of the femur is identified with a longitudinal orientation mark. A transverse mark is made at the level of the lesser trochanter at right angles to the longitudinal orientation mark. This transverse line locates the inferior border of the wedge to be removed. A template composed of adjoining right triangles is placed on the transverse line, and the wedge of bone to be resected is outlined on bone.

Next, a 5.5-mm. hole is made with a drill point in the lateral edge of the anterior cortex of the greater trochanter. With a T-handle chuck, a special threaded holding pin, 6.3 mm. in diameter, is inserted. The line of insertion is parallel and 6.3 mm. proximal to the hypotenuse (oblique line) of the wedge to be removed from the anterior cortex. The holding pin is directed toward the upper margin of the lesser trochanter.

B. The wedge of bone is removed with a sharp osteotome or an electric saw. The surface on the upper segment is oblique, whereas that of the distal shaft segment is transverse. The osteotomy is completed by continuation of the transverse cut through the lesser trochanter. Avoid injury to the soft tissues posteriorly and medially.

A.

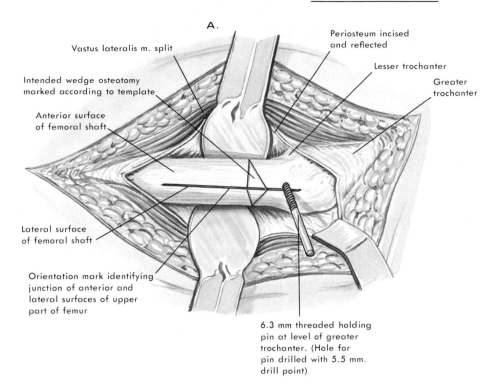

Vastus lateralis m. split

Intended wedge osteotomy marked according to template

Anterior surface of femoral shaft

Lateral surface of femoral shaft

Orientation mark identifying junction of anterior and lateral surfaces of upper part of femur

Periosteum incised and reflected

Lesser trochanter

Greater trochanter

6.3 mm threaded holding pin at level of greater trochanter. (Hole for pin drilled with 5.5 mm. drill point)

B.

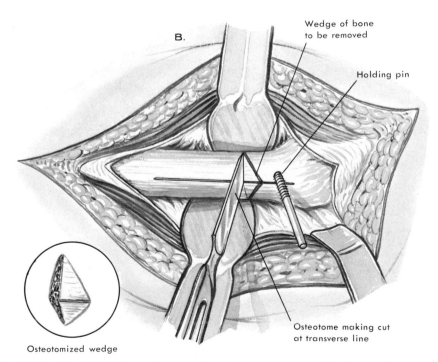

Wedge of bone to be removed

Holding pin

Osteotome making cut at transverse line

Osteotomized wedge

Plate 105. A.–F., Southwick's biplane intertrochanteric osteotomy with internal compression fixation.

C. After completion of the osteotomy, the pin in the proximal fragment is used as a handle to fix the proximal segment; the thigh is abducted and flexed by an assistant until the oblique cut surface of the upper segment fits flush against the transverse cut of the distal segment to correct the lateral rotation deformity to the desired degree. The distal segment is rotated medially the required amount. Once the two fragments are in the desired position, a drill hole, 5.5 mm. in diameter, is made in the distal fragment for the second holding pin. Medial displacement of the distal fragment during drilling and insertion of the pin is prevented with a bone hook, which is inserted into the medullary canal of the shaft. It is crucial that the second holding pin be parallel to the pin in the proximal fragment. Its site should be 3 cm. distal to the osteotomy line. The use of the compression block facilitates placement of the distal pin. If there is any instability of the osteotomized fragments, a third pin may be inserted through a hole in the compression block to control the proximal segment.

D. The knob in the compression block is twisted, compressing the osteotomized segment until the cut surfaces are in stable apposition. All during this procedure, the assistant supports the patient's thigh, preventing slipping or overriding of the osteotomy surfaces.

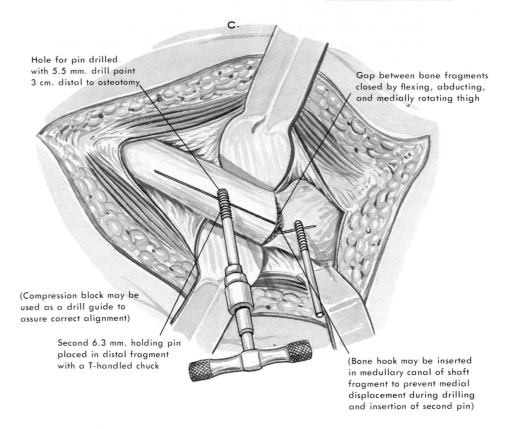

C.

Hole for pin drilled
with 5.5 mm. drill point
3 cm. distal to osteotomy

Gap between bone fragments
closed by flexing, abducting,
and medially rotating thigh

(Compression block may be
used as a drill guide to
assure correct alignment)

Second 6.3 mm. holding pin
placed in distal fragment
with a T-handled chuck

(Bone hook may be inserted
in medullary canal of shaft
fragment to prevent medial
displacement during drilling
and insertion of second pin)

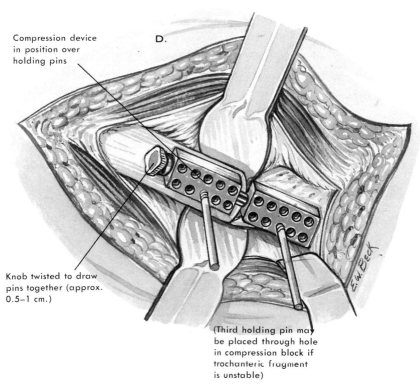

Compression device
in position over
holding pins

D.

Knob twisted to draw
pins together (approx.
0.5–1 cm.)

(Third holding pin may
be placed through hole
in compression block if
trochanteric fragment
is unstable)

Plate 105. (Continued)

E. A specially manufactured compression plate is bent to conform to the contour of the femur and fixed with two cancellous bone screws, 5 cm. in length, that are inserted in the proximal fragment through pre-drilled 5.5 mm. holes. One of the screws should cross the neck of the femur into the calcar. The distal fragment is fixed with 4.2 mm. screws.

Sequence of screw placement is important. First, insert the lower screw in the upper fragment. Second, insert the most distal screw in the lower fragment. Next, place the screw at the top hole of the proximal fragment. Then insert the distal screws in the shaft, as marked in the drawing.

F. The compression plate and holding pins are removed, and the adequacy of the fixation plate is double checked. Anteroposterior and frog-leg lateral radiograms are made to check the position and adequacy of correction of the deformity.

Postoperative Care. Postoperatively, no hip spica cast is required. The patient is placed in bilateral split Russell's traction with the hip in 30 degrees flexion to relax the capsule. Two to three days postoperatively, as soon as he or she is comfortable, the patient is allowed to sit at the edge of the bed. As soon as there is adequate muscle strength, the patient can flex the hip and extend the knee. A three-point crutch gait is permitted with toe touch on the affected side. Crutch protection is continued until bony union has taken place, about two to three months postoperatively.

REFERENCES

Southwick, W. O.: Osteotomy through the lesser trochanter for slipped capital femoral epiphysis. J. Bone Joint Surg., 49–A:807, 1967.

Southwick, W. O.: Treatment of severely slipped upper femoral epiphysis by trochantric osteotomy. A.A.O.S. Instructional Course Lectures, 21:200, 1972.

Southwick, W. O.: Compression fixation after biplane intertrochanteric osteotomy for slipped capital femoral epiphysis. A technical improvement. J. Bone Joint Surg., 66–A:1218, 1973.

Southwick, W. O.: Biplane osteotomy for very severe slipped capital femoral epiphysis. In: The Hip. Proceedings of the Hip Society. St. Louis, C. V. Mosby, 1975, pp. 105–114.

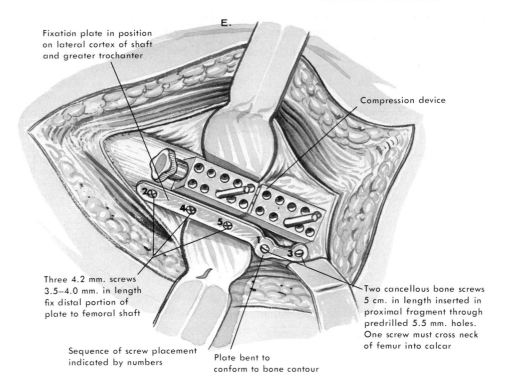

E.

Fixation plate in position on lateral cortex of shaft and greater trochanter

Compression device

Three 4.2 mm. screws 3.5–4.0 mm. in length fix distal portion of plate to femoral shaft

Two cancellous bone screws 5 cm. in length inserted in proximal fragment through predrilled 5.5 mm. holes. One screw must cross neck of femur into calcar

Sequence of screw placement indicated by numbers

Plate bent to conform to bone contour

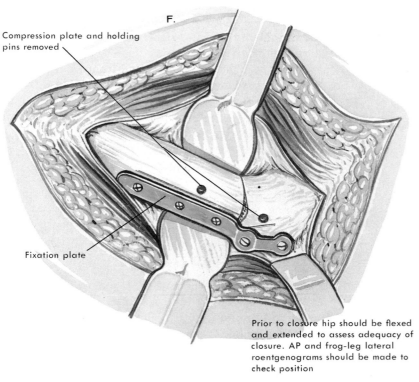

F.

Compression plate and holding pins removed

Fixation plate

Prior to closure hip should be flexed and extended to assess adequacy of closure. AP and frog-leg lateral roentgenograms should be made to check position

Plate 105. (Continued)

PLATE 106   Kramer's Compensatory Osteotomy of the Base of the Femoral Neck for a Slipped Capital Femoral Epiphysis

Indications. Proponents of this technique use it as a primary means to correct lateral rotation. This author does not recommend its use because of the necessity of multiple pin fixation and the danger of avascular necrosis and varus deformity in chronic slipped capital femoral epiphysis.

Blood for Transfusion. Yes.

Radiographic Control. Image intensifier.

Patient Position. Supine on a fracture table.

Operative Technique

A. and **B.** The skin incision begins 2 cm. distal and lateral to the anterior superior iliac spine and curves distally and posteriorly over the lateral aspect of the greater trochanter and the femoral shaft to a point 10 cm. distal to the base of the greater trochanter. The subcutaneous tissue and deep fascia are incised longitudinally. The interval between the gluteus medius and tensor fasciae latae is developed. The hip joint capsule is exposed along the anterior superior surface of the femoral neck. The vastus lateralis muscle is detached at its origin and reflected distally. An incision is made in the capsule along the anterior intertrochanteric line. With the hip joint opened, the degree of slip is assessed by inspection. Also, the amount of callus between the cartilage of the femoral head and the normal cortex of the femoral neck is determined. In general, the wedge of bone to be removed is two thirds of the width of the callus as measured directly anteriorly. The inferior osteotomy line is made first, perpendicular to the femoral neck following the anterior intertrochanteric line from above downward. The osteotomies extend posteriorly, leaving the posterior cortex intact. The vessels in the intertrochanteric fossa should be protected from injury.

Next, a threaded Steinmann pin is drilled into the proximal part of the femoral neck to control the upper fragment. The second, or upper, osteotomy line is made with the blade of the osteotome or saw directed obliquely and posteriorly. Again, the posterior cortex should be left intact. This will permit making a greenstick fracture in the posterior cortex when the osteotomy site is closed.

C. and **D.** Three threaded Steinmann pins are drilled along the outer cortex of the upper femoral shaft toward the osteotomy site. The osteotomy site is closed by medial rotation and abduction of the distal segment. The three pins are then drilled into the femoral head.

Kramer recommends apophyseodesis of the greater trochanteric growth plate to prevent overgrowth of the greater trochanter. This is done in a child who is relatively young—under 14 years of age in boys and under 12 years of age in girls.

Postoperative Care. The patient is placed in split Russell's traction with a medial rotation strap at the thigh. As soon as the patient is comfortable, he or she may stand and ambulate with a three-point crutch gait. The pins are removed when the osteotomy is healed and the physis is closed.

REFERENCES

Barmada, R., Bruch, R. F., Gimbel, J. S., and Ray, R. D.: Base of the neck extracapsular osteotomy for correction of deformity in slipped capital femoral epiphysis. Clin. Orthop., 132:98, 1978.
Kramer, W. G., Craig, W. A., and Noel, S.: Compensating osteotomy at the base of the femoral neck for slipped capital femoral epiphysis. J. Bone Joint Surg., 58–A:796, 1976.

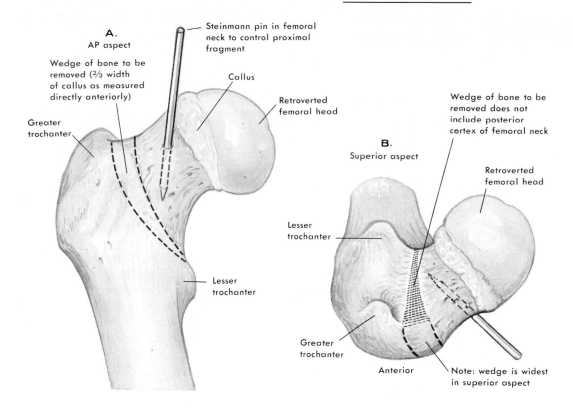

A.
AP aspect

Steinmann pin in femoral neck to control proximal fragment

Wedge of bone to be removed (⅔ width of callus as measured directly anteriorly)

Callus

Retroverted femoral head

Greater trochanter

Lesser trochanter

B.
Superior aspect

Wedge of bone to be removed does not include posterior cortex of femoral neck

Retroverted femoral head

Lesser trochanter

Greater trochanter

Anterior

Note: wedge is widest in superior aspect

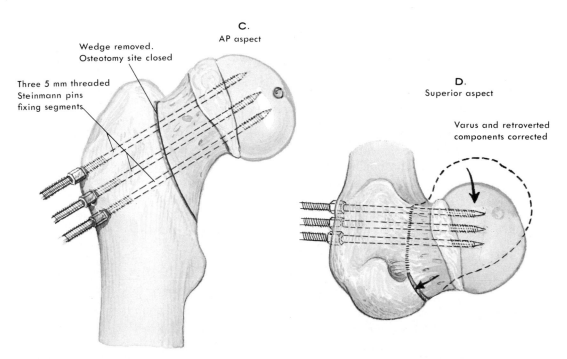

C.
AP aspect

Wedge removed. Osteotomy site closed

Three 5 mm threaded Steinmann pins fixing segments

D.
Superior aspect

Varus and retroverted components corrected

Plate 106. A.–D., Kramer's compensatory osteotomy of the base of the femoral neck for a slipped capital femoral epiphysis.

PLATE 107   Hip Arthrodesis

Indications. Marked destruction of articular cartilage due to chondrolysis or septic arthritis with pain in an adolescent or an adult or occasionally in a child eight years of age or older with marked instability and pain in the hip.

Advantages

1. Compression across the fusion.
2. The hip abductor muscles are not disturbed.
3. Bone stock is preserved.
4. The subtrochanteric femoral osteotomy reduces the length of the lever arm and promotes early fusion.

Disadvantages

1. Possibility of loss of position in the spica cast in the immediate postoperative period and the necessity of wedging or changing the cast. This author circumvents this problem by temporary internal fixation with criss-cross Steinmann pins.
2. Immobilization in a hip spica cast.
3. Malalignment of the femoral canal produced by the subtrochanteric osteotomy, which could interfere with later conversion to a total hip arthroplasty.

Caution! Long-term results have shown that patients with hip arthrodesis will develop osteoarthritis of the L5 spine and the knee with increasing pain and disability. If this problem arises, the patient will require mobilization of the hip with total joint replacement. Total joint arthroplasty is not performed in the young adult or adolescent patient because of loosening of the components of the total joint. Hip arthrodesis in these young patients will buy several decades of time and allow the benefit of improved future technology. It behooves the surgeon to remember that hip arthrodesis may have to be converted to total joint replacement; therefore, he or she should not employ methods of fixation that will destroy hip abductor muscles or bone stock and should not alter normal anatomy of the femur.

Blood for Transfusion. Yes.

Radiographic Control. Image intensifier.

Patient Position. The patient is placed in supine position on a radiolucent operating table. The operative procedure is performed under image intensifier radiographic control. The perineum is shielded with Ioben drape. Both lower limbs, the hips, the pelvis, and the lower abdomen are prepared sterile with povidone-iodine soap and painted with tincture of povidone-iodine solution. Both lower limbs are draped sterile so that they can be manipulated freely and the Thomas test can be performed accurately. The anterosuperior iliac spine is marked with a sterile ink pen; the pelvis should be horizontal and even.

Operative Technique

A. The surgical exposure is through Salter's so-called bikini anterolateral incision (see Plate 82). The cartilaginous iliac apophysis is split into halves, and the medial and lateral walls of the ilium are exposed subperiosteally. The tensor fasciae latae, gluteus minimus, and anterior part of the gluteus medius are retracted laterally. The sartorius muscle is detached at its origin from the anterosuperior iliac spine and retracted distally. Divide the direct and reflected (indirect) heads of rectus femoris. The iliopsoas muscle–tendons are retracted medially.

The anterior capsule of the hip joint is exposed and divided by a T-shaped incision.

B. The femoral head is dislocated anteriorly. With the help of rongeurs and reamers, the acetabulum and femoral head are denuded of articular cartilage.

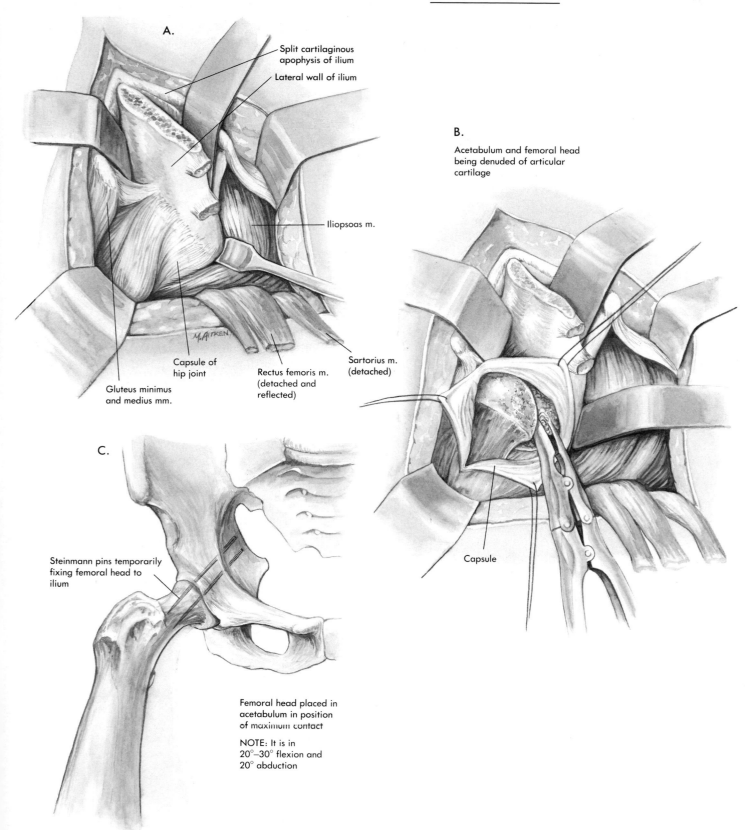

A.

Split cartilaginous apophysis of ilium

Lateral wall of ilium

Iliopsoas m.

Capsule of hip joint

Gluteus minimus and medius mm.

Rectus femoris m. (detached and reflected)

Sartorius m. (detached)

M. AITKEN

B.

Acetabulum and femoral head being denuded of articular cartilage

Capsule

C.

Steinmann pins temporarily fixing femoral head to ilium

Femoral head placed in acetabulum in position of maximum contact

NOTE: It is in 20°–30° flexion and 20° abduction

Plate 107. A.–G., Hip arthrodesis.

C. Place the femoral head in the acetabulum in the position of maximum contact (see p. 525). This is usually 20 to 30 degrees of flexion and 20 degrees of abduction and variable degrees of rotation. Temporarily transfix the femur and innominate bone with two smooth Steinmann pins, and make radiograms to confirm the position of the femoral head. Insert the Steinmann pins superoinferiorly from inside the pelvis; the pins also serve as a guide for insertion of cancellous screws.

D. Insert two large cancellous screws with washers from inside the pelvis through the acetabulum and into the femoral head and neck using the usual AO technique. It is important to achieve a lag effect. Pre-drill under image intensifier radiographic control, aiming at the base of the femoral neck. *Do not penetrate or protrude through the inferior cortex of the femoral neck!*

Determine the length of screw necessary, and insert a screw of the appropriate length. Remove the previously inserted Steinmann pins. The hip wound is irrigated and closed in the usual fashion.

At this point, perform a Thomas test and determine the position of the arthrodesed hip. It is usually in flexion, abduction, and lateral rotation. Ideally, it should be in 20 degrees of flexion, 5 to 10 degrees of lateral rotation, and 5 degrees of adduction.

E. Next, expose the anterolateral surface of the proximal femoral shaft (see Plate 92). Incise the periosteum, and perform a transverse corticotomy at the subtrochanteric level. Holes are drilled into the anterior, medial, and lateral cortices. The drill should not penetrate the medullary cavity or damage the marrow and intramedullary circulation.

With a small sharp osteotome, connect the drill holes. Complete the osteotomy by greenstick fracturing of the posterior cortex. Close the periosteum. The repaired periosteal sleeve provides some degree of stability. After complete hemostasis is obtained, the wound is irrigated and closed in the routine fashion.

F. The subtrochanteric femoral osteotomy allows motion. Carefully transfer the patient to the fracture table, and place the operated lower limb in the optimal desired position. Apply a one-and-one-half hip spica cast. Radiograms are made to double check the alignment of the subtrochanteric osteotomy.

G. This author prefers fixation of the subtrochanteric femoral osteotomy with criss-cross Steinmann pins or internal fixation at initial surgery to prevent loss of alignment in the hip spica cast.

Postoperative Care. Immobilization in a hip spica cast is continued until there is radiographic evidence of healing of the subtrochanteric femoral osteotomy and fusion of the hip. When there is loss of alignment of the subtrochanteric osteotomy, the cast is wedged or the hip spica cast is changed as required.

REFERENCE

Mowery, C. A., Houkom, J. A., Roach, J. W., and Sutherland, D. H.: A simple method of hip arthrodesis. J. Pediatr. Orthop., 6:7, 1986.

D.

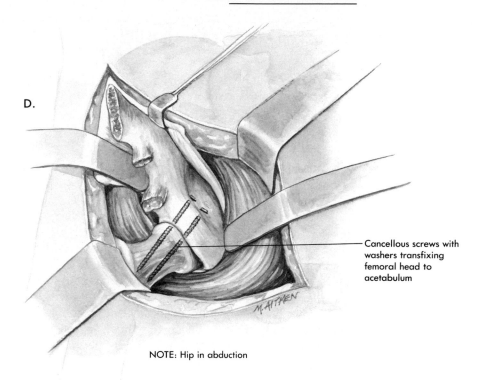

Cancellous screws with washers transfixing femoral head to acetabulum

NOTE: Hip in abduction

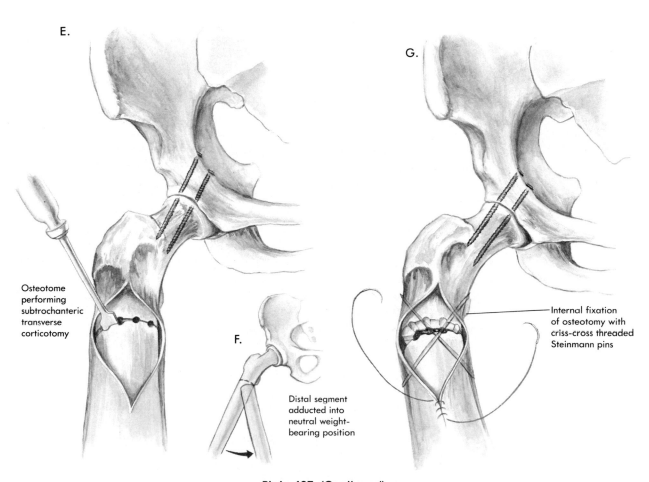

E.

Osteotome performing subtrochanteric transverse corticotomy

F.

Distal segment adducted into neutral weight-bearing position

G.

Internal fixation of osteotomy with criss-cross threaded Steinmann pins

Plate 107. (Continued)

PLATE 108   ## Thompson Arthrodesis of the Hip

Indications

1. Marked destruction of the hip joint due to avascular necrosis of the femoral head with or without chondrolysis.
2. Pain.
3. Instability.

Requisites. Age—adolescent or young adult.

Note. An avascular femoral head may not fuse. Bone grafting with the onlay technique will enhance fusion.

Caution! Long-term results have shown that patients with hip arthrodesis will develop osteoarthritis of the L5 spine and the knee with increasing pain and disability. If this problem arises, the patient will require mobilization of the hip with total joint replacement. Total joint arthroplasty is not performed in the young adult or adolescent patient because of loosening of the components of the total joint. Hip arthrodesis in these young patients will buy several decades of time and allow the benefit of improved future technology. It behooves the surgeon to remember that hip arthrodesis may have to be converted to total joint replacement; therefore, he or she should not employ methods of fixation that will destroy hip abductor muscles or bone stock and should not alter normal anatomy of the femur.

Blood for Transfusion. Yes.

Radiographic Control. Image intensifier.

Patient Position. The patient is placed supine on a radiolucent operating table. Image intensifier radiographic control is used during surgery. The involved hip, ilium, and entire lower limb are prepared sterile and draped so that the limb can be moved without contaminating the operative field.

Operative Technique

A. The surgical exposure is through an anterolateral Smith-Peterson incision. The cartilaginous iliac apophysis is split into halves, and the periosteum is elevated from the medial and lateral walls of the ilium. The interval between sartorius and tensor fasciae femoris is developed by blunt dissection, and the sartorius muscle is divided at its origin from the anterior superior iliac spine and reflected distally. The direct and indirect heads of rectus femoris are detached at their origin and reflected distally. The iliacus muscle is elevated and reflected medially from the anterior aspect of the hip joint and pubic ramus. Divide the psoas tendon, if necessary, to obtain adequate anteromedial exposure of the hip. The Bigelow (iliofemoral) ligament is sectioned, and the capsule of the hip joint is excised anteriorly and superiorly.

A large, broad iliac bone graft, consisting of both medial and lateral cortices, is harvested from the anterior 6 to 7 cm. of the iliac wing and crest.

B. The ligamentum teres is sectioned, and the femoral head is dislocated. All articular cartilage is excised from the acetabulum and head. The acetabulum and wound are thoroughly irrigated to remove all cartilaginous debris.

C. The femoral head is reduced into the acetabulum and maintained in a position of maximum apposition; the position of maximal bony contact will ensure fusion of the joint; however, the limb will not be in good functional position. The resultant deformed functional position of the hip is corrected by osteotomy.

The graft is laid flatly against the anterior surface of the pubic ramus, acetabulum, and head–neck of the femur, extending distally to the intertrochanteric line. In order for the graft to appose evenly on the broad surface of the graft bed, it is often necessary to excise the anteroinferior iliac spine and the prominence

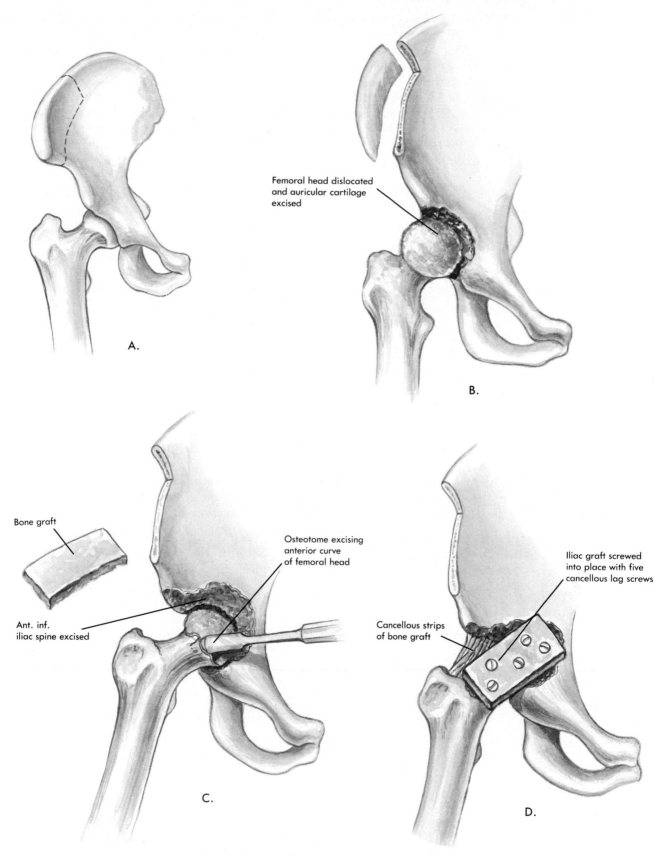

A.

B.

Femoral head dislocated
and auricular cartilage
excised

Bone graft

Ant. inf.
iliac spine excised

Osteotome excising
anterior curve
of femoral head

C.

Iliac graft screwed
into place with five
cancellous lag screws

Cancellous strips
of bone graft

D.

Plate 108. A.–G., Thompson arthrodesis of the hip.

of the pubic ramus and remove a part of the anterior curve of the femoral head. It is vital for the graft to make firm, even contact throughout its extent.

D. The onlay iliac graft is screwed in place into its bed with five cancellous lag screws. The middle screw secures the femoral head into the posterior wall of the acetabulum. The upper two screws are inserted through the graft into the pubic ramus and deep into the substance of the ilium in the direction of the posteroinferior spine. The distal two screws secure the graft to the femoral neck.

E. and **F.** Additional strips of cancellous bone graft are taken from the lateral wall of the ilium and placed along the denuded superior surface of the femoral neck extending to the outer wing of the ilium. The hip is in abduction and some medial rotation.

G. The soft tissues are elevated and retracted distally, and the intertrochanteric and subtrochanteric region of the upper femur is subperiosteally exposed. A transverse osteotomy is performed immediately above the lesser trochanter with the help of an oscillating electric saw. Verify the level of osteotomy by image intensifier radiographic control. *Do not perform the osteotomy below the lesser trochanter because it will take longer to heal!*

Be sure that the line of osteotomy is transverse and not oblique; an oblique osteotomy is more likely to slip and displace. Do not displace the femoral shaft medially (as is done routinely with the McMurray osteotomy); such displacement will cause delayed union or non-union.

The wound and skin are closed in the usual fashion. A single or one-and-one-half hip spica cast is applied. The best position of the hip for fusion is 5 degrees of adduction, neutral rotation, and 20 degrees of flexion. *Be sure that the pelvis and anterior superior iliac spine are level!*

When the lumbar spine is flattened, the hip will be in 20 degrees of flexion. Do not elevate the affected lower limb from the floor, since this will result in a greater degree of hip flexion and cause unsightly gait with exaggerated asymmetric lumbar lordosis and prominence of the buttocks. The ankle and foot are left free. When the affected lower limb is short, it may be compensated by fusion of the hip in the appropriate degree of abduction. Ordinarily a one-and-one-half hip spica cast is applied when the patient is obese or uncooperative.

Postoperative Care. Ambulation with crutch or walker support is begun as soon as the patient is comfortable, usually within a week. To prevent a stiff knee, the posterior part of the leg and lower thigh of the cast is bivalved. Active assisted and gentle passive exercises are performed several times a day with the patient lying prone in bed. At other times, the bivalved leg part of the cast is firmly secured in place with straps and buckles. The hip spica cast is removed in eight to 12 weeks when radiograms in various projections disclose solid fusion and stability of the hip.

REFERENCES

Price, C. T., and Lovell, W. W.: Thompson arthrodesis of the hip in children. J. Bone Joint Surg., 62–A:1118, 1980.

Thompson, F. R.: Combined hip fusion and subtrochanteric osteotomy allowing early ambulation. J. Bone Joint Surg., 38–A:13, 1956.

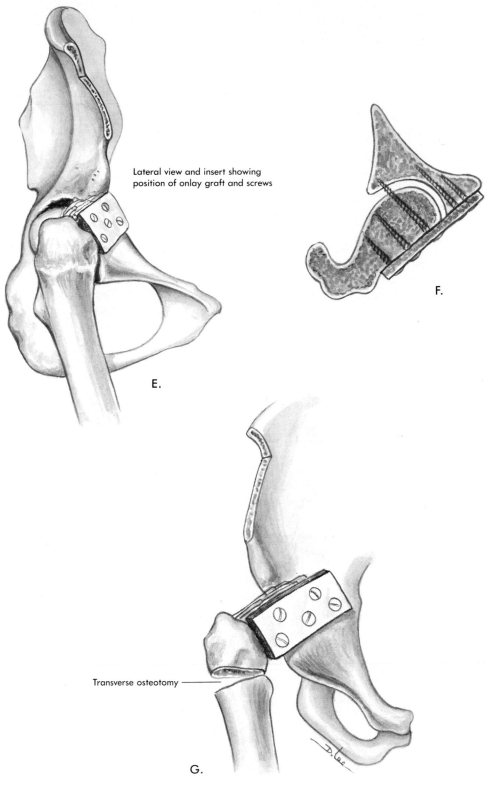

Lateral view and insert showing
position of onlay graft and screws

E.

F.

Transverse osteotomy

G.

Plate 108. (Continued)

PLATE 109 ## Hip Arthrodesis Using the AO Technique and Internal Fixation with a Cobra Plate

Indications

1. Heavy patient with chondrolysis and marked destruction of the hip.
2. Pain.

Advantages. Immobilization in a cast is not necessary.

Disadvantages. The procedure distorts the normal anatomy of the hip and upper femur and causes fibrosis of the gluteus medius and minimus.

Blood for Transfusion. Yes.

Radiographic Control. Image intensifier.

Patient Position. The patient is placed in supine position, and both lower limbs, the pelvis, hips, and lower abdomen are prepared and draped sterile in the usual orthopedic fashion. It is crucial that a Thomas test be performed on the operating table without contaminating the operative field. The patient should be placed on a radiolucent operating table for appropriate radiolucent control.

Operative Technique

A. Make a 20- to 30-cm. longitudinal straight lateral incision; it begins at the juncture of the anterior and middle thirds of the iliac crest, extends distally to the anterior margin of the greater trochanter, and then extends distally along the femoral shaft for a distance of 10 to 15 cm. The subcutaneous tissue is divided in line with the skin incision. Superficial and deep fascia are incised and reflected, and the greater trochanter is exposed. The fascia lata is split longitudinally in the direction of its fibers.

B. The insertion of gluteus medius and minimus at the greater trochanter is identified, and its anterior and posterior margins are delineated. The vastus lateralis is detached proximally from the abductor tubercle of the greater trochanter by an L-shaped incision and elevated in its entire width subperiosteally from the lateral and anterior surfaces of the femoral shaft for a distance of 10 cm.

C. With a power saw, perform an osteotomy of the greater trochanter about 1½ cm. distal to its tip. The gluteus medius and minimus muscles are elevated proximally and laterally, exposing the lateral wall of the ilium. A large Chandler elevator is inserted into the greater sciatic notch, protecting the sciatic nerve.

A.

Incision

B.

Gluteus medius
and minimus mm.

Line of osteotomy
of greater trochanter

Greater trochanter

Vastus lateralis elevated
and reflected anteriorly

C.

Chandler retractor in
greater sciatic notch
protecting sciatic nerve

Gluteus medius and minimus mm.
reflected proximally

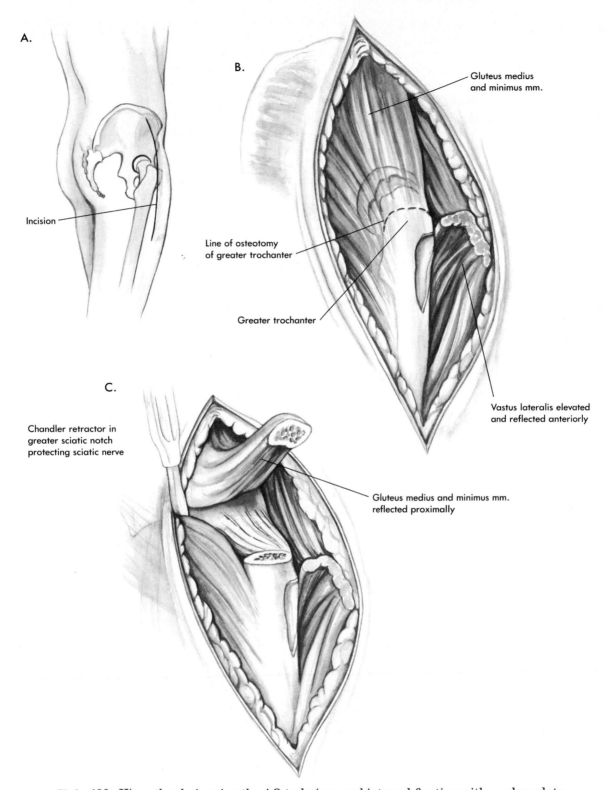

Plate 109. Hip arthrodesis using the AO technique and internal fixation with a cobra plate.

D. The hip is dislocated anterolaterally, and the articular cartilage is reamed out of the acetabulum. Also, the femoral head is denuded of all articular cartilage until raw cancellous bone is exposed. Remove enough bone from the hip joint in order to medialize the femoral head deep into the acetabulum.

E. and **F.** If adequate medialization of the femoral head into the deepened acetabulum cannot be achieved, medial displacement of the pelvis is carried out following the technique of Chiari's osteotomy (see Plate 89).

Next, place the femoral head into the denuded acetabulum and check the position of the hip. The ideal position of the hip should be about 10 degrees of adduction, 5 to 10 degrees of lateral rotation and about 15 to 25 degrees of hip flexion depending on the age of the patient, sex, and future occupation.

Perform a Thomas test on the operating table to determine the degree of hip flexion. Make radiograms of both hips and the pelvis to assess the degree of hip adduction. The femoral head is transfixed by two threaded Steinmann pins into the acetabulum in the desired degree of hip flexion, and adduction and lateral rotation. A cobra plate is contoured onto the lateral wall of the ilium and the lateral proximal femoral shaft.

D.

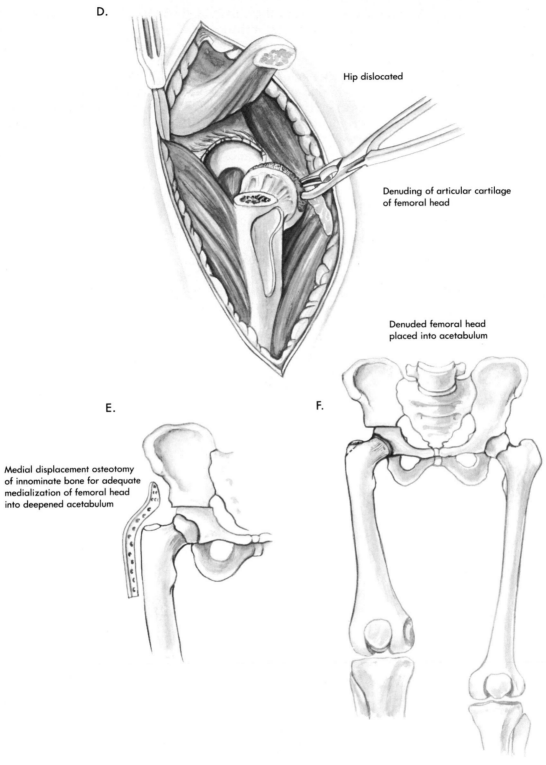

Hip dislocated

Denuding of articular cartilage
of femoral head

Denuded femoral head
placed into acetabulum

E.

Medial displacement osteotomy
of innominate bone for adequate
medialization of femoral head
into deepened acetabulum

F.

Plate 109. (Continued)

G. The plate is fixed to the pelvis by first screwing the head and neck of the cobra plate to the lateral wall of the ilium. Then, a large tensioning device is fixed distally to the femur and is tautened bringing the femoral head and acetabulum under compression.

H. and I. The position of the hip is rechecked. When it is satisfactory, the plate portion of the cobra plate is fixed distally to the femoral shaft.

The protruded portion of the greater trochanter is resected and used as a bone graft in front of the plate, transfixing it into the ilium and the femoral head. The proximal segment of the greater trochanter is reattached to the upper femoral shaft and transfixed with two cancellous screws. The plate must be deep to the gluteus medius and minimus muscles, and the hip abductor muscle mass must be preserved.

Ideally, the limb length should be 1.5 to 1.0 cm. shorter on the fused side compared with the contralateral normal hip. The wound is irrigated, and a closed Hemovac suction drain inserted. The wound is closed in the usual fashion.

Postoperative Care. Immobilization in cast is not necessary. This is a definite advantage of the cobra plate hip fusion. The patient is allowed to ambulate using three-point crutch protection on the affected lower limb until solid fusion has taken place; this may require three to four months.

REFERENCE

Muller, M. E., Allgower, M., Schneider, R., and Willenegger, H.: Manual of Internal Fixation. 2nd ed. Berlin, Springer-Verlag, 1979.

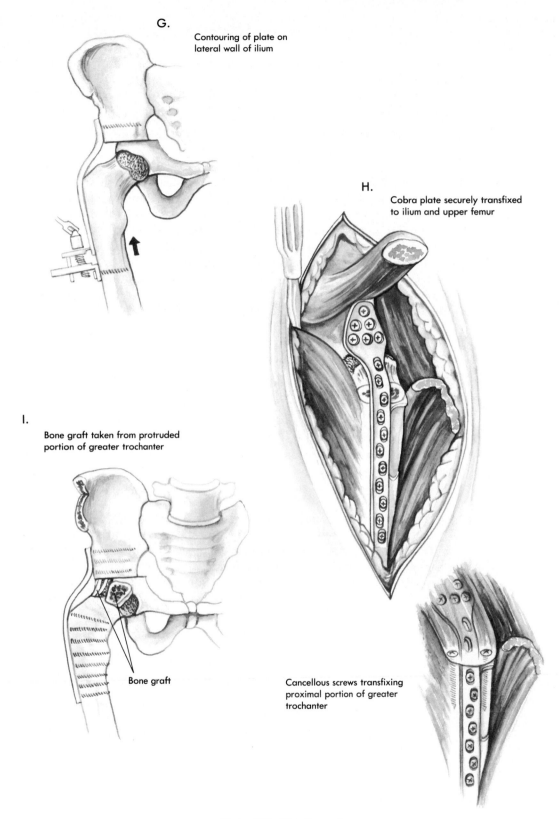

G.
Contouring of plate on
lateral wall of ilium

H.
Cobra plate securely transfixed
to ilium and upper femur

I.
Bone graft taken from protruded
portion of greater trochanter

Bone graft

Cancellous screws transfixing
proximal portion of greater
trochanter

Plate 109. (Continued)

PLATE 110   ## Hemipelvectomy (Banks and Coleman Technique)

Indications. Malignant tumor of the hip region in which limb salvage is not possible because of the extent of involvement.

Note. Be sure that patient has a consultation with a competent prosthetist prior to surgery.

Blood for Transfusion. Yes.

Radiographic Control. Image intensifier.

Patient Position. The patient lies on the unaffected side and is maintained in position by sandbags and kidney rests, which are placed well above the iliac crests. The normal limb lying underneath is flexed at the hip and knee and fastened to the table by wide adhesive straps. The uppermost arm is supported on a rest. The perineal area and, in the male, the scrotum and penis are shielded away from the operative field by sterile, self-adhering skin drapes. The operative area is prepared and draped so that the proximal thigh, the inguinal and gluteal regions, and the abdomen are sterile. It should be possible to turn the patient on his or her back and side without contaminating the surgical field.

Operative Technique

A. The outlines of the skin flaps, consisting of ilioinguinal, iliogluteal, and posterior incisions, are marked with methylene blue. With the patient placed on his or her back, the ilioinguinal incision is made first. It begins at the pubic tubercle and passes upward and backward parallel to Poupart's ligament to the anterior superior iliac spine and then posteriorly on the iliac crest. Its posterior limit depends on the desired level of section of the innominate bone.

B. The subcutaneous tissue and fascia are divided along the line of the skin incision. The periosteum over the iliac crest is incised between the attachments of the abdominal muscles superiorly and the tensor fasciae latae and the gluteus medius inferiorly.

C. The abdominal muscles are detached from the iliac crest and medial wall of the ilium. The tributaries of deep circumflex vessels are ligated.

D. Next, the inguinal ligament is divided and, along with the spermatic cord and abdominal muscles, is retracted superiorly. The lower skin flap is retracted inferiorly, and by blunt dissection the inner pelvis is freed. The inferior epigastric artery and lumboinguinal nerve are exposed, ligated, and divided.

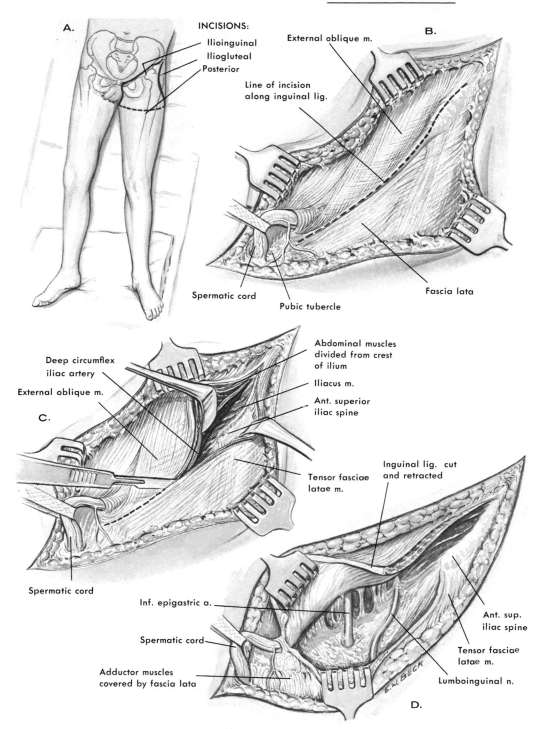

A.   INCISIONS:
— Ilioinguinal
— Iliogluteal
— Posterior

B.   External oblique m.

Line of incision
along inguinal lig.

Spermatic cord

Pubic tubercle

Fascia lata

C.   Deep circumflex
iliac artery

External oblique m.

Abdominal muscles
divided from crest
of ilium

Iliacus m.

Ant. superior
iliac spine

Tensor fasciae
latae m.

Spermatic cord

Inguinal lig. cut
and retracted

Inf. epigastric a.

Spermatic cord

Adductor muscles
covered by fascia lata

Ant. sup.
iliac spine

Tensor fasciae
latae m.

Lumboinguinal n.

D.

E. W. BECK

Plate 110. A.–O., Hemipelvectomy (Banks and Coleman technique).

E. In the loose areolar tissue, the external iliac vessels and femoral nerve are gently dissected out. The external iliac artery and vein are individually clamped, severed, and doubly ligated with 0 Tycron passed through the vessel with a needle.

F. The rectus abdominis and adductor muscles are detached from the pubic bone, which is subperiosteally exposed. The bladder is retracted superiorly. The pubic bone is osteotomized 1.5 cm. lateral to the symphysis. Depending on the proximity of the tumor, the osteotomy may have to be at the symphysis pubis. Injury to the bladder or urethra should be avoided. Any bleeding from the retropubic venous plexus is controlled by coagulation and packing with warm laparotomy pads.

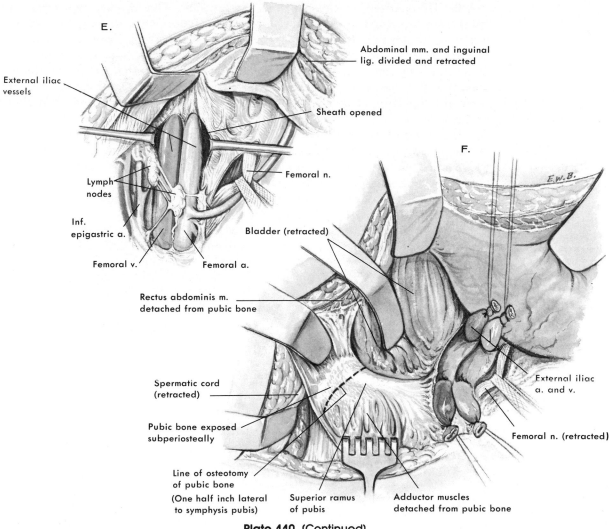

E.

External iliac
vessels

Abdominal mm. and inguinal
lig. divided and retracted

Sheath opened

Femoral n.

Lymph
nodes

Inf.
epigastric a.

Femoral v.   Femoral a.

Bladder (retracted)

Rectus abdominis m.
detached from pubic bone

Spermatic cord
(retracted)

Pubic bone exposed
subperiosteally

Line of osteotomy
of pubic bone

(One half inch lateral
to symphysis pubis)

Superior ramus
of pubis

Adductor muscles
detached from pubic bone

External iliac
a. and v.

Femoral n. (retracted)

F.

E.W.B.

Plate 110. (Continued)

G. The patient is then turned to the side. The drapes are adjusted and reinforced to ensure sterility of the operative field. First, the anterior incision is extended posteriorly to the posterior superior iliac spine. From the upper end of the anterior incision, the second or iliogluteal incision is started. It extends to the thigh, curving forward to an area about 5 cm. distal to the greater trochanter. It then passes backward around the posterior aspect of the thigh to meet the anterior incision. The subcutaneous tissue and fascia are divided in line with the skin incision.

H. By blunt and sharp dissection the gluteus maximus is separated from the gluteus medius and tensor fasciae latae to the depth of the greater trochanter. The gluteus maximus is transected at its insertion, mobilized by blunt dissection, and retracted posteriorly. Vessels and nerves to the gluteus maximus muscle are preserved. (The inferior gluteal nerve and artery emerge distal to the piriformis muscle and the superior gluteal artery proximal to it.)

I. The sciatic nerve is clamped, ligated, and sharply divided distal to the origin of the inferior gluteal nerve. The piriformis, gemelli, and obturator internus muscles are transected near their insertion.

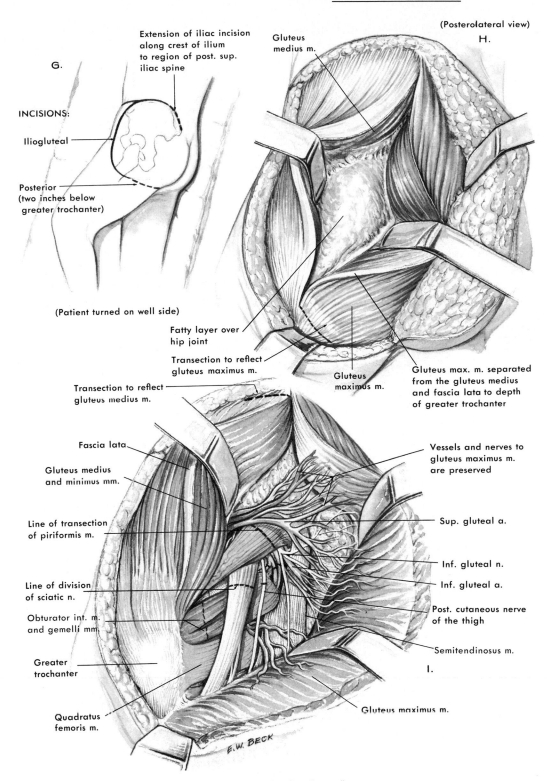

G.

INCISIONS:

Extension of iliac incision along crest of ilium to region of post. sup. iliac spine

Iliogluteal

Posterior (two inches below greater trochanter)

(Patient turned on well side)

(Posterolateral view)

H.

Gluteus medius m.

Fatty layer over hip joint

Transection to reflect gluteus maximus m.

Gluteus maximus m.

Gluteus max. m. separated from the gluteus medius and fascia lata to depth of greater trochanter

Transection to reflect gluteus medius m.

Fascia lata

Gluteus medius and minimus mm.

Line of transection of piriformis m.

Line of division of sciatic n.

Obturator int. m. and gemelli mm.

Greater trochanter

Quadratus femoris m.

Vessels and nerves to gluteus maximus m. are preserved

Sup. gluteal a.

Inf. gluteal n.

Inf. gluteal a.

Post. cutaneous nerve of the thigh

Semitendinosus m.

I.

Gluteus maximus m.

E.W. BECK

Plate 110. (Continued)

J. The ilium is subperiosteally exposed by elevation and detachment of the latissimus dorsi and sacrospinalis muscles, the posterior portion of the gluteus medius, and the anterior fibers of the gluteus maximus. The inner wall of the ilium is also subperiosteally exposed anteriorly to the sacroiliac joint. Chandler retractors are placed in the sciatic notch, and with a Gigli saw the ilium is osteotomized about 5 cm. anterior to the posterior gluteal line. The site of osteotomy of the ilium depends on the location of the tumor; it is carried out farther posteriorly if the neoplasm is adjacent to the gluteal line.

K. Next, the patient is repositioned on the back, and the hip is maximally flexed in 20 to 30 degrees of abduction. The posterior incision is completed.

L. The hip is manipulated into maximal abduction and external rotation, laying open the pelvic area and giving wide exposure to the remaining intrapelvic structures to be severed.

M. Superoinferiorly, the femoral nerve, iliopsoas muscle, obturator vessels, obturator nerve, levator ani, and coccygeus muscles are sectioned. The vessels are doubly ligated prior to division to prevent troublesome bleeding.

N. The gluteus maximus muscle is sutured to the divided margin of the external oblique muscle and lateral abdominal wall. A couple of perforated silicone catheters are inserted and connected to Hemovac suction.

O. Fascia, subcutaneous tissue, and skin are closed in layers in the usual manner. A pressure dressing is applied.

Postoperative Care. Compression dressings are applied. When the patient is comfortable, the wound is healed, and swelling has subsided, the appropriate prosthesis is fitted.

REFERENCES

Brittain, H. A.: Hindquarter amputation. J. Bone Joint Surg., 31–B:104, 1949.
Gordon-Taylor, G., and Monro, R. S.: Technique and management of "hindquarter" amputation. Br. J. Surg., 39:536, 1952.
King, D., and Steelquist, J.: Transiliac amputation. J. Bone Joint Surg., 25:351, 1943.
Sorondo, J. P., and Ferre, R. L.: Amputation interilioabdominal. An. Ortop. Traumatol., 1:143, 1948.

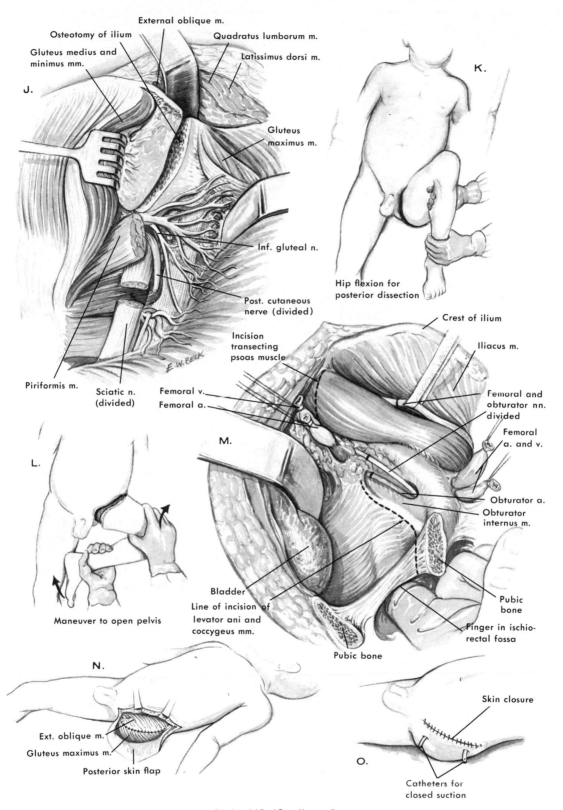

J.

Osteotomy of ilium

External oblique m.

Quadratus lumborum m.

Gluteus medius and minimus mm.

Latissimus dorsi m.

Gluteus maximus m.

Inf. gluteal n.

Post. cutaneous nerve (divided)

Piriformis m.

Sciatic n. (divided)

E.W. BECK

K.

Hip flexion for posterior dissection

Incision transecting psoas muscle

Crest of ilium

Iliacus m.

Femoral v.

Femoral a.

M.

Femoral and obturator nn. divided

Femoral a. and v.

Obturator a.

Obturator internus m.

L.

Maneuver to open pelvis

Bladder

Line of incision of levator ani and coccygeus mm.

Pubic bone

Pubic bone

Finger in ischiorectal fossa

N.

Ext. oblique m.

Gluteus maximus m.

Posterior skin flap

Skin closure

O.

Catheters for closed suction

Plate 110. (Continued)

| PLATE 111 | **Hip Disarticulation** |

Indications. Malignant tumor of the femur or thigh in which limb salvage is not possible.

Blood for Transfusion. Yes.

Note. Be sure that patient has a consultation with a competent prosthetist prior to surgery.

Patient Position. Supine.

Operative Technique

A. An anterior racquet type of incision is made, starting at the anterior superior iliac spine and extending medially and distally, parallel with Poupart's ligament, to the middle of the inner aspect of the thigh about 2 inches distal to the origin of the adductor muscles; and then it is continued around the back of the thigh at a level about 2 inches distal to the ischial tuberosity. Next, the incision is carried along the lateral aspect of the thigh about 3 inches distal to the base of the greater trochanter and is curved proximally and medially to join the first incision at the anterior superior iliac spine.

B. The subcutaneous tissue and the fascia are divided in line with the skin incision. Expose and ligate the long saphenous vein after tracing it to its junction with the femoral vein. If lymph node dissection is indicated, it can be performed at this stage. The sartorius muscle is divided at its origin from the anterior superior iliac spine and is reflected distally. The origins of the two heads of the rectus femoris, one from the anterior inferior iliac spine and the other from the superior margin of the acetabulum, are detached and reflected distally. The femoral nerve is isolated, ligated with 00 Tycron or nonabsorbable sutures, and divided on a tongue blade with a sharp scalpel or razor blade just distal to the ligature. The femoral artery and vein are isolated, doubly ligated with 00 Tycron sutures proximally and distally and severed in between.

C. The hip is abducted to expose its medial aspect, and the adductor longus is detached at its origin from the pubis and reflected distally. The anterior branch of the obturator nerve is exposed deep to the adductor longus and is traced proximally.

D. The adductor brevis is retracted posteriorly. The posterior branch of the obturator nerve is isolated and dissected proximally to the main trunk of the obturator nerve, which is sharply divided. Next, the obturator vessels are isolated and ligated. One should be careful not to sever the obturator artery inadvertently as it will retract into the pelvis and cause bleeding that is difficult to control.

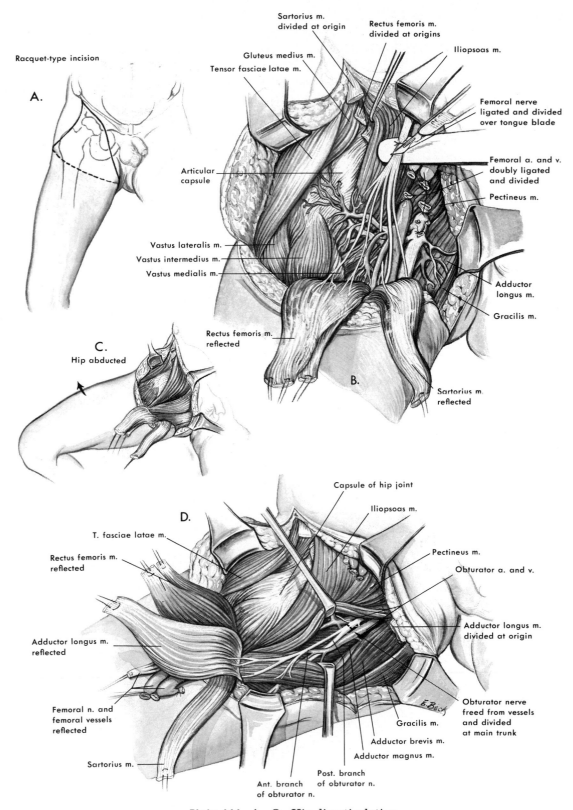

Racquet-type incision

A.

Sartorius m. divided at origin

Rectus femoris m. divided at origins

Iliopsoas m.

Gluteus medius m.

Tensor fasciae latae m.

Femoral nerve ligated and divided over tongue blade

Articular capsule

Femoral a. and v. doubly ligated and divided

Pectineus m.

Vastus lateralis m.

Vastus intermedius m.

Vastus medialis m.

Adductor longus m.

Gracilis m.

C.

Hip abducted

Rectus femoris m. reflected

Sartorius m. reflected

B.

D.

Capsule of hip joint

Iliopsoas m.

T. fasciae latae m.

Rectus femoris m. reflected

Pectineus m.

Obturator a. and v.

Adductor longus m. reflected

Adductor longus m. divided at origin

Femoral n. and femoral vessels reflected

Obturator nerve freed from vessels and divided at main trunk

Sartorius m.

Gracilis m.

Adductor brevis m.

Adductor magnus m.

Ant. branch of obturator n.

Post. branch of obturator n.

Plate 111. A.–O., Hip disarticulation.

E. The pectineus, adductor brevis, gracilis, and adductor magnus are severed near their origin. It is best to use a coagulation knife.

F. The hip is then flexed, externally rotated, and abducted, bringing into view the lesser trochanter. The iliopsoas tendon is exposed, isolated, and divided at its insertion and reflected proximally.

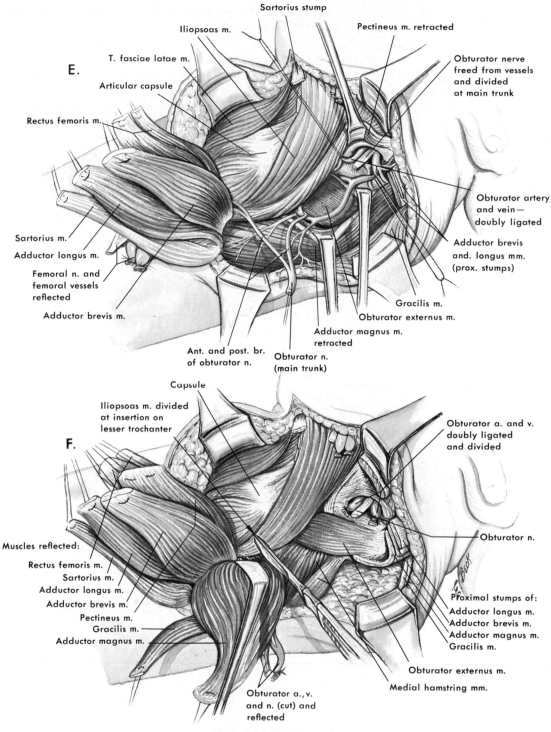

E.

Sartorius stump

Iliopsoas m.

T. fasciae latae m.

Articular capsule

Rectus femoris m.

Pectineus m. retracted

Obturator nerve
freed from vessels
and divided
at main trunk

Obturator artery
and vein—
doubly ligated

Adductor brevis
and. longus mm.
(prox. stumps)

Sartorius m.

Adductor longus m.

Femoral n. and
femoral vessels
reflected

Adductor brevis m.

Ant. and post. br.
of obturator n.

Obturator n.
(main trunk)

Adductor magnus m.
retracted

Obturator externus m.

Gracilis m.

F.

Capsule

Iliopsoas m. divided
at insertion on
lesser trochanter

Obturator a. and v.
doubly ligated
and divided

Obturator n.

Muscles reflected:

Rectus femoris m.
Sartorius m.
Adductor longus m.
Adductor brevis m.
Pectineus m.
Gracilis m.
Adductor magnus m.

Proximal stumps of:
Adductor longus m.
Adductor brevis m.
Adductor magnus m.
Gracilis m.

Obturator externus m.

Medial hamstring mm.

Obturator a., v.
and n. (cut) and
reflected

Plate 111. (Continued)

G. Next, to facilitate surgical exposure, a sterile sandbag is placed under the pelvis and the patient is turned onto the side away from the site of operation. The hip is medially rotated.

H. The gluteus medius and gluteus minimus muscles are divided at their insertion into the greater trochanter and, together with the tensor fasciae latae muscle, are reflected proximally. The gluteus maximus muscle is detached at its insertion and retracted upward. The free ends of the gluteus maximus, medius, and minimus muscles and the tensor fasciae latae muscle are marked with 0 Tycron suture for reattachment.

I. The muscles to be detached at their insertion through the posterior incision are shown. The short rotators of the hip, i.e., quadratus femoris, obturator externus, gemelli, and obturator internus, are detached from their insertion into the femur.

J. The sciatic nerve is identified, dissected free, pulled distally, and crushed with a Kocher hemostat at a level 2 inches proximal to the ischial tuberosity, and it is ligated with 00 Tycron suture to prevent hemorrhage from its accompanying vessels. Then the nerve is sharply divided just distal to the ligature.

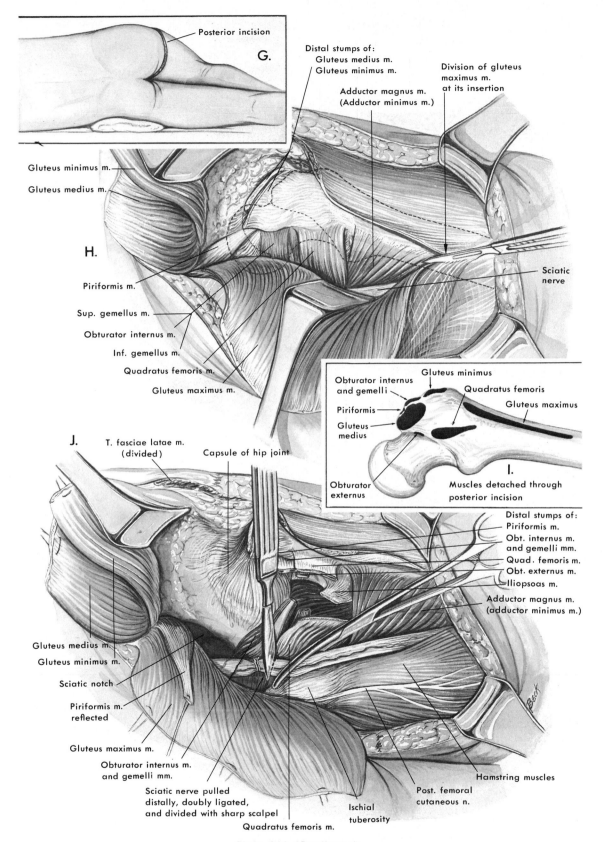

G.

Posterior incision

H.

Gluteus minimus m.

Gluteus medius m.

Piriformis m.

Sup. gemellus m.

Obturator internus m.

Inf. gemellus m.

Quadratus femoris m.

Gluteus maximus m.

Distal stumps of:
Gluteus medius m.
Gluteus minimus m.

Adductor magnus m.
(Adductor minimus m.)

Division of gluteus
maximus m.
at its insertion

Sciatic
nerve

I.

Obturator internus
and gemelli

Piriformis

Gluteus
medius

Obturator
externus

Gluteus minimus

Quadratus femoris

Gluteus maximus

Muscles detached through
posterior incision

J.

T. fasciae latae m.
(divided)

Capsule of hip joint

Gluteus medius m.

Gluteus minimus m.

Sciatic notch

Piriformis m.
reflected

Gluteus maximus m.

Obturator internus m.
and gemelli mm.

Sciatic nerve pulled
distally, doubly ligated,
and divided with sharp scalpel

Quadratus femoris m.

Ischial
tuberosity

Post. femoral
cutaneous n.

Hamstring muscles

Distal stumps of:
Piriformis m.
Obt. internus m.
and gemelli mm.
Quad. femoris m.
Obt. externus m.
Iliopsoas m.

Adductor magnus m.
(adductor minimus m.)

Plate 111. (Continued)

K. The hamstring muscles are detached at their origin from the ischial tuberosity.

L. The capsule of the hip joint is divided near the acetabulum, and the ligamentum teres is severed, completing the disarticulation.

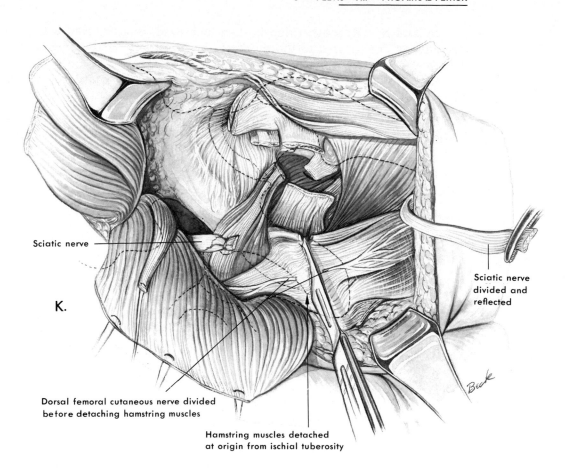

Sciatic nerve

Sciatic nerve
divided and
reflected

K.

Dorsal femoral cutaneous nerve divided
before detaching hamstring muscles

Hamstring muscles detached
at origin from ischial tuberosity

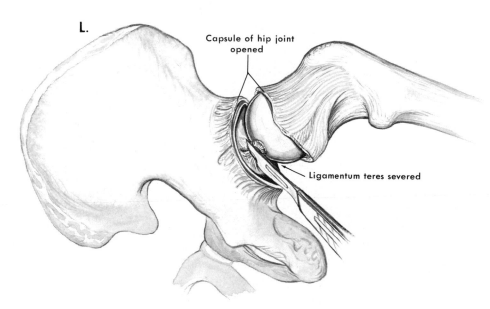

L.

Capsule of hip joint
opened

Ligamentum teres severed

Plate 111. (Continued)

M. and **N.** The gluteal flap is then mobilized, brought forward, and the free distal ends are sutured to the pubis at the origin of the adductor and pectineus muscles.

O. The wound is closed in the routine manner. Hemovac closed suction is placed in the inferior portion of the wound. It is removed in one to two days.

Postoperative Care. Compression dressings are applied. When the patient is comfortable, the wound is healed, and swelling has subsided, the appropriate prosthesis is fitted.

REFERENCE

Boyd, H. B.: Anatomic disarticulation of the hip. Surg. Gynecol. Obstet., 84:346, 1947.

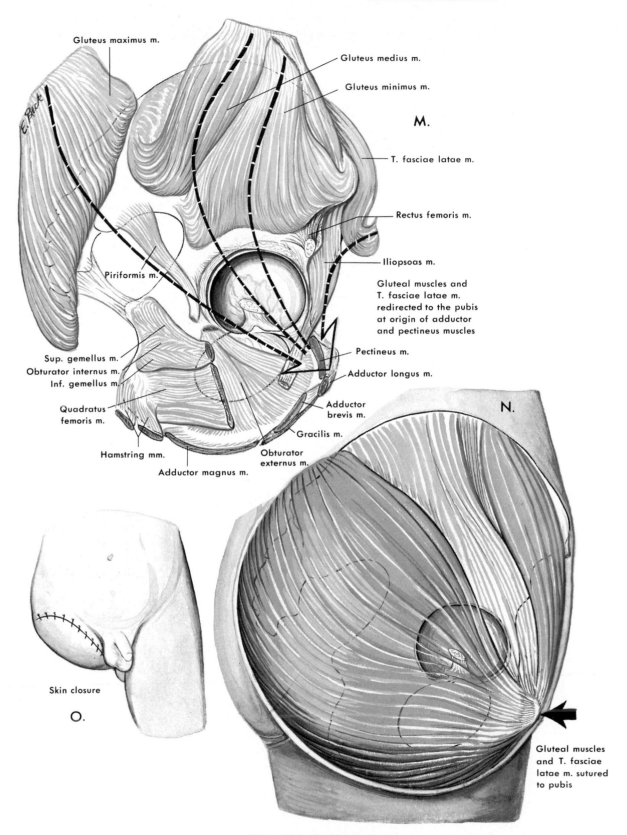

Gluteus maximus m.

Gluteus medius m.

Gluteus minimus m.

M.

T. fasciae latae m.

Rectus femoris m.

Iliopsoas m.

Gluteal muscles and
T. fasciae latae m.
redirected to the pubis
at origin of adductor
and pectineus muscles

Piriformis m.

Pectineus m.

Adductor longus m.

Sup. gemellus m.
Obturator internus m.
Inf. gemellus m.

Adductor
brevis m.

Quadratus
femoris m.

Gracilis m.

Hamstring mm.

Obturator
externus m.

Adductor magnus m.

N.

Skin closure

O.

Gluteal muscles
and T. fasciae
latae m. sutured
to pubis

Plate 111. (Continued)

PLATE 112 · Surgical Drainage of the Hip Through the Posterior Approach (Ober Technique)

Objectives of Open Arthrotomy

1. To halt tissue destruction by débridement of all inflammatory products exuded by the live bacteria, liberated by the cell wall fragments of the dead bacteria, leukocytes, and destroyed tissue. Thick, fibrous exudate cannot be evacuated by aspiration.

2. To create an environment in which antibiotics work more effectively.

3. To decompress the distended hip. Increased articular pressure causes tamponade of retinacular vessels and avascular necrosis of the femoral head. Drainage of the hip through the arthroscope is not recommended because the distension of the joint required for arthroscopy may cause greater tamponade of the retinacular vessels and increase the risk of avascular necrosis.

4. To prevent subluxation or dislocation of the hip.

Indication. Sepsis in the hip.

Requisites. Absence of subluxation or dislocation of the hip. When the femoral head is displaced, use the anterolateral approach for drainage.

Radiographic Control. Image intensifier radiographic control for aspiration prior to drainage.

Patient Position. Prone.

Operative Technique

A. Make the skin incision in line with the middle of the femoral neck, starting 1 inch distal to the tip of the greater trochanter and extending proximally toward the posterior superior iliac spine.

B. With scissors the fibers of the gluteus maximus muscle are bluntly separated in line with the skin incision. If branches of the gluteal vessels are encountered, they are ligated and divided. The sciatic nerve, lying in a layer of fatty tissue in the medial angle of the incision, is identified and protected from injury. The distended capsule is exposed by retracting the short rotator muscles. If wider exposure is necessary, the short rotator muscles can be detached from the trochanter.

C. and **D.** The capsule and synovial membrane are incised throughout their posterosuperior length, and, if necessary, also transversely in the superomedial portion. The joint is thoroughly irrigated with normal saline and then with appropriate antibiotic solution to remove all fibrinous debris. The synovial membrane and capsule are sutured with 00 Vicryl to the surrounding soft tissues and gluteal fascia. One or two plastic tubes of small diameter are sutured with 00 Vicryl to the "marsupialized" capsule. The tubes are placed into the joint, but not between the femoral head and the acetabulum.

E. The soft tissues and skin are closed primarily. The egress tube is connected to a low Gomko wall suction unit or to a Hemovac evacuator. Closed suction irrigation of the joint with antibiotics is not recommended; therefore, I do not insert an ingress tube as shown in the illustration.

On leaving the operating room, the infant is immediately placed in counterpoised bilateral split Russell's traction with the hips in wide abduction.

Postoperative Care. Active and passive exercises should be performed by the patient several times a day while in traction to gradually develop motion of the hip joint. Periodic radiograms are taken with the hip in traction to determine the relationship of the femoral head to the acetabulum and also the subsidence of effusion and synovial thickening. Traction is continued for at least three weeks

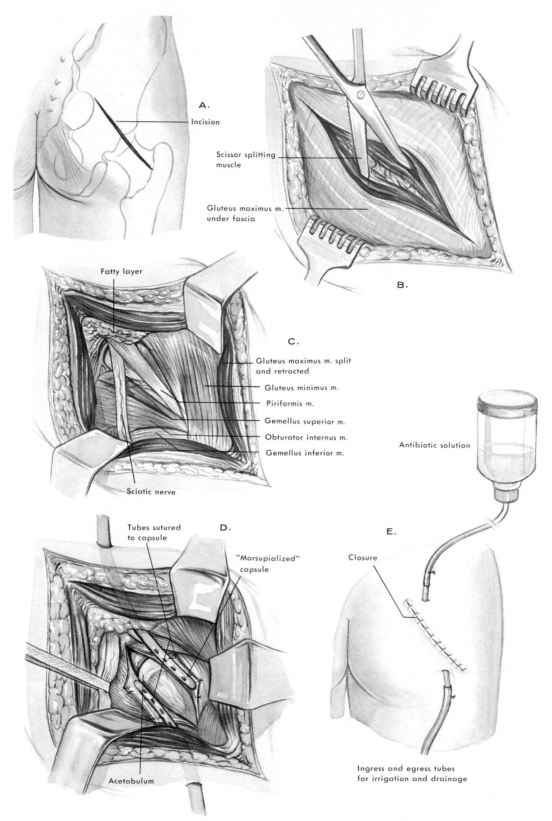

A.

Incision

Scissor splitting
muscle

Gluteus maximus m.
under fascia

B.

Fatty layer

C.

Gluteus maximus m. split
and retracted

Gluteus minimus m.

Piriformis m.

Gemellus superior m.

Obturator internus m.

Gemellus inferior m.

Sciatic nerve

Antibiotic solution

Tubes sutured
to capsule

D.

"Marsupialized"
capsule

E.

Closure

Acetabulum

Ingress and egress tubes
for irrigation and drainage

Plate 112. A.–E., Surgical drainage of the hip through the posterior approach (Ober
technique).

postoperatively until the affected hip has full range of motion and synovial thickening has subsided.

The patient is discharged home in a bivalved one-and-one-half hip spica cast, maintaining the affected hip in 30 to 40 degrees of abduction and neutral rotation. Active and passive range-of-motion exercises are performed out of the cast several times a day, and the periods out of the cast are gradually increased. Weight-bearing, such as crawling or standing, is not permitted for six weeks; then walking is resumed gradually, the hip being protected with a three-point crutch gait. Early weight-bearing causes compression of the softened hyaline cartilage and consequent degenerative arthritis in later life.

REFERENCE

Ober, R.: Posterior arthrotomy of the hip joint. Report of five cases. J.A.M.A., 83:1500, 1924.

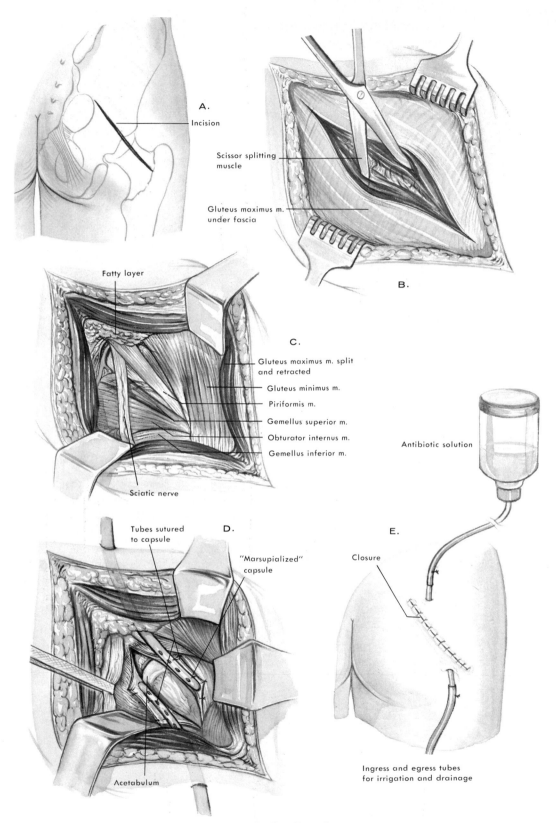

A.

Incision

Scissor splitting
muscle

Gluteus maximus m.
under fascia

B.

Fatty layer

C.

Gluteus maximus m. split
and retracted

Gluteus minimus m.

Piriformis m.

Gemellus superior m.

Obturator internus m.

Gemellus inferior m.

Antibiotic solution

Sciatic nerve

D.

Tubes sutured
to capsule

"Marsupialized"
capsule

E.

Closure

Acetabulum

Ingress and egress tubes
for irrigation and drainage

Plate 112. (Continued)

PLATE   113   ## Surgical Drainage of the Hip Through the Anterior and Anterolateral Approaches

Objectives of Open Arthrotomy

1. To halt tissue destruction by débridement of all inflammatory products exuded by the live bacteria, liberated by the cell wall fragments of the dead bacteria, leukocytes, and destroyed tissue. Thick, fibrous exudate cannot be evacuated by aspiration.

2. To create an environment in which antibiotics work more effectively.

3. To decompress the distended hip. Increased articular pressure causes tamponade of retinacular vessels and avascular necrosis of the femoral head. Drainage of the hip through the arthroscope is not recommended because the distension of the joint required for arthroscopy may cause greater tamponade of the retinacular vessels and increase the risk of avascular necrosis.

4. To prevent subluxation or dislocation of the hip.

Indication. Sepsis in the hips, particularly if there is a suspicion of associated osteomyelitis of the femoral neck or if the hip is subluxated or dislocated. Some surgeons prefer the anterolateral approach over the posterior approach because it provides more adequate exposure and there is no risk of injury to the sciatic nerve.

Radiographic Control. Image intensifier.

Patient Position. The patient is placed in supine position on the operating table. The entire lower limb and lower pelvis are prepared and draped to allow free motion of the hip.

Operative Technique

Anterior Approach

A. A transverse incision 5 to 7 cm. long is made 2 cm. distal to the inguinal ligament beginning 2 cm. inferior and lateral to the anterosuperior iliac spine. The subcutaneous tissue is divided in line with the skin incision. Complete hemostasis is obtained by electrocautery. The skin margins are undermined and retracted.

B. The sartorius muscle is identified, and the superficial fasciae and the fascia lata are divided longitudinally on the medial border of the sartorius muscle. *Do not injure the lateral femoral cutaneous nerve!*

C. The sartorius muscle is retracted laterally, and the iliacus muscle is identified and elevated from the underlying capsule of the hip joint.

D. The iliacus muscle and psoas tendon are retracted medially, the hip joint capsule is exposed, and a T-shaped incision is made in the capsule of the hip.

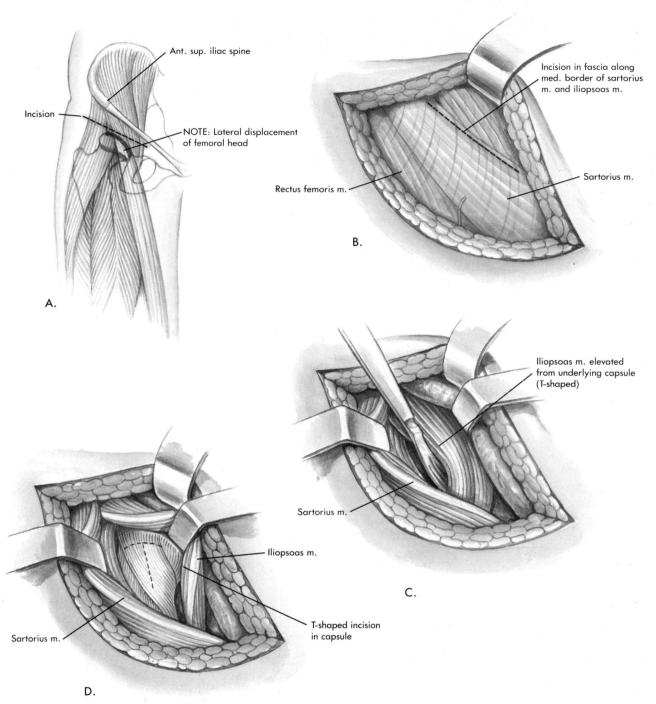

Ant. sup. iliac spine

Incision

NOTE: Lateral displacement of femoral head

A.

Incision in fascia along med. border of sartorius m. and iliopsoas m.

Rectus femoris m.

Sartorius m.

B.

Iliopsoas m. elevated from underlying capsule (T-shaped)

Sartorius m.

C.

Sartorius m.

Iliopsoas m.

T-shaped incision in capsule

D.

Plate 113. A.–H., Surgical drainage of the hip through the anterior and anterolateral approaches.

E. The joint is thoroughly irrigated with normal saline, and all fibrous debris is removed. The synovial membrane and capsule are sutured to the surrounding tissues with 00 Vicryl to leave them open. Plastic tubes are placed into the joint, but not in between the femoral head and the acetabulum.

The soft tissues and skin are closed primarily, and closed Hemovac suction is applied to the plastic tubes.

Anterolateral Approach. An alternate way to drain the hip joint anteriorly is through a longitudinal incision approaching the hip joint in the interval between the sartorius and tensor fasciae femoris muscles.

F. The incision begins 2 cm. proximal to the anterosuperior iliac spine and extends distally and inferiorly in the groove between the tensor fasciae femoris and sartorius muscles for a distance of 5 to 7 cm.

G. Subcutaneous tissue is divided in line with the skin incision, the superficial fasciae is incised, and the wound margins are mobilized and retracted with the help of self-retaining retractors. The deep fascia is divided over the interval between the tensor fasciae latae and sartorius muscle and the iliac crest.

H. The iliac apophysis immediately proximal to the anterosuperior iliac spine is split with a sharp scalpel, and the anterior part of the gluteus medius–minimus and tensor fasciae latae muscles is retracted laterally and the sartorius muscle medially, exposing the capsule of the hip joint. A T-shaped incision is made in the capsule, and the hip is drained (see Step **E.**).

Postoperative Care. Immobilize the hip in abduction, medial rotation, and slight flexion for three weeks in a hip spica cast to prevent anterior dislocation. The cast is removed, and active and passive exercises are performed to restore range of motion and motor strength of the muscles controlling the hip and knee.

REFERENCES

Griffin, P. P.: Bone and joint infections in children. Pediatr. Clin. North Am., 14:533, 1967.

Griffin, P. P., and Green, W. T.: Hip joint infections in infants and children. Orthop. Clin. North Am., 9:123, 1978.

Morrey, B. F., Bianco, A. J., and Rhodes, K. H.: Suppurative arthritis of the hip in children. J. Bone Joint Surg., 78–A:338, 1976.

Morrissy, R. T.: Bone and joint sepsis in children. A.A.O.S. Instructional Course Lectures, 31:49, 1982.

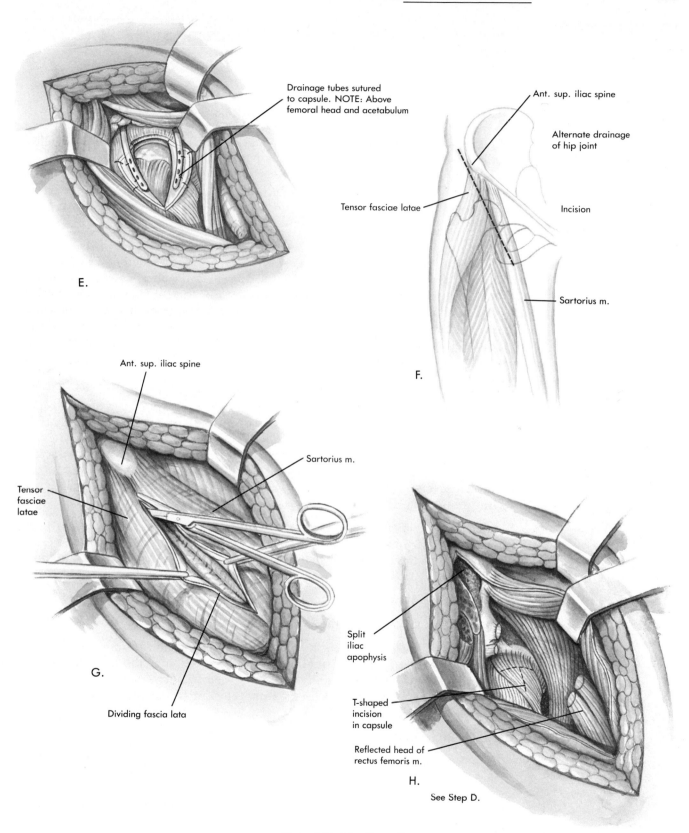

E.

Drainage tubes sutured to capsule. NOTE: Above femoral head and acetabulum

Ant. sup. iliac spine

Alternate drainage of hip joint

Tensor fasciae latae

Incision

Sartorius m.

F.

Ant. sup. iliac spine

Sartorius m.

Tensor fasciae latae

G.

Dividing fascia lata

Split iliac apophysis

T-shaped incision in capsule

Reflected head of rectus femoris m.

H.

See Step D.

Plate 113. (Continued)

PLATE 114 ## Adductor Myotomy of the Hip. Gracilis Myotomy and Section of the Psoas Tendon at Its Insertion

Indications

1. Adduction contracture of the hip causing scissoring and difficulty with stance and ambulation in walkers.

2. Hip at risk for subluxation and dislocation in non-ambulators. Often adduction contracture of the hip is associated with flexion contracture of the hip. In non-ambulators, the psoas tendon is sectioned at its insertion via the medial approach. In ambulators, it is best to recess the psoas tendon at the pelvic rim through a separate subinguinal incision (see Plate 115). The gracilis muscle is almost always divided simultaneously with hip adductor myotomy.

Caution!

1. Preoperatively, meticulously examine the patient for asymmetry of involvement. Also, when the patient is anesthetized prior to draping, determine passive range of motion of each hip. Look for asymmetry of the contracture. On the less affected side, perform adductor myotomy and iliopsoas lengthening to a lesser extent. It is imperative to immobilize the hips in a bilateral below-knee hip spica cast and not in bilateral below-knee casts with a bar; the latter permit the pelvis to tilt. If these precautions are not taken, pelvic obliquity may result in the postoperative period.

2. Do not perform overzealous myotomy of the hip adductors and flexors. This is particularly important in the non-ambulatory child with a strong startle reflex, with the upper limbs assuming an abducted, laterally rotated posture. In these patients, divide only the adductor longus and gracilis and do not section the obturator nerve. If these precautionary measures are not taken, an abduction, lateral rotation, extension contracture of the hips will develop, making sitting difficult. In severe cases, the hip may subluxate or dislocate anteriorly, which may be painful and very disabling.

I do not recommend neurectomy of the anterior branch of the obturator nerve because it causes muscle fibrosis. The procedure is illustrated because some surgeons still perform obturator neurectomy with adductor myotomy of the hip.

Blood for Transfusion. Yes, particularly if the psoas tendon is divided at its insertion. Inadvertent injury to the obturator nerve or medial circumflex vessels may occur.

Radiographic Control. Yes, if hip is subluxated.

Patient Position. With the patient in supine position, both lower limbs and hips are prepared and carefully draped to allow full manipulation of the hips. Meticulous attention should be paid to avoiding contamination from the perineal area. In the groin, the prepared area should be proximal enough to include the origin of the adductor longus muscle.

Operative Technique

A. With both hips in flexion, abduction, and lateral rotation, a longitudinal incision is made over the posterior border of the adductor longus, beginning about ½ inch below the pubis and extending distally for about 3 inches. An alternate incision is horizontal about 5 cm. long centered over the adductor longus and about 1 cm. distal to the inguinal crease (not illustrated).

B. The subcutaneous tissue and deep fascia are incised in line with the skin incision. Any bleeding vessels are clamped and coagulated.

C. With a blunt instrument or finger, the interval between the adductor longus (anteriorly) and the adductor brevis (posteriorly) is developed.

D. Next, the adductor longus is retracted forward and the anterior branch of

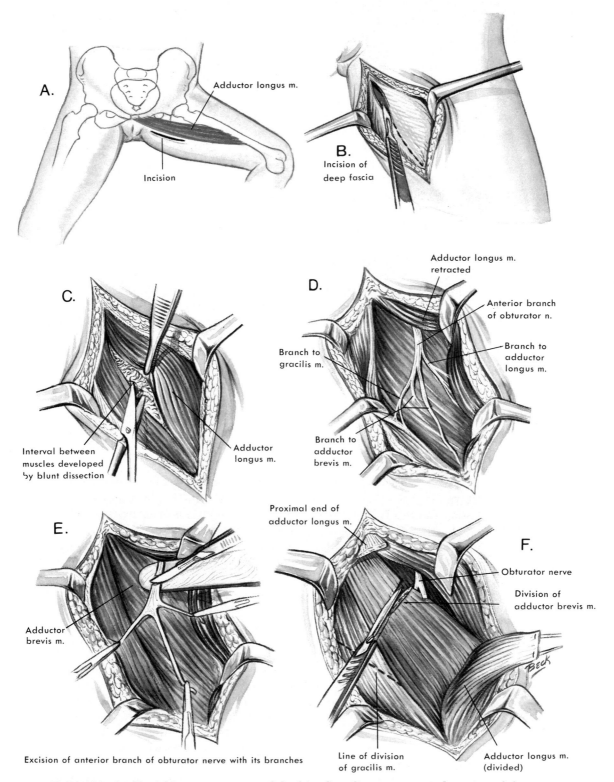

A.

Adductor longus m.

Incision

B.

Incision of deep fascia

C.

Interval between muscles developed by blunt dissection

Adductor longus m.

D.

Adductor longus m. retracted

Anterior branch of obturator n.

Branch to gracilis m.

Branch to adductor longus m.

Branch to adductor brevis m.

E.

Adductor brevis m.

Excision of anterior branch of obturator nerve with its branches

F.

Proximal end of adductor longus m.

Obturator nerve

Division of adductor brevis m.

Line of division of gracilis m.

Adductor longus m. (divided)

Plate 114. A.–K., Adductor myotomy of the hip. Gracilis myotomy and section of the psoas tendon at its insertion.

the obturator nerve is identified. The motor branches to the adductor longus, adductor brevis, and gracilis muscles are isolated.

E. I do not recommend neurectomy, but if the surgeon prefers to perform it, the motor branches are individually clamped distally with hemostats and dissected proximally to their origin, where they are sectioned, an approximately 2 cm. segment of the nerve being excised. Do not damage the posterior branch of the obturator nerve (see p. 565).

F. The adductor longus is then sectioned transversely in its tendinous portion over a blunt instrument close to its origin from the pubis. The adductor brevis is divided obliquely at a lower level to minimize the extent of dead space. (The author uses a coagulation knife, sectioning the muscle over a nonconductive object such as plastic tubing.) Next, the gracilis muscle is isolated in the posteromedial portion of the wound. With the knees in extension, the gracilis is sectioned obliquely in an opposite direction to that of the adductor brevis and at a lower level (see p. 565).

G. At this time, the degree of correction obtained is checked by abducting both hips in extension. If there is still some limitation to complete hip abduction, the most anterior fibers of the adductor magnus may be divided.

H. If iliopsoas lengthening is indicated, the hips are again flexed, laterally rotated, and abducted. This position of the hip rotates the proximal femur, bringing the lesser trochanter anteriorly and making it more accessible. The interval between the pectineus and adductor brevis is developed and widened by blunt dissection to expose the lesser trochanter and the iliopsoas tendon. If the pectineus muscle is hypertrophic and covers the iliopsoas tendon, it may be released or retracted medially with the adductor brevis.

I. A small periosteal or staphylorrhaphy elevator is inserted deep to the iliopsoas tendon, bringing it into view. With a curved hemostat, the iliopsoas tendon is dissected free of its adjacent tissues. Care should be taken not to injure the sciatic nerve.

Next, with the elevator under the iliopsoas tendon, two transverse incisions are made 1.5 to 2 cm. apart, dividing only its tendinous fibers, not its muscle fibers. The hip is hyperextended and the tendon is lengthened 2 to 4 cm.

J. All bleeding vessels should be clamped and coagulated, establishing complete hemostasis. The author routinely uses suction tubes, which are connected to a Hemovac. The deep fascia is not sutured. Only subcutaneous tissue and skin are closed.

K. A plaster of Paris hip spica cast is applied with the hips in full abduction and extension and in 10 to 15 degrees of lateral rotation. If there is flexion contracture of the knees, the patellae should be well padded. Toe-to-groin casts joined by an abduction bar should not be used, as pelvic obliquity may result.

Postoperative Care. One or two days after operation, the suction catheters are removed. The period of immobilization in solid casts varies. Ordinarily in three weeks, the solid casts are removed and bilateral above-knee bivalved hip spica casts are made, in which the hips are kept in the desired amount of abduction, extension, and lateral rotation. In the presence of subluxation or dislocation of the hip, immobilization in a solid cast is continued for two to three months. When the patient is cooperative and has a good motor picture, the casts may be bivalved and exercises instituted as early as the fifth to seventh postoperative day.

Active hip abduction, adduction, and extension exercises are performed, first in the supine position. The range of motion of joints is maintained by gentle passive stretching exercises. As muscle strength increases, exercises are performed, first against gravity and then against resistance. As soon as functional range of motion in the weight-bearing joints is developed, standing and walking are allowed under supervision and appropriate external support; reverse walkers may be used. Forward flexion of the trunk should be avoided. Gait training is continued until as normal a gait pattern as is possible is obtained. External support is discontinued

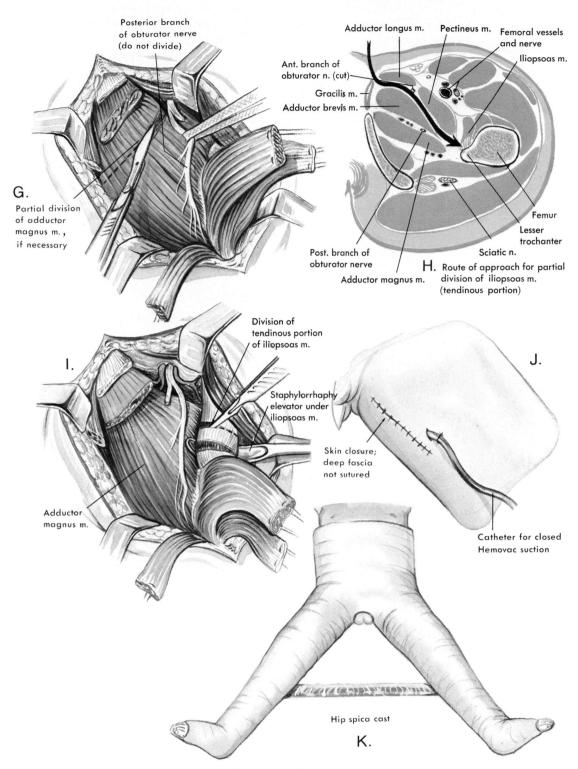

G. Partial division of adductor magnus m., if necessary

Posterior branch of obturator nerve (do not divide)

Adductor longus m.   Pectineus m.   Femoral vessels and nerve

Ant. branch of obturator n. (cut)

Gracilis m.

Adductor brevis m.

Iliopsoas m.

Post. branch of obturator nerve

Adductor magnus m.

Sciatic n.

Femur

Lesser trochanter

H. Route of approach for partial division of iliopsoas m. (tendinous portion)

I.

Division of tendinous portion of iliopsoas m.

Staphylorrhaphy elevator under iliopsoas m.

Adductor magnus m.

J.

Skin closure; deep fascia not sutured

Catheter for closed Hemovac suction

Hip spica cast

K.

Plate 114. (Continued)

when good balance is present. Some patients, especially severe quadriplegics, have to use reverse walkers for support indefinitely.

The length of time that bivalved casts should be worn at night is variable. As a rule, they are used for at least six months to a year. They are not discontinued until the patient has effective full active abduction of the hips against gravity. If there is any tendency to recurrence of contracture, bivalved night casts are reapplied.

REFERENCES

Banks, H. H., and Green, W. T.: Adductor myotomy and obturator neurectomy for the correction of adduction contracture of the hip in cerebral palsy. J. Bone Joint Surg., 42–A:111, 1960.
Bleck, E. E.: Orthopaedic Management of Cerebral Palsy. Philadelphia, J. B. Lippincott Co., 1987.

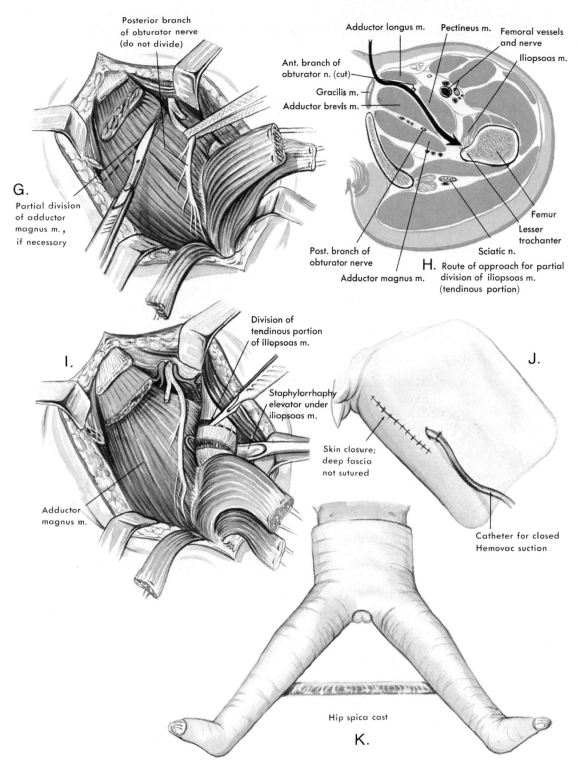

G.

Posterior branch of obturator nerve (do not divide)

Partial division of adductor magnus m., if necessary

H. Route of approach for partial division of iliopsoas m. (tendinous portion)

Adductor longus m.   Pectineus m.   Femoral vessels and nerve

Ant. branch of obturator n. (cut)

Iliopsoas m.

Gracilis m.

Adductor brevis m.

Femur

Lesser trochanter

Post. branch of obturator nerve

Sciatic n.

Adductor magnus m.

I.

Division of tendinous portion of iliopsoas m.

Staphylorrhaphy elevator under iliopsoas m.

Adductor magnus m.

J.

Skin closure; deep fascia not sutured

Catheter for closed Hemovac suction

K.

Hip spica cast

Plate 114. (Continued)

PLATE 115 ### Recession (Musculotendinous Lengthening) of the Psoas Tendon at the Pelvic Brim (Carroll Technique)

Indications

1. When the flexion deformity of the hip is caused by spasticity and contracture of the iliopsoas, as shown by the Thomas test performed with the patient supine, prone (with the opposite hip dangling off the edge of the table [Staheli test], and side lying. Distinguish between the iliopsoas and rectus femoris as the cause of hip flexion deformity by performing the Thomas test with the knee in extension and flexion. When the rectus femoris is the deforming force, hip flexion deformity is increased with the knee in flexion and decreased with the knee in extension.

2. A decreased sacrofemoral angle, as determined in a standing lateral radiogram. The lower limit of normal is 50 degrees. The contracted psoas is lengthened if it is 40 degrees or less.

3. Leaning forward while walking when the knees are immobilized in extension in above-knee casts or splints. Forward posture of the trunk at the hips indicates that the psoas is contracted. If the hamstrings are short and the cause of the crouch gait, the patient will walk upright with the knees extended.

Blood for Transfusion. Yes.

Radiographic Control. Image intensifier.

Special Instrumentation. Nerve stimulator. The surgical approach is in close proximity to femoral nerve and vessels. Inadvertent injury may occur. Ask the anesthesiologist not to paralyze the patient.

Patient Position. The patient is placed in supine position, and the perineal region is draped. The entire lower limb and adductor region of the hip and lower pelvis are prepared and draped to allow free motion of the hip. The anterosuperior iliac spine, inguinal crease, and pubic tubercle should be sterile in the operating field.

Operative Technique

Using general anesthesia, determine the degree of the range of extension of the hip, first with the knee in extension and then with the knee in flexion. When the degree of hip flexion deformity does not change with the knee in flexion and extension, the pelvic origin of the rectus femoris is not a pathogenic factor in flexion deformity of the hip; however, when the degree of hip flexion deformity is increased with the knee in flexion and decreased with the knee in extension, contracture and spasticity of the rectus femoris are contributing factors. If the prone rectus or Ely test, when conducted properly, is strongly positive, proximal release of the rectus femoris can be performed through the same incision. Place the operated hip in about 20 degrees of abduction, 30 degrees of lateral rotation, and about 20 to 30 degrees of flexion. Palpate the pulse of the femoral artery and mark its location.

A. A transverse incision, about 4 to 5 cm. long, is made 2 cm. distal to the inguinal crease. It begins below the anterior superior iliac spine and extends medially. The subcutaneous tissue is divided in line with the skin incision. Complete hemostasis is obtained by clamping and coagulating all bleeding vessels. Branches of the femoral circumflex artery and vein will be in the superficial fascia layer. Isolate and cauterize them. The wound flaps are undercut and retracted.

B. The sartorius muscle lies in the lateral part of the wound. The lateral femoral cutaneous nerve is identified and kept out of harm's way. It is usually 1 cm. medial to the anterior superior iliac spine and passes anterior to the sartorius muscle.

C. The sartorius muscle is retracted laterally, exposing the deep fascia covering the iliacus muscle. The femoral nerve lies superficial to the iliacus muscle

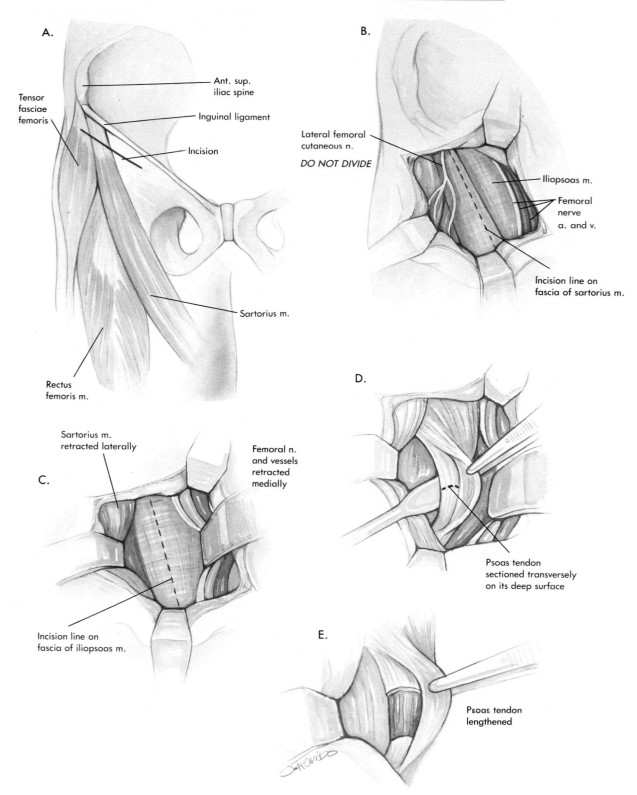

A.

Tensor
fasciae
femoris

Ant. sup.
iliac spine

Inguinal ligament

Incision

Sartorius m.

Rectus
femoris m.

B.

Lateral femoral
cutaneous n.

DO NOT DIVIDE

Iliopsoas m.

Femoral
nerve
a. and v.

Incision line on
fascia of sartorius m.

C.

Sartorius m.
retracted laterally

Femoral n.
and vessels
retracted
medially

Incision line on
fascia of iliopsoas m.

D.

Psoas tendon
sectioned transversely
on its deep surface

E.

Psoas tendon
lengthened

Plate 115. A.–E., Recession (musculotendinous lengthening) of the psoas tendon at the pelvic brim (Carroll technique).

and deep to the iliacus fascia at the medial part of the wound. The femoral vessels are superficial to this fascia and medial to the femoral nerve. Divide the iliacus fascia and identify the femoral nerve, which is usually surrounded by perineural fat. The femoral nerve and vessels are retracted medially.

D. The hip is flexed and slightly abducted and laterally rotated. The iliacus muscle is everted by rolling the muscle laterally.

Note: In the illustration, the psoas muscle is rotated medially. It should be lateral.

The psoas tendon is exposed on its posterolateral surface. The tendon is pulled with a nerve hook and sectioned transversely with a scalpel.

E. The hip is extended, and the psoas tendon will slide over the underlying muscle. The Thomas test is performed to determine range of extension of the hip joint. A medium Hemovac is inserted. The superficial fascia and subcutaneous tissues are closed with 00 Vicryl interrupted sutures, and the skin is closed with 00 subcutaneous nylon sutures.

Postoperative Care. Usually, this procedure is performed in conjunction with hip adductor and gracilis myotomy. Follow the same procedures as outlined for Plate 114.

REFERENCES

Carroll, N. C.: Personal communication, 1993.

Salter, R.: Salter, R. B.: Innominate osteotomy in the treatment of congenital dislocation and subluxation of the hip. J. Bone Joint Surg., 43–B:518, 1961.

Sutherland, D. H., Santi, M., and Abel, M. F.: Treatment of stiff-knee gait in cerebral palsy: A comparison by gait analysis of distal rectus femoris transfer versus proximal rectus release. J. Pediatr. Orthop., 10:433, 1990.

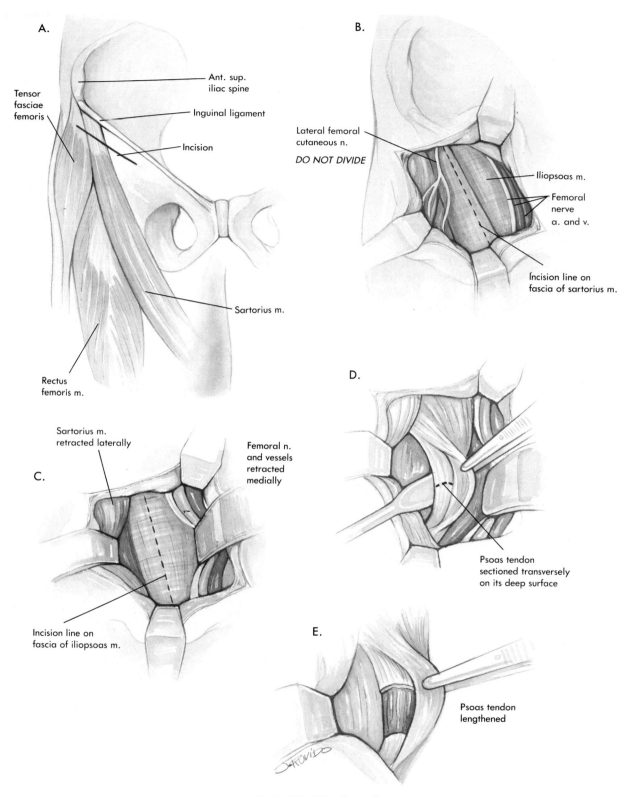

A.

Tensor
fasciae
femoris

Ant. sup.
iliac spine

Inguinal ligament

Incision

Sartorius m.

Rectus
femoris m.

B.

Lateral femoral
cutaneous n.

DO NOT DIVIDE

Iliopsoas m.

Femoral
nerve
a. and v.

Incision line on
fascia of sartorius m.

C.

Sartorius m.
retracted laterally

Femoral n.
and vessels
retracted
medially

Incision line on
fascia of iliopsoas m.

D.

Psoas tendon
sectioned transversely
on its deep surface

E.

Psoas tendon
lengthened

Plate 115. (Continued)

| PLATE 116 | Rectus Femoris Release at Its Origin |

Indications. Moderate extension contracture of the knee associated with flexion contracture of the hip caused by spasticity of the rectus femoris. The procedure may be combined with recession of the psoas at the pelvic brim.

Requisites

1. Ability to walk independently. The gait is stiff knee with the hip in varying degrees of flexion posture and excessive lumbar lordosis.
2. Dynamic electromyogram and gait analysis demonstrating continuous abnormal activity of the rectus femoris in both swing and stance phases of gait.
3. Spasticity and contracture of the rectus femoris, as shown by the following clinical tests:
   a. Determine the degree of knee flexion with the leg dangling at the edge of the table, first with the hip extended and the patient lying supine and second with the hip flexed and the patient sitting. If the rectus femoris is contracted, the degree of knee flexion is decreased with the hip in extension.
   b. On the side-lying Thomas test, increase in the degree of hip flexion when the knee is flexed.
   c. A positive Ely or prone rectus test. The patient is placed prone with the hips in complete extension; the knee is passively flexed. When the test is positive, the quadriceps muscle will grab first; on further knee flexion, the pelvis will be elevated off the table. The Ely test is not reliable for distinguishing between spasticity of the iliopsoas and rectus femoris because dynamic EMG studies have demonstrated that the test will stimulate contracture of the psoas.
4. Normal or good motor strength of quadriceps femoris muscle. When the quadriceps femoris is fair or less in motor strength, the patient may be unable to walk independently.

Patient Position. Supine.

Operative Technique

    A. Make a longitudinal incision beginning 1 cm. distal to the anterior-superior iliac spine and extending distally for a distance of 5 cm. between the tensor fasciae latae and sartorius muscles. Subcutaneous tissues and superficial fascia are divided in line with the skin incision. Identify the lateral femoral cutaneous nerve, and retract it out of harm's way.

    B. Retract the tensor fasciae latae muscle laterally and the iliopsoas muscle medially. Identify the reflected and oblique heads of rectus femoris muscle. Insert a Freer elevator deep to the tendons of rectus femoris, and with a sharp scalpel divide the tendons. Do not open the capsule of the hip joint.

    The wound is irrigated, and hemostasis is achieved with electrocautery. The subcutaneous tissue is closed with 000 Vicryl interrupted sutures and the skin with 00 subcuticular nylon. An above-knee cast is applied, with the knee in flexion of about 30 to 45 degrees.

Postoperative Care. Often this procedure is performed simultaneously with other soft tissue releases around the hip. Passive stretching exercises of the hip are performed as soon as the patient is comfortable. The cast is removed in two to three weeks postoperatively.

REFERENCE

Bleck, E. E.: Orthopaedic Management of Cerebral Palsy. Philadelphia, J. B. Lippincott Co., 1987.

A.

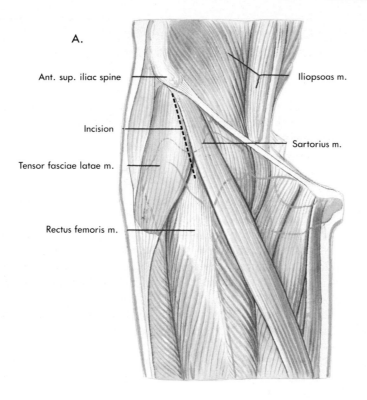

Ant. sup. iliac spine

Iliopsoas m.

Incision

Sartorius m.

Tensor fasciae latae m.

Rectus femoris m.

B.

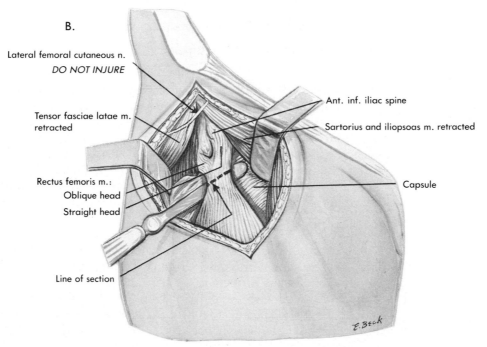

Lateral femoral cutaneous n.
DO NOT INJURE

Ant. inf. iliac spine

Tensor fasciae latae m.
retracted

Sartorius and iliopsoas m. retracted

Rectus femoris m.:
Oblique head
Straight head

Capsule

Line of section

E. Beck

Plate 116. A. and **B.,** Rectus femoris release at its origin.

PLATE 117   ## Schanz Abduction Osteotomy for Chronic, Painful Dislocation of the Hip in Spastic Cerebral Palsy

Indications

1. Painful subluxation and dislocation of the hip with a shallow acetabulum in a total body-involved cerebral palsy patient who has no potential for ambulation.
2. Difficulty with perineal care.
3. Difficulty with assisted sitting.

Requisites

1. Adequate range of hip adduction so that following abduction osteotomy the hip will adduct 15 to 20 degrees and abduct enough for sitting.
2. Preoperative anteroposterior radiograms of the hip, with the hips in neutral rotation and maximal extension, and in varying degrees of adduction and abduction are made. In the adduction views, determine the degree of abduction osteotomy required to adequately displace the femoral head from the acetabulum and lateral wall of the ilium.
3. Absence of adhesions and scarring between the femoral head and margin of the acetabulum and lateral wall of the ilium. If adhesions are present, release scar adhesions by open surgery.
4. Correct antetorsion of the proximal femur to neutral. Be sure that the laterally tilted femoral head does not become prominent anteriorly or posteriorly.

Blood for Transfusion. Yes.

Radiographic Control. Image intensifier.

Special Instrumentation. AO equipment/limited contact–dynamic compression plate (LC-DCP).

Patient Position. The patient is placed supine on a radiolucent operating table. It is best to position the obese adolescent on a fracture table because it is simpler to apply a bilateral hip spica cast. The entire lower limb, hip, and ipsilateral pelvis are prepared and draped to permit free passive motion of the hip without contamination of the hip. In the presence of severe adduction deformity of the hip, a limited adductor myotomy (longus and part of brevis) is performed to increase range of passive hip abduction. It is vital to preserve hip adductor motor strength; the patient should be able to abduct the hip following osteotomy.

Operative Technique

A. A straight, wide, lateral longitudinal incision is made; it begins at the tip of the greater trochanter and extends distally for a distance of 12 to 15 cm., depending on the size of the patient. The subcutaneous tissue and superficial fascia are divided in line with the skin incision. The fascia lata is split longitudinally in line with its fibers. The vastus lateralis is detached from the abductor tubercle by a horseshoe-shaped incision based proximally and elevated subperiosteally from the femoral shaft for a distance of 7 to 10 cm. and retracted anteriorly. The exposure should be wide enough to enable the surgeon to palpate the base of the femoral neck and the lesser trochanter.

B. The level of osteotomy is immediately distal to the lesser trochanter. It is a laterally based closing wedge. For a femur that is 5 to 6 cm. in diameter, a rule of thumb is 1 degree of correction for each millimeter of width of the base of the wedge. The degree of valgization is determined by the preoperative adduction views.

With a power drill, first insert a large threaded Steinmann pin from the tip of the greater trochanter, directing it medially and distally toward the lesser trochanter. Second, percutaneously drill a large threaded Steinmann pin at the

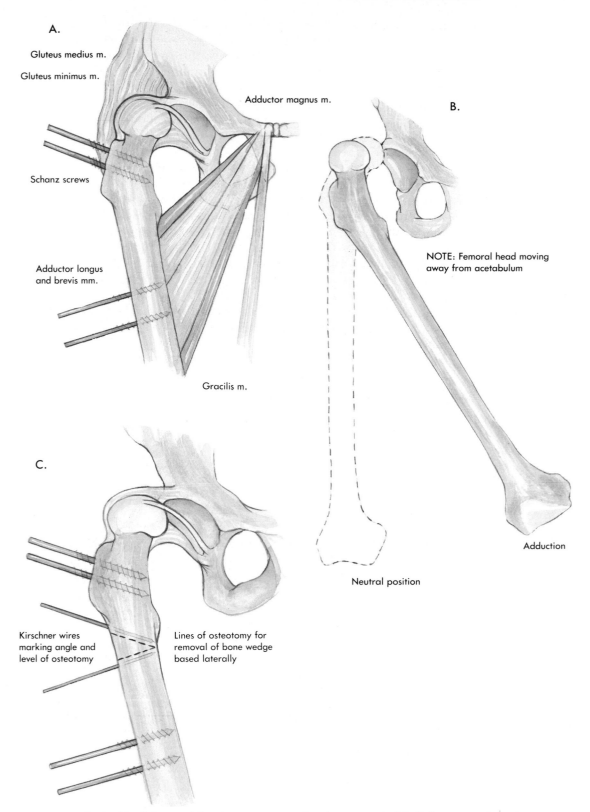

A.

Gluteus medius m.

Gluteus minimus m.

Adductor magnus m.

B.

Schanz screws

Adductor longus
and brevis mm.

Gracilis m.

NOTE: Femoral head moving
away from acetabulum

C.

Kirschner wires
marking angle and
level of osteotomy

Lines of osteotomy for
removal of bone wedge
based laterally

Neutral position

Adduction

Plate 117. A.–F., Schanz abduction osteotomy for chronic, painful dislocation of the hip in spastic cerebral palsy.

midshaft of the femur, directing it superiorly and medially. The angle between the two Steinmann pins should be equal to the angle of valgization. The site of insertion of the pins should not interfere with internal fixation with a bent plate on the lateral aspect of the femur. The Steinmann pins should be firmly anchored in bone.

Under image intensifier radiographic control, insert two smooth Kirschner wires at the intended level of the osteotomy. The apex of the osteotomy is at the lower border of the lesser trochanter. The Kirschner wires will serve as a guide for the wedge of bone to be resected.

C. With an oscillating saw, resect the wedge of bone.

D. With the large Steinmann pins used as a lever, the proximal and distal segments of the femur are abducted and the osteotomy gap is closed. The Steinmann pins are temporarily fixed with an external fixator.

Under image intensifier control, the hip joint is visualized; the femoral head should be tilted away from the lateral wall of the ilium.

If the femoral head is adherent to the lateral wall of the ilium, capsular adhesions must be released through an anterior approach before the osteotomy is performed.

E. and **F.** The femoral fragments are fixed with either two criss-cross threaded Steinmann pins or a six-hole or seven-hole bent AO plate; this author prefers to use the LC-DCP.

The wound is closed in the usual fashion. A double hip spica cast is applied. It is important to provide symmetry to both lower limbs.

Postoperative Care. With the hip spica cast on, the patient is placed in prone position most of the time. The patient is also positioned upright with weight-bearing on both lower limbs with the cast on to prevent disuse atrophy of the bones.

The cast is removed when the osteotomy is solidly healed, usually six weeks postoperatively. Physical therapy is prescribed.

REFERENCE

Schanz, A.: Zur Behandlung der veralteten angeborenen Huftverrenkung. Munch. Med. Wochenschr., 69:930, 1922.

D.

E.

Release of soft tissues
if necessary

External
fixation
fixing bone
fragments

Alternative method of
temporary internal fixation
with threaded Steinmann pins

F.

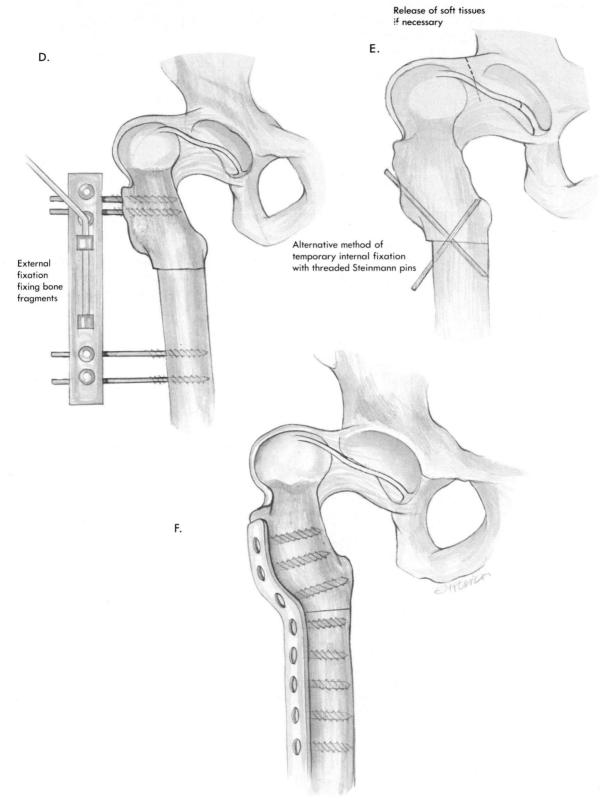

Plate 117. (Continued)

PLATE 118 ## Posterolateral Transfer of the Tensor Fasciae Latae and Sartorius and Proximal Advancement of the Gluteus Medius and Minimus

Indications. Medial rotation gait with gluteus medius limp and Trendelenburg lurch in an ambulatory (independent walker) spastic cerebral palsy patient who is ten years of age or older.

Requisites

1. Normal passive range of hip abduction, extension, and lateral rotation (with the hip in extension). There should be no hip flexion, adduction, or medial rotation contracture.
2. Concentrically reduced and stable hip.
3. Normal or good motor strength of hip flexors; previous iliopsoas lengthening may have weakened power of hip flexion.
4. Normal or good motor strength of the tensor fasciae latae and sartorius.
5. Femoral torsion should be less than 40 degrees as determined by CT scan.
6. Motivated patient who is cooperative in the postoperative training program.

Blood for Transfusion. Yes.

Special Instrumentation. Nerve stimulator.

Patient Position. The patient is placed supine, with a small sandbag under the buttock of the operated hip tilting him or her 20 degrees toward the opposite hip. The lower abdomen, the pelvis, and the entire lower limb are prepared and draped to allow free motion of the hip. Ask the anesthesiologist not to paralyze the patient.

The range of abduction of the hip is tested. A vital requisite for the posterolateral transfer of the tensor fasciae latae and sartorius is full range of hip abduction; if it is limited by spastic contracted hip adductors, an adductor myotomy is performed first.

Operative Technique

A. and **B.** The incision begins at the junction of the posterior and middle thirds of the iliac crest, extends forward to the anterior superior iliac spine, and then is carried distally into the thigh for about 7 to 10 cm. in the groove between the tensor fasciae latae and the sartorius muscles. The subcutaneous tissue and superficial and deep fasciae are incised over the iliac crest, and the fascia lata is divided in line with the skin incision. The lateral femoral cutaneous nerve is identified, mobilized by sharp dissection, and protected by retracting with a vascular tape.

C. The groove between the tensor fasciae latae laterally and sartorius and rectus femoris muscles medially is opened by blunt dissection, and the deep fascia is divided. The ascending branches of the lateral femoral circumflex vessels cross the midpoint of the intermuscular groove; they are identified, isolated, and protected from inadvertent injury.

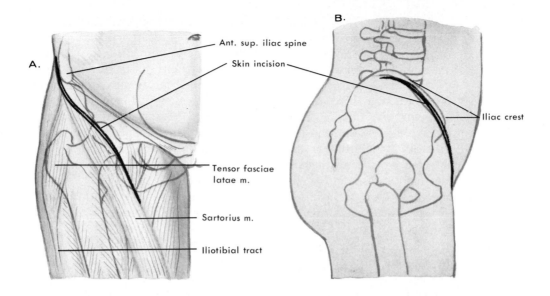

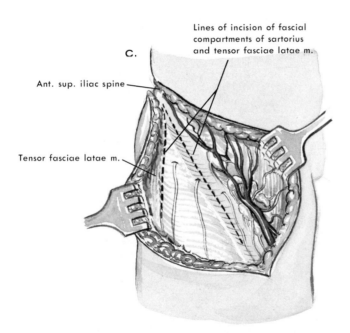

Plate 118. A.–J., Posterolateral transfer of the tensor fasciae latae and sartorius and proximal advancement of the gluteus medius and minimus.

D. and **E.** The origin of the sartorius is detached from the anterior superior iliac spine, and its free end is marked with 0 Tycron or nonabsorbable suture. The sartorius is reflected distally and medially by blunt dissection; the muscle is freed and mobilized distally as far as possible without disturbing its nerve supply.

F. Next, with a scalpel the cartilaginous iliac apophysis is sharply divided into its lateral one third and medial two thirds down to bone from the junction of its posterior and middle thirds to the anterior superior iliac spine. With a broad periosteal elevator, the lateral part of the iliac apophysis and the tensor fasciae latae and the gluteus medius and minimus are subperiosteally stripped and reflected as a continuous sheet to the superior rim of the acetabulum. It is not necessary to extend the dissection posteriorly to the greater sciatic notch. With a periosteal elevator, the medial half of the cartilaginous iliac apophysis with the periosteum on the inner wall of the ilium is stripped in a continuous sheet for a distance of 3 cm.

The intermuscular interval between the tensor fasciae latae anteriorly and the gluteus minimus posteriorly is identified and gently developed. The boundary between the two muscles is not definite; a Bovie electrocautery knife is used to separate the two muscles. The nerve and blood supply to the muscles by the superior gluteal nerve and vessels should not be disturbed.

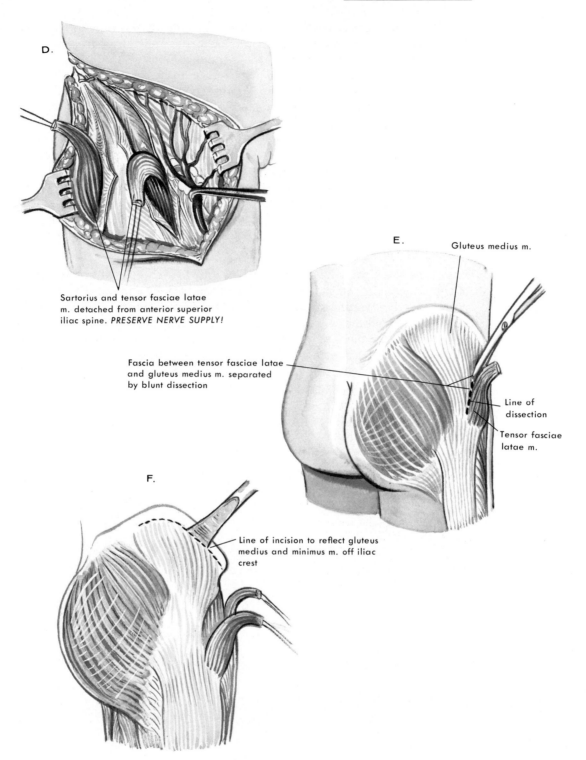

D.

Sartorius and tensor fasciae latae
m. detached from anterior superior
iliac spine. *PRESERVE NERVE SUPPLY!*

E.

Gluteus medius m.

Fascia between tensor fasciae latae
and gluteus medius m. separated
by blunt dissection

Line of
dissection

Tensor fasciae
latae m.

F.

Line of incision to reflect gluteus
medius and minimus m. off iliac
crest

Plate 118. (Continued)

G. With a power drill, four holes are made in the middle third of the iliac crest, two for the reattachment of the sartorius and tensor fasciae latae and two for the proximal advancement of the gluteus medius and minimus.

H. The hip is fully abducted. The tensor fasciae latae is firmly reattached to the iliac crest as far posteriorly as possible in the posterior part of the middle third of the iliac crest, and the sartorius is reattached to the anterior part of the middle third of the iliac crest.

I. With the hip in full abduction, the gluteus medius and minimus are reattached to the inner aspect of the iliac crest. The medial two thirds of the iliac apophysis is resutured to the gluteal fasciae and muscles over the iliac crest.

The procedure is usually performed bilaterally in the cerebral palsied child with spastic diplegia.

J. The wound is closed in the usual fashion. A bilateral long-leg hip spica cast is applied with the hips in 40 degrees of abduction, neutral extension, and 15 degrees of lateral rotation.

Postoperative Care. The cast is bivalved four to six weeks after surgery (the length of time depending on the age and size of the patient and security of fixation of the muscle tendon transfers), and a physical therapy program is begun. Active assisted exercises are performed to develop hip abduction, lateral rotation, and flexion. It is important for these patients to sleep prone in a bivalved hip spica cast or splint. Standing with assistance is allowed when the transferred tensor fasciae latae and sartorius muscles are fair in motor strength. Walking is begun gradually. Meticulous postoperative care is crucial for success.

REFERENCES

Barr, J. S.: Muscle transplantation for combined flexion–internal rotation deformity of the thigh in spastic paralysis. Arch. Surg., 46:605, 1943.

Green, W. T., and McDermott, L. J.: Operative treatment of cerebral palsy of spastic type. J.A.M.A., 118:434, 1942.

Legg, A. R.: Transplantation of tensor fasciae femoris in cases of weakened gluteus medius. J.A.M.A., 80:242, 1923.

Legg, A. T.: Transplantation of tensor fasciae femoris in cases of weakened gluteus medius. N. Engl. J. Med., 209:61, 1933.

G. Four 3/16″ drill holes below sectioned cartilaginous apophysis of ilium. Holes emerge on inner wall of ilium

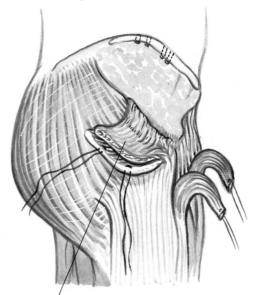

Gluteus medius and minimus m. reflected distally to level of hip capsule

H. Sartorius and tensor fasciae latae m. attached to whip sutures through drill holes to middle third of iliac crest

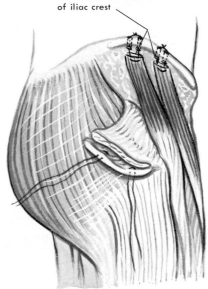

I. Gluteal mm. advanced proximally and attached by whip sutures through drill holes to inner wall of iliac crest—overlapping tensor fasciae latae and sartorius m.

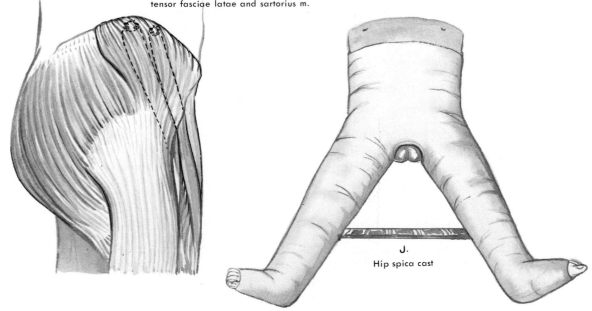

J.
Hip spica cast

Plate 118. (Continued)

PLATE 119 ### Steel's Anterior Advancement of the Gluteus Medius and Minimus for Correction of Medial Rotation Gait

Principle. Anterior advancement of the insertion of the gluteus medius–minimus from the greater trochanter to the anterior aspect of the upper femoral shaft will change the function of these muscles from medial rotators of the hip to that of lateral rotators.

Indications. Medial rotation gait in spastic cerebral palsy caused by spastic hypertonic gluteus medius–minimus muscles.

Preoperative Assessment

1. Gait analysis and dynamic EMG to delineate abnormal activity of deforming muscles: the gluteus medius–minimus, the medial hamstrings, and the anterior hip abductors.
2. CT scan for femoral torsion, tibial torsion, and acetabular torsion.
3. Manual muscle testing by a physical therapist.

Requisites

1. Passive range of lateral rotation of the hip in extension (tested prone) of at least 30 degrees.
2. Normal passive range of hip abduction and absence of hip adduction contracture.
3. Absence of hip flexion contracture. When the hip is in adduction-flexion, iliopsoas will aggravate medial rotation of the hip.
4. Absence of stretch reflex or contracture of the rectus femoris. If it is present, release the rectus femoris proximally; this can be performed simultaneously.
5. Femoral torsion, as determined by CT scan, less than 40 to 45 degrees. If it is greater, perform derotation osteotomy of the femur.
6. Normal or good motor strength of hip abductors. A Trendelenburg test should be negative. There should be no gluteus medius lurch.
7. A congruous and stable hip joint that is concentrically reduced.

Blood for Transfusion. Yes.

Radiographic Control. Image intensifier.

Patient Position. The patient is supine. The pelvis and both lower limbs are prepared and draped. One should be able to manipulate the lower limbs freely during surgery without contamination of the wound. There should be complete surgical access to the hip adductor region superomedially, to the iliac crest, and to 5 cm. posterior to the greater trochanter.

Operative Technique

A. A curvilinear incision (slightly convex anteriorly) is centered over the lateral aspect of the greater trochanter. It begins at the anterior border of gluteus maximus far enough superiorly to expose the muscle bellies of the gluteus medius and minimus; it is extended distally curving anteriorly toward the greater trochanter, and posteriorly toward the linea aspera of the femur for a distance of about 5 cm. By palpation, identify the fascia overlying the gluteus medius–minimus muscle bellies. The deep fascia lying between the gluteus maximus posteriorly and tensor fasciae latae anteriorly is divided.

Next, carefully develop the plane between the gluteus minimus and hip joint capsule. Both the gluteus medius and minimus should be transposed as one functional unit, taking great care to preserve their nerve and blood supply. Do not confuse the plane between the gluteus medius and minimus with the interval between the gluteus minimus and the hip joint capsule.

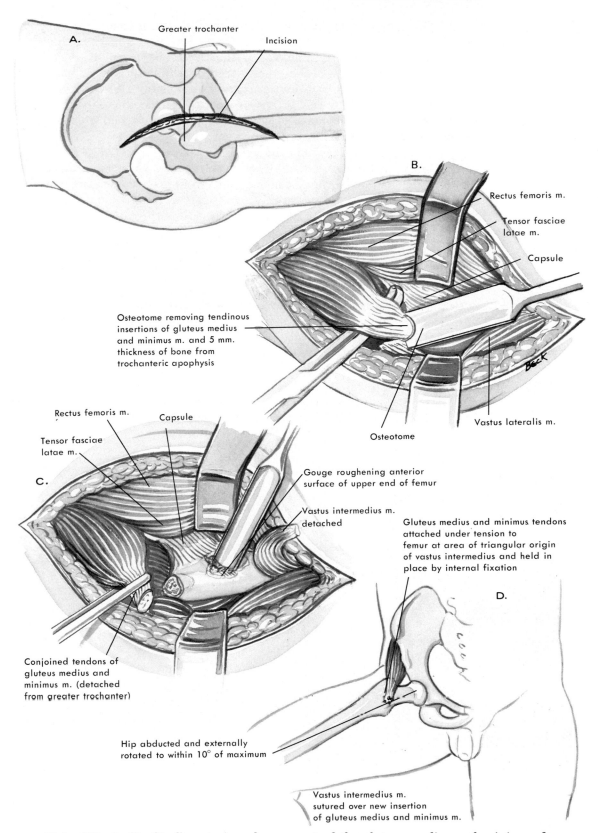

A.

Greater trochanter

Incision

B.

Rectus femoris m.

Tensor fasciae latae m.

Capsule

Osteotome removing tendinous insertions of gluteus medius and minimus m. and 5 mm. thickness of bone from trochanteric apophysis

Vastus lateralis m.

Osteotome

Rectus femoris m.

Capsule

Tensor fasciae latae m.

C.

Gouge roughening anterior surface of upper end of femur

Vastus intermedius m. detached

Gluteus medius and minimus tendons attached under tension to femur at area of triangular origin of vastus intermedius and held in place by internal fixation

D.

Conjoined tendons of gluteus medius and minimus m. (detached from greater trochanter)

Hip abducted and externally rotated to within 10° of maximum

Vastus intermedius m. sutured over new insertion of gluteus medius and minimus m.

Plate 119. A.–D., Steel's anterior advancement of the gluteus medius and minimus for correction of medial rotation gait.

B. The conjoined tendons of gluteus medius and minimus are detached from their insertion to the tip of the greater trochanter with a piece of the trochanteric apophysis and bone; one may use a sharp osteotome or an electric saw. The apophyseal growth plate of the greater trochanter should not be disturbed.

C. Identify the intertrochanteric and subtrochanteric surfaces of the femur anteriorly, and elevate the origin of vastus intermedius and reflect distally. Exposure should be adequate to accommodate the detached greater trochanteric wafer. The femoral cortex is roughened with a gouge.

D. At this point, the hip is abducted and laterally rotated to within 10 degrees of maximum. (If the hip adductors are taut, they are released by myotomy at this time.) Next, the tendons of gluteus medius–minimus are anchored with a wafer of trochanteric bone to the anterior surface of the roughened femur by use of a cancellous screw, a staple or staples, or criss-cross, threaded Steinmann pins. The vastus intermedius is resutured over the new insertion of gluteus medius–minimus to bone.

The fasciae latae and the wound are closed in layers. A double hip spica cast is applied to include the foot and leg.

Postoperative Care. The hip spica cast is removed in six weeks, and the hip is mobilized and ambulation commenced. The internal fixation device is removed two to three months postoperatively.

REFERENCE

Steel, H. H.: Gluteus medius and minimus insertion advancement for correction of internal rotation gait in spastic cerebral palsy. J. Bone Joint Surg., 62–A:919, 1980.

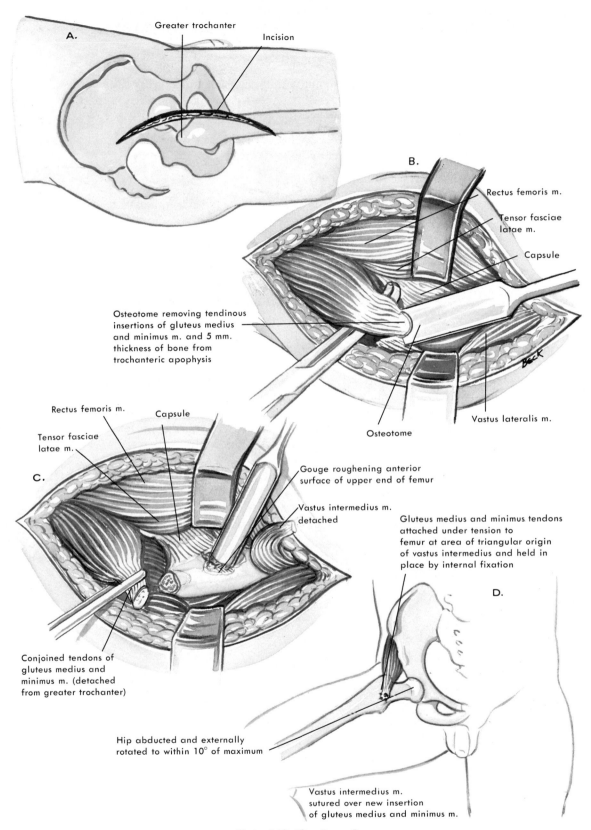

A.

Greater trochanter

Incision

B.

Rectus femoris m.

Tensor fasciae latae m.

Capsule

Osteotome removing tendinous insertions of gluteus medius and minimus m. and 5 mm. thickness of bone from trochanteric apophysis

Osteotome

Vastus lateralis m.

Rectus femoris m.

Capsule

Tensor fasciae latae m.

C.

Gouge roughening anterior surface of upper end of femur

Vastus intermedius m. detached

Gluteus medius and minimus tendons attached under tension to femur at area of triangular origin of vastus intermedius and held in place by internal fixation

D.

Conjoined tendons of gluteus medius and minimus m. (detached from greater trochanter)

Hip abducted and externally rotated to within 10° of maximum

Vastus intermedius m. sutured over new insertion of gluteus medius and minimus m.

Plate 119. (Continued)

PLATE 120   Iliopsoas Muscle Transfer for Paralysis of the Hip Abductors

Objectives

1. To provide active abduction power of the hip in stance phase.
2. To take away toe flexion power of the iliopsoas across the hip joint—a deforming force.

Indications. Progressive instability of the hip in a young child with myelomeningocele with an L3, L4 neurosegmental lesion.

Requisites

1. Stable, concentric reduction of the hip. First, correct the anatomic factors causing instability of the hip.
   a. Tauten the lax capsule by capsulorrhaphy.
   b. Correct coxa valga and excessive femoral antetorsion by derotation varus osteotomy of the proximal femur at the intertrochanteric level.
   c. Correct superolateral posterior deficiency of the acetabulum by modified Albee shelf, Staheli slotted augmentation shelf or Chiari's innominate osteotomy.
2. Passive range of hip abduction of at least 45 to 50 degrees. When hip adduction contracture is present, perform hip adductor myotomy to obtain adequate passive range of hip abductors.
3. Motor strength of iliopsoas—at least good, preferably normal.
4. Adequate motor strength of the sartorius, pectineus, and rectus femoris muscles to flex the hip against gravity. Otherwise, do not transfer the iliopsoas. Consequent hip flexion weakness will make the patient unable to climb steps. When the sartorius and pectineus muscles are weak, transfer the external oblique muscle.
5. Adequate knee control, a good or normal quadriceps femoris, and preferably hamstring muscle function.
6. A community ambulator or a child with that potential.
7. Adequate intelligence, motivation, and cooperation in the postoperative training program.
8. An experienced pediatric orthopedic hip surgeon; the procedure is technically demanding.

Problems and Complications

1. A greater than ordinary risk of hematoma or infection because the wound is near the perineum.

2. Detachment of the transferred iliopsoas tendon from the greater trochanter, necessitating reattachment. Use secure fixation.

3. Disuse osteoporosis while the child is in the cast. There is a possibility of multiple stress fractures after cast removal.

4. Stiff hip joint with abduction contracture because of fibrosis of denervated iliopsoas muscle.

5. Avascular necrosis of the femoral head due to inadvertent injury to medial circumflex femoral artery.

6. Decreased power of hip flexion causing difficulty in climbing steps.

Caution! Do not perform bilateral iliopsoas transfer until power of hip flexors against gravity on the operated side is achieved.

Blood for Transfusion. Yes.

Radiographic Control. Image intensifier.

Patient Position. The patient lies supine with a small sandbag under the sacrum and a larger sandbag under the ipsilateral scapula. The entire involved lower limb, the hip, the lower abdomen and chest, and the iliac and sacral regions are prepared sterile and draped so that the limb that is to be operated on can be freely manipulated and the incision extended to the posterior third of the iliac crest without contamination.

Operative Technique

A. The skin incision extends forward from the junction of the posterior and middle thirds of the iliac crest to the anterior superior iliac spine; it is then carried distally into the thigh along the medial border of the sartorius muscle for a distance of 10 to 12 cm., ending 2 cm. distal to the lesser trochanter.

B. The deep fascia is incised over the iliac crest, and the fascia lata is opened in line with the skin incision.

The lateral femoral cutaneous nerve is identified; it usually crosses the sartorius muscle 2.5 cm. distal to the anterior superior iliac spine and lies in close proximity to the lateral border of the sartorius. The nerve is mobilized by sharp dissection and protected by retracting it medially with a moist hernia tape. The wound flaps are undermined and retracted. The anterior medial margin of the tensor fasciae latae muscle is identified, and by blunt dissection the groove between the sartorius and rectus femoris muscles medially and the tensor fasciae latae muscle laterally is opened. The dissection is carried deep through the loose areolar tissue that separates these structures, and the adipose tissue that covers the front of the capsule of the hip joint is exposed. The ascending branch of the lateral femoral circumflex artery and the accompanying vein cross the midportion of the wound; they are isolated, clamped, cut, and ligated.

The origin of the sartorius muscle from the anterior superior iliac spine is detached and the muscle is reflected distally and medially. The free end is marked with a Tycron or nonabsorbable whip suture for later reattachment. The origins of the two heads of the rectus femoris are divided and reflected distally. The femoral nerve and its branches to the sartorius and rectus femoris are identified. A moist hernia tape is passed around the femoral nerve for gentle handling. The femoral vessels and nerve are retracted medially.

C. The cartilaginous apophysis of the ilium is split, and the dissection is deepened along the iliac crest down to bone. With a broad periosteal elevator, the tensor fasciae latae and the gluteus medius and minimus muscles are stripped subperiosteally from the lateral surface of the ilium and reflected in one continuous mass laterally and distally to the superior margin of the acetabulum. Bleeding is controlled by packing the interval between the reflected muscles and ilium with laparotomy pads.

D. With a large periosteal elevator, the iliacus muscle is subperiosteally elevated and reflected medially, exposing the inner wall of the wing of the ilium from the greater sciatic notch to the anterior superior iliac spine.

By careful blunt dissection with a periosteal elevator, the iliacus muscle is freed, elevated, and mobilized from the inner wall of the ilium and the anterior capsule of the hip joint. It is important to stay lateral and deep to the iliacus muscle and work in a proximal to distal direction.

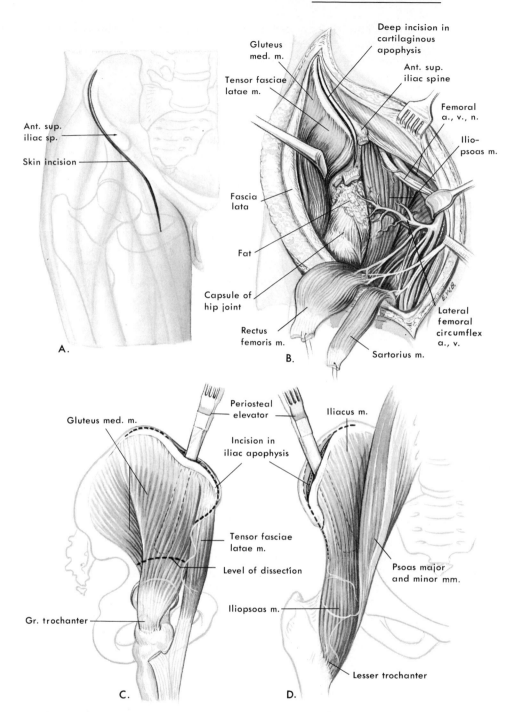

Ant. sup. iliac sp.

Skin incision

A.

Gluteus med. m.

Tensor fasciae latae m.

Deep incision in cartilaginous apophysis

Ant. sup. iliac spine

Femoral a., v., n.

Ilio-psoas m.

Fascia lata

Fat

Capsule of hip joint

Rectus femoris m.

Lateral femoral circumflex a., v.

Sartorius m.

B.

Gluteus med. m.

Periosteal elevator

Incision in iliac apophysis

Iliacus m.

Tensor fasciae latae m.

Level of dissection

Psoas major and minor mm.

Gr. trochanter

Iliopsoas m.

Lesser trochanter

C.

D.

Plate 120. A.–R., Iliopsoas muscle transfer for paralysis of the hip abductors.

E.–G. The hip is flexed, abducted, and laterally rotated; with the index finger, the lesser trochanter is cleared of soft tissues proximally, posteriorly, and distally. The index finger is then placed on the posteromedial aspect of the lesser trochanter and is used to direct a curved osteotome to the superior and deep aspect of the base of the lesser trochanter.

The lesser trochanter is osteotomized, and the distal insertion of the iliacus muscle on the linea aspera of the femur is freed with a periosteal elevator.

H. The iliacus and psoas muscles are reflected proximally by sharp and dull dissection. It is very essential not to injure the nerve to the iliacus, which at times enters the muscle belly quite distally; also, the femoral nerve should not be damaged. The author finds the use of a nerve stimulator of great help. Circumflex vessels are clamped, cut, and ligated as necessary.

I. In the middle third of the wing of the ilium, a rectangular hole, usually 1½ to 2 inches, is cut with drill holes and osteotomes. The hole should be large enough to accommodate the transferred muscle. It should be located as far posteriorly as possible to allow a more direct line of muscle action. The limiting factor is the nerve supply to the iliacus, which should not be stretched.

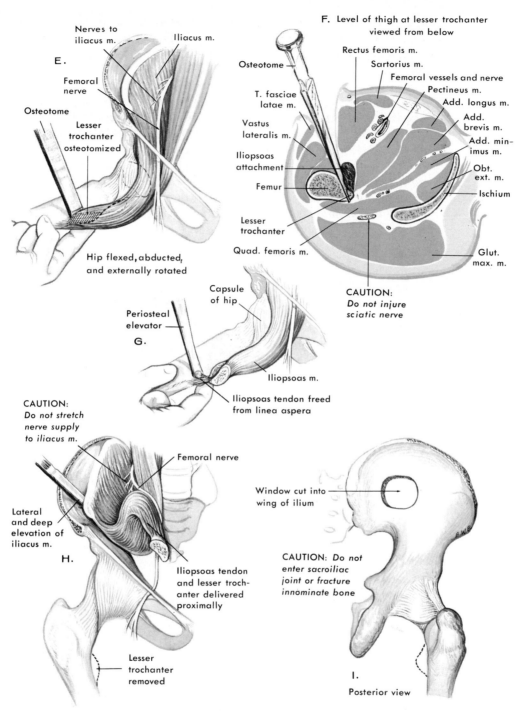

E.

Nerves to iliacus m.

Iliacus m.

Femoral nerve

Osteotome

Lesser trochanter osteotomized

Hip flexed, abducted, and externally rotated

F. Level of thigh at lesser trochanter viewed from below

Osteotome

Rectus femoris m.

Sartorius m.

Femoral vessels and nerve

Pectineus m.

Add. longus m.

Add. brevis m.

Add. minimus m.

Obt. ext. m.

Ischium

T. fasciae latae m.

Vastus lateralis m.

Iliopsoas attachment

Femur

Lesser trochanter

Quad. femoris m.

Glut. max. m.

CAUTION: Do not injure sciatic nerve

G.

Capsule of hip

Periosteal elevator

Iliopsoas m.

Iliopsoas tendon freed from linea aspera

CAUTION: Do not stretch nerve supply to iliacus m.

Lateral and deep elevation of iliacus m.

H.

Femoral nerve

Iliopsoas tendon and lesser trochanter delivered proximally

Lesser trochanter removed

Window cut into wing of ilium

CAUTION: Do not enter sacroiliac joint or fracture innominate bone

I.

Posterior view

Plate 120. (Continued)

J. With the hip in extension and medial rotation, the greater trochanter is exposed by a longitudinal lateral incision. The vastus lateralis muscle is split and the lateral surface of the proximal 4 to 5 cm. of femoral shaft is subperiosteally exposed.

K. Do not damage the greater trochanteric apophyseal growth plate.

L. Next, a large Ober tendon passer is inserted through the hole in the wing of the ilium, directed deep to the glutei, and brought out in the greater trochanteric region by splitting the insertion of the fibers of the gluteus medius muscle.

M. and N. The iliopsoas muscle is then transferred laterally by this route with the Ober tendon passer. The nerve supply to the iliacus is again checked to be sure that it is not under great tension. The hip is abducted at least 45 to 60 degrees and medially rotated 10 to 15 degrees. The site of insertion of the iliopsoas tendon on the femoral shaft is determined and is roughened with curved osteotomes. The muscle should be under proper tension.

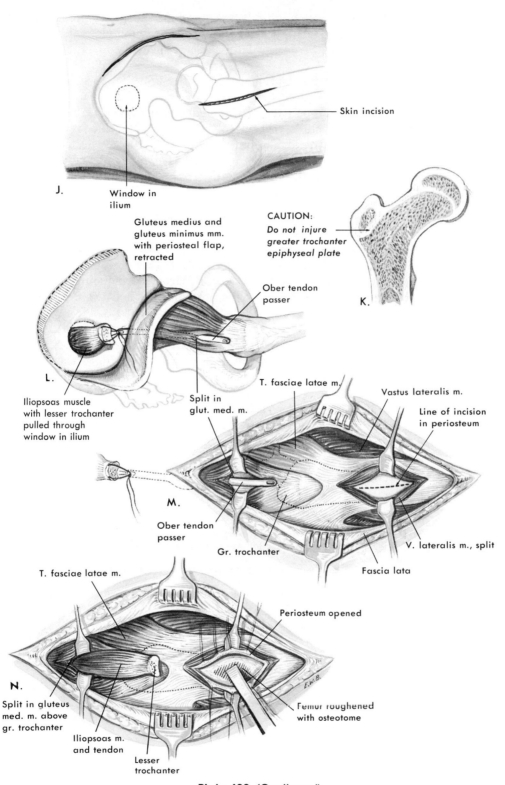

J. Window in ilium

Skin incision

Gluteus medius and gluteus minimus mm. with periosteal flap, retracted

Ober tendon passer

CAUTION:
Do not injure greater trochanter epiphyseal plate

K.

L.

Iliopsoas muscle with lesser trochanter pulled through window in ilium

Split in glut. med. m.

T. fasciae latae m.

Vastus lateralis m.

Line of incision in periosteum

M.

Ober tendon passer

Gr. trochanter

V. lateralis m., split

Fascia lata

T. fasciae latae m.

Periosteum opened

N.

Split in gluteus med. m. above gr. trochanter

Iliopsoas m. and tendon

Lesser trochanter

Femur roughened with osteotome

E.W.B.

Plate 120. (Continued)

O. The lesser trochanter is anchored to the proximal femur by one or two transversely placed small staples. Mustard recommends making a trap door in the femur into which the lesser trochanter is drawn and anchored by heavy wire sutures.

P. The periosteum and vastus lateralis muscle are sutured to the edges and over the iliopsoas tendon.

Q. and **R.** The rectus femoris and sartorius muscles are sutured to the inferior and superior iliac spines, respectively. The tensor fasciae latae, the gluteus medius and minimus, and the abdominal muscles are sutured to the iliac crest.

The wound is closed in layers in routine manner. A one-and-one-half hip spica cast is applied, with the hip in 60 degrees of abduction, 10 to 15 degrees medial rotation, and slight flexion.

Postoperative Care. Four to six weeks following surgery, the patient is readmitted to the hospital. The cast is removed, and a new bivalved hip spica cast made. This should be cut low on the lateral side so that hip abduction exercises can be performed in the posterior half of the cast. Radiograms of the hips are made to determine the stability of the hip joint. Great care should be exercised so that a pathologic fracture of the femur is not caused when the child is lifted out of the cast.

Training of the iliopsoas transfer follows the same general principles as those for training tendon transfers in poliomyelitis. In myelomeningocele, however, there is extensive paralysis of the lower limb, necessitating orthotic support, and the patient is much younger. Thus, as soon as the transferred iliopsoas has fair motor strength and the lower limbs can be adducted to neutral position, weight-bearing is permitted in bilateral above-knee orthoses. The butterfly pelvic band will keep the hips in 5 to 10 degrees of abduction during locomotion. At night, the hips and the transfer are protected in the bivalved hip spica cast or plastic hip-knee-ankle-foot orthosis (HKAFO).

REFERENCES

Carroll, N. C., and Sharrard, W. J.: Long-term followup of posterior iliopsoas transplantation for paralytic dislocation of the hip. J. Bone Joint Surg., 54–A:551, 1972.

Mustard, W. T.: Iliopsoas transfer for weakness of the hip abductors. J. Bone Joint Surg., 34–A:647, 1952.

Mustard, W. T.: A follow-up study of iliopsoas transfer for hip instability. J. Bone Joint Surg., 41–B:289, 1959.

Sharrard, W. J. W.: Posterior iliopsoas transplantation in the treatment of paralytic dislocation of the hip. J. Bone Joint Surg., 46–B:426, 1964.

Sharrard, W. J. W.: Long-term follow-up of posterior transplant for paralytic dislocation of the hip. J. Bone Joint Surg., 52–B:779, 1970.

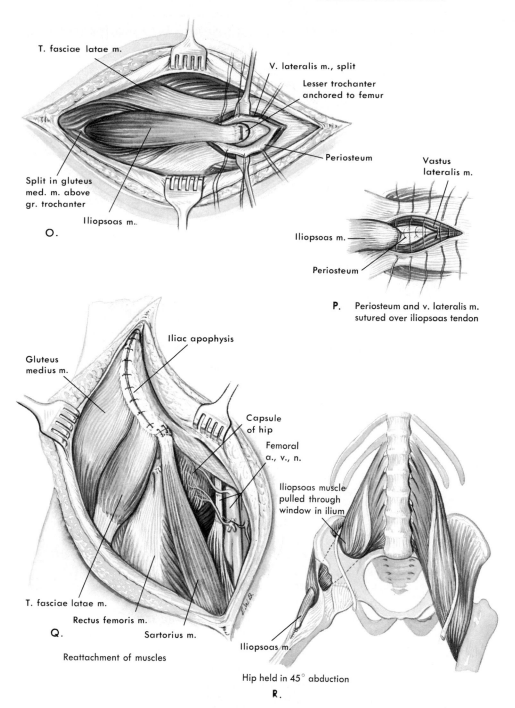

T. fasciae latae m.

V. lateralis m., split

Lesser trochanter anchored to femur

Periosteum

Split in gluteus med. m. above gr. trochanter

Iliopsoas m.

O.

Vastus lateralis m.

Iliopsoas m.

Periosteum

P. Periosteum and v. lateralis m. sutured over iliopsoas tendon

Gluteus medius m.

Iliac apophysis

Capsule of hip

Femoral a., v., n.

Iliopsoas muscle pulled through window in ilium

T. fasciae latae m.

Rectus femoris m.

Sartorius m.

Q.

Reattachment of muscles

Iliopsoas m.

Hip held in 45° abduction

R.

Plate 120. (Continued)

PLATE 121 ## Correction of Hip Flexion Contracture by Anterior Soft-Tissue Release in High-Level Myelomeningocele

Objectives. To provide full motion of the hips and to correct anterior pelvic tilt and excessive lumbar lordosis. In these patients, the prognosis for functional walking is poor.

Indications. Fixed flexion deformity of the hip 25 degrees or greater that has failed to respond to conservative measures of treatment—passive exercises, prone posturing, and splinting.

Hip flexion deformity causes anterior pelvic tilt and compensatory excessive lumbar lordosis. Often hip flexion deformity is accompanied by knee flexion deformity. Both deformities impede walking, with or without orthosis. Correct hip flexion deformity and knee flexion deformity simultaneously. They may be accompanied by lateral rotation and abduction contracture of the hip; when they are significant, correct them simultaneously with hip flexion deformity by soft tissue release.

Caution! In the preoperative assessment, determine the cause of hip flexion deformity. Is it static forces of malposture in a child with myelomeningocele with a high level lesion who is primarily a sitter? Is it fibrotic contracture of paralyzed hip flexor muscles? Or is it muscle imbalance when there is hip flexion power in the absence of hip extension strength? Rectify the etiologic factor in order to prevent recurrence. Provide standing orthosis in sitters and encourage standing. In muscle imbalance, restore muscle balance by release or muscle-tendon transfer.

Blood for Transfusion. Yes.

Patient Position. Ordinarily, the procedure is performed on both hips. The patient is placed in supine position, and both lower limbs, hips, pelvis, and lower abdomen are prepared and draped sterile. The surgeon should be able to perform the Thomas test without contaminating the operative field.

Operative Technique

A. and **B.** The surgical exposure is through the anterior part of the incision utilized for Salter's innominate osteotomy (see Plate 82). It extends obliquely medial 2 cm. distal to the inguinal crease.

In order to prevent recurrence of deformity, excise segments of the contracted tendons and fibrosed muscles; *do not simply divide!*

First, identify and detach the sartorius muscle from its origin from the anterior superior iliac spine. Then reflect the muscle distally and medially.

In the lateral part of the wound, identify the tensor fasciae latae. By blunt dissection, separate the muscle fibers from the fascia and transversely section the fascia as far posteriorly as the gluteus minimus–medius muscle. Divide the fibrotic and contracted muscle fibers of the tensor fasciae latae and the anterior part of the gluteus minimus–medius muscles with an electrocautery knife.

C. Next, the hip is flexed, abducted, and laterally rotated. The femoral nerve and vessels are gently retracted medially. The iliacus muscle fibers and iliopsoas tendon are exposed, and 1.5 to 2 cm. of the tendon are resected.

A.

B.

Ant. sup. iliac spine

Incision

Line of division
of fascia and
contracted fibrotic
muscle fibers

Tensor fasciae femoris

Sartorius m. detached

C.

Iliopsoas tendon resected

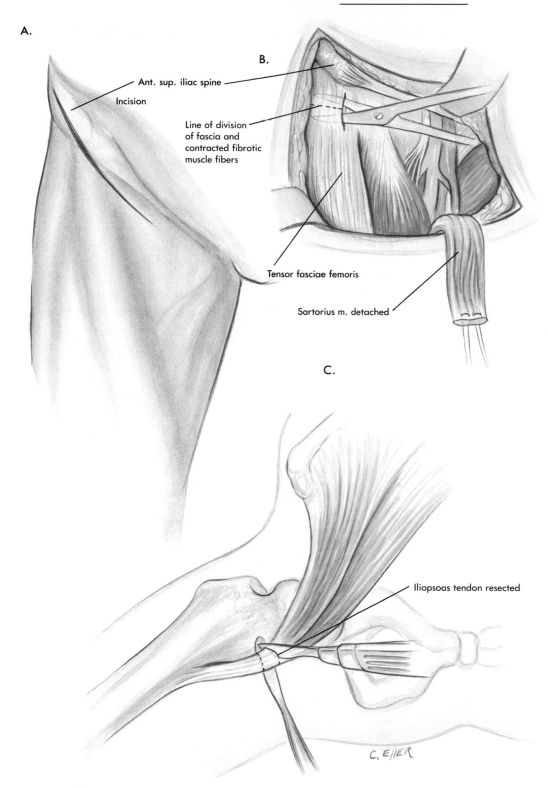

Plate 121. A.–E., Correction of hip flexion contracture by anterior soft-tissue release in high-level myelomeningocele.

D. The two heads of the rectus femoris—the direct from the anterior-inferior iliac spine and the reflected from the superior margin of the acetabulum—are identified. Excise both heads of the rectus femoris.

Perform a Thomas test, and determine the degree of correction of hip flexion deformity. The hip should hyperextend 20 degrees. Avoid incomplete correction.

E. If possible, do not section the anterior capsule of the hip joint because of the risk of anterior dislocation of the hip. If absolutely necessary, divide the anterior capsule of the hip transversely 2.0 cm. distal to the acetabular labrum.

Insert a closed suction drain into the wound. Do not close the fascia. The subcutaneous tissue and skin are closed in the usual fashion. A bilateral hip spica cast is applied with the hips in full extension and 15 to 20 degrees of abduction and neutral rotation.

Postoperative Care. The period of immobilization in a spica cast should not exceed two weeks. When in the cast, the patient is placed upright in weight-bearing position several hours a day to minimize disuse atrophy and osteoporosis of the paralyzed limb bones and to prevent stress fractures. After removal of the cast, the patient is fitted with a total-body orthosis; this encourages standing and walking several times a day. Hip extension and range of motion exercises are performed gently. The child should not sit for prolonged periods but should be placed in prone position to maintain the hips and knees in extension.

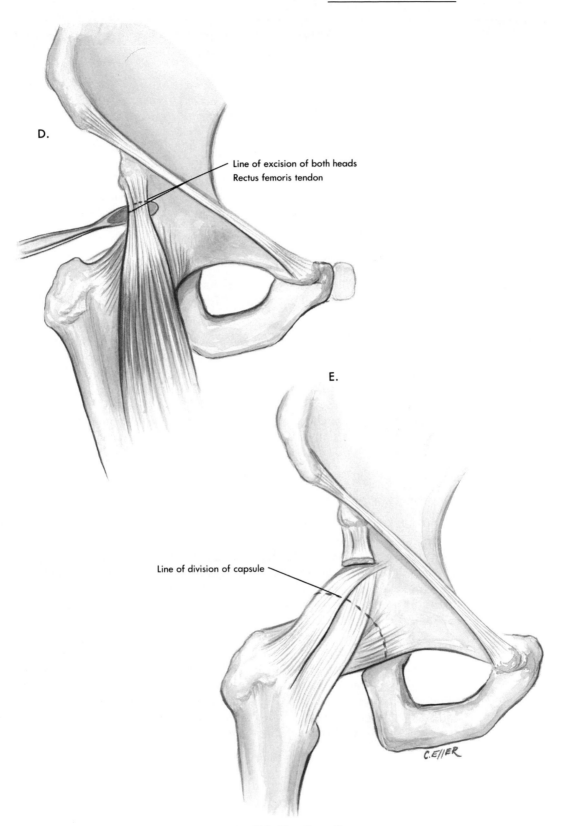

D.

Line of excision of both heads
Rectus femoris tendon

E.

Line of division of capsule

Plate 121. (Continued)

PLATE 122 ## Subtrochanteric Extension Osteotomy of the Proximal Femur to Correct Flexion Deformity of the Hip

Indications. Severe hip flexion deformity (exceeding 50 degrees) in an older child or adolescent near skeletal maturity. First perform anterior soft tissue release to decrease the degree of fixed flexion deformity and then extension osteotomy. The two procedures can be combined.

Caution! Avoid the following pitfalls:

1. When there is fixed lumbar lordosis and restricted range of hip flexion, excessive extension osteotomy will impede sitting posture.
2. Correct muscle imbalance to prevent recurrence of deformity.

Blood for Transfusion. Yes.

Radiographic Control. Image intensifier.

Special Instrumentation. An external fixator of the surgeon's preference for temporary fixation and AO plate/limited contact–dynamic compression plate (LC-DCP).

Principle. Extension osteotomy of the proximal femur is performed when hip flexion deformity cannot be corrected by simple soft tissue release.

The anterior, lateral, and posterior aspects of the proximal femur are subperiosteally exposed from the level of the greater trochanteric apophyseal plate (which should not be disturbed) for a distance of 7 to 10 cm. distal to the greater trochanter. The surgical approach is through an anterolateral approach if the bent AO or reconstruction plate manufactured by Synthes for internal fixation is to be placed anteriorly.

Patient Position. Prone.

Operative Technique

A. A posterior approach is used if the bent plate is to be placed posteriorly. With the patient in prone position, a 12- to 15-cm.-long incision is made over the posterolateral aspect of the hip and upper thigh. The incision begins 4 to 5 cm. proximal to the tip of the greater trochanter in line with the fibers of the gluteus maximus. At the greater trochanter, the longitudinal incision extends distally straight along the lateral aspect of the femur. The subcutaneous tissue and fascia are divided in line with the skin incision.

B. Rotate the hip medially and identify (1) the greater trochanter, (2) the origin of vastus lateralis, (3) the tendinous attachment of the gluteus maximus, (4) the quadratus femoris muscle, and (5) the upper portion of linea aspera. Detach the origin of vastus lateralis with electrocautery through a "hockey stick" incision—a transverse cut at the base of the greater trochanter and a longitudinal cut along the lateral aspect of the linea aspera. By subperiosteal dissection, elevate and reflect the vastus lateralis anteriorly.

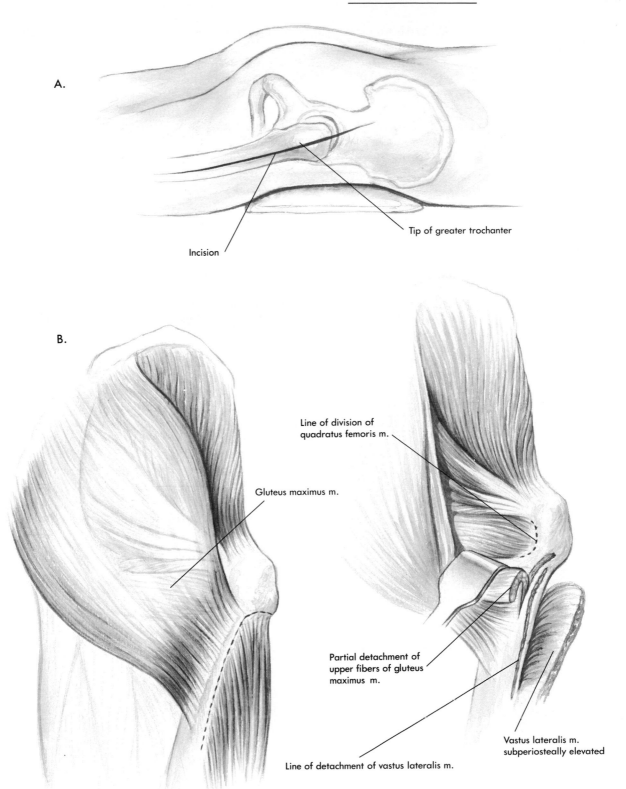

A.

Incision

Tip of greater trochanter

B.

Line of division of
quadratus femoris m.

Gluteus maximus m.

Partial detachment of
upper fibers of gluteus
maximus m.

Vastus lateralis m.
subperiosteally elevated

Line of detachment of vastus lateralis m.

Plate 122. A.–E., Subtrochanteric extension osteotomy of the proximal femur to correct flexion deformity of the hip.

C. With an electrocautery knife, make a cut through the periosteum and the fibers of quadratus femoris at the superior margin of the lesser trochanter. By subperiosteal dissection, the quadratus femoris is elevated and reflected medially. Insert Chandler or Homan retractors subperiosteally, exposing the upper shaft of the femur posteriorly, laterally, and anteriorly.

D. With an electric drill, two threaded Steinmann pins are drilled into the upper and lower segments of the proposed osteotomy in an anteroposterior direction at an angle determining the degree of flexion deformity to be corrected. The wedge of bone to be resected is based posteriorly. There should be enough bone in the upper segment for screw insertion into the two or three holes of a pre-bent five-hole or six-hole AO or reconstruction semiflexible plate. The bone is then cut with an electric oscillating saw. The wedge of bone is removed. The two bone surfaces are apposed by extending the distal segment.

Caution! Pay attention to rotational alignment.

The osteotomy is then temporarily fixed with criss-cross pins or an external fixator (such as Wagner tibia-lengthening apparatus) applied on the threaded Steinmann pins.

E. Internal fixation is carried out with a bent five-hole or six-hole AO plate or a six-hole or eight-hole reconstruction semiflexible plate. The wounds are closed in the usual fashion.

Postoperative Care. When in doubt as to the security of internal fixation, a bilateral long-leg hip spica cast is applied for external immobilization for three to four weeks. The child is allowed to stand several times a day in the cast in order to prevent disuse atrophy, osteoporosis of the lower limb bones, and stress fractures. After cast removal, the child is fitted with appropriate orthosis for support and ambulation. When internal fixation is secure, cast immobilization may be avoided. The child is fitted with an HKAFO immediately after surgery. Splinting at night with the hips in extension and prone posturing are crucial to prevent recurrence of the hip flexion deformity.

A pitfall of extension osteotomy of the proximal femur is excessive extension; in such a case, the combined fixed lumbar lordosis and restricted hip flexion impede sitting posture.

REFERENCES

Menelaus, M. B.: The hip in myelomeningocele—management directed towards a minimum number of operations and a minimum period of immobilization. J. Bone Joint Surg., 58–B:448, 1976.

Menelaus, M. B.: The Orthopedic Management of Spina Bifida Cystica. 2nd ed. Edinburgh: Churchill Livingstone, 1980.

Schafer, M. F., and Dias, L. S.: Myelomeningocele. Orthopaedic Treatment. Baltimore: Williams & Wilkins, 1983.

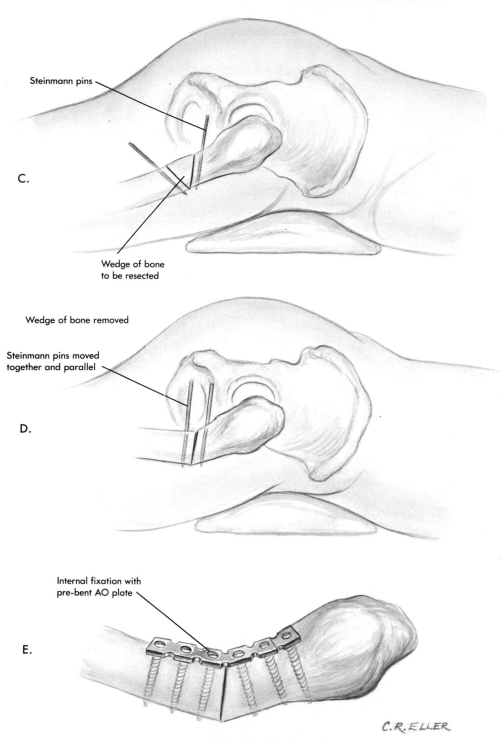

Steinmann pins

Wedge of bone
to be resected

C.

Wedge of bone removed

Steinmann pins moved
together and parallel

D.

Internal fixation with
pre-bent AO plate

E.

C.R.ELLER

Plate 122. (Continued)

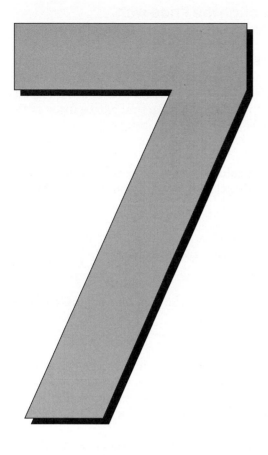

Thigh–Knee

PLATE 123 **Rotation-Plasty of the Lower Limb Through the Knee with Simultaneous Knee Fusion (Torode and Gillespie Technique)**

In this operation the lower limb is rotated 180 degrees on a vertical axis at the knee, turning the foot posteriorly and using the ankle joint as a knee. Thus, dorsiflexion of the foot in the prosthesis will flex the prosthetic knee, and plantar flexion will extend it. The purpose of this conversion surgery is to provide a stump that can be fitted with a conventional prosthesis and managed as a below-knee amputation.

Indications

1. Unilateral proximal femoral focal deficiency with severe lower limb length disparity in which limb elongation and equalization is not feasible or advisable.
2. Limb salvage surgery.

Requisites

1. An ankle joint with normal range of motion and motor power.
2. Unilateral involvement.
3. A stable hip.
4. A predicted lower limb length inequality that would place the ankle of the deficient limb at the level of the opposite normal knee.

Disadvantages

1. Without the prosthesis, the child's appearance with the posteriorly rotated foot is unnatural, bizarre, and cosmetically objectionable. Before surgery, the child and parents should see another patient who has had the procedure, without the prosthesis. They should observe the other child walk and play while wearing the prosthesis. If possible, show this on videotape.
2. Ambulatory function of the patient is decreased markedly without the prosthesis. To minimize neurovascular compromise, the limb is shortened while being rotated. Also, to make the ankle of the deficient limb level with the knee of the contralateral lower limb, epiphyseodesis of the distal femur and/or the proximal tibia is performed at the appropriate skeletal age.
3. Following surgery, there is a gradual derotation of the leg by the twisted musculature in the growing child. The spiral torque of the tautened tissues can be diminished by appropriate muscle-tendon release or transfer. Despite this, the parents and the child should understand preoperatively the probability of recurrence and the need for repeat derotation later in life.
4. Neurovascular compromise can occur.

Blood for Transfusion. Yes.

Radiographic Control. Image intensifier.

Patient Position. The patient is placed supine on the operating table, and the entire affected lower limb, hip, and pelvis are prepared and draped free. It is vital to be able to palpate the contralateral lower limb through the drapes in order to estimate the amount of shortening required to level the ankle of the deficient limb with the knee of the opposite normal limb.

Operative Technique

A. An anterolateral longitudinal skin incision is made. It begins proximally below the hip. At the knee it curves medially and extends distally along the line of the tibia, terminating 2.5 cm. above the medial malleolus. The subcutaneous tissue is divided in line with the skin incision.

B. The capsule of the knee and the patellar tendon are exposed. The tendon is sectioned and the knee capsule is incised. The patellar and quadriceps muscles are retracted upward, exposing the joint. On the medial aspect of the distal thigh the

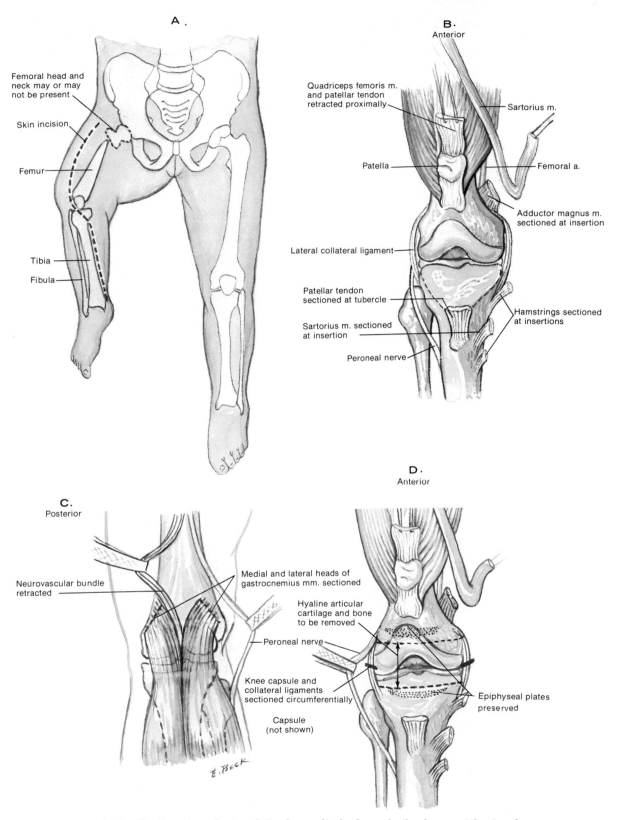

Plate 123. A.–G., Rotation-plasty of the lower limb through the knee with simultaneous knee fusion (Torode and Gillespie technique).

insertion of the adductor magnus is located, and the adductor hiatus with the neurovascular bundle is identified. In proximal femoral focal deficiency, the adductor magnus usually traverses from the pubis at a 70- to 80-degree angle to insert into the femur. The adductor magnus insertion is sectioned distal to the adductor hiatus, facilitating distal exposure of the femoral and popliteal arteries. The sartorius and medial hamstrings are sectioned near their insertions.

C. The lateral aspect of the distal thigh and knee is exposed. Dissection should be done carefully. If there is associated fibular hemimelia, the peroneal nerve will abut the proximal tibia rather than taking its normal course around the fibular neck. Dissect the peroneal nerve, and trace it proximally to its junction with the sciatic nerve.

D. The neurovascular structures both medially and laterally are retracted, and the capsule is divided all around the knee joint. Next, the medial and lateral heads of the gastrocnemius are sectioned, freeing the knee of all muscle and ligamentous attachments. The proximal tibial physis and the distal femoral physis are identified under radiographic control. With an oscillating saw, the hyaline articular cartilage of the proximal tibia and of the distal femoral epiphysis is removed. The level of division of the distal femur is governed by the overall length of the limb and by the length that is required to make the ankle of the affected limb level with the normal knee at skeletal maturity.

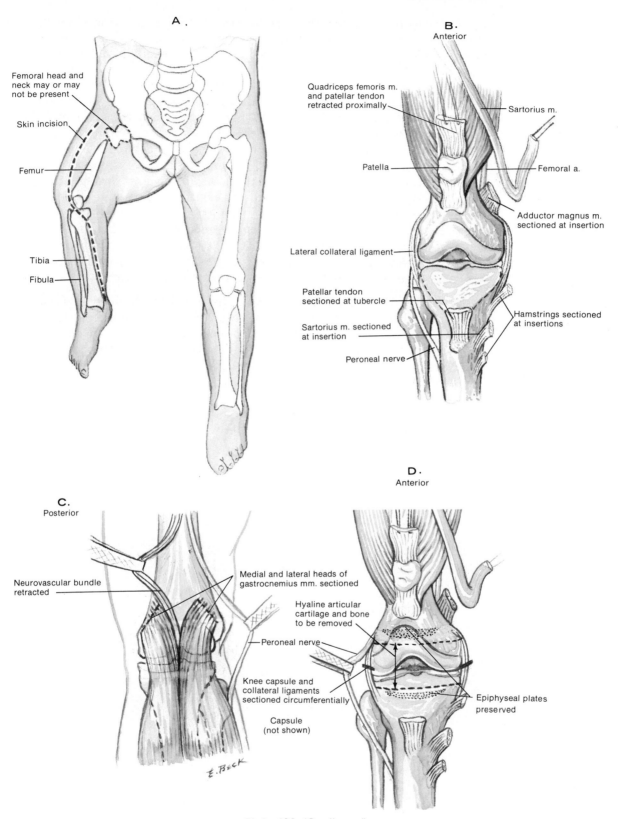

A.

Femoral head and neck may or may not be present

Skin incision

Femur

Tibia

Fibula

B.
Anterior

Quadriceps femoris m. and patellar tendon retracted proximally

Sartorius m.

Patella

Femoral a.

Adductor magnus m. sectioned at insertion

Lateral collateral ligament

Patellar tendon sectioned at tubercle

Hamstrings sectioned at insertions

Sartorius m. sectioned at insertion

Peroneal nerve

C.
Posterior

Neurovascular bundle retracted

Medial and lateral heads of gastrocnemius mm. sectioned

Peroneal nerve

Knee capsule and collateral ligaments sectioned circumferentially

Capsule (not shown)

D.
Anterior

Hyaline articular cartilage and bone to be removed

Epiphyseal plates preserved

E. Beck

Plate 123. (Continued)

E. Insert an intramedullary rod into the distal femur, bring it out through the gluteal region, and hammer it distally into the level of the resected knee. Then, rotate the leg laterally at the resected knee level gradually, as much as possible. With care, 120 to 140 degrees of rotation may be possible. At this stage the femoral vessels will slide forward anteromedial to the distal femur.

F. Next, expose the tibia and fibula subperiosteally and perform fasciotomies of all compartments. With an oscillating electric saw, the tibia and fibula are sectioned at the middle of their shafts. Segments of bone may be excised from the tibia and fibula if necessary to elevate the foot to the desired level.

G. The lower segment is rotated so that the foot points posteriorly, and the intramedullary rod is driven across the knee fusion and through the osteotomy site. The rod provides stability in both the sagittal and coronal planes; a hip spica cast incorporating the foot is applied to maintain rotary stability.

If postoperative swelling and vascular embarrassment dictate that the degree of rotation be decreased, the hip spica cast is removed and rotation is reduced. When the swelling subsides, the lower segment is rotated to the desired degree. This safety measure is not provided by internal fixation with plate and screws.

Postoperative Care. By six to eight weeks union is obtained at both the knee fusion and tibial osteotomy levels. The cast is removed and the prosthesis is fitted. Physical therapy is instituted to develop motor power of the triceps surae muscle and increase range of plantar flexion of the ankle and foot. The child is instructed in how to move the below-knee section of the modified prosthesis.

REFERENCE

Torode, I. P., and Gillespie, R.: Rotationplasty of the lower limb for congenital defects of the femur. J. Bone Joint Surg., 65-B:569, 1983.

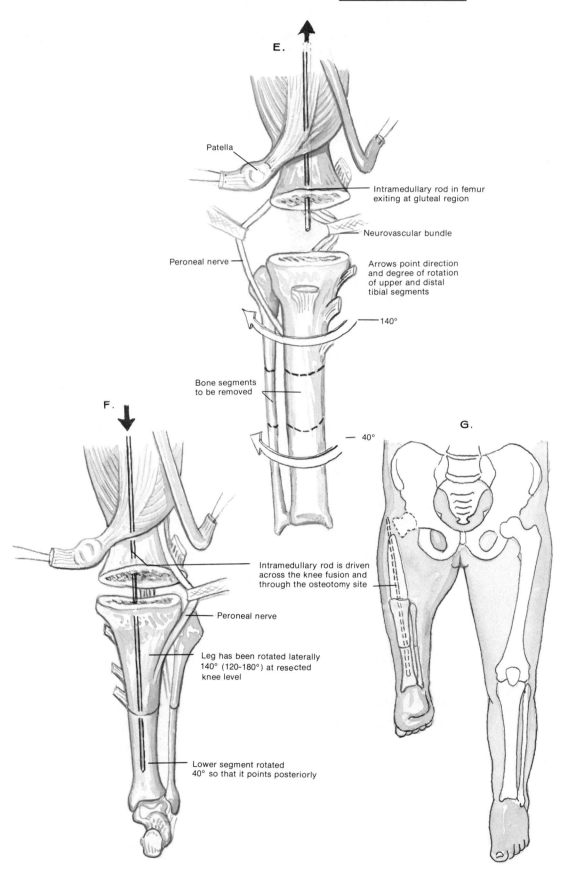

E.

Patella

Intramedullary rod in femur exiting at gluteal region

Neurovascular bundle

Peroneal nerve

Arrows point direction and degree of rotation of upper and distal tibial segments

140°

Bone segments to be removed

40°

F.

Intramedullary rod is driven across the knee fusion and through the osteotomy site

Peroneal nerve

Leg has been rotated laterally 140° (120-180°) at resected knee level

Lower segment rotated 40° so that it points posteriorly

G.

Plate 123. (Continued)

PLATE 124 **Knee Fusion and Syme Amputation for Prosthetic Conversion Surgery in Above-Knee Proximal Femoral Focal Deficiency (King Technique)**

Indications

1. Types B and C proximal femoral focal deficiency in which limb length equalization is not feasible or advisable.
2. Limb salvage in malignant tumors of the lower limb.

Advantages

1. Cosmetically, the appearance of the stump is more pleasing than with rotation-plasty.
2. The procedure converts the lower limb by knee fusion into a single skeletal lever, which makes the muscles function more effectively across the hip joint, decreasing the fixed flexion deformity.
3. Technically, the procedure is simpler than rotation-plasty. Both procedures require epiphyseodesis of the distal femur or proximal tibia to level the knees.

Disadvantages. The disadvantages of amputation and conversion to an above-knee stump as compared with a turnabout procedure and conversion into a below-knee stump are as follows:

1. There is a lack of position sense in amputation. In the turnabout procedure (rotation-plasty) with preservation of the foot, position sense is maintained with an added sensory feedback.
2. In rotation-plasty and conversion to below-knee stump, the gait is more stable and more effectively controlled in the swing phase. In the above-knee stump (i.e., after knee fusion and Syme amputation), the gait in the prosthesis is awkward because stability and control of the knee are poor.
3. In the below-knee stump (converted after rotation-plasty), the patient is able to actively flex and extend the knee during sitting or bicycle riding. This is a definite advantage over the above-knee stump with extension prosthesis in which the patient cannot actively flex the knee during walking or sitting.

Blood for Transfusion. Yes.

Radiographic Control. Image intensifier.

Special Instrumentation. Intramedullary rod, preferably smooth. The type depends on the surgeon's preference.

Principle. King's method converts the proximal femoral focal deficient limb into a single skeletal lever arm by arthrodesis of the knee in extension and Syme's ankle disarticulation.

Patient Position. Supine.

Operative Technique

A. An anterior S-shaped incision is made to expose the anterior aspect of the lower femur and upper tibia. If there is a definite pseudarthrosis in the metaphyseal-diaphyseal subtrochanteric region, King recommends repairing it by excision of its fibrocartilaginous site. Proximally, the incision is extended laterally to expose the lateral aspect of the upper femur.

B. The capsule and synovium of the knee joint are opened, and the articular cartilage of the lower end of the femur and the upper end of the tibia is excised with an oscillating electric saw until the ossific nucleus of the epiphysis is seen. Avoid injury to the growth plates.

C. Insert an 8-mm. Küntscher or similar nail in retrograde fashion. First, insert it distally into the tibia, exiting from the sole of the foot.

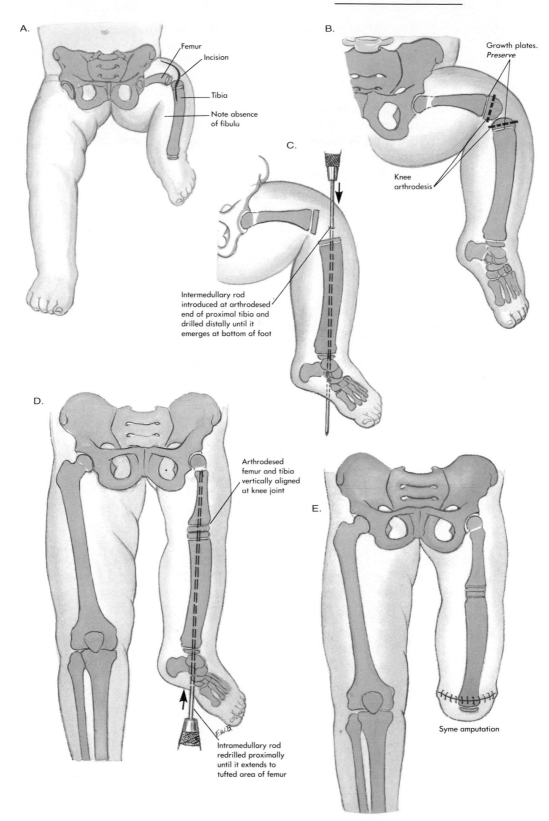

A. Femur
Incision
Tibia
Note absence of fibula

B. Growth plates. *Preserve*
Knee arthrodesis

C. Intermedullary rod introduced at arthrodesed end of proximal tibia and drilled distally until it emerges at bottom of foot

D. Arthrodesed femur and tibia vertically aligned at knee joint
Intramedullary rod redrilled proximally until it extends to tufted area of femur

E. Syme amputation

Plate 124. A.–E., Knee fusion and Syme amputation for prosthetic conversion surgery in above-knee proximal femoral focal deficiency (King technique).

D. The nail is then passed proximally into the femur, impacting the lower end of the femur and the upper epiphysis of the tibia in extension. Take care to provide proper rotational alignment of the lower limb and ensure that the fused knee is not in flexion. The intramedullary nail should be in the center of the physes of the distal femur and the proximal tibia to avoid growth retardation.

If the pseudarthrosis site is excised, the intramedullary nail is inserted to fix the upper femoral segments internally (not shown in the drawing).

The wound is closed in routine fashion. A one-and-one-half hip spica cast is applied for immobilization.

E. Six weeks postoperatively, when the intramedullary nail is removed, a Syme's amputation is performed. (See Plate 171).

Postoperative Care. Three weeks later, when adequate wound healing has taken place, the amputated, fused limb is fitted with a prosthesis, and the patient is instructed in gait training. Active and passive exercises are performed to maintain range of hip motion and prevent development of hip flexion deformity.

REFERENCES

King, R. E.: Providing a single skeletal lever in PFFD. Int. Clin. Inform. Bull., 6:23, 1966.

King, R. E.: Some concepts of proximal femoral focal deficiency. J. Bone Joint Surg., 49-A:1470, 1967.

King, R. E.: Some concepts of proximal femoral focal deficiency. In: Aitken, G. T. (ed.): Proximal Femoral Focal Deficiency: A Symposium. Washington, D.C., National Academy of Sciences, 1969, pp. 23–49.

King, R. E.: Proximal femoral focal deficiencies. In: Tronzo, R. G. (ed.): Surgery of the Hip Joint. Philadelphia, Lea & Febiger, 1975.

King, R. E.: Proximal femoral focal deficiency. In: Harris, N. (ed.): Clinical Orthopedics. Bristol, Wright, 1983, pp. 184–193.

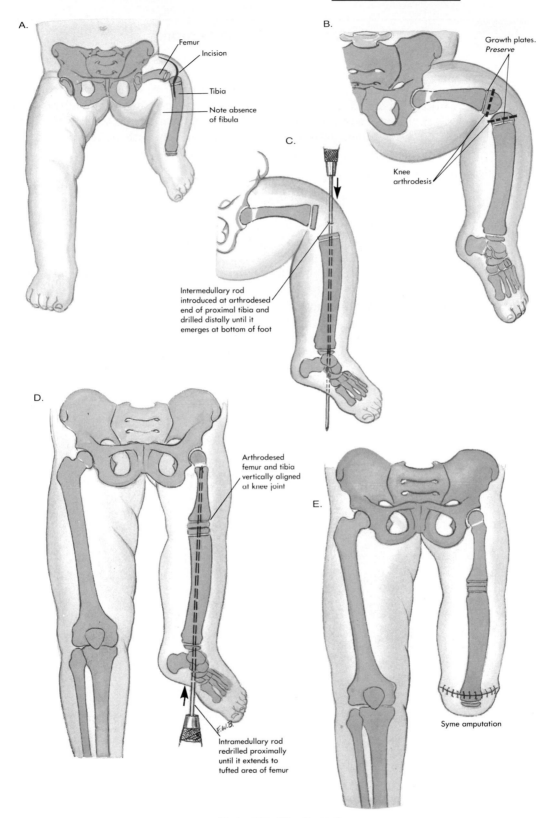

A.
Femur
Incision
Tibia
Note absence of fibula

B.
Growth plates. *Preserve*
Knee arthrodesis

C.
Intermedullary rod introduced at arthrodesed end of proximal tibia and drilled distally until it emerges at bottom of foot

D.
Arthrodesed femur and tibia vertically aligned at knee joint
Intramedullary rod redrilled proximally until it extends to tufted area of femur

E.
Syme amputation

Plate 124. (Continued)

PLATE   125   ## Proximal Recession of the Rectus Femoris

Indications

1. Moderate or severe extension contracture of the knee in a patient who walks with a stiff-knee gait due to spasticity and contracture of the rectus femoris.

2. Presence of associated hip flexion deformity due to a short rectus femoris.

3. Continuous activity of the rectus femoris both in stance and swing phases of gait as shown by gait analysis with dynamic electromyography.

Patient Position. Supine

Operative Technique

A. A 5- to 6-cm. longitudinal incision is made, beginning 1 cm. distal to the anterior superior iliac spine, and is extended distally between the sartorius and tensor fasciae latae muscles. The subcutaneous tissue is divided in line with the skin incision, and the superficial and deep fascia are incised longitudinally.

B. Identify the lateral femoral cutaneous nerve, and retract it with silicone (Silastic) tubing. Do not injure the nerve. The medial and lateral borders of the rectus femoris are identified and, with a blunt instrument, dissected free of adjacent tissues. A curved hemostat is inserted under the origin of the rectus femoris, and its tendon and muscle fibers are divided with electrocautery.

A medium Hemovac suction tube is inserted, and the wound is closed in layers in the usual fashion.

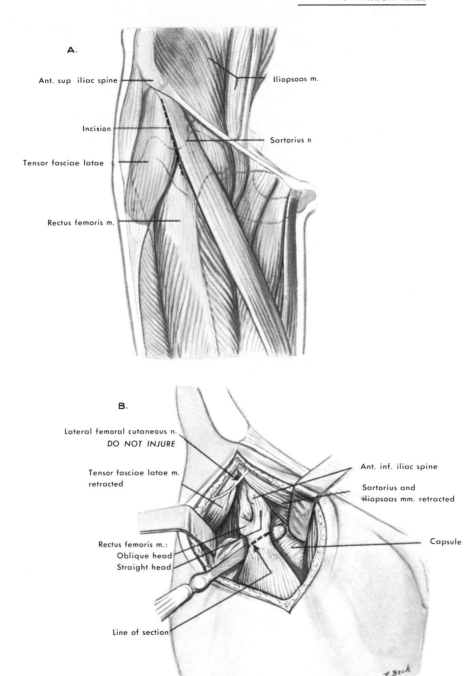

Plate 125. A.–F., Proximal recession of the rectus femoris.

C. A rectus femoris recession can be performed distally if there is no associated hip flexion deformity. Make a midline, longitudinal incision beginning at the superior pole of the patella and extending proximally for a distance of 4 to 5 cm. Subcutaneous tissue and superficial fascia are divided in line with the skin incision.

D. Identify the rectus femoris tendon. A Freer elevator is inserted deep to the rectus tendon, separating it from the underlying vastus intermedius. With a scalpel, section the rectus tendon transversely.

E. Flex the knee acutely.

F. Displace the rectus femoris tendon proximally. The wound is irrigated, the tourniquet is released, and complete hemostasis is achieved. The wound is closed in routine fashion. An above-knee cast is applied with the knee in about 45 to 60 degrees of flexion and the foot-ankle in neutral position.

Postoperative Care. The cast is removed in 10 to 14 days. Exercises are begun to restore full flexion and extension of the knee and to develop motor function of the quadriceps femoris and hamstring muscles. Other details of postoperative care depend upon the severity of involvement and whether other simultaneous surgical procedures have been performed.

REFERENCE

Bleck, E. E.: Orthopaedic Management of Cerebral Palsy. Philadelphia, J.B. Lippincott Co., 1987.

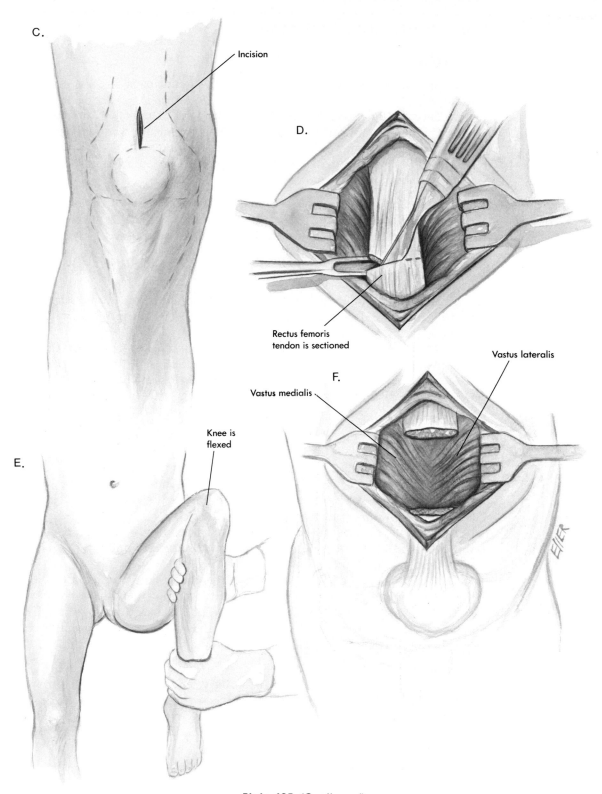

C.

Incision

D.

Rectus femoris
tendon is sectioned

Vastus lateralis

Vastus medialis

F.

Knee is
flexed

E.

Plate 125. (Continued)

PLATE 126   Distal Transfer of the Rectus Femoris

Indications

1. Stiff-knee gait with cospasticity of the quadriceps femoris and hamstring muscles.
2. Zero to 15 degrees of knee flexion on swing phase (short stride length).
3. Prolonged and out-of-phase abnormal potentials of quadriceps and hamstring muscles on dynamic gait electromyography.
4. Good or normal motor strength of quadriceps femoris muscle.
5. In-toeing or out-toeing gait.

When the stiff-knee gait is accompanied by lateral foot progression angle (out-toeing gait), the rectus femoris is transferred to the medial hamstring. When the foot progression angle is medial (in-toeing gait), the muscle is transferred to the biceps femoris tendon.

Requisites

1. Adequate quadriceps femoris motor strength to extend the knee fully against gravity and to maintain the knee extended at the initial and midstance phases of gait.
2. The hamstrings should be strong enough to flex the knee in the initial swing phase of 35 degrees and complete swing phase of 60 to 70 degrees.
3. Absence of fixed knee flexion deformity. When there is stiff, flexed knee gait, combine distal transfer of the rectus femoris with hamstring lengthening.

Patient Position. Supine position with a sterile tourniquet on the proximal thigh.

Operative Technique

A. and **B.** A midline longitudinal incision is made over the lower thigh, beginning at the superior pole of the patella and extending proximally for 5 to 7 cm. The subcutaneous tissue and fasciae are divided in line with the skin incision. The wound edges are undermined.

The rectus femoris tendon is identified and divided at its insertion at the patella. Longitudinal incisions are made over the medial and lateral borders of the rectus tendon.

C. The tendon is dissected free from the underlying vastus lateralis muscles. The rectus tendon is mobilized and elevated proximally and sutured into a tube.

D. The vastus lateralis and vastus medialis are sutured together. The rectus tendon is transferred subcutaneously and sutured either to the medial hamstrings or to the biceps femoris tendon. The wound is closed in routine fashion.

Postoperative Care. An above-knee cast is applied with the knee in 20 to 30 degrees of flexion for two or three weeks. Active and passive exercises are performed to develop balance of motor strength between the knee flexors and extensors and reciprocal hip-knee flexion in gait. Some surgeons prefer to use a postoperative knee immobilizer and begin exercises as soon as the patient is comfortable, a few days following surgery.

REFERENCE

Gage, J. R., Perry, J., Hicks, R. R., Koop, S., and Werntz, J. R.: Rectus femoris transfer as a means of improving knee function in cerebral palsy. Dev. Med. Child Neurol., 29:159, 1987.

Ounpuu, S., Muik, E., Davis, R. B., III, Gage, J. R., and DeLuca, P. A.: Rectus femoris surgery in children with cerebral palsy. Part I: The effect of rectus femoris transfer location on knee motion. J. Pediatr. Orthop., 13:325, 1993.

Ounpuu, S., Muik, E., Davis, R. B., III, Gage, J. R., and DeLuca, P. A.: Rectus femoris surgery in children with cerebral palsy. Part II: A comparison between the effect of transfer and release of the distal rectus femoris on knee motion. J. Pediatr. Orthop., 13:331, 1993.

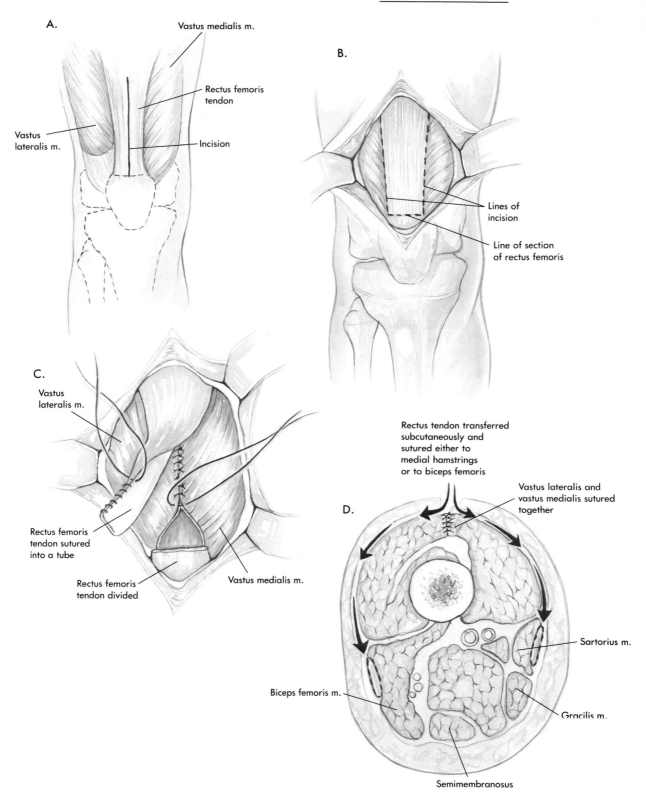

A.
Vastus medialis m.
Rectus femoris tendon
Vastus lateralis m.
Incision

B.
Lines of incision
Line of section of rectus femoris

C.
Vastus lateralis m.
Rectus femoris tendon sutured into a tube
Rectus femoris tendon divided
Vastus medialis m.

D.
Rectus tendon transferred subcutaneously and sutured either to medial hamstrings or to biceps femoris
Vastus lateralis and vastus medialis sutured together
Sartorius m.
Biceps femoris m.
Gracilis m.
Semimembranosus

Plate 126. A.–D., Distal transfer of the rectus femoris.

PLATE 127   Fractional Musculotendinous Lengthening of the Hamstrings Distally

Indications. Flexion deformity of the knee caused by spasticity and contracture of the hamstrings. Failure to respond to conservative measures, such as passive exercises, splinting, and prone posturing.

Requisites

1. Normal or good motor strength of hamstrings and gluteus maximus. Ability to flex the knees against gravity and resistance in the prone position. Ability to extend the hips against gravity with the knees flexed.

2. Absence of hip flexion deformity. Spasticity and contracture of iliopsoas inhibit function of the gluteus minimus. Hamstrings supply one third of the hip extensor torque and provide posterior stability of the hip. Lengthening of hamstrings will decrease hip extensor strength, decrease posterior pelvic support, tilt the pelvis forward, and result in excessive low lumbar lordosis and compensatory thoracolumbar kyphosis. Patients may lose the ability to stand independently and thus may require crutches or a walker for support. Lengthening of the hamstrings is contraindicated in the presence of hip flexion deformity and weak gluteus maximus motor strength.

3. Absence of genu recurvatum. This will be aggravated by hamstring lengthening.

4. Absence of equinus deformity. The short contracted soleus will tilt the proximal tibia posteriorly into genu recurvatum at heel strike. The combination of excessive lumbar lordosis and genu recurvatum is functionally disabling.

Patient Position. The patient is placed in prone position with a pneumatic tourniquet high on the proximal thigh.

Operative Technique

A. A 7 to 10 cm. longitudinal midline incision is made, starting just proximal to the popliteal crease. The subcutaneous tissue is divided, and the incision is carried to the deep fascia. The posterior femoral cutaneous nerve will be in the proximal aspect of the wound and should not be damaged.

B. The deep fascia is incised, and the hamstring tendons are identified by blunt dissection. It is imperative to divide the tendon sheath of each hamstring tendon separately.

C. In the lateral compartment of the wound, the biceps femoris tendon is exposed. It should be gently dissected away from the common peroneal nerve, which lies on its posteromedial surface. A blunt instrument, such as a staphylorrhaphy probe, is passed deep to the biceps tendon.

D. With a sharp scalpel, the tendinous portion of the biceps femoris is incised transversely at two levels, 3 cm. apart, leaving the muscle fibers intact. The tendon is lengthened in continuity by straight leg raising with the knee in extension.

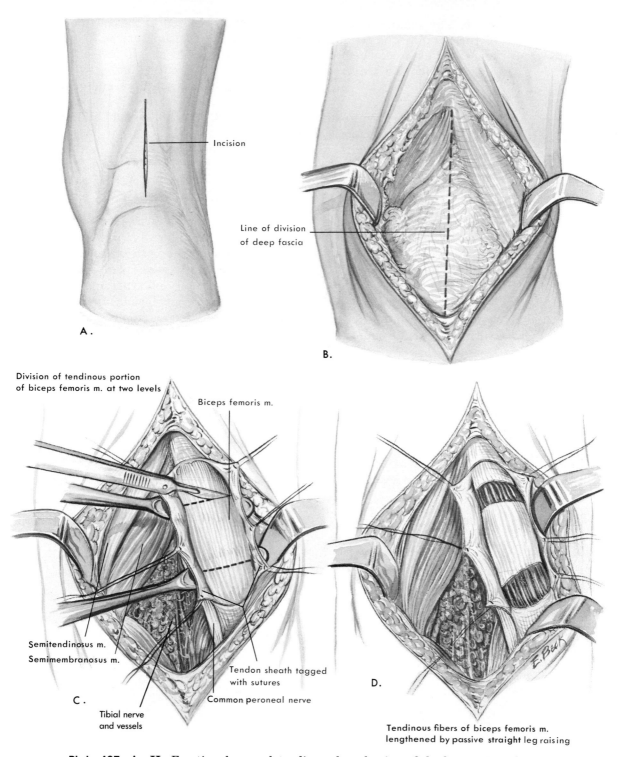

A.

Incision

B.

Line of division of deep fascia

Division of tendinous portion of biceps femoris m. at two levels

Biceps femoris m.

C.

Semitendinosus m.
Semimembranosus m.

Tibial nerve and vessels

Tendon sheath tagged with sutures

Common peroneal nerve

D.

Tendinous fibers of biceps femoris m. lengthened by passive straight leg raising

E.Beck

Plate 127. A.–H., Fractional musculotendinous lengthening of the hamstrings distally.

E. The semimembranosus tendon is then isolated in the medial compartment of the wound. The tendinous portion lies on its deep surface; to expose it, the muscle is everted. The tendinous fibers are divided at two levels (similar to the biceps tendon), leaving the muscle fibers in continuity. Again, by extending the knee and flexing the hip, a sliding lengthening of the semimembranosus is performed.

F. Next, the semitendinosus is exposed. The tendinous portion is divided proximal to the musculotendinous junction.

G. If the semitendinosus tendon inadvertently is ruptured, perform a Z-plasty.

H. The tendon sheath of each tendon is meticulously closed. The deep fascia is not sutured. The subcutaneous tissue and skin are closed in routine manner, and bilateral above-knee casts are applied with the knees in full extension.

Postoperative Care. While the patient is in the solid cast, straight leg raising exercises are performed 15 times, once a day, for further stretching of the hamstrings. At the end of three to four weeks, the casts are removed and new above-knee bivalved casts are made. Active and passive exercises are performed to develop knee flexion, first side-lying with gravity eliminated and then against gravity. The motor strength of the quadriceps is developed. Whenever functional range of motion of the knees is present, the patient is allowed to be ambulatory with appropriate support.

REFERENCE

Green, W. T., and McDermott, L. J.: Operative treatment of cerebral palsy of spastic type. J.A.M.A., 118:434, 1942.

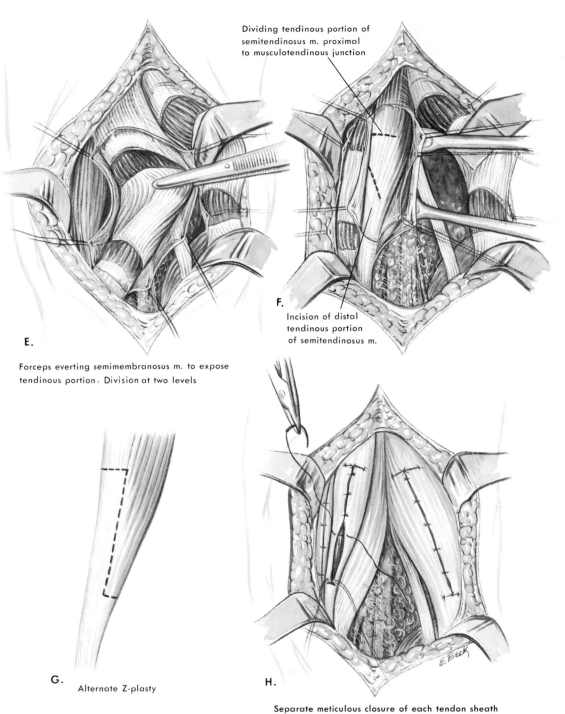

Dividing tendinous portion of
semitendinosus m. proximal
to musculotendinous junction

E.

Forceps everting semimembranosus m. to expose
tendinous portion. Division at two levels

F.

Incision of distal
tendinous portion
of semitendinosus m.

G.   Alternate Z-plasty

H.

Separate meticulous closure of each tendon sheath
Deep fascia is not sutured

Plate 127. (Continued)

PLATE 128 ## Posterior Soft-Tissue Release to Correct Paralytic Knee Flexion Deformity in Myelomeningocele

Indications. Fixed knee flexion deformity that interferes with stance and gait.

Patient Position. The patient is in prone position.

Note: If hip flexion deformity requires surgical correction, first perform the hip surgery with the patient supine, and then turn the patient prone and prepare and redrape for the posterior knee release.

A sterile pneumatic tourniquet is applied on the upper thigh—as high as possible—to minimize blood loss.

Operative Technique

A. Make two longitudinal incisions, one posterolaterally centered over the biceps femoris and the other located posteromedially over the medial border of the semitendinosus. The incisions begin at the popliteal crease and extend proximally for 7 to 10 cm. The subcutaneous tissue and superficial fascia are divided in line with the skin incision.

B. and **C.** Through the lateral incision, identify the common peroneal nerve, medial and deep to the biceps femoris, and gently retract it to prevent injury. Resect two or three long segments of the tendon of biceps femoris and the iliotibial band.

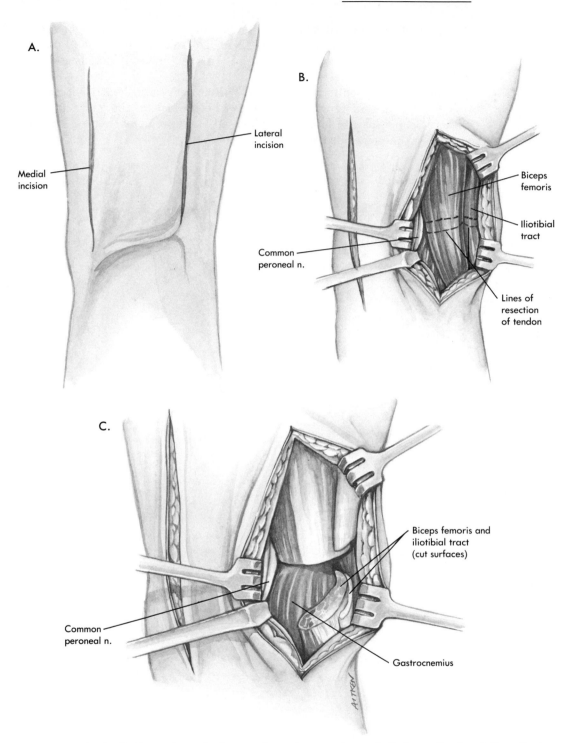

Plate 128. A.–I., Posterior soft-tissue release to correct paralytic knee flexion deformity in myelomeningocele.

D. and **E.** Next, through the medial incision, the tendons of semitendinosus, semimembranosus, and gracilis are identified and isolated, and a 2- to 3-cm. portion of the tendons is resected. Function of the sartorius, if not paralyzed, should be preserved.

Identify the popliteal vessels and tibial nerve and gently retract them.

F. The musculotendinous origins of both heads of the gastrocnemius from the femoral condyles are identified, elevated extraperiosteally, and recessed distally, exposing the posterior capsule of the knee joint.

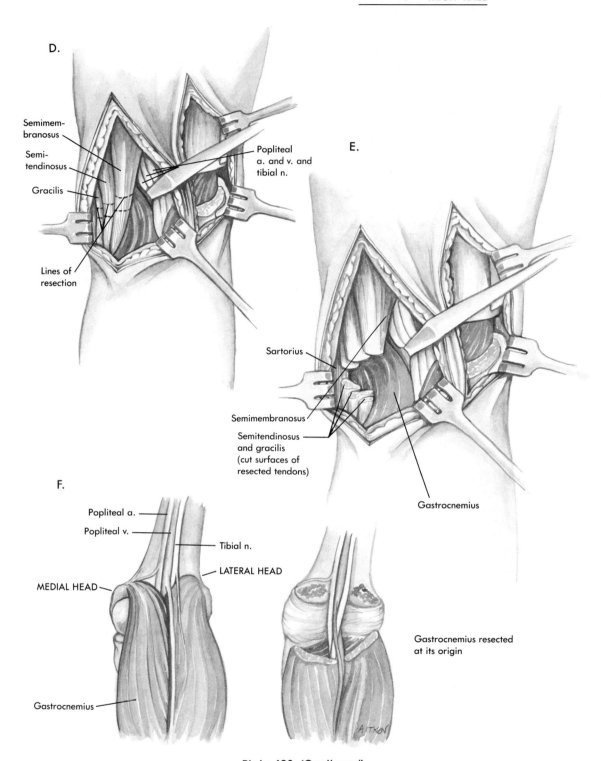

D.

Semimem-
branosus

Semi-
tendinosus

Gracilis

Lines of
resection

Popliteal
a. and v. and
tibial n.

E.

Sartorius

Semimembranosus

Semitendinosus
and gracilis
(cut surfaces of
resected tendons)

Gastrocnemius

F.

Popliteal a.

Popliteal v.

Tibial n.

LATERAL HEAD

MEDIAL HEAD

Gastrocnemius

Gastrocnemius resected
at its origin

Plate 128. (Continued)

G. and **H.** Excise a segment of the posterior capsule of the knee; that is, perform a capsulectomy and *not* a capsulotomy.

Caution! Do not injure the growth plate of the distal femur or proximal tibia.

I. Manipulate the knee joint into maximal extension. If it cannot be extended fully, divide the posterior one third to one half of the medial and lateral collateral ligaments. Identify and carefully section the posterior cruciate ligament. Remanipulate the knee into extension.

At this time, take a true lateral radiograph of the knee in maximal extension in order to confirm and document the degree of correction obtained. Remember, the objective is to achieve full correction of the deformity with 5 to 10 degrees of hyperextension of the knee.

The tourniquet is released, and after complete hemostasis, the wound is closed in routine fashion with Hemovac suction drainage.

Postoperative Care. In the immediate postoperative period, a compression dressing with a plaster posterior splint is applied with the knee in 10 to 30 degrees of flexion to prevent vascular compromise resulting from the postoperative development of hematoma and swelling in the popliteal region. Three to four days after surgery, an above-knee cast is applied, and the knee is maintained in complete extension for two or three weeks. An above-knee posterior night orthosis is then made with the knee in full extension. The night splint is worn for several years.

REFERENCES

Abraham, E., Verinder, D. G. R., and Sharrard, W. J. W.: The treatment of flexion contracture of the knee in myelomeningocele. J. Bone Joint Surg., 59-B:433, 1977.

Birch, R.: Surgery of the knee in children with spina bifida. Dev. Med. Child Neurol. (Suppl. 37), 18:111, 1976.

Dias, L. S.: Surgical management of knee contractures in myelomeningocele. J. Pediatr. Orthop., 2:127, 1982.

Dupré, P. H., and Walker, G. L.: Knee problems associated with spina bifida. Dev. Med. Child Neurol. (Suppl.), 27:152, 1972.

Menelaus, M. B.: The Orthopedic Management of Spina Bifida Cystica. 2nd ed. Edinburgh, Churchill Livingstone, 1980.

G.

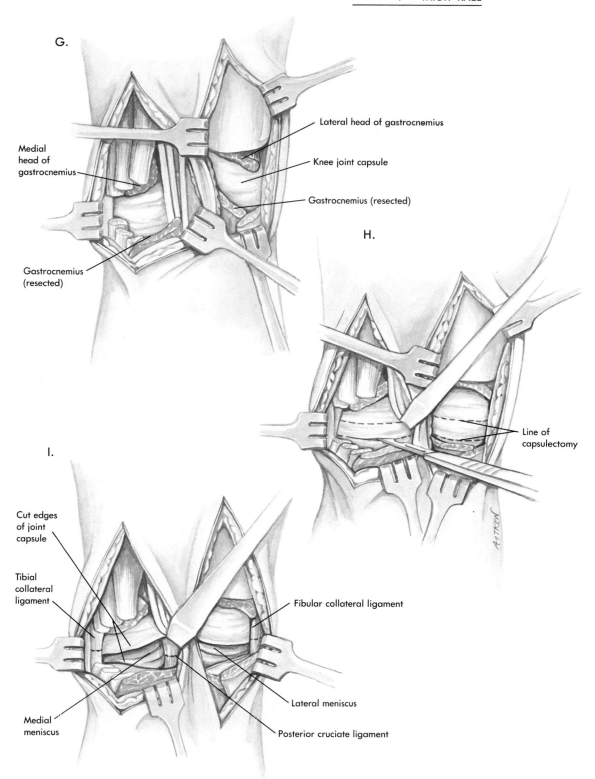

Medial
head of
gastrocnemius

Gastrocnemius
(resected)

Lateral head of gastrocnemius

Knee joint capsule

Gastrocnemius (resected)

H.

Line of
capsulectomy

I.

Cut edges
of joint
capsule

Tibial
collateral
ligament

Medial
meniscus

Fibular collateral ligament

Lateral meniscus

Posterior cruciate ligament

Plate 128. (Continued)

PLATE 129   ## Supracondylar Distal Femoral Extension Osteotomy to Correct Paralytic Flexion Deformity of the Knee in Myelomeningocele

Indications

1. Fixed knee flexion deformity of 20 degrees or more that cannot be corrected by thorough radical soft-tissue release and conservative measures of splinting, posturing, and passive exercise regimens. Soft-tissue release should always be performed first, and then extension osteotomy, to minimize the degree of vertical tilting of the distal femoral articular plane.

2. The patient should be skeletally mature. Do not perform extension osteotomy in the growing child because the chance of recurrence of flexion deformity is great.

Objective

1. The objective of surgery is to correct the flexion deformity fully and to hyperextend the knee.

Caution!

1. Do not be satisfied with partial correction! Document the degree of correction by true lateral radiograms of the knee on the operating table. Use a sterile tourniquet for ischemia to make adequate radiograms.

2. Hip flexion deformity often coexists with knee flexion deformity. Correct the hip flexion deformity first, and knee flexion deformity second. Combine the two procedures so that they are performed with the patient under the same anesthesia episode.

3. Do not transfer the hamstrings anteriorly to the patella. The results are poor.

4. Do not employ stretching-wedging casts because of the hazard of fractures and problems with pressure sores under the cast.

Blood for Transfusion. Yes.

Radiographic Control. Image intensifier.

Patient Position. Supine.

Operative Technique. Soft-tissue release should be performed first and then extension osteotomy if the degree of knee flexion deformity exceeds 20 degrees. Initial soft-tissue release will minimize the degree of vertical tilting of the distal femoral articular plane. Supracondylar distal femoral osteotomy is performed in the adolescent patient who is near skeletal maturity and ambulatory in the community. If the patient is not fully ambulatory, do not intervene surgically because knee flexion contracture will recur with sitting posture.

A. The distal femoral metaphysis and shaft of the femur are exposed through a lateral approach. The incision begins 1 cm. above the joint line and extends proximally for a distance of 7 to 10 cm. Subcutaneous tissue is divided in line with the skin incision. Superficial fascia is incised, and the wound flaps are mobilized and retracted anteriorly and posteriorly. The fascia lata is incised with the skin incision.

B. The vastus lateralis muscle is exposed and elevated and retracted anteriorly.

C. Identify the distal femoral physis with a Keith needle. Do not injure the growth plate. Make a T-shaped incision in the periosteum with its horizontal limb immediately above the growth plate.

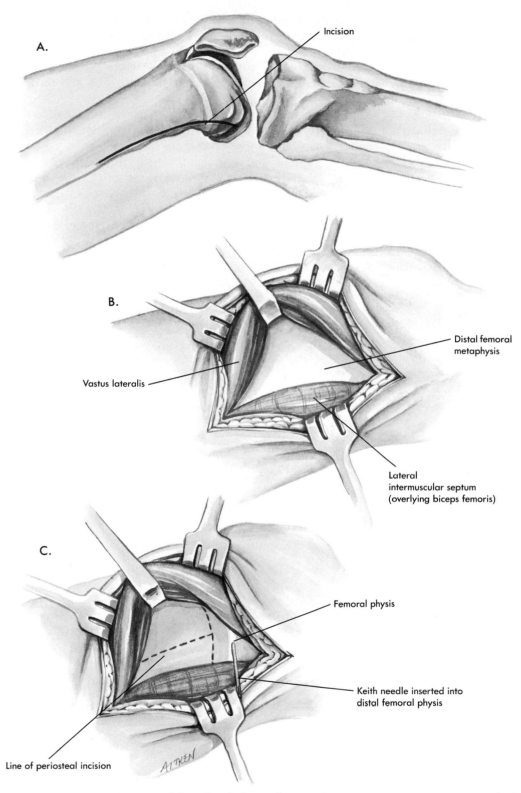

Plate 129. A.–F., Supracondylar distal femoral extension osteotomy to correct paralytic flexion deformity of the knee in myelomeningocele.

D. Expose the distal femoral shaft and metaphysis subperiosteally.

A valgus or varus deformity can be simultaneously corrected by an appropriate modification of the wedge.

E. The wedge of bone is removed, and the bone surfaces are apposed and temporarily fixed with two criss-cross pins. Radiograms are made to verify the degree of correction.

F. If adequate correction of deformity is achieved, internal fixation is carried out with a laterally placed AO or reconstruction plate. Some surgeons may prefer to use internal fixation with three criss-cross large threaded Steinman pins. This allows fixation to be more distal without interfering with growth. This author recommends screw fixation with an AO plate because it allows early mobilization of the knee joint and weight-bearing. Disuse osteoporosis, stress fractures, and knee joint stiffness are thereby circumvented.

The wound is closed in the usual fashion, and a hip spica cast is applied.

Postoperative Care. The cast is removed in two weeks if the fixation is very secure. If fixation is carried out with threaded Steinmann pins, the pins are removed after four weeks, and another cast is applied for an additional two weeks.

REFERENCES

Dias, L. S.: Surgical management of knee contractures in myelomeningocele. J. Pediatr. Orthop., 2:127, 1982.

Menelaus, M. B.: The Orthopedic Management of Spina Bifida Cystica. 2nd ed. Edinburgh, Churchill Livingstone, 1980.

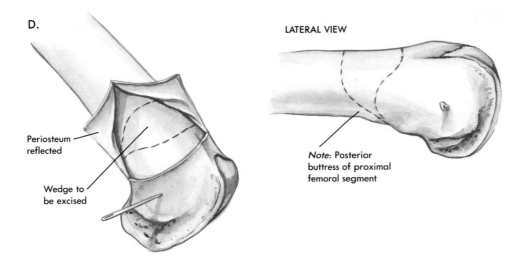

D.

Periosteum reflected

Wedge to be excised

LATERAL VIEW

Note: Posterior buttress of proximal femoral segment

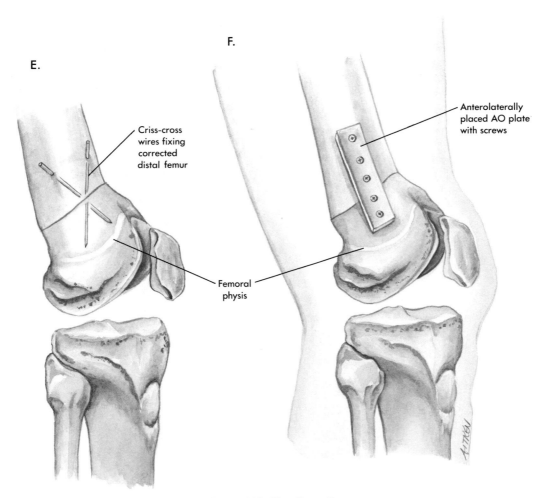

E.

F.

Criss-cross wires fixing corrected distal femur

Femoral physis

Anterolaterally placed AO plate with screws

Plate 129. (Continued)

PLATE 130 ## Ischial-Bearing, Above-Knee (Mid-Thigh) Amputation

Indications

1. Malignant tumor of the limb in which limb salvage is not possible because of the extent of involvement.

2. Major congenital malformation of the leg, such as congenital absence of the tibia, in which a prosthetic conversion is much more functionally desirable.

Preoperative Requisites. The level of amputation is determined by use of a Bell Thompson ruler when the preoperative radiograms are taken. Measurements are made from the top of the greater trochanter and from the knee joint line. If the level of amputation permits, a pneumatic tourniquet or an Esmarch bandage is employed for hemostasis. A sandbag is placed under the ipsilateral buttock.

Blood for Transfusion. Yes.

Patient Position. Supine.

Operative Technique

With methylene blue the following areas are marked: (1) the intended bone level of amputation; (2) the midpoints of the medial and lateral aspects of the thigh 1 cm. above the bony level; and (3) the distal border of the anterior and posterior incisions. The latter is determined by the rule of thumb that the combined length of the anterior and posterior flaps is slightly longer than the diameter of the thigh at the intended bone level and that the length of the anterior flap is 2.5 cm. longer than the posterior flap.

A.–C. The skin incision begins at the midpoint of the medial aspect of the thigh, gently curves anteriorly and inferiorly to the distal border of the anterior incision, and then passes convexly to the midpoint on the lateral aspect of the thigh. The posterior incision starts at the same medial point, extends to the distal margin of the posterior flap, and swings proximally to end at the midpoint of the lateral thigh.

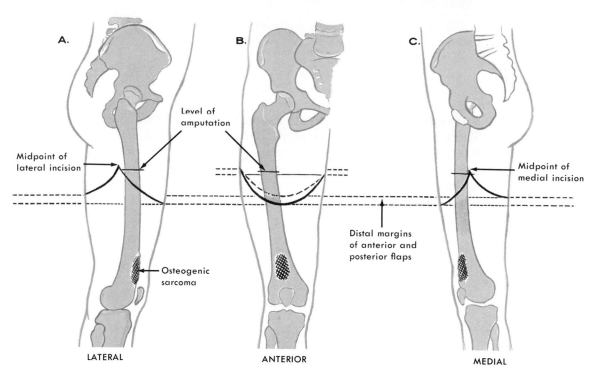

Plate 130. A.–R., Ischial-bearing, above-knee (mid-thigh) amputation.

D. The subcutaneous tissue and deep fascia are divided in line with the skin incision, and the anterior and posterior flaps are reflected proximally to the amputation level.

E.–G. The femoral vessels and saphenous nerve are identified. They are located deep to the sartorius muscle, between the adductor longus and the vastus medialis muscles. The *deep femoral vessels* are found adjacent to the femur in the interval between the adductor magnus, adductor longus, and vastus medialis muscles. There are variations in the origin of the deep femoral artery, as shown in G. The femoral artery and vein are isolated, doubly ligated with heavy nonabsorbable sutures, and divided. The saphenous nerve is pulled distally and divided with a sharp scalpel. If the amputation level is high, the deep femoral vessels may be ligated and divided through this anteromedial approach.

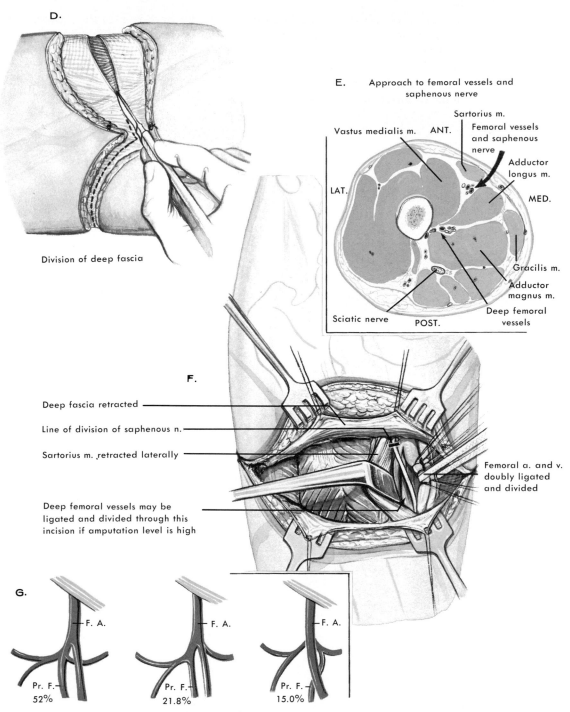

D.

Division of deep fascia

E.   Approach to femoral vessels and saphenous nerve

Vastus medialis m.   ANT.   Sartorius m.

Femoral vessels and saphenous nerve

Adductor longus m.

LAT.   MED.

Gracilis m.

Adductor magnus m.

Sciatic nerve   POST.   Deep femoral vessels

F.

Deep fascia retracted

Line of division of saphenous n.

Sartorius m. retracted laterally

Deep femoral vessels may be ligated and divided through this incision if amputation level is high

Femoral a. and v. doubly ligated and divided

G.

F. A.   F. A.   F. A.

Pr. F.— 52%   Pr. F.— 21.8%   Pr. F.— 15.0%

Variations in origin of deep femoral artery.

Plate 130. (Continued)

H. and **I.** Next, the hip is acutely flexed for approach to the posterior structures. The sciatic nerve is exposed in the interval between the medial hamstrings medially and the long head of the biceps femoris laterally. With a Kocher forceps, it is pulled distally, doubly ligated, and sharply divided over a tongue blade.

J. and **K.** The posterior approach to the deep femoral vessels is used when the level of amputation is distal.

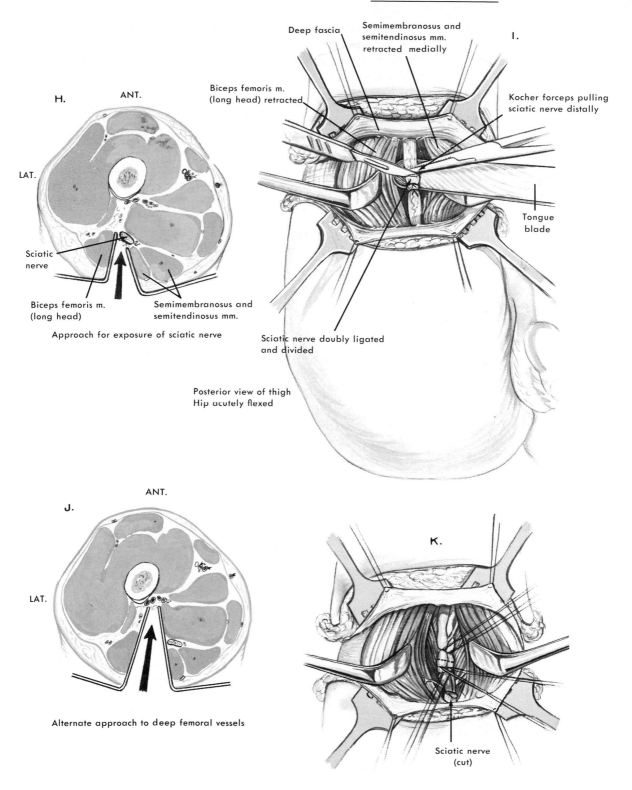

H.

ANT.

LAT.

Sciatic nerve

Biceps femoris m. (long head)

Semimembranosus and semitendinosus mm.

Approach for exposure of sciatic nerve

Deep fascia

Semimembranosus and semitendinosus mm. retracted medially

Biceps femoris m. (long head) retracted

I.

Kocher forceps pulling sciatic nerve distally

Tongue blade

Sciatic nerve doubly ligated and divided

Posterior view of thigh Hip acutely flexed

J.

ANT.

LAT.

Alternate approach to deep femoral vessels

K.

Sciatic nerve (cut)

Deep femoral vessels doubly ligated and lines of division

Plate 130. (Continued)

L. With an amputation knife, the quadriceps and adductor muscles are sectioned and beveled upward to the site of bone division so that the anterior myofascial flap is approximately 1.5 cm. thick. The posterior muscles are divided transversely. Muscular branches of the femoral vessels are clamped and ligated, as necessary.

M. The proximal muscles are retracted upward with an amputation shield, and the periosteum is incised circumferentially.

N. The femur is sectioned with a saw immediately distal to the periosteal incision.

O. With a rongeur, the prominence of the linea aspera is excised, and the bone end is made smooth with a file. The wound is irrigated with normal saline solution to wash away all loose fragments of bone.

L.   Division of muscles

M.

Circular incision of periosteum of femur

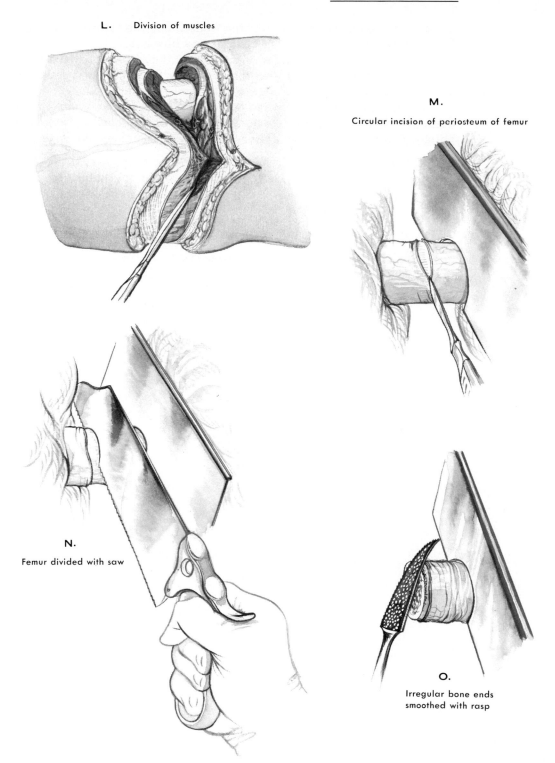

N.

Femur divided with saw

O.

Irregular bone ends
smoothed with rasp

Plate 130. (Continued)

P. Hot packs are applied over the wound, and the tourniquet is released. After five minutes, the stump is inspected for any bleeders.

Q. The anterior and posterior myofascial flaps are pulled distally and approximated with interrupted sutures through their fascial layer. Suction catheters are placed in the wound and connected to a Hemovac evacuator.

R. The subcutaneous tissue and skin are closed in the usual manner. Immediate prosthetic fitting in the operating room is employed by the author, and the patient is allowed to be ambulatory on the first postoperative day.

Postoperative Care. The patient is fitted with a temporary prosthesis as soon as possible. When the wound is healed and the stump is comfortable, usually within four to six weeks, the patient is fitted with a permanent prosthesis.

REFERENCE

Slocum, D. B.: An Atlas of Amputations. St. Louis, C.V. Mosby, 1949.

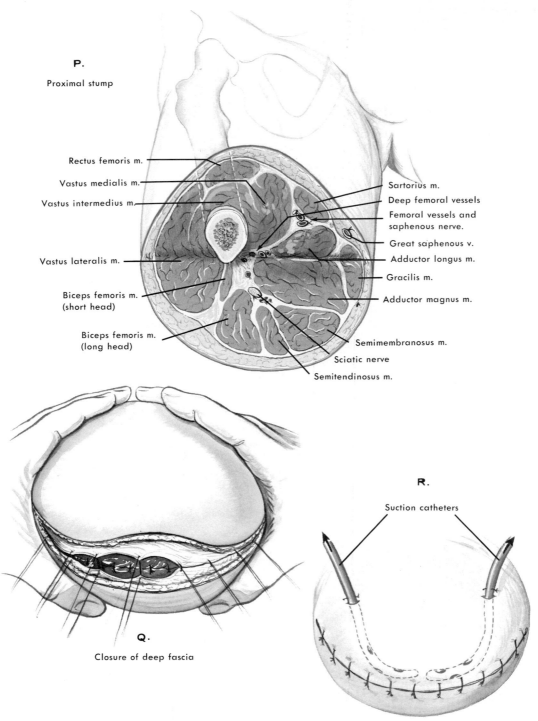

P.

Proximal stump

Rectus femoris m.

Vastus medialis m.

Vastus intermedius m.

Vastus lateralis m.

Biceps femoris m.
(short head)

Biceps femoris m.
(long head)

Sartorius m.

Deep femoral vessels

Femoral vessels and
saphenous nerve.

Great saphenous v.

Adductor longus m.

Gracilis m.

Adductor magnus m.

Semimembranosus m.

Sciatic nerve

Semitendinosus m.

Q.

Closure of deep fascia

R.

Suction catheters

Skin edges approximated and closed

Plate 130. (Continued)

PLATE 131   Disarticulation at the Knee Joint

Indications. Malignant tumor of the lower limb in which limb salvage is not possible because of the extent of involvement. Unilateral or bilateral congenital absence of the tibia.

Blood for Transfusion. Yes.

Patient Position. The patient is placed in the lateral position, which allows easy turning into a supine, prone, or semilateral posture. The operation is performed under pneumatic tourniquet ischemia.

Operative Technique

A. The skin incisions are placed in such a manner that they provide a long anterior flap and a short posterior flap; thus, the operative scar is posterior and away from the weight-bearing skin. Measuring from the distal pole of the patella to the distal border, the length of the anterior flap is equal to the anteroposterior diameter of the knee, whereas the posterior flap is half the length of the anterior flap. The medial and lateral proximal points of the incisions are at the joint line at the junction of the anterior two thirds and posterior one third of the diameter of the knee. The anterior and posterior wound flaps are raised, including the subcutaneous tissue and the deep fascia.

B. The medial aspects of the knee joint and the proximal tibia are exposed. Tendons of the sartorius, gracilis, semimembranosus, and semitendinosus muscles are identified and marked with 00 Tycron whip sutures, then sectioned near their insertions on the tibia. The ligamentum patellae is detached at the proximal tibial tubercle. The anterior and medial joint capsule and synovial membrane are divided proximally near the femoral condyles.

C. Next, the lateral aspect of the knee joint is exposed. The iliotibial tract is divided and the biceps femoris tendon is sectioned from its attachment to the head of the fibula. The lateral part of the joint capsule and synovial membrane is divided above the joint line.

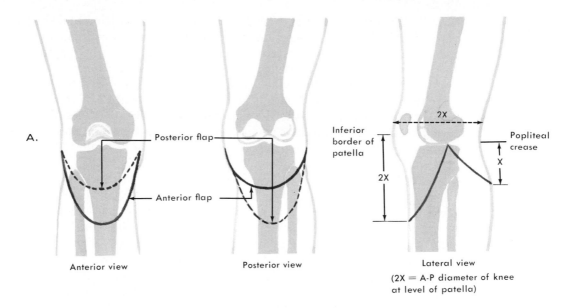

A.

Posterior flap

Anterior flap

Anterior view

Posterior view

Inferior border of patella

2X

Popliteal crease

X

2X

Lateral view
(2X = A-P diameter of knee
at level of patella)

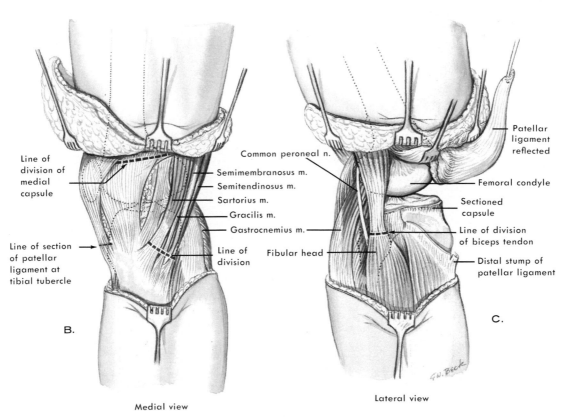

Line of division of medial capsule

Line of section of patellar ligament at tibial tubercle

B.

Common peroneal n.

Semimembranosus m.

Semitendinosus m.

Sartorius m.

Gracilis m.

Gastrocnemius m.

Line of division

Medial view

Patellar ligament reflected

Femoral condyle

Sectioned capsule

Line of division of biceps tendon

Fibular head

Distal stump of patellar ligament

C.

Lateral view

Plate 131. A.–G., Disarticulation at the knee joint.

D. Now the patient is turned to the semiprone position and the popliteal fossa is exposed. By blunt dissection the popliteal vessels are identified; the popliteal artery and vein are separately doubly ligated distal to the origin of the superior genicular branches and divided. The tibial nerve and common peroneal nerve are pulled distally, sharply divided with a scalpel, and allowed to retract proximally. The medial and lateral heads of the gastrocnemius are extraperiosteally elevated and stripped from the posterior aspect of the femoral condyles. The distal femoral epiphyseal plate should not be damaged. The plantaris and popliteus muscles, the oblique popliteal ligament, the posterior part of the capsule of the knee joint, and the meniscofemoral ligaments are completely divided.

E. Next, the patient is turned to a semisupine position and the knee is acutely flexed. The cruciate ligaments are identified and sectioned, completing the amputation. The pneumatic tourniquet is released and complete hemostasis is secured.

F. The patellar ligament is sutured to the medial and lateral hamstrings in the intercondylar notch. In children, the patella is usually not removed and reshaping of the femoral condyles should not be performed because of the danger of damage to the growth plate. Synovectomy is not indicated.

G. Two catheters are placed in the wound for closed suction. The deep fascia and subcutaneous tissue of the anterior and posterior flaps are approximated with interrupted sutures, and the skin is closed in routine fashion.

Postoperative Care. The patient is fitted with a temporary prosthesis as soon as possible and is placed on active and passive exercises to develop motor strength of the muscles controlling the thigh and hip. A permanent prosthesis is fitted when the wound is healed, the swelling has subsided, and the patient is comfortable.

REFERENCES

Batch, J. W., Spittler, A. W., and McFaddin, J. G.: Advantages of the knee disarticulation over amputations through the thigh. J. Bone Joint Surg., 36-A:921, 1954.

Mazet, R., Jr., and Hennessy, C. A.: Knee disarticulation: A new technique and a new knee-joint mechanism. J. Bone Joint Surg., 48-A:126, 1966.

Rogers, S. P.: Amputation at the knee joint. J. Bone Joint Surg., 22:973, 1940.

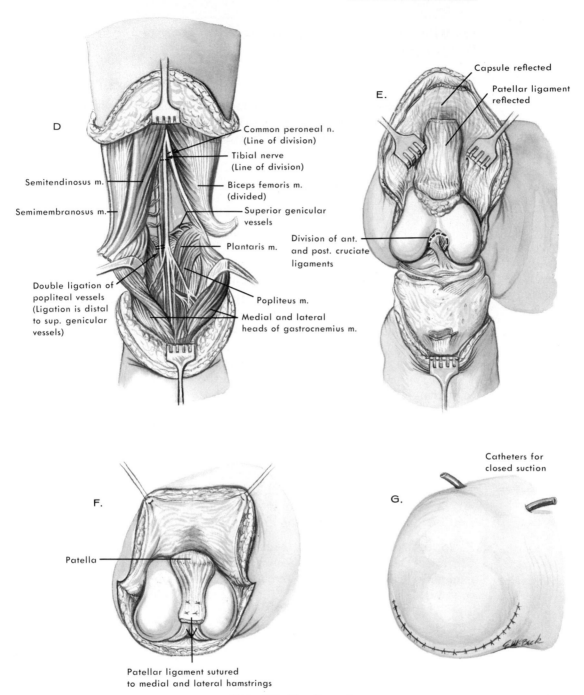

D

Semitendinosus m.

Semimembranosus m.

Double ligation of popliteal vessels (Ligation is distal to sup. genicular vessels)

Common peroneal n. (Line of division)

Tibial nerve (Line of division)

Biceps femoris m. (divided)

Superior genicular vessels

Plantaris m.

Popliteus m.

Medial and lateral heads of gastrocnemius m.

E.

Capsule reflected

Patellar ligament reflected

Division of ant. and post. cruciate ligaments

F.

Patella

Patellar ligament sutured to medial and lateral hamstrings

G.

Catheters for closed suction

Plate 131. (Continued)

PLATE 132   **Excision of Osteochondroma from the Medial Aspect of the Distal Femoral Metaphysis**

Indications

1. Interference with knee joint motion because of pressure and irritation of the vastus medialis or medial hamstrings.
2. Painful adventitious bursa because of overlying osteochondroma.
3. Progressive enlargement and pain.
4. Deformity.
5. Suspicion of sarcomatous transformation.

The mere presence of osteochondroma is not an indication for surgery.

Patient Position. Supine with a pneumatic tourniquet on the proximal thigh.

Operative Technique

A. A longitudinal incision is made over the protruding mass. Subcutaneous tissue and deep fascia are divided in line with the skin incision.

Caution! Do not injure the saphenous nerve.

B. The vastus medialis muscle is split in the direction of its fibers.

C. By blunt dissection, the tumor is exposed, leaving the bursal sac and the perichondrium attached to the osteochondroma undisturbed.

D. The periosteum is incised around the base of the tumor. Next, with curved and straight osteotomes, the exostosis with its perichondrium is excised. Drill holes may be made to delineate the base of the tumor. Anteroposterior and lateral radiograms are made to verify that the exostosis is excised completely. The base of the tumor is curetted. With electrocautery the raw cancellous bone is burned to destroy possible cartilaginous growth cells. Bone wax is applied for hemostasis. The tourniquet is released, and complete hemostasis is achieved. A medium Hemovac suction tube is inserted.

E. The vastus medialis muscle and fascia are sutured. The skin is closed in routine manner. A compression dressing or an above-knee cylinder cast is applied.

Postoperative Care. The cast is removed 3 to 4 weeks after surgery. Active assisted exercises are performed to restore range of knee motion. Progressive resistive exercises are performed to strengthen the quadriceps femoris and hamstring muscles.

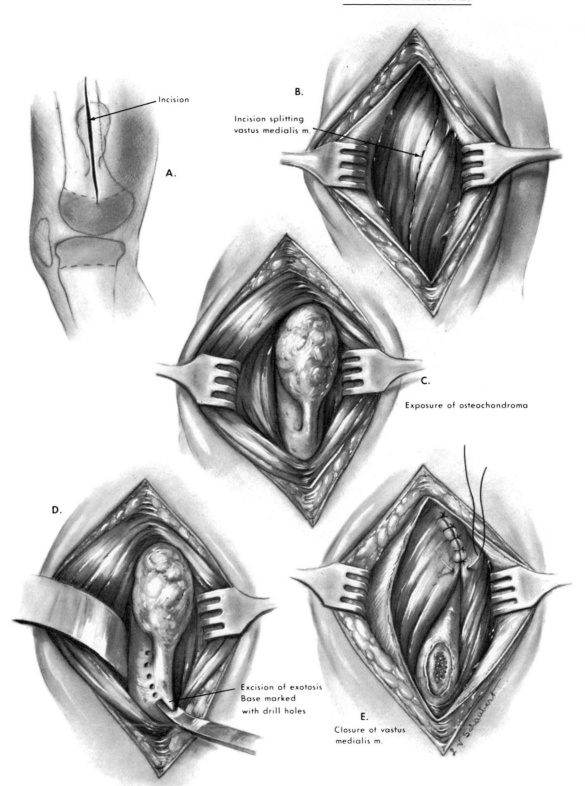

Incision

A.

B.

Incision splitting
vastus medialis m.

C.

Exposure of osteochondroma

D.

Excision of exotosis
Base marked
with drill holes

E.

Closure of vastus
medialis m.

Plate 132. **A.–E.,** Excision of osteochondroma from the medial aspect of the distal femoral
metaphysis.

PLATE   133   ## Epiphyseodesis of the Distal Femur (Green Modification of Phemister Technique)

Indications. Projected leg length inequality of 5 cm. or less at skeletal maturity in a person of average stature.

Radiographic Control. Image intensifier.

Patient Position. Supine with pneumatic tourniquet on proximal thigh.

Operative Technique

A. The knee is supported in 20 to 30 degrees of flexion, and the joint line is identified. First, the medial aspect of the distal femur is exposed. Beginning 1 cm. superior to the joint line, a longitudinal incision about 5 to 7 cm. long is made midway between the anterior and posterior margins of the femoral condyles. The subcutaneous tissue and deep fascia are divided in line with the skin incision.

B. Following the anterior surface of the medial intermuscular septum, the vastus medialis muscle is lifted anteriorly with a blunt periosteal elevator. The suprapatellar pouch should not be entered. In the inferior margin of the wound, the capsule and reflected synovial membrane of the knee joint are gently elevated and retracted with blunt instruments distally.

Caution! Do not open the joint. If the synovial membrane is inadvertently divided, which will be indicated by oozing of synovial fluid, it is closed by 00 Vicryl continuous suture. The superior medial genicular vessels traverse the wound; it is best to coagulate them to prevent troublesome bleeding later.

C. A midline longitudinal incision is made in the periosteum, starting proximally and extending throughout the extent of the wound.

D. The medial distal femoral physis is exposed by raising anterior and posterior flaps of periosteum by subperiosteal dissection; it appears as a white, glistening transverse line that is softer than adjacent cancellous bone. Some surgeons prefer to make a longitudinal I-shaped incision in the periosteum to expose the growth plate; the author, however, prefers a simple longitudinal incision, as it permits a more taut periosteal closure. The periosteum is gently retracted by 00 Tycron sutures on its borders. Rough traction and shredding of the periosteum should be avoided. If necessary, Chandler elevators are placed subperiosteally on the anterior and posterior aspects of the distal femur for adequate exposure. Dull right-angled retractors are used for proximal and distal retraction.

E. and F. With matched pairs of osteotomes, a rectangular piece of bone 1⅛ to 1½ inches long and ½ to ⅝ inch wide is excised. The epiphyseal plate should be at the junction of the distal one third and proximal two thirds of the length of bone graft resected, at a point equidistant between the anterior and posterior surfaces of the femur. The posterior cortex of the femur should not be broken. The depth of the bone graft is ½ to ¾ inch (the blood at the tip of the osteotome will mark its depth of penetration into bone). Because of the flare of the femoral condyles, the anterior and posterior osteotomes should be tilted somewhat distally so that they are perpendicular to the medial surface of the femur. Following removal of the osteotomes, the completeness of osteotomy is checked with a thin (⅜- or ¼-inch) osteotome. Then, the graft is removed with curved osteotomes. Breakage of the graft at the physis is prevented by straddling the growth plate with the osteotomes.

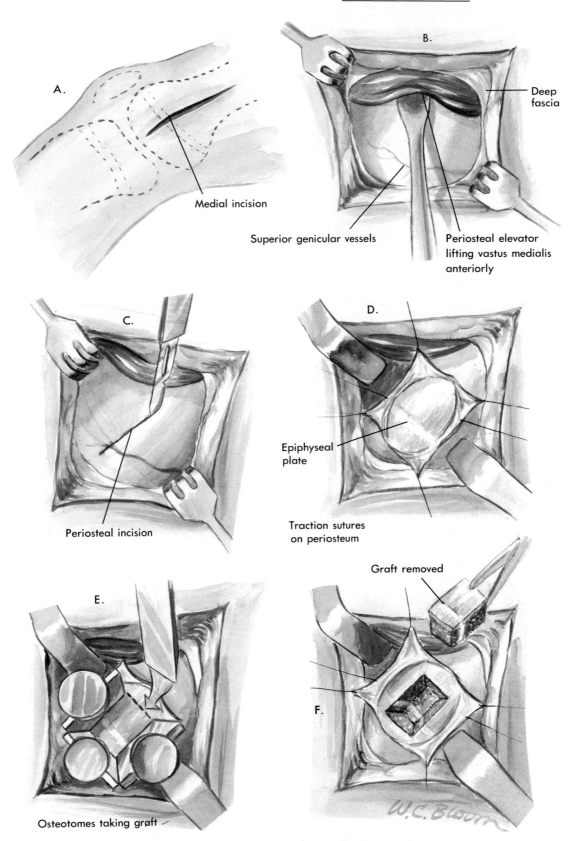

A.

Medial incision

B.

Deep fascia

Superior genicular vessels

Periosteal elevator lifting vastus medialis anteriorly

C.

Periosteal incision

D.

Epiphyseal plate

Traction sutures on periosteum

E.

Osteotomes taking graft

F.

Graft removed

W.C.Bloom

Plate 133. A.–L., Epiphyseodesis of the distal femur (Green modification of Phemister technique).

G. The growth plate is drilled with diamond-shaped drills of increasing size in anterior, posterior, and distal directions. A hand drill provides better control and feel of depth. It should be remembered that the distal femoral physis is pointed inferiorly. The softness of the cartilaginous plate serves as a guide to its direction. Then, with a small curet, removal of the growth plate is completed, the debris of cartilage and bone being saved for later packing around the proximal end of the graft. Curettage should extend to the periphery of the growth plate, avoiding the popliteal vessels posteriorly.

H. Cancellous bone graft is taken from the proximal bed and packed into the defect created by removal of the growth plate.

I. The bone graft is then reinserted into its original bed, with its ends reversed by 180-degree rotation.

J. With an impacter and mallet, the bone graft is securely seated in the bony defect. It should be tapped in a distal direction, as the growth plate is inferior in location.

K. The periosteum is tightly closed with interrupted sutures. It is important not to include the patellar retinaculum with the periosteum, as this will bind it down, restricting knee motion. Suture the periosteum with the knee in complete extension.

L. The same procedure is repeated on the lateral side. Before closure of the wounds, the position of the medial bone graft is checked to be sure it has not been dislodged by the tapping on the opposite side. The tourniquet is released. Complete hemostasis is achieved with electrocautery. The wound is closed in the usual fashion.

Postoperative Care. The limb is immobilized in an above-knee cylinder cast with the knee in neutral position or 5 degrees of flexion for a total of four weeks. The foot and ankle are left out of the cast and the patient is allowed to walk with crutches (three-point gait) as soon as he or she is comfortable. Because the long leg is in an extended position in the cast, appropriate lifts are placed on the shoe on the short side so that the patient can clear the leg with the cast.

Before the patient is discharged, it is best to make radiograms of the distal femur, taken through the cast, to record the integrity of bony continuity and the position of the reversed bone plugs. The cast usually becomes loose in 10 to 14 days. The cast and sutures are removed two weeks after surgery, and a new snug cast is applied. A common pitfall is the failure to extend the cast proximally enough on the the thigh. Torsional stress on the distal femur should be prevented.

Following removal of the cast, the knee is mobilized by side-lying flexion-extension exercises to develop motor strength in the quadriceps femoris muscle. Crutch support is discontinued when there is 90 degrees of knee flexion and the quadriceps muscle is fair in motor power. Radiograms of the distal femur are made six weeks and three months following surgery to be sure that fusion of the growth plate has taken place. Lower limb length studies are performed at three-month intervals during the first year, and then at six-month intervals until completion of growth.

REFERENCES

Green, W. T., and Anderson, M.: Experiences with epiphyseal arrest in correcting discrepancies in length of the lower extremities in infantile paralysis. J. Bone Joint Surg., 29:659, 1947.

Green, W. T., and Anderson, M.: Discrepancy in length of the lower extremities. A.A.O.S. Instructional Course Lecture, 8:294, 1951.

Green, W. T., and Anderson, M.: Epiphyseal arrest for the correction of discrepancies in length of the lower extremities. J. Bone Joint Surg., 39-A:353, 1957.

Phemister, D. B.: Operative arrestment of longitudinal growth of bones in the treatment of deformities. J. Bone Joint Surg., 15:1, 1933.

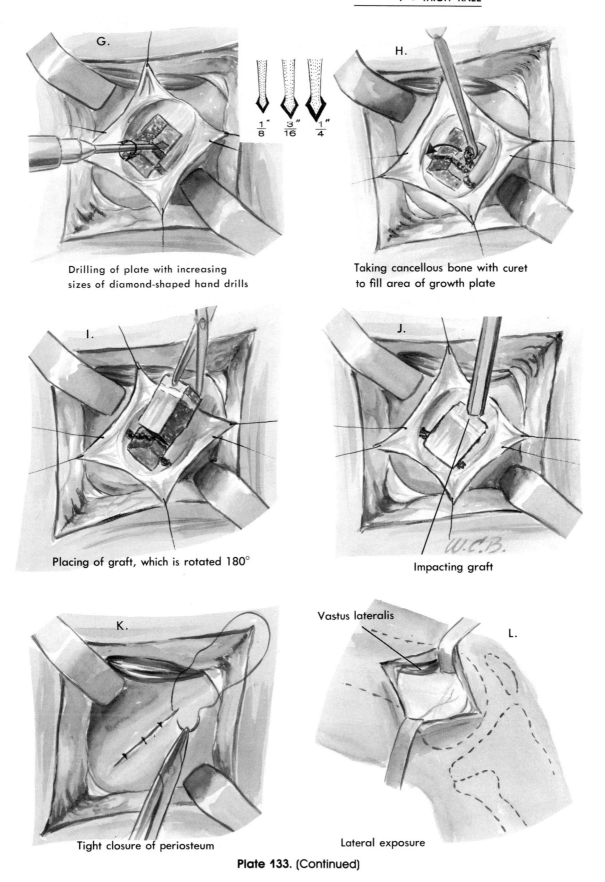

G.

Drilling of plate with increasing
sizes of diamond-shaped hand drills

$\frac{1}{8}"$ $\frac{3}{16}"$ $\frac{1}{4}"$

H.

Taking cancellous bone with curet
to fill area of growth plate

I.

Placing of graft, which is rotated 180°

J.

Impacting graft

K.

Tight closure of periosteum

L.

Vastus lateralis

Lateral exposure

Plate 133. (Continued)

PLATE 134   Percutaneous Epiphyseodesis

Indications. Limb length inequality of less than 5 cm.

Advantages. The percutaneous approach is preferred by surgeons because the scar is small and cosmetically more pleasing and the surgical dissection is of a lesser magnitude than that used in the classic Phemister-Green epiphyseodesis. Postoperatively, cast immobilization is ordinarily not required.

Disadvantages. There is a higher incidence of failure of fusion and asymmetrical growth arrest with consequent genu varum, genu valgum, or genu recurvatum deformity. The patient and parents should understand the potential for these complications and the possibility that future surgery will be necessary for correction.

Radiographic Control. Image intensifier.

Special Instrumentation. Cannulated reamer, power drill, and dental bur.

Choice of Procedure. At present, the Canale technique and the Bowen technique are used in North America. The Macnicol tube saw technique is used in Great Britain.

CANALE TECHNIQUE

Patient Position. The patient is placed supine on a radiolucent operating table or a fracture table. The procedure is performed with image-intensifier radiographic control, visualizing the growth plate in several planes by rotation of the image intensifier.

Operative Technique

A. Under image-intensifier radiographic control, identify the level of the distal femur or proximal tibial growth plates medially and laterally with a guide pin. With a scalpel, make a longitudinal incision, 5 to 10 mm. in length, medially and laterally centered over the growth plate.

Subcutaneous tissue and superficial fascia are divided in line with the skin incision, and with Metzenbaum or blunt scissors, the soft tissues are split down to the bone.

B. A drill sleeve is inserted through the stab wound, straight down to the growth plate, and its exact position is determined by image intensifier radiograms. Through the drill sleeve, a small Kirschner wire is drilled into the growth plate as deep as its midportion.

C. Remove the drill sleeve and introduce a 4-mm. cannulated reamer over the Kirschner wire and ream the physis to its midportion.

D. Remove the reamer and the Kirschner wire, and insert various sizes and angles of pneumatic burs, that is, dental drills or Hall air drills, up to 3 mm. in size. Remember the undulation of the growth plate: the distal femur points distally and the proximal tibial plate points proximally. Drill not only from outside in but also superiorly and inferiorly. Use image-intensifier radiographic control.

Caution! Do not violate the cortex and injure neurovascular structures!

The objective is to create a bony bridge to stop growth across the physis. It is not necessary to drill the entire physis anterior to posterior, especially as visualized in the lateral projection on the image intensifier.

The wound is irrigated copiously with saline, and one small absorbable suture is used for closure of the skin.

A similar technique is used to obliterate the distal femoral physis laterally.

Postoperative Care. The knee is immobilized in a knee immobilizer or a cylinder cast for three weeks. Weight-bearing is allowed as soon as the patient is comfortable.

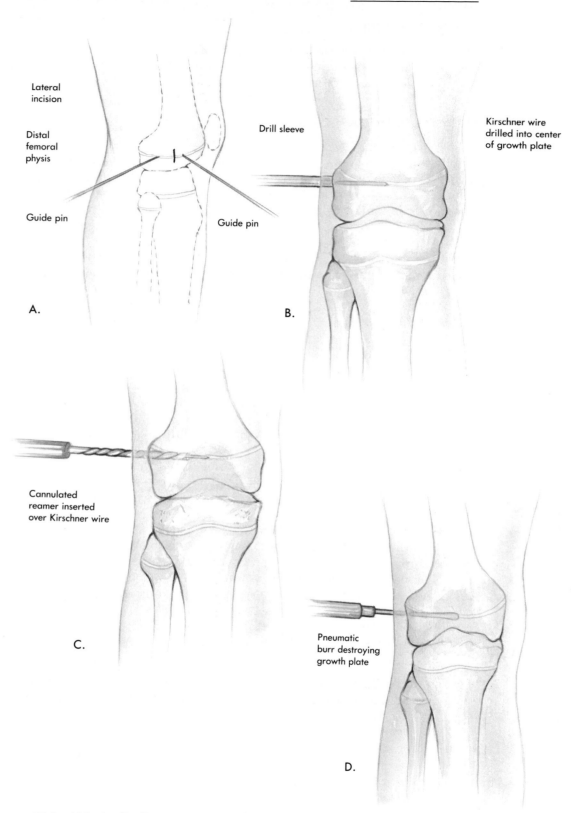

A.

Lateral incision

Distal femoral physis

Guide pin

Guide pin

B.

Drill sleeve

Kirschner wire drilled into center of growth plate

C.

Cannulated reamer inserted over Kirschner wire

D.

Pneumatic burr destroying growth plate

Plate 134. A.–O., Percutaneous epiphyseodesis. Canale technique, Bowen technique, and epiphyseodesis by tube saw (Macnicol technique).

BOWEN TECHNIQUE

Patient Position. The patient is placed supine on a radiolucent operating table, and the procedure is performed under image-intensifier radiographic control. The objective of the surgery is to ablate the medial and lateral thirds of the growth plate and to preserve the central one third for stability.

Operative Technique

E. Rectangular pieces of growth plate with the adjoining metaphysis and epiphysis are removed, with the peripheral side being the bony cortex and the deep side extending to the depth of one third of the growth plate. The superior and inferior sides of the rectangle extend equidistant into the epiphysis or one half the distance from the articular surface to the growth plate.

F. With the knee in complete extension, under image-intensifier radiographic control, make a 3-mm. stab incision medially and laterally at the level of the growth plate. First, the lateral side is operated upon, and then the medial side. Introduce a 3-mm. wide osteotome into the stab wound. Verify its level under image intensification and drive it 1 cm. into the growth plate.

G. Rotate the osteotome 180 degrees and create a hole in the cortex.

H. A 3 mm. wide oval curet is introduced through the hole in the cortex to the depth of the rectangular area as shown in **E**.

Forcefully ablate the rectangular area by sweeping the curet superiorly and inferiorly across the growth plate. Withdraw the curet slowly during the sweeping action. Verify each sweep of the curet by image intensifier to ensure that the growth plate is ablated. Be sure that the cortical margins are thoroughly removed. The anteroposterior width of the rectangular area ablated should be at least 1 cm. wide. Ordinarily, three passes of the curet will achieve the proper width and depth of the desired area of ablation.

Caution! Do not penetrate the posterior cortex and damage the neurovascular structures!

I. Inject 3 ml. of radiopaque contrast material (Renografin 60) into the ablated area. The purpose of this step is to determine the amount of growth plate ablated in both the anteroposterior and mediolateral planes.

The technique of injection of Renografin is as follows: Place a 21-gauge spinal needle through the center of the longitudinal axis of a piece of rolled gauze, 5 cm. long. The needle should protrude beyond the edge of the gauze. Insert the needle through the stab wound into the depth of the ablated rectangular area. Press the gauze against the skin over the stab wound incision to prevent leakage of the contrast material into the subcutaneous tissue, and slowly inject the contrast material into the ablated growth plate. Make permanent radiograms. The stab wound is closed with one absorbable suture. A compression dressing is applied.

Postoperative Care. A knee immobilizer is used, and full weight-bearing is allowed with three-point crutch protection. Knee immobilization is continued for at least three or four weeks.

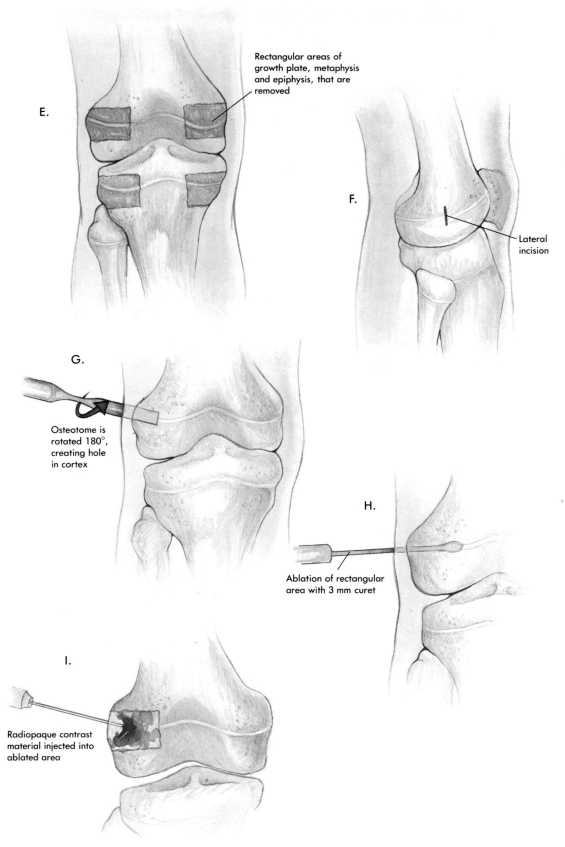

E.

Rectangular areas of
growth plate, metaphysis
and epiphysis, that are
removed

F.

Lateral
incision

G.

Osteotome is
rotated 180°,
creating hole
in cortex

H.

Ablation of rectangular
area with 3 mm curet

I.

Radiopaque contrast
material injected into
ablated area

Plate 134. (Continued)

EPIPHYSEODESIS BY TUBE SAW (MACNICOL TECHNIQUE)

Patient Position. The patient is placed supine on a radiolucent operating table, and image-intensifier radiographic control is used during the procedure. Tourniquet ischemia is used to control bleeding.

Operative Technique

J. Make a 2-cm. longitudinal incision over the lateral aspect of the distal femur centered over the growth plate and midway between the anterior and posterior cortices of the bone. Subcutaneous tissue is divided in line with the skin incision. Superficial and deep fascia are incised, and with the help of dull Metzenbaum scissors, the soft tissues are separated and the distal femoral physis is identified under image-intensifier radiographic control.

K. The perichondrium over the growth plate and the adjoining periosteum are incised, and a 3.2-mm. guide wire is inserted with a hand drill across the physis. The growth plate offers the least resistance as compared to bone. The position of the guide wire is double-checked by anteroposterior, lateral, and oblique radiographic projections of the distal femur.

L. A centralizing cylinder is applied over the guide wire to help direct the 10-mm. diameter cannulated tube saw along the extent of the growth plate.

M. A cylinder of cancellous bone and growth plate is cored out until the opposite cortex is breached. The tube saw is inserted by hand using a Jacobs chuck and not a power drill. The contralateral medial cortex of the femur is carefully palpated as the tube saw is advanced across the growth plate.

N. The guide wire is then removed, and the tube saw is withdrawn. A plunger is used to extrude a column of contained bone and cartilage.

O. With a curet, remove a portion of growth plate and adjoining cancellous and metaphyseal bone. The plug of bone is replaced into the defect. The subcutaneous tissue is closed with 000 Vicryl interrupted sutures, and the skin is closed with Steri-Strips. The proximal tibial and fibular physes are arrested through a lateral incision centered over their growth plates.

Postoperative Care. Immobilization is not required. A removable knee immobilizer may be applied for a few days for comfort. Knee motion and strength are rapidly restored, and disability is minimal.

REFERENCES

Bowen, J. R., and Johnson, W. J.: Percutaneous epiphyseodesis. Clin. Orthop., 190:170, 1984.

Canale, S. T., Russell, T. A., and Holcomb, R. I.: Percutaneous epiphyseodesis. J. Pediatr. Orthop., 6:150, 1986.

Macnicol, M. F.: Epiphyseodesis by tube saw. Personal communication. 1992.

Ogilvie, J. W.: Epiphysiodesis: Evaluation of a new technique. J. Pediatr. Orthop., 6:147, 1986.

Timperlake, R. W., Bowen, J. R., Guille, J. T., and In Ho Choi: Prospective evaluation of fifty-three consecutive percutaneous epiphysiodeses of the distal femur and proximal tibia and fibula. J. Pediatr. Orthop., 11:350, 1991.

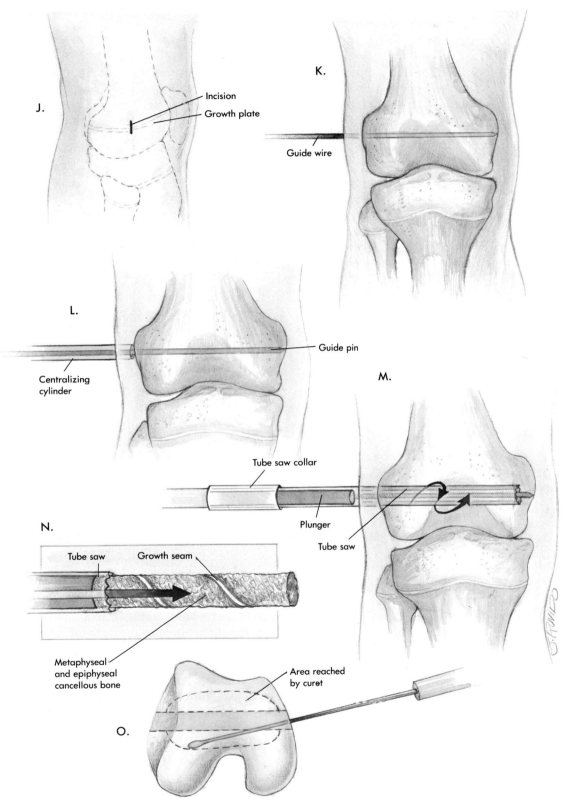

J.

Incision

Growth plate

K.

Guide wire

L.

Centralizing
cylinder

Guide pin

M.

Tube saw collar

Plunger

Tube saw

N.

Tube saw   Growth seam

Metaphyseal
and epiphyseal
cancellous bone

Area reached
by curet

O.

Plate 134. (Continued)

PLATE 135

Angular Osteotomy of the Distal Femur to Correct Genu Valgum or Varum

Indications. Moderate or severe angular deformity with significant loss of anatomic-biomechanical axis of the lower limb due to asymmetrical growth disturbance as a result of trauma, bone dysplasia or rickets, or infection.

Requisites. Meticulous preoperative planning is vital.

1. Make standing, weight-bearing films with the lower limbs as straight and symmetrical as possible. Make long radiograms that include hips, knees, and ankles. In difficult problems, the surgeon should personally supervise accurate positioning of the patient. Determine the exact degree of angular deformity and deviation from the mechanical axis. (See Appendix, Plate 251.)

2. Rule out anterior or posterior angulation deformity of one or both femoral condyles. What is the exact degree of genu recurvatum or flexion deformity of the knee? Each component of deformity should be corrected.

3. Is there rotational alignment? Inspect the foot progression angle. Is the child toeing-in or toeing-out? Often it is advisable to determine the exact degree of femoral antetorsion and tibial torsion by computed tomography (CT).

4. Joint laxity should be ruled out clinically and by medial and lateral stress anteroposterior radiograms of the knee. Failure to assess the ligamentous laxity component of angular deformity at the knee is a common pitfall. Stress views of the knee may be combined with arthrography. When internal derangement of the knee is suspected, magnetic resonance imaging (MRI) of the knees may be indicated.

5. Determine lower limb length. Varus or valgus deformity at the knee will functionally shorten the lower limb length. Restoration of alignment to normal will functionally elongate the limb. The type of osteotomy that is performed affects limb length; that is, an opening-wedge osteotomy will elongate, whereas a closing-wedge osteotomy will shorten. Geometrically the limb length alteration is equal to the height at the center of the wedge.

This author recommends the preoperative drawing of templates on transparent long films or paper before and after correction to determine the gain or loss in limb length.

6. The health of the distal femoral physis should be carefully determined. Is it open or closed? Is there premature asymmetrical fusion? Is there an osseous bar that can be excised to restore growth? It is vital to preserve growth and not cause physeal injury by fixation devices or extension of the osteotomy line into the growth plate. The level of osteotomy should be as close to the deformity as possible. In the child with an open growth plate, osteotomy is performed at the diaphyseal-metaphyseal junction, and internal fixation is achieved by two or three criss-cross threaded Steinmann pins with additional support of a single hip spica cast. In the skeletally mature patient, the level of osteotomy is often at the metaphyseal region with rigid internal fixation with blade-plate, AO plate, or T-plate with screws. In both skeletally immature and skeletally mature patients, external fixation may be preferred, particularly if translation, rotation, and angulation are required to correct complex deformities. The Ilizarov technique is more versatile than the Orthofix; however, the Ilizarov apparatus is clumsier in the thigh, making if difficult for the patient to sit or lie down.

Radiographic Control. Image intensifier.

Blood for Transfusion. Yes.

Special Equipment. Equipment depends upon the type of fixation used—Steinmann pins, blade-plate or AO plate, external fixators, Orthofix (articulating) or Ilizarov fixators.

CORRECTION OF GENU VALGUM WITH LATERAL TORSION OF THE DISTAL FEMUR

An anterolateral approach is used to expose the distal femoral metaphysis and diaphysis.

Patient Position. The posture of the patient is supine, lying on a translucent operating table with a bag under the ipsilateral pelvis to maintain the lower limb in neutral position. The entire lower limb and hip are prepared and draped sterile in the usual orthopedic fashion. The anterosuperior iliac spine should be in the sterile field. Use the sterile Bovie cord to drop the line distally; after correction of the deformity, it should fall between the first and second metatarsals.

TECHNIQUE IN A CHILD WITH OPEN PHYSIS USING CRISS-CROSS STEINMANN PINS FOR INTERNAL FIXATION

Operative Technique

A. and **B.** Make an anterolateral skin incision beginning 1 cm. proximal to the knee joint line and extend it proximally for a distance of 7 to 10 cm. Subcutaneous tissue is divided in line with the skin incision.

C. Expose the iliotibial band. It is a deforming force in longstanding genu valgum. If it is taut, it is elongated to a long oblique or Z-cut. When the iliotibial band is not contracted, it is divided longitudinally. The underlying vastus lateralis is identified, freed from its attachments to the intermuscular septum with the femur, and reflected anteriorly.

Caution! Carefully identify and coagulate the perforating vessels and the branches of superior genicular artery.

ANTERIOR VIEW

ANTEROLATERAL VIEW

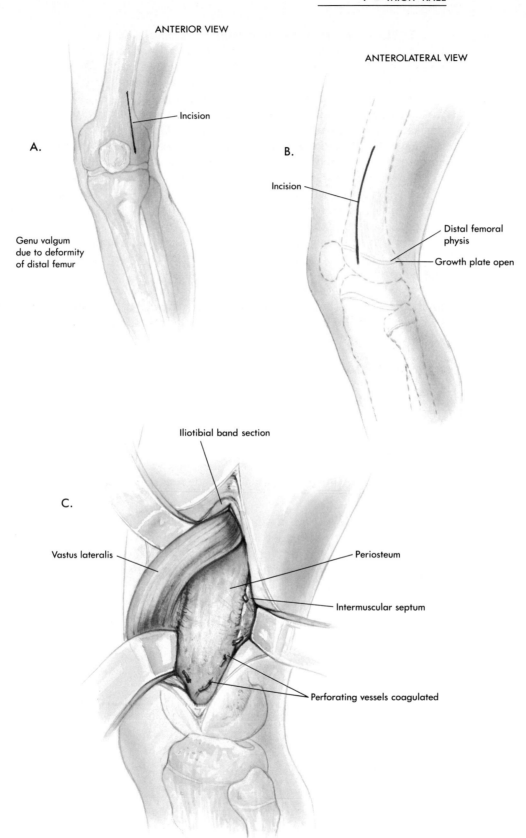

A.

— Incision

Genu valgum
due to deformity
of distal femur

B.

Incision —

Distal femoral
physis

Growth plate open

Iliotibial band section

C.

Vastus lateralis —

Periosteum

Intermuscular septum

Perforating vessels coagulated

Plate 135. Angular osteotomy of the distal femur to correct genu valgum or varum.

D. Next, insert a Keith needle or a small Kirschner wire into the distal femoral physis under image-intensifier radiographic control. It is vital to keep away from the growth plate to avoid injury. Make a transverse incision parallel and 1 cm. proximal to the distal femoral physis. Then make a 6- to 7-cm. longitudinal incision in the periosteum bisecting the distal transverse periosteal incision. If necessary for exposure, make another transverse incision in the periosteum proximally, converting it to an "H."

E. With drill holes (made with a power drill), mark the line of the dome osteotomy—the concave part in the proximal segment and the convex part in the distal segment of the femur. The medial part of the dome is shallow, whereas the lateral part is deep. This will prevent translation of the osteotomized fragments. It may be necessary to take a wedge of bone from the apex and medial part of the convex segment of the osteotomy.

F. With sharp osteotomes, connect the drill holes and complete the osteotomy.

Flex the knee (to prevent tension on the common peroneal nerve) and correct the deformity.

Under image-intensifier radiographic control, transfix the osteotomized fragments with two threaded Steinmann pins inserted from the lateral aspect of the proximal segment and directed medially and distally to engage the distal segment, stopping short of the physis.

One threaded Steinmann pin is inserted from the lateral side of the distal fragment and directed medially and superiorly to firmly engage the proximal segment. The wedge of bone resulting is used as a local bone graft.

The tourniquet is released and complete hemostasis is achieved. The knee is extended and the degree of correction achieved is checked clinically and by a long film radiogram. The Steinmann pins are cut subcutaneously; do not leave the pins protruding outside the skin because of potential risk of infection. The wound is drained by medium-sized Hemovac suction and closed in the routine fashion.

A single or one-and-one-half hip spica cast is applied for more secure immobilization.

Postoperative Care. Four weeks after surgery, the patient is taken to the operating room and the hip spica cast is removed. Radiograms are then made out of cast. The pins are removed through small stab wounds, and the sutures are removed. Ordinarily, there will be adequate healing by then and a high, above-knee cast (molded at the greater trochanter) is applied with the foot and ankle free. Partial weight-bearing is allowed with three-point crutch support.

The cylinder cast is removed in two or three weeks. Active, assisted, and passive exercises are performed to restore range of motion of the knee and motor strength of muscles controlling the knee.

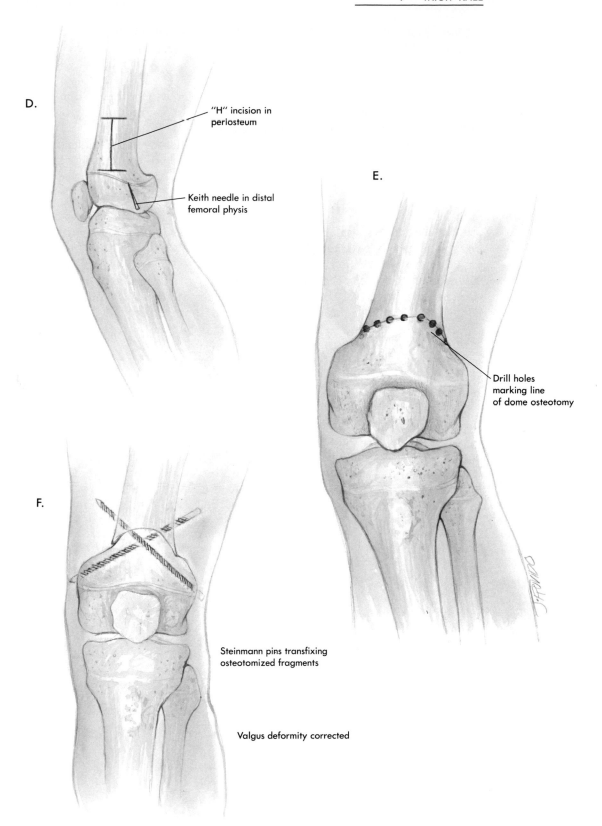

D.

"H" incision in periosteum

Keith needle in distal femoral physis

E.

Drill holes marking line of dome osteotomy

F.

Steinmann pins transfixing osteotomized fragments

Valgus deformity corrected

Plate 135. (Continued)

CORRECTION OF GENU VALGUM AND LATERAL TORSION OF THE DISTAL FEMUR BY USE OF THE ORTHOFIX EXTERNAL FIXATOR

Indications

1. Severe valgus deformity of the knees in which there is a great risk of stretching and injury to the common peroneal nerve. Gradual controlled correction minimizes the possibility of such nerve damage.

2. Personal preference of the surgeon in moderate valgus deformity.

3. Limb is short and simultaneous lengthening of the limb is desired.

Requisite. Emotional maturity of the patient.

Radiographic Control. Image intensifier.

Special Instrumentation. Basic Orthofix fixation equipment. Orthofix self-aligning, articulating body with template.

Two sizes of Orthofix fixator with articulated body are used, depending upon the size of the limb: the standard (10.000) with articulated body (10.036) and related templates (10.101 and 11.136); or the small fixator (30.000) with articulated body (30.0036) and related templates (13.101 and 13.136).

Note: The numbers refer to the Orthofix apparatus parts as designated in their catalog.

First prepare the self-aligning articulating body.

G. and **H.** For the standard fixator, first remove the male part (10.018) and replace it with the articulated body (10.036).

I. Remove the cam (10.004) and bush (10.005) from the male part (10.018) of the standard body fixator, and attach them to the articulated body.

J. Next, fit the T-clamp (10.007) to the articulated body. Then the compression-distraction unit (10.008) is applied by inserting one shank into the cam of the female part of the standard body and the other shank into the seat on the articulated body. It is important that the joint be free to move.

K. Next, the template (11.101) is prepared by removing the male body and the clamp.

G.

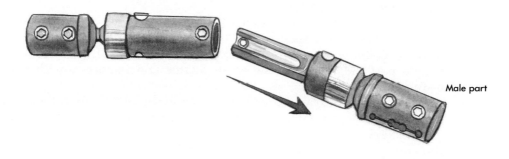

Male part

Articulated body

H.

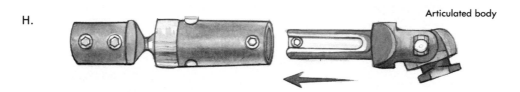

I.

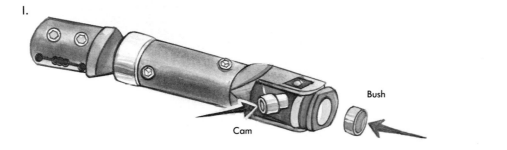

Bush

Cam

Compression-distraction unit

J.

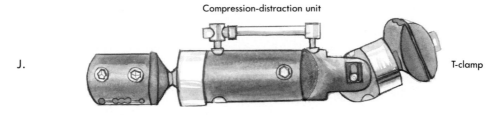

T-clamp

K.

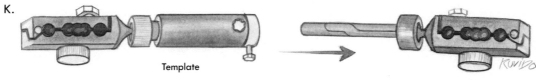

Template

Male body and clamp

Plate 135. (Continued)

L. Replace the inner male body with the guide template for the self-aligning articulated body (11.136).

Next, rotate the clamp template for use with the T-clamp (10.007).

M. and **N.** For preparation of the small fixator (30.000) with the articulated body (30.036) and related templates (13.101 and 13.136), first remove the external female part (30.019) from the small fixator and replace it with the articulated body.

O. Remove the cam body (30.004) and bush (30.005) from the external female part (30.019) of the small body, and attach them to the articulating body (30.036).

P. Next, fit the T-clamp (30.007) on the articulating body. Insert one shank of the compression-distraction unit (30.008) into the cam of the main part of the small body and the other into the seat of the articulated body. The position and fit of the compression-distraction unit is such that the joint is free to move.

Clamp template rotated

L.

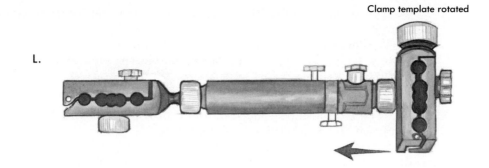

M.

Small fixator

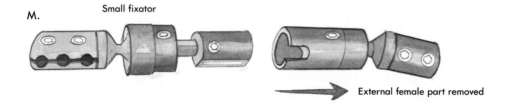

External female part removed

Articulated body

N.

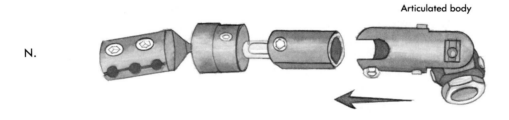

O.

Cam

Bush

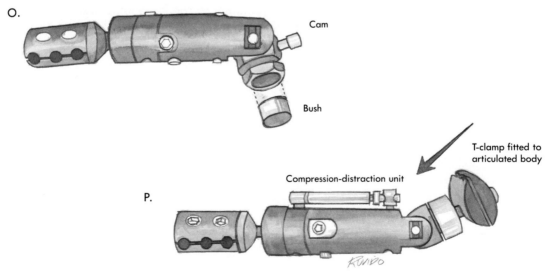

Compression-distraction unit

T-clamp fitted to articulated body

P.

Plate 135. (Continued)

Q. The template (30.101) is prepared by removing the inner male body and the clamp.

R. The inner male body is replaced by the guide template for the self-aligning articulated body (13.136). Next, rotate the clamp template for use with the T-clamp (30.007).

S. Apply these rules and principles:

1. The fixator is positioned on the concave side of the deformity, that is, in genu valgum on the lateral side of the thigh.

2. First, the cancellous screws in the epiphysis are inserted—they should be parallel to the articular surface of the knee joint. Confirm this by radiogram.

3. The body of the fixator should be parallel to the longitudinal axis of the femoral shaft. Confirm this by radiogram.

4. The angle between the axis of the fixator and the axis of the self-aligning body must be equal to the degree of the angular deformity.

5. The arc of movement of the articulated body should be in the coronal plane.

6. The slide pivot of the self-aligning body provides automatic compression for minimal transverse movement of the epiphysis; position it at the end of the slot nearest to the bone segment so that it allows movement of the articulated component away from the bone during distraction.

7. The level of the osteotomy is through the distal metaphysis of the femur. The medial cortex is left intact; only the lateral, anterior, and posterior surfaces of the femur are cut.

8. The angle between the longitudinal axis of the fixator and the longitudinal axis of the self-articulating body is equal to the angle of the angular deformity.

9. Self-articulating body. Note its arc of movement is in the frontal plane.

10. T-clamp.

Operative Technique

T. First, insert cancellous screws in the epiphysis. The technique of insertion of screws is described and illustrated in femoral lengthening (see Plate 138).

Under image-intensifier radiographic control, first insert the anterior screw. The site of the screw is 2 cm. proximal to the knee joint and 1 cm. posterior to the edge of the lateral condyle. The screw should not pass through the intercondylar notch and should not rub against the patella.

Q.   Inner male body and clamp

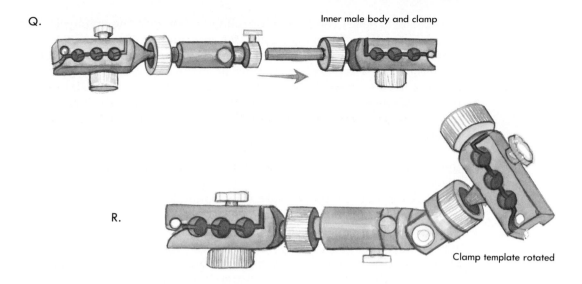

R.

Clamp template rotated

Body of fixator
parallel to long axis of femur

T.

S.

First cancellous screw

Note: Cancellous screws
parallel to
articular surface
of distal femur

1 cm.

2 cm.

Line of
osteotomy

Note: Medial cortex intact

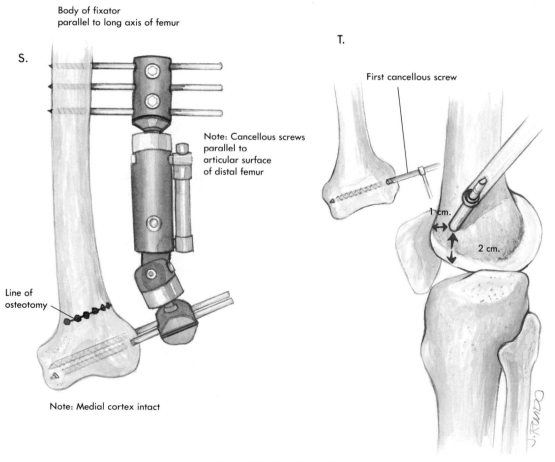

Plate 135. (Continued)

U. Next, insert the second cancellous screw into the epiphysis. Use the clamp template in the "T" configuration for positioning. To achieve a balanced load, provide maximal distance between the cancellous screws in the epiphysis; that is, the second screw is placed in the third or fourth seat of the clamp template posterior to the anterior screw. Be sure the second screw is also parallel to the knee joint. It is desirable for the posterior screw not to traverse through the posterior intercondylar notch; if it passes through, however, it does not cause serious problems.

Try to insert both screws at the first attempt. Avoid making multiple holes in the epiphysis because this will weaken the bone and secure fixation will not be provided.

V. Next use the appropriate body template for insertion of the two (or three in the heavy, older patient) cortical screws. The level of insertion of proximal screws is important—determine it by using the body templates of the body fixator, self-articulating body, and T-clamp all attached. Be sure the body template is parallel to the femoral diaphysis. Fully close the body template, and insert the two or three cortical screws of the appropriate length.

W. Next, determine the level of osteotomy in the distal metaphysis of the femur under image-intensifier radiographic control as follows:

1. Temporarily mount the fixator assembly on the cortical and cancellous bone screws. Be sure the body of the fixator is parallel to the longitudinal axis of the femur.

2. Pass a Steinmann pin or trocar through the cam of the self-aligning, articulating body straight down to the lateral cortex of the femur. This level of the osteotomy will permit angular opening without axis deviation.

Through a 5- to 6-cm. longitudinal direct lateral surgical approach, expose the anterolateral surfaces of the distal femoral metaphysis-diaphysis.

Remove the fixator and perform an osteotomy of the lateral, anterior, and posterolateral cortices by drilling holes and joining them with an osteotome as described and illustrated in Plate 138. Leave the medial cortex intact.

X. Apply the fixator assembly. Make radiograms to ensure that the body of the fixator is parallel to the femoral shaft.

Insert the compression-distraction unit and distract it to make sure that the osteotomy opens laterally and that correction can be achieved. Document this by clinical observation and by radiograms.

Compress and bring the osteotomized segments back into contact.

Close the wound in the usual fashion.

Seven to ten days postoperatively, begin to distract by turning one quarter of a turn four times per day.

Once adequate correction is achieved and normal anatomic-mechanical axis is provided, the fixator assembly is locked and the patient is allowed partial to full weight-bearing with three-point crutch support.

The fixator assembly and screws are removed when there is solid union of the osteotomy, ordinarily eight to ten weeks after surgery.

Genu valgum due to distal femoral angulation can be corrected by the Ilizarov technique and frame.

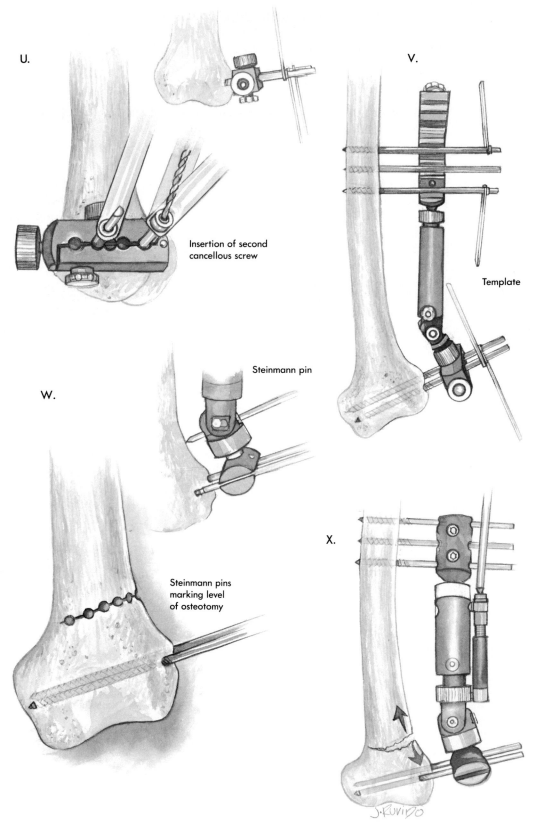

U.

Insertion of second
cancellous screw

V.

Template

W.

Steinmann pin

Steinmann pins
marking level
of osteotomy

X.

J·RUVIDO

Plate 135. (Continued)

CORRECTION OF GENU VALGUM WITH LATERAL TORSION OF THE DISTAL FEMUR IN THE SKELETALLY MATURE (DISTAL FEMORAL PHYSIS CLOSED WITH INTERNAL FIXATION WITH CONDYLAR BLADE-PLATE)

Blood for Transfusion. Yes.

Patient Position. The patient lies supine on a translucent operating table. The whole lower limb and hip are prepared and draped sterile. A sterile tourniquet is used for ischemia.

Operative Technique. A straight lateral surgical approach is used for exposure of the distal femur. The incision begins at the knee joint line and extends proximally for a distance of 10 to 12 cm. The subcutaneous tissue is incised in line with the skin incision. The iliotibial band is identified and divided longitudinally. The vastus lateralis muscle is elevated anteriorly, exposing the anterior and lateral surface of the distal femur. As the distal femoral physis is closed, the lateral condyle, distal femoral metaphysis, and diaphysis are surgically explored with no fear of growth plate injury.

A1. Determine the location and direction for the insertion of the seating chisel. It is vital to place the blade in the correct position—it is 1.5 cm. proximal and parallel to the knee joint line and in the axis (in line with) of the middle of the femoral shaft.

First, flex the knee at a right angle, and under image-intensifier radiographic control insert a smooth Steinmann pin of appropriate diameter over both femoral condyles parallel to the joint line.

Second, determine the inclination of the femoral condyles in the sagittal plane by inserting a smooth pin over the anterior surface of the femoral condyles through the patellofemoral joint.

Third, drill a threaded Steinmann pin as a guide for insertion of the seating chisel using the first pin (parallel to the knee joint line) and the second pin for orientation as to the inclination of the femoral condyles. The third pin is drilled into the lateral femoral condyle 1 cm. proximal to the joint line and in line with the middle of the femoral shaft. Verify its position by radiogram, and remove the first two pins.

B1. Make a small window in the cortex 0.5 cm. superior to the guide pins for insertion of the chisel and control its direction. Using the threaded pin as a guide, make three holes with a 4.5-mm. drill bit 0.5 cm. superior to the pin. Connect the drill holes with a small rongeur.

C1. Using the seating chisel guide and the slotted hammer, drive the seating chisel into the femoral condyles. Use image-intensifier radiographic control. Maintain proper rotation of the chisel.

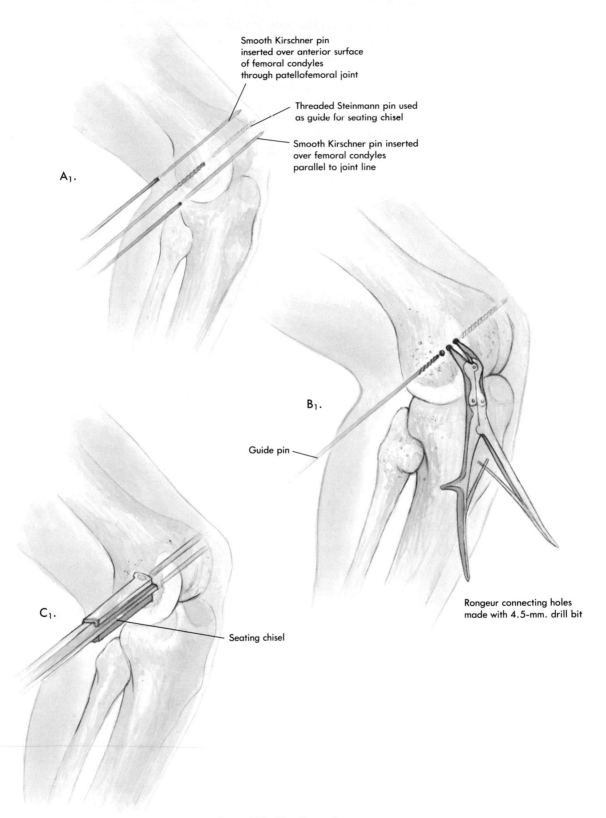

Smooth Kirschner pin inserted over anterior surface of femoral condyles through patellofemoral joint

Threaded Steinmann pin used as guide for seating chisel

Smooth Kirschner pin inserted over femoral condyles parallel to joint line

A₁.

B₁.

Guide pin

Rongeur connecting holes made with 4.5-mm. drill bit

C₁.

Seating chisel

Plate 135. (Continued)

D1. and **E1.** When the limb is short and additional length is desired, an opening wedge osteotomy is performed. Make a transverse osteotomy in the supracondylar region. The distal segment is adducted and the blade of the blade-plate is inserted into the channel created by the seating chisel. Two cancellous screws of appropriate length are inserted into the two distal holes of the condylar plate; this provides secure fixation of the distal fragment. The plate is held to the femoral shaft with a clamp and fixed with screws. The open osteotomy site is grafted with autogenous bone harvested from the ilium.

F1. and **G1.** When lower limb length disparity is not a consideration, a wedge of bone of appropriate width is removed from the medial half of the proximal fragment. Fixation of the condylar blade-plate is the same as earlier. Bone grafting is not required.

A Hemovac suction tube is placed in the wound, which is closed in the usual fashion. Immobilization in a cast is not necessary.

Postoperative Care. As soon as the patient is comfortable, he or she is allowed to be up and around, supporting and protecting the operated lower limbs with a three-point crutch, partial weight-bearing gait. Active assisted exercises are performed to restore range of joint motion and motor strength of muscles.

When the osteotomy is solidly healed (usually in two months), full weight-bearing is allowed.

An alternative method of fixation of the osteotomy of the distal femur in the skeletally mature patient is by the use of a T-plate. This is not as secure a fixation as the condylar blade-plate, but it is simpler and technically less demanding. Because of this advantage, it is performed by some surgeons. When using a T-plate for fixation, it is best to protect the limb in an above-knee cylinder cast or single hip spica cast.

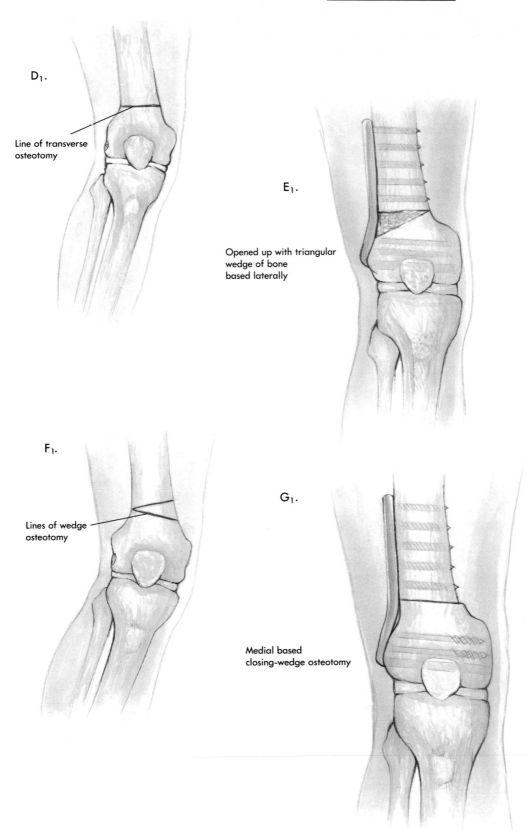

D₁.

Line of transverse
osteotomy

E₁.

Opened up with triangular
wedge of bone
based laterally

F₁.

Lines of wedge
osteotomy

G₁.

Medial based
closing-wedge osteotomy

Plate 135. (Continued)

PLATE 136 | Asymmetrical Medial Stapling of the Distal Femur and Proximal Tibia to Correct Genu Valgum

Indications. Correction of severe genu valgum in patients in whom growth prediction is difficult to calculate because of skeletal dysplasia, such as multiple hereditary exostoses and when a surgical procedure of lesser magnitude than osteotomy is preferred by the parents and patient. They must have full understanding of all the possible problems and complications.

Disadvantages

1. The unpredictability of growth after the staples have been removed.
2. The possibility of asymmetrical growth retardation in the stapled growth region, as a result of which genu valgum, varum, or recurvatum or flexion deformity of the knee may develop.
3. Extrusion of staples.
4. Irregular pattern of initial growth retardation after stapling, which may result in overcorrection or undercorrection.
5. The necessity of a second procedure to remove the staples.
6. The possibility of large and unsightly operative scars.

Radiographic Control. Image intensifier.

Patient Position. Supine on a radiolucent operating table.

Operative Technique

A.–C. The distal femoral epiphysis is approached through a 5-cm. longitudinal incision between the anterior and posterior margins of the femoral condyles (see Plate 133). The subcutaneous tissue is divided in line with the skin incision. The deep fascia and patellar retinaculum are incised, and the growth plate is identified by probing with a straight Keith needle under image-intensifier radiographic control in both anteroposterior and lateral views.

D. With a staple holder, first insert the central staple. It is best to use Vitallium staples because they cause minimal reaction, do not bend, and almost never break. Remember that the growth plate of the distal femur is convex distally and the staples should be directed 5 to 10 degrees distally. After driving the central staple into bone and verifying that it is straddling the growth plate and not going into the joint, insert an anterior staple at the juncture of the anterior one fourth and posterior three fourths and a posterior staple at the juncture of the posterior one fourth and anterior three fourths. The cross-member of the staples must be parallel to the bone surface and perpendicular to the growth plate. The legs of the staple must be equidistant from the physis and joint and directed to the center of the bone. Be sure both legs of the staple are placed in bone. A common error is to have one leg buried in soft tissue and the other in bone. Verify the position of the staples by anteroposterior and lateral radiograms.

E. The wound closure is important. The patellar retinaculum should be closed by interrupted sutures, and the deep fascia should be closed separately with continuous running sutures. The importance of separate closure of the patellar retinaculum and the deep fascia cannot be overemphasized. Otherwise, the patellar retinaculum may be bound down and can cause restriction of knee motion, local swelling, and pain. The subcutaneous tissue and skin are closed in the usual fashion.

A similar technique is used for asymmetrical stapling of the proximal tibia, but it is important to dissect and free the pes anserinus and medial hamstrings and to be sure that the staples are not straddling or anchored across the medial hamstrings.

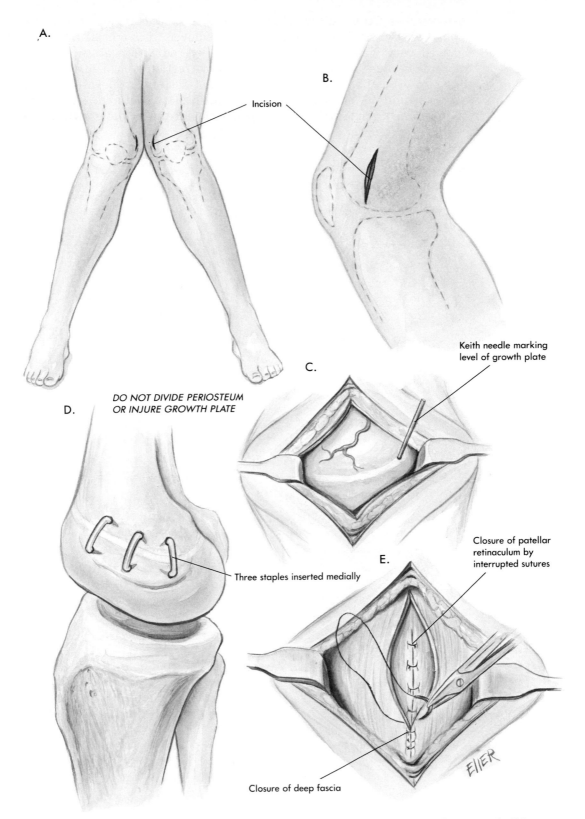

A.

B.

Incision

Keith needle marking
level of growth plate

C.

D.

*DO NOT DIVIDE PERIOSTEUM
OR INJURE GROWTH PLATE*

Three staples inserted medially

Closure of patellar
retinaculum by
interrupted sutures

E.

Closure of deep fascia

ELLER

Plate 136. A.–E., Asymmetrical medial stapling of the distal femur and proximal tibia to correct genu valgum.

Postoperative Care. Full weight-bearing is allowed as tolerated. A cylinder cast is applied for two or three weeks and then removed. It is crucial that the patient be followed very closely both clinically and by radiogram at two- to three-month intervals because of the possibility of overcorrection. When removing the staples, it is also crucial that the periosteum is not incised or elevated. The epiphyseal vessels should not be injured, and the growth plate should be left intact.

Caution! Simple stripping of the perichondrium at the growth plate may stop growth prematurely.

REFERENCES

Bowen, J. R., Torres, R. R., and Forlin, E.: Partial epiphysiodesis to address genu varum or genu valgum. J. Pediatr., 12:359, 1992.

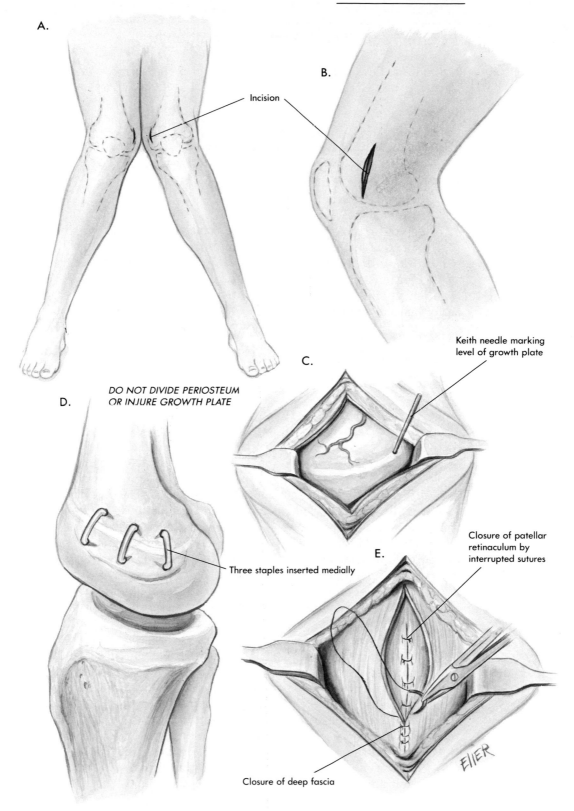

A.

B.

Incision

Keith needle marking
level of growth plate

C.

*DO NOT DIVIDE PERIOSTEUM
OR INJURE GROWTH PLATE*

D.

Three staples inserted medially

Closure of patellar
retinaculum by
interrupted sutures

E.

Closure of deep fascia

ELLER

Plate 136. (Continued)

PLATE 137 ## Wagner Technique of Femoral Lengthening

Indications. Lower limb length disparity of 5 cm. or more in a patient of normal stature.

Requisites

1. Stable joints proximal and distal to the elongated bone. In femoral lengthening, the hip and knee must be stable. If the acetabulum is dysplastic, the femoral head should be covered prior to lengthening. The absence of cruciate ligaments is a relative contraindication.

2. Normal neuromuscular function.

3. Normal circulation.

4. Skin and soft tissues should be relatively normal.

5. Bone structure should be normal and strong.

6. Mentally stable patient with no psychological dysfunction.

7. Patient should be of sufficient age to be cognizant of the complications of limb lengthening and to be cooperative in the postoperative regimen (preferably eight years of age or older).

Special Instrumentation. Wagner femoral lengthening apparatus. Schanz screws.

Blood for Transfusion. Yes.

Patient Position. Supine on a radiolucent operating table.

Operative Technique

A. and **B.** The Wagner limb-lengthening external distraction apparatus can be distracted or compressed by turning the handle at its upper end counterclockwise or clockwise. Screws inserted into the holding pieces of the apparatus are anchored by bolts and washers. By tilting the holding pieces, realignment of 20 degrees in each direction is possible, for a total of 40 degrees. The screws (Schanz screws) act as a cantilever; they transmit force from the fixator body (which is not bulky) to the bone—in this specific case, the femur, osteotomized in its mid-diaphysis by open surgery. The use of unilateral pins decreases the extent of soft-tissue trapping and muscle fixation by the screws. Well tolerated by most patients, the apparatus permits daily lengthening of the femur.

The Wagner limb-lengthening apparatus is available in two sizes. The large size is used for the femur in children and for the tibia in adults, and the small size is used for the tibia or upper limb in children.

C. After the desired length is achieved, the bone is plated with a specially designed rigid osteosynthesis plate, and the elongated segment is grafted with autogenous bone from the ilium. The external fixator is removed. When there is sufficient evidence of cortex formation on the opposite side of the plate and of medullary canalization, the rigid plate is removed and the elongated segment is internally fixed with a flexible semitubular plate. The final step of the Wagner technique is removal of the semitubular plate.

There are four phases of Wagner limb-lengthening:

The *first phase* entails insertion of the Schanz screws; application of the distraction apparatus; mid-diaphyseal osteotomy; and lengthening.

The *second phase* involves plating with the rigid osteosynthesis plate; grafting of autogenous iliac bone; and removal of the external distractor apparatus.

The *third phase* consists of exchanging the rigid plate for a flexible semitubular plate.

(The *fourth phase,* removal of the semitubular plate, is not illustrated here.)

Note. Limb-lengthening surgery should be preceded by extensive soft-tissue releases in the congenitally short limb (three to six months prior to lengthening).

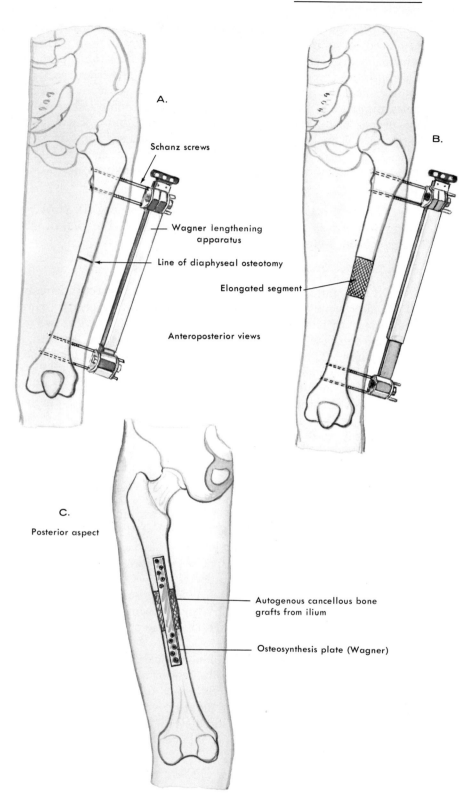

A.

Schanz screws

Wagner lengthening
apparatus

Line of diaphyseal osteotomy

Anteroposterior views

B.

Elongated segment

C.

Posterior aspect

Autogenous cancellous bone
grafts from ilium

Osteosynthesis plate (Wagner)

Plate 137. A.–II., Wagner technique of femoral lengthening.

In preparation for the first phase of Wagner femoral lengthening, the patient is placed in supine position, and the entire lower limb and ipsilateral pelvis are surgically prepared. The patient is so draped that the hip and knee can be freely manipulated through their full range of motion without contamination. A sterile folded sheet is placed under the knee to hold it in flexion, and to facilitate determination of the knee joint axis. Radiographic image intensification is used for proper orientation in the placement of Schanz screw sites and the level of osteotomy. The larger Wagner apparatus is used for femoral lengthening; it is placed on the lateral aspect of the thigh, where there is more space (and where the skin and soft tissues are relatively less sensitive) than on the medial side of the thigh.

The first phase of Wagner limb lengthening (D. *to* W.) *consists of screw insertion* (D. *to* K.); *apparatus application* (L.); *osteotomy* (M. *to* S.); *and actual bone lengthening* (T. *to* W.).

Percutaneous Insertion of Schanz Screws (D. to K.)

D. Two pairs of Schanz screws are inserted percutaneously, one pair distally at the supracondylar region of the femur, the other pair proximally at the level of the lesser trochanter. The screws should be far enough away from the center of the bone to allow adequate space for internal fixation later on.

Caution! Do not disturb the growth of the distal femoral physis or the greater trochanteric apophysis, if they are still open.

Another factor to consider is the stability of screw anchorage on the cortex; the cortical thickness in the metaphyseal area should be at least one half of the thickness of the diaphyseal cortex. The direction of the screws is parallel to the knee joint axis. The most distal screw is inserted first. A 1- to 1½-cm.-long incision is made through the skin and subcutaneous tissues.

E. A second clean scalpel is used to divide the fascia lata longitudinally in the direction of its fibers. Upon flexion of the knee, the fascia lata moves posteriorly; therefore, a transverse incision extending anteriorly for 2 cm. is made in the fascia lata to provide adequate space for the screw, and to prevent mechanical pressure on the soft tissues. With Metzenbaum scissors or blunt scissors, the muscle fibers of the vastus lateralis are split longitudinally, deep to the bone. With a periosteal elevator, the aperture in the fascia lata and muscle fibers is enlarged, and the periosteum is split. The importance of the provision of adequate space around the screws cannot be overemphasized. Without such space, factors such as soft-tissue shift and mechanical pressure by the screw(s) will cause soft-tissue necrosis, and outside contamination of the necrotic tissue by the pin tract will lead to sepsis and drainage.

F. Now a drill sleeve is introduced through the incision. By touching the bone and identifying the anterior and posterior margins of the femoral cortex, the drill sleeve is placed exactly in the midlateral position. The posterior part of the femur should be left free for internal fixation with a plate. Because the lower Schanz screws will move distally with elongation of the limb, they are to be placed through the proximal end of the wounds. The drill sleeve should therefore be at the upper margin of the incision.

First distal skin incision—1.5 cm. long

D.

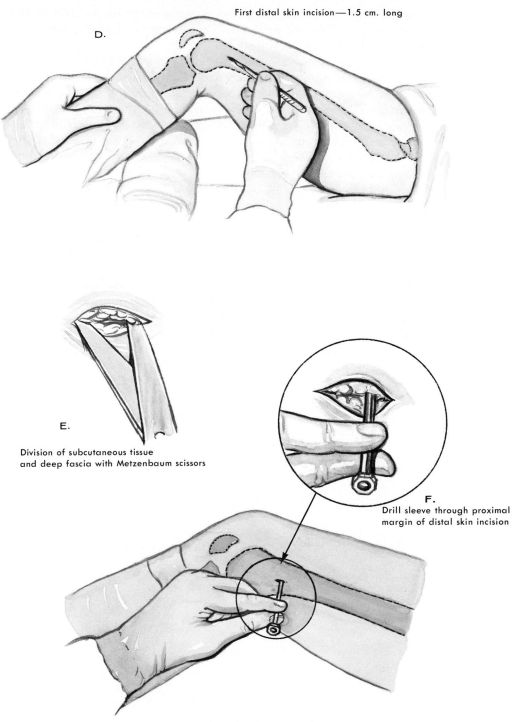

E.

Division of subcutaneous tissue
and deep fascia with Metzenbaum scissors

F.
Drill sleeve through proximal
margin of distal skin incision

Plate 137. (Continued)

G. A hole for a Schanz screw is made with an electric drill through both cortices with a 3.6-mm. drill bit. The direction of the Schanz screw should be parallel to the axis of the knee joint.

H. A Schanz screw of adequate length is secured on a universal chuck. The end of this screw and of each succeeding screw should be 6 to 7 cm. away from the skin to allow 3 cm. of space between the skin and the holding piece of the Wagner apparatus. The ends of the screws should protrude 1 to 2 cm. from the holding piece to facilitate later removal. The Schanz screws are self-tapping. The "T" part of the handle of the universal chuck should be exactly parallel to the tip of the screw. Upon penetration of the medial cortex, the tip of the screw should be vertical (i.e., parallel to the longitudinal axis of the femur) for adequate anchorage of the threads of the screw on the medial femoral cortex in the direction of the distraction forces. Because the screw has no threads on its flat side, the screw should *not* be inserted in a horizontal position, in that the screw will have to penetrate deeper by two or three turns to have adequate bony purchase above and below. An additional problem is that the tip of the screw will irritate soft tissues and cause discomfort.

The drill hole is located blindly by moving the Schanz screw up and down. The Schanz screw is inserted. On penetration of the medial cortex, one can feel the tapping of the tip of the screw; as it goes through the cortex, two additional turns are made and the chuck handle is removed.

I. With a drill guide, determine the correct site for placement of the second Schanz screw. There are three holes in the drill guide; it is best to use the holes farthest apart for greatest stability. The holes in the drill guide are large enough to accommodate the Schanz screws. With a drill sleeve, the skin is marked for the site of insertion of the second screw. The drill guide is removed. An incision 1½ cm. long is made with the hole for the second Schanz screw in its upper end.

J. Following the details of technique just described, the second Schanz screw is inserted, parallel to the first screw, through the drill guide.

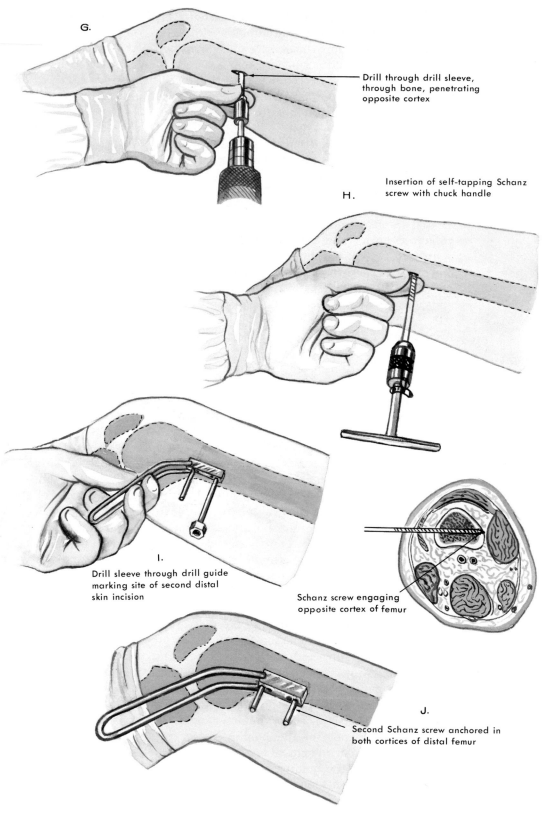

G.

Drill through drill sleeve, through bone, penetrating opposite cortex

H.

Insertion of self-tapping Schanz screw with chuck handle

I.

Drill sleeve through drill guide marking site of second distal skin incision

Schanz screw engaging opposite cortex of femur

J.

Second Schanz screw anchored in both cortices of distal femur

Plate 137. (Continued)

K. The preceding technique is utilized for the second pair of Schanz screws. The screws are anchored through the proximal femur at the level of the lesser trochanter. The uppermost screw is level with the upper half of the lesser trochanter. It should not penetrate too deeply, as it may hook the iliopsoas tendon and cause the patient to be made to sit. The position and length of the screw are double-checked by radiographic image intensification in anteroposterior and lateral projections, and adjustments are made if necessary.

The distal screws are always parallel to the axis of the knee joint, and normally, the proximal pair of screws are parallel to the distal pair. However, if rotational deformities are present, they can be corrected by changing the direction of the proximal pair of screws, keeping the distal pair always parallel to the knee joint axis. Angular deformities, valgus and varus, or anterior or posterior bowing can be corrected at the same time that the limb is lengthened, provided they are located in the center of the femoral shaft. As stated before, major deformities of valgus or varus, and those located near the hip or knee, should be realigned one or two years before limb lengthening to enable the soft tissues, muscle function, and bone structure to be restored to normal. When rotational realignment is corrected, the apparatus is applied after the osteotomy. In all other situations, the apparatus is applied *before* the osteotomy.

Application of the Wagner Lengthening Apparatus (L.)

L. Screws are inserted through the holes of the holding piece, preferably with the lateral tips of the screws protruding out of the lateral margin of the holding piece by 1½ to 2 cm. When fluid gets inspissated between the holding piece and the screws, it may be difficult to disconnect them unless the tips of the screws are protruding. Also, there should be enough space (2 to 3 cm.) between the skin and the apparatus to prevent skin pressure. *Remember*: When the patient is awake and sits down, the soft tissues become more protuberant and bulkier than when the patient is positioned for surgery and under anesthesia. One must be sure that the skin does not touch the apparatus. Proximally, the handle of the apparatus should be well clear of the greater trochanter and pelvis.

Next, the lengthening apparatus is connected to the holding piece and covered with the washer, and the bolt tightened. Attention should be paid to the length of the apparatus and to whether there is the required distance between the two holding pieces for telescoping when the limb is lengthened. For femoral lengthening, the apparatus is applied anteriorly with the holes for the screws posteriorly, giving adequate space for posterior exposure of the femur. The bolts are tightened to prevent sliding of the holding piece. The Schanz screws have a diameter of 6 mm.; if subjected to distraction forces, the screws may bend. Upon elongation, the upper screw is subjected to tension forces and the lower screw to compression forces; elongation may thus cause the screws to move or at least shift. Therefore, it is imperative to tighten the nuts firmly to increase stability and guarantee the security of the fixation of the screws to the apparatus. To achieve this, an AO screwdriver (with a 5.6-mm. diameter) or a long Schanz screw is placed into the additional free hole of the holding piece; with a wrench on the nut the two instruments are firmly closed together manually. This provides a very firm fixation of the screws to the holding piece and to the apparatus. The bolts are tightened. Sterile gauze (moistened with povidone-iodine [Betadine] solution) is split and straddled around the screws. Blood should not seep into the holes of the apparatus.

To liberate entrapped tissues such as the vastus lateralis and the fascia lata from the screws, the knee is manipulated into full flexion. This is very important, because otherwise active exercise will be painful. Distraction is applied on the apparatus by turning the handle counterclockwise three to five times, and again the knee is flexed fully.

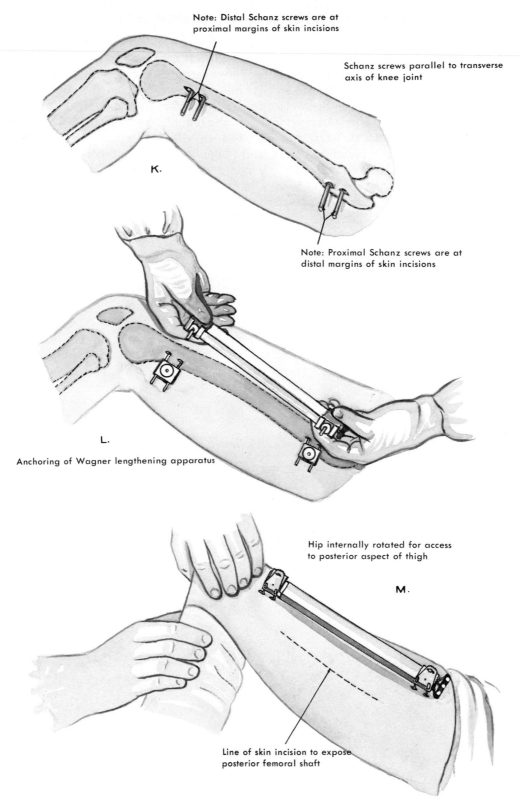

Note: Distal Schanz screws are at proximal margins of skin incisions

Schanz screws parallel to transverse axis of knee joint

K.

Note: Proximal Schanz screws are at distal margins of skin incisions

L.

Anchoring of Wagner lengthening apparatus

Hip internally rotated for access to posterior aspect of thigh

M.

Line of skin incision to expose posterior femoral shaft

Plate 137. (Continued)

Transverse Osteotomy of the Femoral Shaft (M. to S.)

M. With the knee at 45 to 90 degrees of flexion, the hip is flexed, medially rotated, and adducted for a posterolateral approach to the femoral shaft. If the hip is ankylosed, it cannot be flexed and medially rotated; in such a case, the patient is appropriately draped so that he or she can be turned from the supine position, which allows the Schanz screws and apparatus to be applied, to a lateral position, permitting a posterior approach to the femur. (A prone position is not recommended for the patient because the soft tissues will shift when he or she is turned back to the supine position and cause problems.) A 7- to 10-cm. longitudinal incision is made, centered between the upper and lower pairs of Schanz screws over the interval between the vastus lateralis and the biceps femoris, about four finger-breadths posterior to the Schanz screws. The linea aspera is almost subcutaneous in this location. The subcutaneous tissue and deep fascia are divided in line with the skin incision.

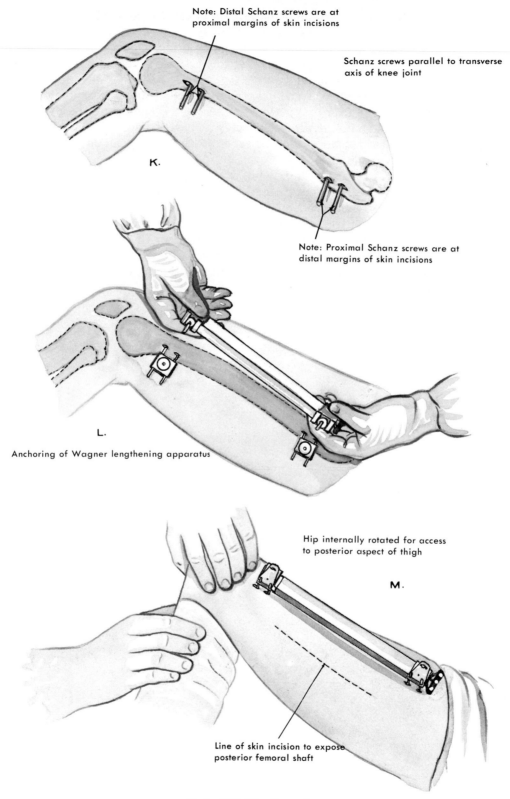

Note: Distal Schanz screws are at proximal margins of skin incisions

Schanz screws parallel to transverse axis of knee joint

K.

Note: Proximal Schanz screws are at distal margins of skin incisions

L.

Anchoring of Wagner lengthening apparatus

Hip internally rotated for access to posterior aspect of thigh

M.

Line of skin incision to expose posterior femoral shaft

Plate 137. (Continued)

N. The vastus lateralis muscle is gently elevated from the lateral intermuscular septum and retracted anteriorly with two Hibbs retractors. The periosteum is divided longitudinally. With the help of a sharp periosteal elevator, two large Chandler elevators are inserted subperiosteally to expose the anterior and lateral aspects of the femoral shaft.

O. Exposure of the posterior aspect of the femur may cause troublesome hemorrhage from the perforating vessels. Bleeding can be avoided if sharp osteotomes and a mallet are used to elevate part of the cortical wall with the periosteum. Exposure of the posterior aspect of the femur by such decortication prevents injury to the vessels.

P. Two large Chandler elevators are placed posteriorly; adequate space is provided for a reciprocating saw by twisting the elevators. The level of femoral osteotomy should be midway between the two pairs of Schanz screws. This is measured with a ruler to ensure that there are equally long bone fragments for internal fixation. The periosteum is thin in the adolescent and not important in bone healing; it is sectioned transversely at the level of the osteotomy. If the periosteal tube is left intact, it will tear during distraction and may be the source of pain.

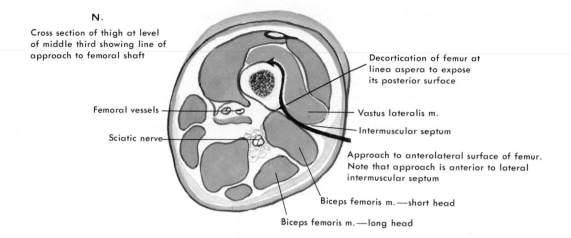

N.

Cross section of thigh at level of middle third showing line of approach to femoral shaft

Decortication of femur at linea aspera to expose its posterior surface

Femoral vessels

Sciatic nerve

Vastus lateralis m.

Intermuscular septum

Approach to anterolateral surface of femur. Note that approach is anterior to lateral intermuscular septum

Biceps femoris m.—short head

Biceps femoris m.—long head

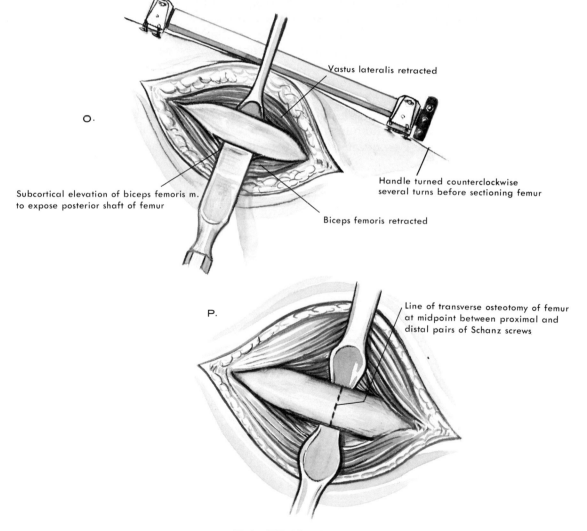

Vastus lateralis retracted

O.

Subcortical elevation of biceps femoris m. to expose posterior shaft of femur

Handle turned counterclockwise several turns before sectioning femur

Biceps femoris retracted

P.

Line of transverse osteotomy of femur at midpoint between proximal and distal pairs of Schanz screws

Plate 137. (Continued)

Q. To put the femur under further tension just before the osteotomy is performed, the handle at the upper end of the apparatus is turned counterclockwise a couple of turns. Then, with an electrical reciprocating saw, a transverse osteotomy is made through the femoral shaft under normal saline irrigation. Z-pattern osteotomies or other complicated geometric configurations are not recommended. Upon completion of the osteotomy, the previously applied tension on the femur provides further stability and prevents malalignment. In the past, the handle on the limb-lengthening apparatus was turned counterclockwise several more turns, elongating the femur by 10 to 15 mm. The resulting soft-tissue tension further stabilized the osteotomized fragments and prevented painful contact between bone ends.

At present, this author recommends corticotomy as described by Ilizarov (Plate 138) and DeBastiani (Plate 117) and not osteotomy with a reciprocating saw. Do not disturb the endosteal blood supply! The lengthening of the femur is begun three to five days after surgery.

R. and **S.** The knee is flexed fully once or twice. The osteotomy site is drained by two closed-suction tubes. The fascia lata and the wound are closed in the usual fashion; the skin is closed with a subcuticular running 00 nylon suture. A fine mesh gauze is applied over the incision. The soft-tissue channels around the Schanz screws are reinspected to ensure that there is no mechanical pressure. Elastic compression by Ace bandage dressing is applied. Final radiograms are made in the operating room to double-check the anatomic alignment of the femoral fragments. Any angular or axial deviation is corrected by realigning the Schanz screws and the holding piece in their anchorage to the lengthening apparatus. Fixation by the Wagner limb-lengthening apparatus is very stable, and external support by plaster of Paris cast is not necessary. The knee, ankle, and hip can be moved freely.

Q.

Elongation of femur by turning
knob on screw counterclockwise several
turns until soft tissues are taut

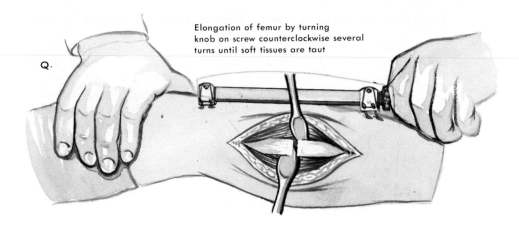

R.
Flex knee fully

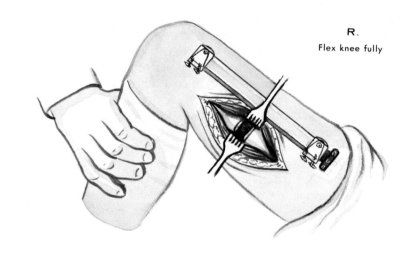

S.

Closed Hemovac suction

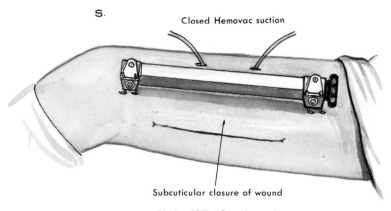

Subcuticular closure of wound

Plate 137. (Continued)

Daily Lengthening of the Femur; Exercise Program; Wound Care (T. to W.)

T. Limb lengthening is carried out by the patient under direct supervision of the surgeon, the orthopedic nurse, or the parents. Initially it is preferable to keep the patient in the hospital for close observation. Three to five days after surgery the patient is discharged from the hospital, provided that he or she is reliable and can be observed closely as an outpatient. If problems and complications develop, the patient is readmitted to the hospital. (No special attire is required; many patients undergoing femoral lengthening can even wear blue jeans, "customized" only in that they are split on the lateral side of the femur.)

The knob is turned counterclockwise a quarter-turn at a time; six quarter-turns per day (to distract) and two quarter-turns clockwise once a day (to compress) provide a gain of 1.5 mm. of length per day, or 1.0 cm. per week. Function of the limb should be maintained during the process of limb lengthening. *Function is never sacrificed for length.*

U.–W. The patient is instructed to walk with crutches in a three-point gait with partial weight-bearing on the lengthened limb. He or she is allowed to be up and around one or two days postoperatively. The amount of body weight borne should not exceed the weight of the limb distal to the site of the osteotomy. Falls should be avoided. Suction-drainage tubes are removed two days after surgery. Physical therapy is directed toward maintaining a functional range of knee motion. If the knee cannot be actively flexed more than 60 degrees, or if loss of complete knee extension is greater than 15 degrees, limb lengthening is discontinued. Exercises are continued to increase range of knee motion; if a range of 60 degrees of knee flexion is regained, limb lengthening is resumed. If functional range of knee motion cannot be restored after two weeks of exercises, limb lengthening is stopped and internal fixation is carried out. (It should be explained to the patient and family that after two or three years, a limb lengthening can be repeated.)

One cannot overemphasize the need for preservation of joint function. Experience has shown that, if the limits of the arc of knee motion (60 degrees of knee flexion to minus 15 degrees of knee extension) are maintained within a year, the full range of knee motion will be recovered. Individuals with ligamentous laxity do not usually present a problem. The difficulty is with those patients with congenital shortening of the femur and those with stiff joints. Should persistent flexion contracture of the knee develop, it may be corrected by fractional lengthening of the hamstrings. A hip adductor myotomy may be required in an occasional case if the hip adductors are very taut and pull the distal femoral segment into varus deformity. These soft-tissue releases are performed with the Wagner apparatus still anchored to the femur. If major soft-tissue contractures are corrected one year prior to femoral lengthening, one usually is not confronted with these problems.

Exercises are performed twice a day. The exercises are active and gravity-assisted; passive and forceful exercises are avoided, because overly aggressive exercise programs will cause irritation of the soft tissues by the Schanz screws, especially the distal ones. Manipulation of the knee with the patient under general anesthesia is fraught with danger and is not recommended except in occasional situations. Side-lying knee flexion-extension utilizes the principle of reciprocal innervation of agonist-antagonist muscles. On active flexion of the knee, the quadriceps muscle relaxes.

The most useful exercise—especially if the patient is relaxed (even listening to music or reading a book)—is sitting knee flexion, assisted by gravity forces.

The channels in the soft tissue around the Schanz screws are kept clean the first three postoperative days by application of povidone-iodine solution three times a day. Thereafter, sponges dipped in normal saline are used for mechanical cleaning three times a day.

There is a large amount of soft-tissue coverage on the lateral aspect of the

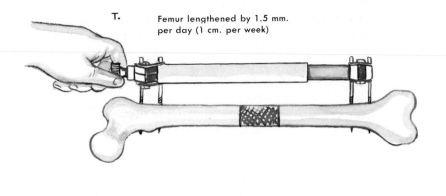

T.   Femur lengthened by 1.5 mm.
per day (1 cm. per week)

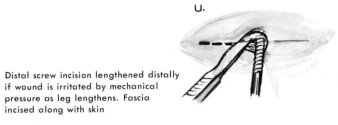

U.

Distal screw incision lengthened distally
if wound is irritated by mechanical
pressure as leg lengthens. Fascia
incised along with skin

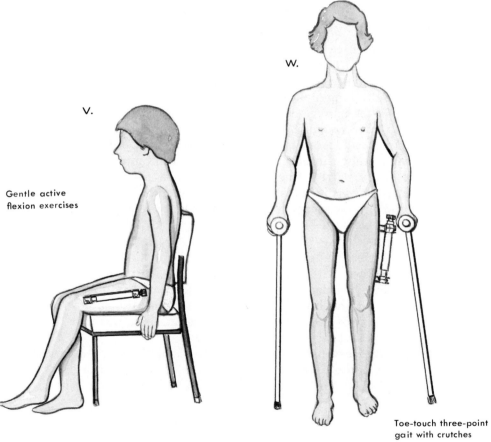

W.

V.

Gentle active
flexion exercises

Toe-touch three-point
gait with crutches

Plate 137. (Continued)

thigh, and soft tissues do shift. The distal screws in the femur can cause trouble by exerting mechanical pressure on the soft tissues. The screws migrate through the incision during the course of distraction. The lower screws migrate distally; the upper screws migrate proximally. As soon as the screws touch or press the opposite ends of the skin, the skin incision should be enlarged.

Any swelling, inflammatory reaction, or pain calls for emergency relief of mechanical pressure and tension in the soft tissues. The problem area is sterilized with a disinfectant such as Betadine solution and anesthetized. An incision then made with a scalpel will relieve pain, allow swelling to subside, and prevent pin tract infection. Limb lengthening is actually not painful; whenever the patient develops pain, the screw tracts must be inspected. Schanz screws removed because of infection should be replaced with screws inserted at more distal or proximal sites. Replacement will require general anesthesia and radiographic control.

Radiograms obtained at weekly intervals may reveal bending of screws due to tension. Commonly, tension pulls the distal femoral segment into adduction, sometimes posteriorly, causing lateral or anterior bowing of the femur. If the angular deformity is less than 20 degrees, realignment can be performed at the time of internal fixation. However, if the varus deformity is greater than 20 degrees, the soft tissues do not elongate on the medial side, becoming instead progressively tauter and causing greater varus. In such an instance, it is best to realign during the period of distraction. In the cooperative and mature patient, general anesthesia is not required. With the patient supine and the knee in full extension, gentle traction (of about 10 to 15 lb.) is applied on the lower leg. Clockwise turns on the handle of the lengthening apparatus will decrease its distraction force to zero. The distal nuts are then opened, and the bone segments are realigned by adjusting the screws and the holding piece of the apparatus. Since straightening makes the femur longer, a further compensatory decrease in distraction force may be necessary. If medial soft tissues are taut, a slight overcorrection into some valgus may be desirable. Realignment is double-checked by radiograms. A long radiopaque pin may be used as an index to radiographic distortion, especially when image intensification is used. Tightening the nuts will once again secure stability of the fragments. If there is medial or lateral displacement of the fragments, the distal nuts are opened and the screws are shifted medially or laterally for proper realignment. When there is anterior or posterior bowing, the distal bolts are loosened and the upper end of the distal segment is tilted posteriorly or anteriorly.

After realignment, distraction is applied gradually; the original length is reobtained within 24 to 48 hours. Measurements of length made with a Bell Thompson ruler on leg-length scanograms are preferred over readings from the scale on the limb-lengthening apparatus (the latter is not reliable because of elasticity of the screws). The true length obtained may be 1 or 2 cm. shorter than the amount registered on the scale.

At the completion of the required lengthening, radiograms are carefully studied for evidence of malalignment (varus or valgus, anterior or posterior bowing) and for clues to the adequacy of the callus at the elongation site.

The second phase of Wagner limb lengthening (X. to EE.) involves osteosynthesis by plating, to which bone grafting may or may not be added.

If there is continuity of bone between the femoral fragments, there is a possibility of spontaneous consolidation. In such an instance, desired length is maintained and physical therapy is continued. The decision as to internal fixation by plating should be made at the end of distraction, and should not be delayed for two or three months, when local wound conditions and bone atrophy may make osteosynthesis by plating very difficult. There are a number of alternatives available: (1) keeping external fixation by the apparatus until spontaneous consolidation has taken place; (2) internal fixation with plating but without bone grafting;

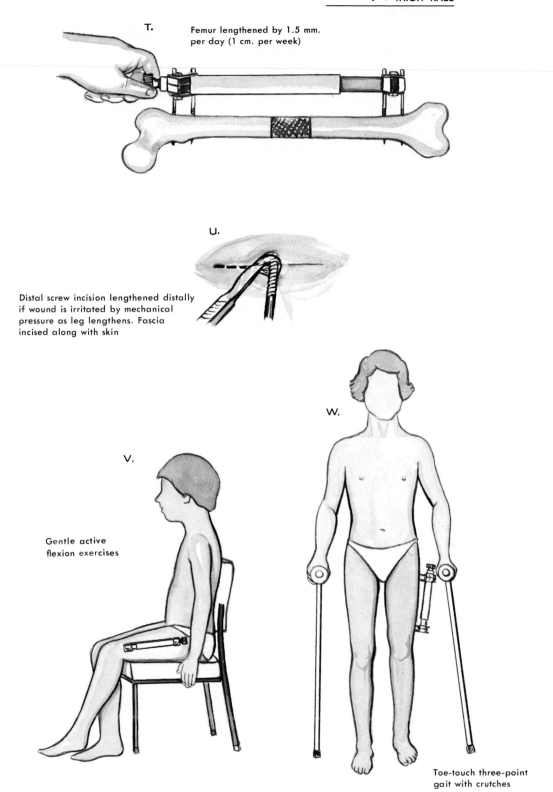

T.

Femur lengthened by 1.5 mm. per day (1 cm. per week)

U.

Distal screw incision lengthened distally if wound is irritated by mechanical pressure as leg lengthens. Fascia incised along with skin

W.

V.

Gentle active flexion exercises

Toe-touch three-point gait with crutches

Plate 137. (Continued)

and (3) internal fixation with plating and with simultaneous bone grafting. Factors determining the option chosen are the surgeon's expertise, local wound conditions, the adequacy of consolidation and callus as seen on the radiograms, and the stability of the fragments.

If it is decided not to plate—that is, to allow spontaneous consolidation with external fixation by the apparatus—minimal compression force is applied by turning the handle clockwise a few quarter-turns. Pin tract care is continued. At four weeks, radiograms are again obtained. If healing and stability are adequate, compression force is applied and increasing weight-bearing permitted. Up to a 2-cm. loss in length is allowed on the scale of the limb-lengthening apparatus. A greater than 2-cm. loss in length will result in instability of fixation, collapse of the callus, and loss of alignment. When there are signs of homogeneous canalization of the medullary cavity and of normal cortication (it will take 9 to 12 months for these signs to appear), the Wagner apparatus and screws are removed. First, the Wagner apparatus is removed; the Schanz screws are left in place. Stress is applied on the screws. If stability of the elongated segment is demonstrated, the screws are removed.

Ordinarily, immediate plating upon completion of limb lengthening is recommended; it is reliable and less fraught with potential problems.

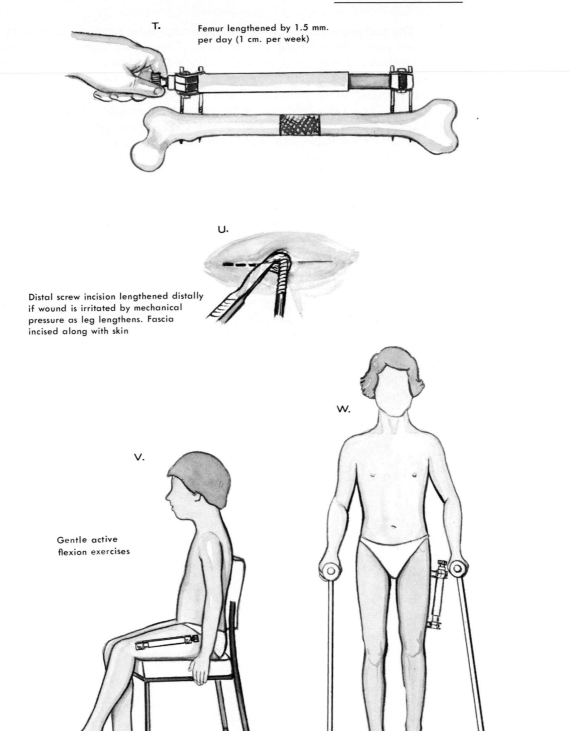

T. Femur lengthened by 1.5 mm. per day (1 cm. per week)

U.

Distal screw incision lengthened distally if wound is irritated by mechanical pressure as leg lengthens. Fascia incised along with skin

V.

Gentle active flexion exercises

W.

Toe-touch three-point gait with crutches

Plate 137. (Continued)

X. The patient is placed in a prone position under general anesthesia. The pin tracts are carefully cleansed and shielded. The entire lower limb is surgically prepared, then the Wagner apparatus is draped out with elastic Ace bandages and self-adhering drapes. For a second time, the entire lower limb and pelvis are surgically prepared; the posterior ilium, from which bone grafts are to be obtained, should be in the sterile field. It is imperative to pay utmost attention to antisepsis. The draping should be done in such a way that the surgeon can reach the handle of the lengthening apparatus and make necessary adjustments during surgery. The previous skin incision is used for exposure of the posterior aspect of the femur. The scar is excised. The subcutaneous tissue and deep fascia are divided in line with the skin incision.

Y. The lateral intermuscular septum and vastus lateralis are gently retracted anteriorly, and the biceps femoris is retracted posteriorly. In the course of the surgical approach *the screw tracts, sealed in fibrous granulation tissue, should not be opened,* as they are potentially contaminated. Excessive callus, if present on the linea aspera, is removed tangentially with an osteotome in order to provide a flat surface for attachment of the plate.

Z. and **AA.** The femoral segments are connected with an osteosynthesis plate. Designed by Professor Wagner, the plate is wide, sturdy, and relatively rigid. The plate has five holes proximally and five holes distally, with an intervening solid segment that straddles the elongated femoral segment. The screw holes are close together and obliquely zigzagged, making it possible to insert five screws instead of four. The intervening solid part comes in varying lengths, depending on the extent of lengthening.

X.

Line of skin incision in line
with previous posterior incision

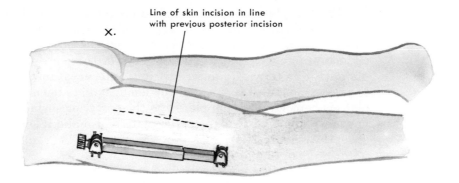

Biceps femoris m.—long head

Biceps femoris m.—short head

Intermuscular septum

Sciatic nerve

Approach to posterior surface of femur.
Note that it is posterior to lateral
intermuscular septum

Femoral vessels

Y.

Vastus lateralis m.

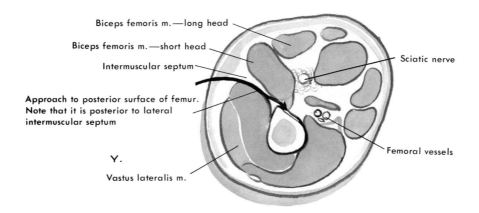

Proximal femoral fragment

Distal femoral fragment

Z.

Elongated femoral segment

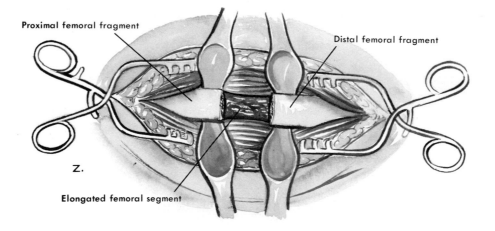

AA.   Wagner osteosynthesis plate

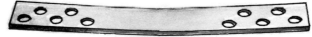

Plate 137. (Continued)

BB. The plate should be applied on the *posterior* aspect of the femur; if the plate is secured on the lateral aspect of the femur, bending into varus deformity will ensue. By application of the plate on the posterior aspect of the femur, the adduction forces are on the lateral edge of the plate. It is important to bend the plate with its convexity anteriorly into antecurvatum. The muscle forces acting at the weak elongated segment of the femur tend to bend the plate posteriorly. If the plate is bent forward and placed on the posterior surface of the femur, the muscle forces will tend to straighten the plate and make it longer, but these effects are offset by the resistance of the soft tissue. The countertensions thus prevent untoward bending of the plate.

CC. The plate is securely fixed to the femur with screws in the usual fashion. If the distraction gap is filled with hyperemic cartilaginous tissue, bone grafting is not necessary. If the tissue in the elongated segment is fibrous and exhibits no hyperemia, it is best to bone graft. This author recommends bone grafting to expedite consolidation.

DD. and **EE**. Strips of autogenous cancellous bone, harvested from the ilium, are used for onlay bone grafting. Closed-suction drainage tubes are inserted, the wound is closed in the usual fashion, and the Wagner elongation apparatus is then removed. Within 24 to 48 hours, the patient is allowed to be up and around with the help of crutches and to begin partial weight-bearing on the lengthened limb. Knee exercises are continued. Increased weight-bearing is permitted as the radiograms disclose progressive healing. Full weight-bearing is allowed when the medullary cavity shows complete homogeneous canalization and when a thick cortex is remodeled in the wall of the elongated segment opposite the plate. Then, after a month or two, the plate is removed. If after one year the cortical wall is not of solid density and the medullary canal is not homogeneously canalized, it is best to replace the rigid plate with a smaller, semiflexible AO plate to prevent a stress fracture at the distal or proximal end of the rigid plate. The rigid plate protects the elastic femur from biological forces, but excessive stress protection may cause fatigue fracture. By exchanging plates, the incidence of fatigue fracture is greatly diminished.

The third phase of Wagner limb lengthening entails exchanging the rigid plate for a flexible semitubular plate.

The Wagner rigid osteosynthesis plate is exchanged for a semitubular plate 9 to 12 months after surgery, provided there is strong cortex formation on the opposite side of the plate and there is canalization of the medulla. It is imperative to change the plate to prevent stress fractures above and below the rigid plate. The semitubular plate is removed three to six months later.

With the patient placed in prone position, the elongated lower limb and hip are prepared and draped sterile in the usual fashion.

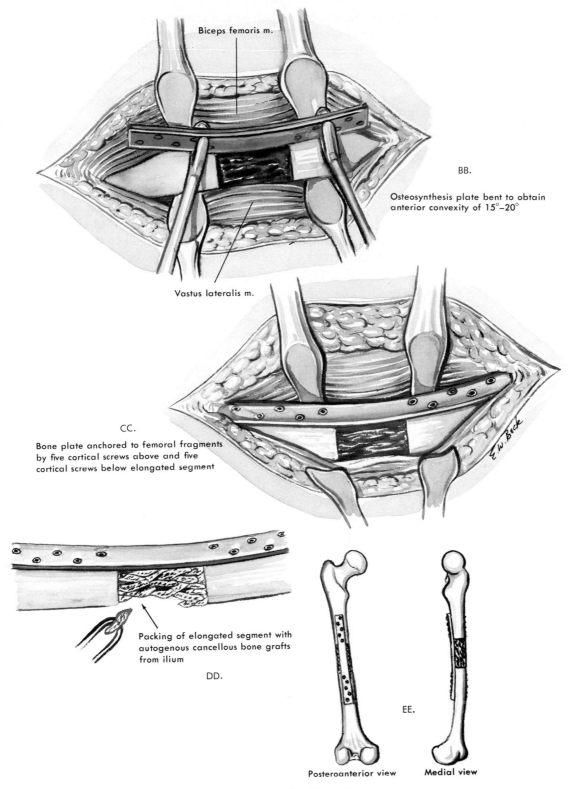

Biceps femoris m.

BB.

Osteosynthesis plate bent to obtain
anterior convexity of 15°–20°

Vastus lateralis m.

CC.

Bone plate anchored to femoral fragments
by five cortical screws above and five
cortical screws below elongated segment

Packing of elongated segment with
autogenous cancellous bone grafts
from ilium

DD.

EE.

Posteroanterior view   Medial view

Plate 137. (Continued)

FF. The previous skin incision on the posterolateral aspect of the femur is used for exposure of the femur. The subcutaneous tissue and deep fascia are divided in line with the skin incision. The lateral intermuscular septum and vastus lateralis are retracted anteriorly. The biceps femoris muscle is retracted and elevated posteriorly, exposing the posterior surface of the femur and the rigid plate and screws. The screws and plate are removed. The screw holes are curetted, and with the help of sharp osteotomes and rongeurs, all the bony ridges are removed, preparing the bed for the semitubular plate.

GG. The semitubular plate is placed on the posterolateral aspect of the femur immediately next to the site of the rigid plate. First, the top screw is inserted, then the distal one.

HH. and II. The other screws are inserted, anchoring the plate to the femur. Anteroposterior and lateral radiograms are made to check the position of the plate and screws. The wound is copiously irrigated with normal saline solution and is closed in the usual fashion. The patient is discharged to home within a few days with a three-point crutch gait protecting the elongated limb.

REFERENCES

Wagner, H.: Operative lengthening of the femur. Clin. Orthop., 136:125, 1978.

Wagner, H.: Surgical lengthening of the femur. Report of fifty-eight cases (author's translation). Ann. Chir. 43:263, 1980.

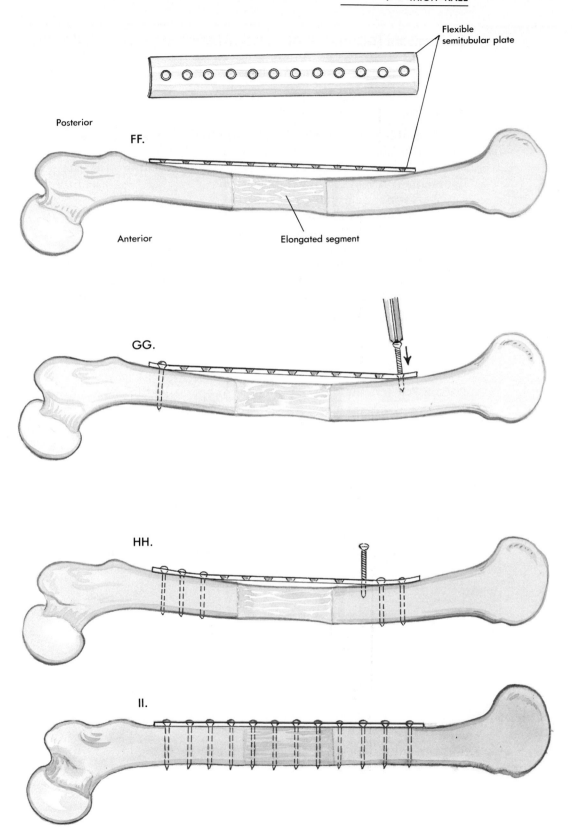

Flexible
semitubular plate

Posterior

FF.

Anterior

Elongated segment

GG.

HH.

II.

Plate 137. (Continued)

PLATE 138   DeBastiani Technique of Femoral Lengthening by Callotasis

Indications. Lower limb length disparity of 5 cm. or more in a patient of normal stature.

Requisites

1. Stable joints proximal and distal to the elongated bone. In femoral lengthening, the hip and knee should be stable. If the acetabulum is dysplastic, the femoral head should be covered prior to lengthening. The absence of cruciate ligaments is a relative contraindication.
2. Normal neuromuscular function.
3. Normal circulation.
4. Skin and soft tissues should be relatively normal.
5. Bone structure should be normal and strong.
6. Patient should be mentally stable with no psychological dysfunction.
7. Patient should be of sufficient age to be cognizant of the complications of limb lengthening and to be cooperative in the postoperative regimen.

Special Instrumentation. Orthofix femoral lengthening device.

Radiographic Control. Image intensifier.

Blood for Transfusion. Yes.

Patient Position. Supine on a radiolucent operating table.

Operative Technique

A. The first stage of the operation is insertion of screws. The most proximal screw is inserted first, immediately above the lesser trochanter and perpendicular to the longitudinal axis of the femur. Under image-intensifier control the proper level of the screw is determined. A 1-cm. longitudinal skin incision is made.

B. With a pair of blunt Metzenbaum scissors the wound is spread apart.

C. The midline of the lateral cortex of the femur is determined with a trocar inserted into the correct screw guide; the screw guide should be placed on bone, perpendicular to the longitudinal axis of the femur and midline in position.

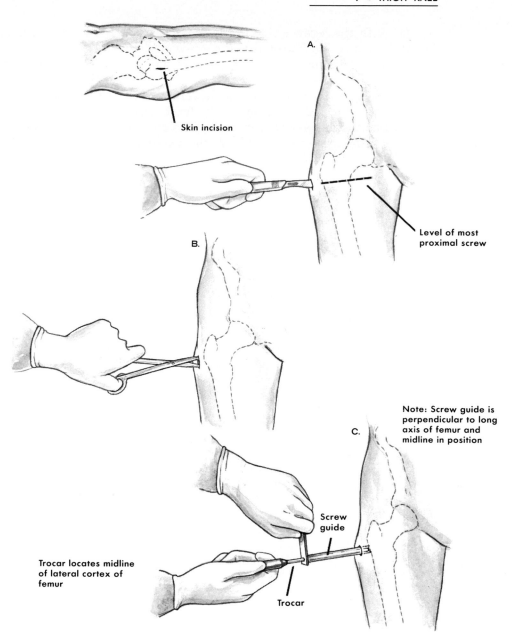

Skin incision

A.

Level of most
proximal screw

B.

Note: Screw guide is
perpendicular to long
axis of femur and
midline in position

C.

Screw
guide

Trocar locates midline
of lateral cortex of
femur

Trocar

Plate 138. A.–Y., Femoral lengthening by callotasis (DeBastiani technique).

D. With the screw guide firmly pressed on bone (by pressure exerted on the handle); remove the trocar from the screw guide.

E. With a hammer, the screw guide is gently tapped to engage its teeth on the cortex.

F. A drill guide is inserted into the screw guide. Drill size should be appropriate to screw size. For cortical screws (used for femoral lengthening), a 4.8-mm. drill is used. When the diameter of the femur is 15 mm. or less, 4.5-mm. or 3.5-mm. screws are used; the correct-size drill for the smaller screws is usually 3.2 mm. For cancellous screws, a 3.2-mm. drill is used.

D.

Note: Keep screw
guide firmly pressed
on bone

Trocar is removed

E.

Note: Teeth of screw
guide penetrate
lateral cortex of femur

F.

Drill guide is inserted
into the screw guide

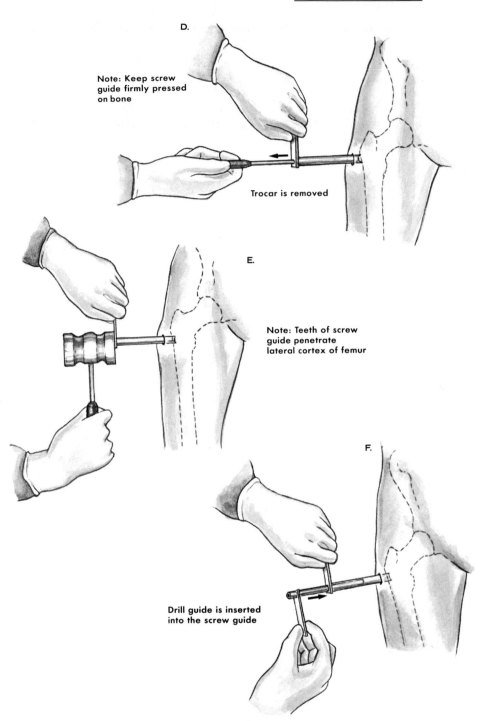

Plate 138. (Continued)

G. A drill bit of the correct size is fitted with a drill stop and inserted into the drill guide. The drill should be perpendicular to the femur.

H. With a low-speed power drill, the first cortex is drilled up to the second cortex.

I. and **J.** Next, the drill stop is offset by 5 mm. for drilling through the second cortex, which should be completely penetrated by the drill. Offsetting the drill stop will prevent overpenetration of the drill and thus protect against damage to the soft tissues.

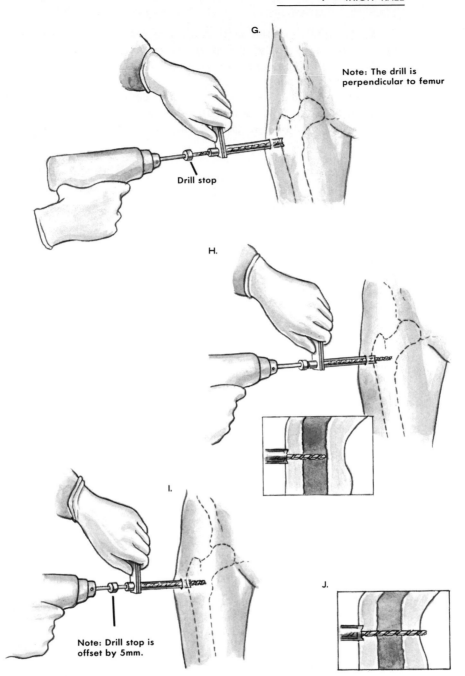

G.

Note: The drill is
perpendicular to femur

Drill stop

H.

I.

Note: Drill stop is
offset by 5mm.

J.

Plate 138. (Continued)

K. The drill bit and drill guide are removed. Be sure to maintain the screw guide in place by applying firm pressure on the screw guide handle.

L. A screw of appropriate size and length is selected, fitted to a "T" wrench, and inserted into the screw guide. The screw is self-tapping and requires minimum force for insertion. The screw should penetrate the first cortex, traverse the medullary canal, and penetrate the second cortex, at which point increased resistance should be felt. Screw penetration should be confirmed on radiographic image intensification.

M. The screw is turned clockwise slowly under image-intensifier x-ray control. By seven or eight further half-turns—be careful not to overpenetrate!—at least two threads of the screw should protrude beyond the second cortex.

Caution! The threads of the screw are tapered; thus, turning the screw counterclockwise will loosen its purchase.

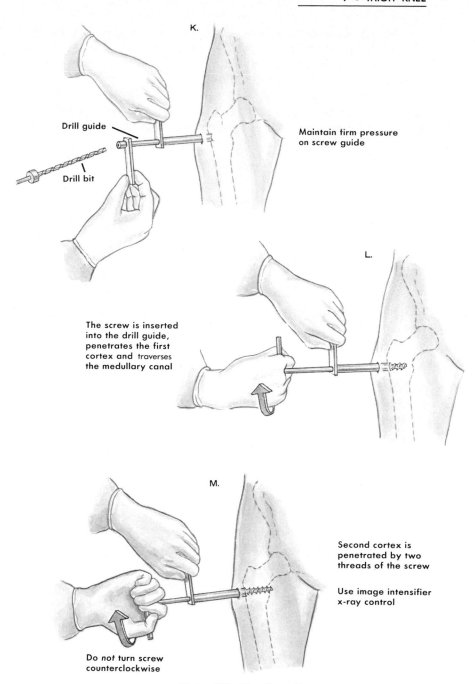

K.

Drill guide

Drill bit

Maintain firm pressure
on screw guide

The screw is inserted
into the drill guide,
penetrates the first
cortex and traverses
the medullary canal

L.

M.

Second cortex is
penetrated by two
threads of the screw

Use image intensifier
x-ray control

Do *not* turn screw
counterclockwise

Plate 138. (Continued)

N. The lengthening device's rigid template is positioned on the lateral side of the thigh, in line with and parallel to the femoral shaft. The screw guide is left in place, and one end of the template is applied to it. The first screw should be in the most proximal hole of the template.

O. The second screw is placed in the most distal hole. The grooves on the template can be used as a guide to mark the second skin incision. The screw insertion follows the steps already spelled out (**A.** to **M.**).

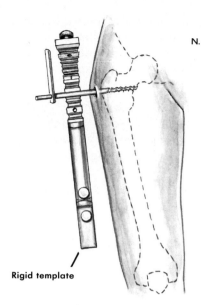

N.

Note: First screw is placed
in the second grooved seat

Rigid template

O.

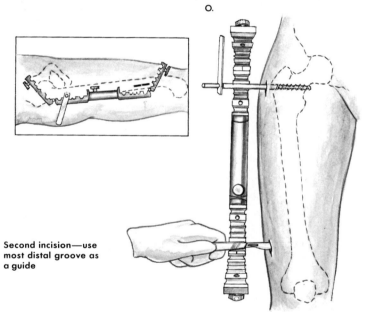

Second incision—use
most distal groove as
a guide

Plate 138. (Continued)

P. The third screw is placed into the fourth hole distal from the first screw.

Q. The fourth screw is placed in the hole closest to the most distal screw. Then the fifth screw is inserted in the distal clamp and the sixth screw into the proximal clamp. Three screws in the proximal clamp and three screws in the distal clamp are recommended.

The next stage of the callotasis is corticotomy. In the femur the level of corticotomy corresponds to the distal point of insertion of the iliopsoas muscle—usually 1 cm. inferior to the most distal of the proximal set of screws. Verify the level on radiographic image intensification.

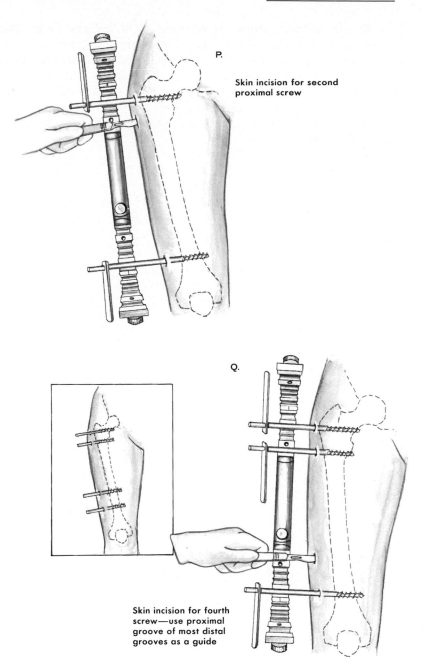

P.

Skin incision for second
proximal screw

Q.

Skin incision for fourth
screw—use proximal
groove of most distal
grooves as a guide

Plate 138. (Continued)

R. and **S.** The template is removed. A 4- to 5-cm. longitudinal skin incision is made on the anterior aspect of the upper thigh. The subcutaneous tissue and fascia are divided in line with the skin incision. The interval between the sartorius muscle and the tensor muscle of the fascia lata is widened. The fibers of the rectus femoris muscle are separated from the vastus intermedialis muscle by gentle blunt dissection, exposing the periosteum on the anterior aspect of the femur. A longitudinal incision is made in the periosteum. Elevating the periosteum exposes the upper femoral diaphysis.

T. A 4.8-mm. drill is inserted into a short Orthofix screw guide. The drill stop is adjusted so that the tip of the drill protrudes 5 mm. beyond the end of the screw guide.

U. Holes are drilled into the medial, anterior, and lateral cortices. The drill stop will prevent the drill from penetrating the medullary cavity and damaging the marrow and intramedullary circulation.

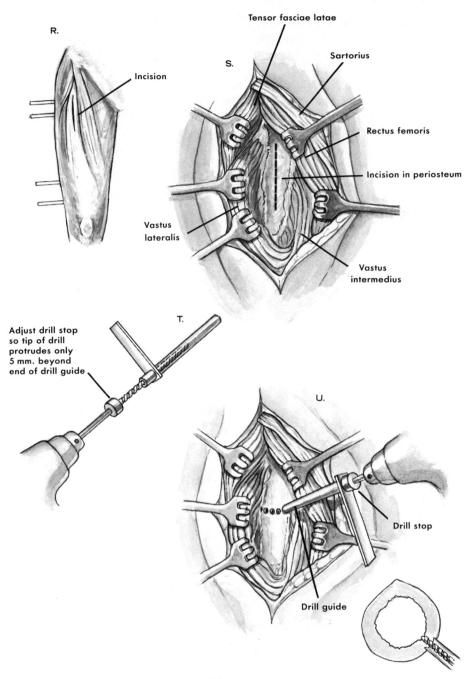

R.

Incision

S.

Tensor fasciae latae

Sartorius

Rectus femoris

Incision in periosteum

Vastus
lateralis

Vastus
intermedius

T.

Adjust drill stop
so tip of drill
protrudes only
5 mm. beyond
end of drill guide

U.

Drill stop

Drill guide

Plate 138. (Continued)

V. By the use of a small sharp-edged bone chisel, the drill holes are joined and the corticotomy completed. The medullary cavity and marrow should not be penetrated. The periosteum on the posterior aspect of the femur usually remains intact.

W. The Orthofix Dynamic Axial Fixator is anchored to the screws. The body-locking screw should be on the outside. The dot and arrow on the cam mechanism and the screws on the clamps should face upward.

The fixator should be 3 cm. away from the skin to allow space for postoperative swelling and cleansing of the screw sites. The body of the lengthening device should be parallel to the diaphysis of the femur. Using an Allen wrench tighten the clamp screws. In order to prevent stresses when locking the clamp screws, it is wise to insert dummy screws in empty (unused) outer clamp holes.

V.

Caution: Do not penetrate
medullary cavity

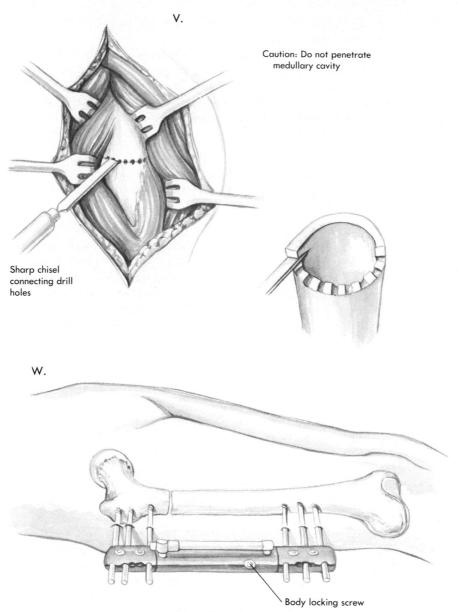

Sharp chisel
connecting drill
holes

W.

Body locking screw

Plate 138. (Continued)

X. The cams and body-locking screw are locked by the use of a torque wrench. A click indicates the correct torque.

Y. The completeness of the corticotomy is confirmed by distracting the bony segments under image-intensifier radiographic control, and the segments are then returned to their original position. The periosteum is sutured, and the wound is closed in the usual fashion. A Hemovac suction drain is left in situ for 24 to 48 hours. Any tension on the skin around the screws is relieved. The range of hip and knee motion is tested to ensure that movement is unrestricted and full.

Postoperative Care. Partial weight-bearing is allowed as soon as the patient is comfortable after surgery. Physical therapy is performed several times a day to maintain the range of hip and knee motion and to preserve motor strength in the muscles of the hip and knee.

Pin Site Care. Immediately postoperatively and several times a day thereafter, the wounds are cleaned with Betadine solution. Three days after surgery the pin sites are cleansed with sterile normal saline solution twice a day. It is important to keep a crust from forming at the pin's junction with the skin. Mechanical cleansing will prevent infection. Sterile gauze, is used for local dressing.

Distraction commences when callus formation is seen on radiograms, about 10 to 15 days postoperatively. With the distraction attachment in place, the body-locking screw is released. Turning the screw 90 degrees (a quarter-turn) counterclockwise achieves 0.25 mm. of distraction. Following completion of distraction, the body locking screw is firmly tightened. The sequence used to achieve a total of 1.00 mm. of distraction is incremental: three successive quarter-turns counterclockwise (distraction), followed by a single quarter-turn clockwise (compression), are spaced over the course of eight hours; three more quarter-turns counterclockwise and a final quarter-turn clockwise then follow, again carried out over eight hours. Thus, in a 16-hour period (the patient's waking hours), six distractive quarter-turns are "countered" by two compressive quarter-turns, yielding four advances in distraction of 0.25 mm. each—for a total gain of 1 mm. of distraction. The rate of distraction is reduced when it causes pain or muscle spasm. Hip and knee range of motion are checked for stiffness and to detect subluxation.

Seven days after distraction is begun, anteroposterior, oblique and lateral radiograms of the upper femur are obtained to confirm the separation of the corticotomy with callus continuity. Follow-up radiograms are obtained at three- to four-week intervals. If the callus response is poor, callus distraction is stopped for seven days and then restarted. If the distraction is excessive and a gap develops in the callus, compression is started at the same rate as that of previous distraction. (To achieve compression, the screw is turned clockwise; a 360-degree clockwise turn achieves 1 mm. of compression.) When callus continuity is re-established, distraction is restarted; in the beginning it is best to distract 1.5 mm. and compress 0.5 mm. With distraction-compression, osteogenesis is enhanced as, gradually, the bone is being lengthened.

When the desired length is obtained, the body-locking screw is tightened and the distraction attachment removed. Full weight-bearing is allowed. When radiograms show good consolidation of the callus, the body-locking screw is loosened; dynamic axial loading is started and continued until adequate cortex is formed all around the elongated segment. At this time the stability of the elongated segment is tested clinically with the fixator removed and the body-locking screw tightened.

If the elongated segment is stable, the screws are left in place for four to six days and then removed. Removal will require appropriate sedation or, in the case of the apprehensive child or adolescent, general anesthesia.

If the elongated segment is mechanically unstable, the fixator is reapplied and dynamic axial loading restarted.

All during this period, physical therapy is performed daily to maintain function of the elongated limb. Again, function is never sacrificed for length.

X.

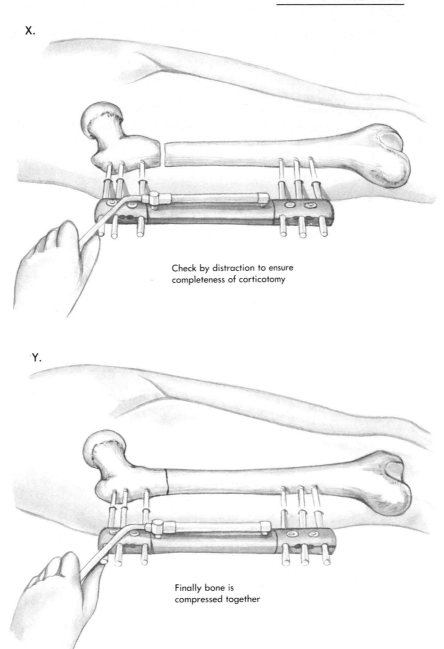

Check by distraction to ensure
completeness of corticotomy

Y.

Finally bone is
compressed together

Plate 138. (Continued)

Healing index is an expression of the number of days required to achieve 1 cm. of lengthening; the figure is obtained by dividing the overall treatment time in days by the total amount of lengthening achieved in centimeters. The healing index, in the experience of Professor DeBastiani, is 36 days for the femur, 41 days for the tibia, and 24 days for the humerus.

Often I recommend protecting the elongated segment of the femur by external support in the form of a hip-knee-ankle-foot orthosis (HKAFO) with an anterior shell on the femur. The HKAFO is worn during the day for a period of two to four months when the patient is walking, depending on the radiographic findings.

REFERENCE

DeBastiani, G., Aldegheri, R., Renzi-Brivio, L., and Trivella, G.: Limb lengthening by callus distraction (callotasis). J. Pediatr. Orthop., 7:129, 1987.

X.

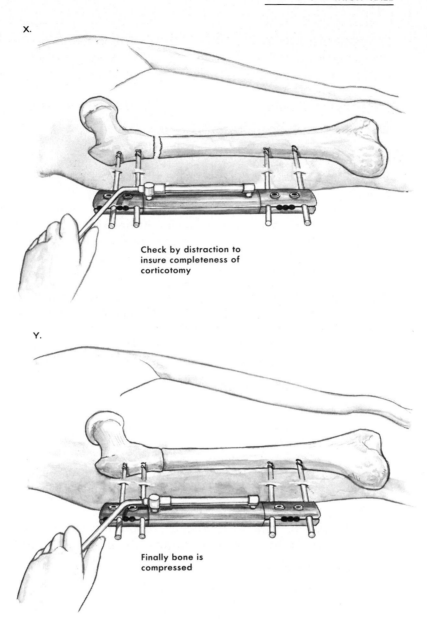

Check by distraction to
insure completeness of
corticotomy

Y.

Finally bone is
compressed

Plate 138. (Continued)

PLATE 139   Fragmentation by Multiple Osteotomies, Realignment, and Intramedullary Solid Rod Fixation in Osteogenesis Imperfecta (Williams Modification of Sofield-Millar Technique)

Indications. Multiple fractures in a child with severe osteogenesis imperfecta.

Blood for Transfusion. Yes.

Radiographic Control. Image intensifier.

Special Instrumentation. Intramedullary rod fixation—surgeon's preference as to type. (e.g., Williams, Rush, Luque, or similar). Prior to surgery, measure the length and width of the bone in which the intramedullary rod is to be inserted. Personally check the availability of a complete set of different diameter rods and a corresponding set of short and long drills for reaming. Other surgical instruments required are an oscillating saw, a heavy bolt cutter, and two parallel-action, heavy-duty pliers for bending the solid rods.

Preoperative Preparation. Children with severe osteogenesis imperfecta present greater than normal anesthesia risk because of their diminished respiratory function due to deformity of their thoracic cage and atrophy of their intercostal muscles. Also, these children are prone to develop hyperthermia during surgery. Preoperatively, the orthopedic surgeon should communicate with the anesthesiologist. Atropine as a preoperative medication should be administered in a minimal dosage, if at all.

Blood should be available for replacement in all cases, as when the bones are subperiosteally exposed, bleeding always occurs, especially during the insertion of femoral and humeral rods where a tourniquet cannot be used. The surgeon should remember that easy bruising is a manifestation of osteogenesis imperfecta. Open surgery on both femora should not be performed at a single operation; death due to excess blood loss can occur. It is best to stage the procedures.

It is vital to use image-intensifier radiographic control.

Patient Position. Supine. The child should be placed on the operating table on a thermally controlled mattress. Draping should be light, preferably sterile paper.

Operative Technique

A. Incision. The femur is approached through a lateral approach, anterior to the intermuscular septum. The tibia is exposed through an anterolateral approach (see **M.**). A pneumatic tourniquet is used for ischemia when the tibia is fixed by an intramedullary rod. The humerus is approached through Henry's anterolateral approach.

A vital surgical requisite for intramedullary rod insertion in osteogenesis imperfecta is adequate exposure of the entire diaphysis; the deformed, bowed bone should be visualized metaphysis to metaphysis. Any attempt to pass a rod blindly through a small incision will end in disaster. Radiograms will be deceiving; there are almost always imperceptible angular and rotational deformations of the long bones in osteogenesis imperfecta.

In this plate intramedullary rod fixation of the femur is illustrated. A straight, lateral, longitudinal incision is made from the tip of the greater trochanter to the lateral condyle of the femur. Subcutaneous tissue and deep fascia are divided in line with the skin incision. Meticulous hemostasis is crucial to minimize blood loss.

B. Reflect and elevate the vastus lateralis at the lateral intermuscular septum. Preservation of muscles is important—they surround and support the fragile bones. Resist the temptation of direct surgical approach and muscle splitting, even when the bone is severely deformed.

A.

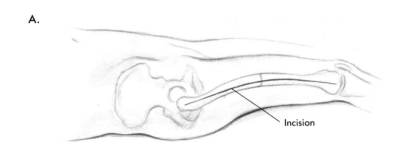

Incision

B.

Gluteus maximus

Greater trochanter

Vastus lateralis reflected

Lateral intermuscular septum

Biceps femoris

CAUTION: *Do not injure growth plates*

Line of incision of periosteum

C.

Fracture site

Keith needle in greater trochanteric apophysis

C. EllER

Keith needle in distal femoral physis

Plate 139. A.–O., Fragmentation by multiple osteotomies, realignment, and intramedullary solid rod fixation in osteogenesis imperfecta (Williams modification of Sofield-Millar technique).

C. Avoid injury to growth plates. Determine the exact level of the distal femoral physis and greater trochanteric apophysis radiographically by inserting Keith needles into the growth plates. Make a horizontal incision in the periosteum immediately proximal and parallel to the distal femoral physis and another horizontal periosteal incision immediately distal to the greater trochanteric apophysis. Connect the two horizontal incisions by a straight longitudinal incision in the periosteum. The incisions in the periosteum are made sharply with a scalpel. Begin elevating the periosteum gently with a Freer elevator and then with a moist sponge rather than a large periosteal elevator. Be gentle! Elevate the periosteum first over intact bone and then proximally toward the fracture site.

A.

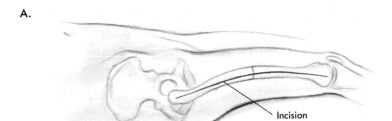

Incision

B.

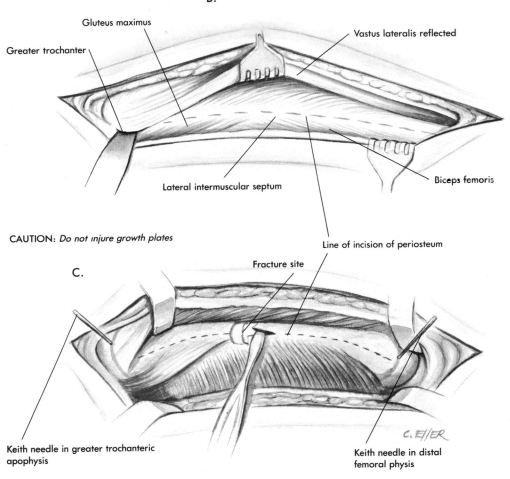

Gluteus maximus

Greater trochanter

Vastus lateralis reflected

Lateral intermuscular septum

Biceps femoris

CAUTION: *Do not injure growth plates*

Line of incision of periosteum

C.

Fracture site

Keith needle in greater trochanteric apophysis

Keith needle in distal femoral physis

C. EILER

Plate 139. (Continued)

D. Place bone retractors (such as Chandler) subperiosteally and expose the entire shaft of the femur—metaphysis to metaphysis.

Caution! The soft bones of osteogenesis imperfecta can easily be crushed by the bone-holding forceps—be gentle!

Inspect and assess the deformity. How many cuts are required to achieve correction? The individual fragments should be as long and as few as possible, yet they should be straight enough to be strung on a rod. The surgeon should understand the principles of carpentry; a vital requisite to rod insertion is the feasibility of placing all of the fragments in a straight line. A common pitfall is failure to resect and discard sufficient bone. It is crucial that everything fall into a straight line without force. Inadequate bone shortening will tauten the soft tissue on the concave side; when correction is attempted, the excessive stress on the bone ends will displace the rods.

Make all the bone cuts with an oscillating saw and not an osteotome. Do not splinter or butterfly fracture the fragile bones. In the femur (as well as in the tibia) the initial cut is made distally, at the metaphyseal-diaphyseal junction, and then the proximal cut is made.

E. Intramedullary reaming is often required. Choose the narrowest bone fragment first and ream with a drill of appropriate diameter. There may be no medullary cavity. Meticulous technique is vital. Time is of the essence to minimize blood loss, the risk of anesthesia, and surgical complications.

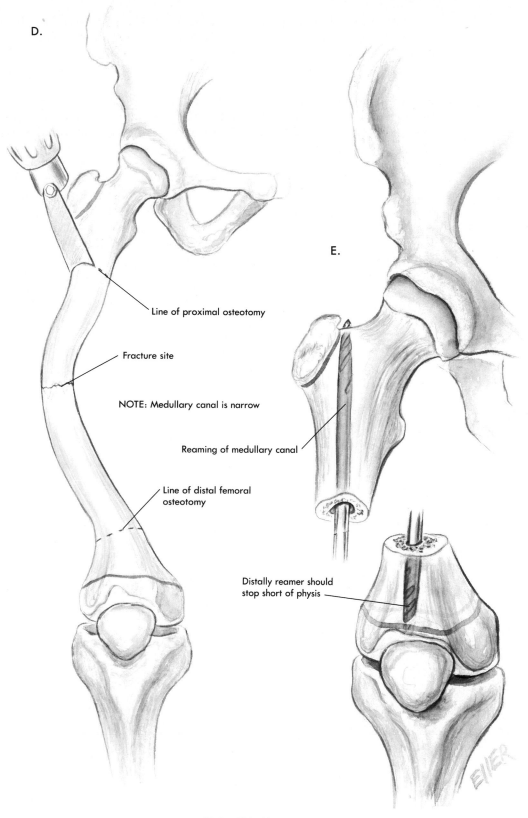

D.

Line of proximal osteotomy

Fracture site

NOTE: Medullary canal is narrow

Line of distal femoral osteotomy

E.

Reaming of medullary canal

Distally reamer should stop short of physis

Plate 139. (Continued)

F.–H. Next, determine the length of the rod to be used. Make three measurements: First, measure the length of the gap between the two ends of the diaphysis with traction applied on the knee.

Note: For the tibia, traction is applied on the foot, and for the humerus, on the flexed elbow. Often there is less than the total length of the fragments, necessitating shortening or discarding a bone fragment. The second and third measurements are the distances between the cuts at the proximal and distal diaphyseal-metaphyseal junction and the growth plate. These measurements are obtained by pushing a rod into the open end of the shaft until the resistance of the physis is felt.

Next, decide whether the rod will extend metaphysis to metaphysis or if it will traverse the physes and extend epiphysis to epiphysis. Ordinarily, a smooth rod that traverses the center of the physis and lies in the epiphysis will not disturb growth. Intramedullary rods that extend epiphysis to epiphysis add length to the rod and delay the problem of relative bone overgrowth than a rod that is too short. Some surgeons, however, prefer to avoid violation of the growth plates. The rods should not enter the joints and should not penetrate the proximal and distal cortices of the metaphyses.

F.

First measurement: Gap distance between 2 ends
of diaphysis with traction applied distally

G.

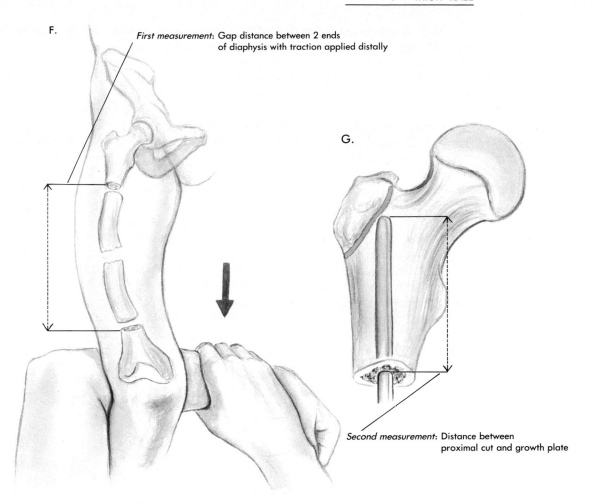

Second measurement: Distance between
proximal cut and growth plate

H.

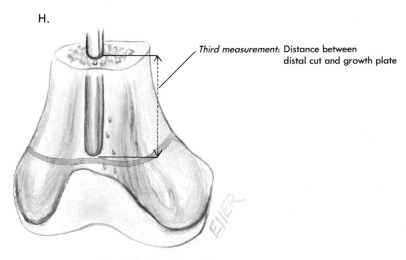

Third measurement: Distance between
distal cut and growth plate

Plate 139. (Continued)

I.–L. A common deformity of the distal part of the femur is anterolateral angulation. To minimize the problem of the rod cutting out of the cortex, it is crucial that during realignment osteotomy this anterolateral angulation be corrected completely and the distal end of the intramedullary rod be placed centrally or slightly anterolaterally into the distal femoral epiphysis. Other factors to consider in placement of the rod in the distal femur are the deformity of the knee joint, angular deformity of the upper tibia, and future plans for surgery of the knee. Proximally, the rod should be in the medial portion of the greater trochanter toward the base of the femoral neck; this is particularly important when there is coxa vara deformity.

In the Williams modification of the Sofield-Millar technique, the femoral rod is inserted as follows: Cut a rod with a female thread to the measured length and a rod of appropriate length with a male thread. The male end is then screwed into the female end. The male end of the joined rods is driven from below into the open proximal femoral metaphysis, up into the greater trochanter, the gluteal muscles, and out of the skin. The osteotomized segments of the femoral shaft are threaded snugly onto the rod with the female threads; the rod is then driven gently into the distal femoral metaphysis or epiphysis by gentle hammering of the male part of the rod. Radiograms in the anteroposterior, lateral, and oblique projections are made to double-check the position of the rod; the unwanted part of the rod is then unscrewed and removed from the gluteal region. A hook is bent into the proximal end of the rod to prevent later migration.

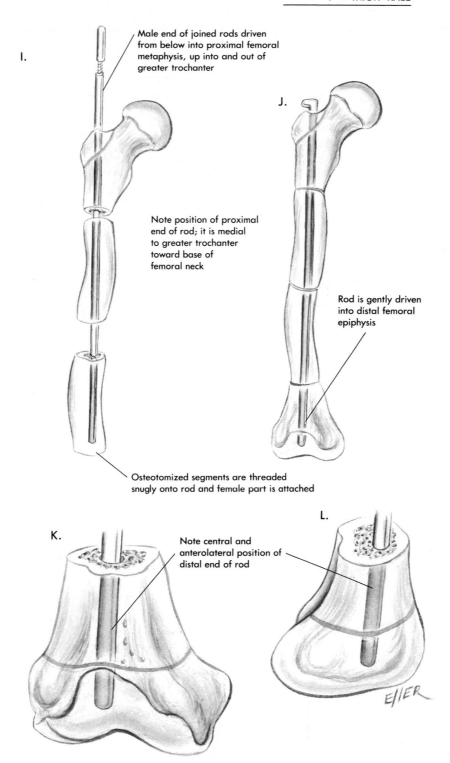

I. Male end of joined rods driven from below into proximal femoral metaphysis, up into and out of greater trochanter

Note position of proximal end of rod; it is medial to greater trochanter toward base of femoral neck

J. Rod is gently driven into distal femoral epiphysis

Osteotomized segments are threaded snugly onto rod and female part is attached

K.

Note central and anterolateral position of distal end of rod

L.

Plate 139. (Continued)

M.–O. In the tibia the male end of the rod is driven into the open lower tibial metaphysis, across the ankle and tarsus, to exit from the sole of the foot. After threading the osteotomized segments onto the rod with the female threads, the rod is gently hammered into the proximal tibial metaphysis or epiphysis. The deformity of the upper part of the tibia is usually anteromedial. The danger is anterior protrusion of the rod; therefore, the rod is anchored securely in the posterior part of the upper tibia.

The periosteum, whenever possible, and the fascia are meticulously closed. After closure of the subcutaneous tissue and skin in the routine fashion, a bilateral, long-leg hip spica cast is applied. The hip, knee, ankle, and foot should be in a functional stance position to allow early weight-bearing in the cast within a day or two after surgery. The cast should be very light, preferably made of plastic. An above-knee cast will exert leverage on the femur and cause angular deformity; thus, it should be avoided.

An alternate method of internal fixation is by a Rush rod. In such an instance, in the femur, the Rush rod is driven distally from the greater trochanter into the proximal femoral metaphysis under image intensifier control. After secure internal fixation, the hook of the Rush rod is anchored into the greater trochanter.

Postoperative Care. The cast is removed when the osteotomized bone fragments and the fracture have healed. Healing usually takes place in six weeks. This author recommends that the cast be removed in the hospital and the child placed in counterpoised bilateral split-Russell's traction. Gentle active assisted and passive exercises are performed by a physical therapist to restore range of motion of the hip, knee, and ankle and to develop motor strength of muscles.

The child is allowed to stand and walk with a walker or crutch support in a bilateral hip-knee-ankle-foot orthosis. Initially, the hips and knees are locked; gradually, the hips and knees are unlocked. Crutch and orthotic support are discontinued when motor power of muscles and weight-bearing bones are strong. This may require six to twelve months or longer, depending on the age of the patient and the degree of severity of osteogenesis imperfecta.

Intramedullary rod fixation may be complicated by extreme osteoporosis, with the bone almost disappearing because of lack of stress. Delayed union and nonunion are other complications that present very different problems of management. External orthotic support in hip-knee-ankle-foot orthosis is continued indefinitely in these children.

Bending and fractures of the rod and fractures adjacent to the rod ends and relative bone longitudinal overgrowth and a short rod require rod replacement.

Growth arrest due to violation of the physes by the rod ends is a definite complication. This problem is managed by excision of the osseous bridges across the physis and interposition with fat following the Langenskiöld technique.

REFERENCES

Millar, E. A.: Observation on the surgical management of osteogenesis imperfecta. Clin. Orthop., 159:154, 1981.

Sofield, H. A., and Millar, E. A.: Fragmentation, realignment, and intramedullary rod fixation of deformities of the long bones of children: a ten-year appraisal. J. Bone Joint Surg., 41-A:1371, 1959.

Tiley, F., and Albright, J. A.: Osteogenesis imperfecta: Treatment by multiple osteotomy and intramedullary rod insertion. Report of thirteen patients. J. Bone Joint Surg., 55-A:701, 1973.

Williams, P. F., Cole, W. H. J., Bailey, R. W., Dubow, H. I., Solomons, C. C., and Millar, E. A.: Current aspects of the surgical treatment of osteogenesis imperfecta. Clin. Orthop., 96:288, 1973.

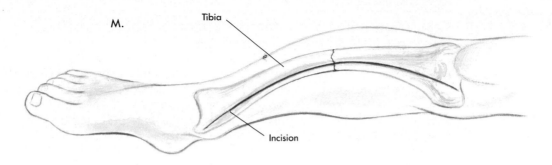

M.

Tibia

Incision

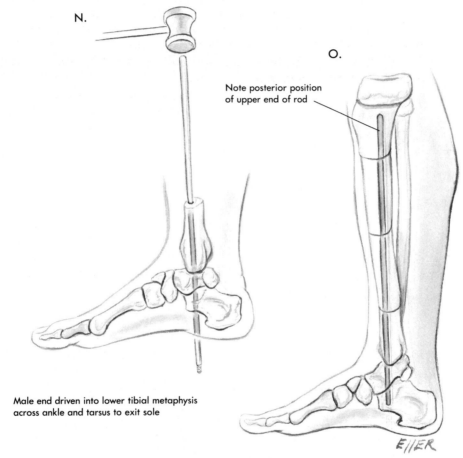

N.

Male end driven into lower tibial metaphysis
across ankle and tarsus to exit sole

O.

Note posterior position
of upper end of rod

E//ER

Plate 139. (Continued)

PLATE 140 **Open Reduction and Internal Fixation of Fractures of the Intercondylar Eminence of the Tibia**

Indications. Type III fractures (Meyers and McKeever) in which the avulsed fragment is completely elevated from its bed with total lack of bone apposition. The avulsed fragment may be rotated or angulated so that its cartilaginous surface is at the base of the intercondylar eminence, making union impossible. The anterior horn of the lateral meniscus may interpose between the avulsed fragment and its bed.

Operative Technique

A. Reduction and internal fixation are usually performed through the arthroscope with the patient anesthetized. First, aspirate and irrigate the tense swollen knee joint. Do not manipulate the knee into hyperextension, because it serves no useful purpose and may in fact further displace the avulsed fragment attached to the distal end of the anterior cruciate ligament.

B. Through the arthroscope, use a dull probe to liberate the entrapped anterior pole of the lateral meniscus.

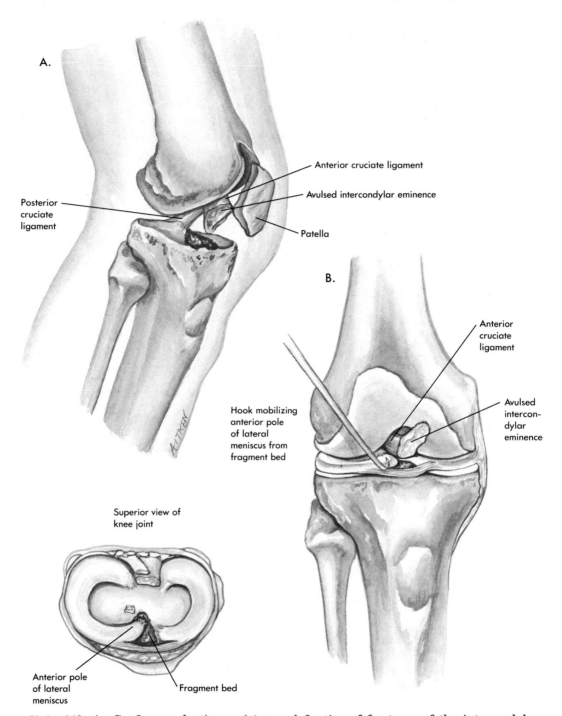

Plate 140. A.–C., Open reduction and internal fixation of fractures of the intercondylar eminence of the tibia.

C. With a large probe, push the fragment down into its bed in anatomic position. Internal fixation is carried out simply by strong absorbable sutures (such as Vicryl), passed with a cutting needle into the anterior cruciate ligament, the margins of the fragment, and the anterior horns of the menisci. Tightening of the suture will firmly hold the fracture fragment anatomically reduced.

Open arthrotomy is occasionally indicated when visualization through the arthroscope and fixation of the fragment are difficult. When open arthrotomy is performed, use the anterolateral approach, as the pathology is lateral. Ordinarily, I do not recommend the use of threaded pins, screws, or wire loops for internal fixation because it is not required for stability of reduction and a second operation is necessary to remove them. However, on occasion, internal fixation with a screw is required in the skeletally mature patient.

Postoperative Care. Following open reduction, the knee is immobilized in an above-knee cast with the knee in 20 to 30 degrees of flexion. Immobilization is continued until there is radiographic evidence of healing, usually six to eight weeks.

REFERENCES

Garcia, A., and Neer, C. S., II: Isolated fractures of the intercondylar eminence of the tibia. Am. J. Surg., 95:593, 1958.

McLennan, J. G.: The role of arthroscopic imaging in the treatment of fractures of the intercondylar eminence of the tibia. J. Bone Joint Surg., 64-B:477, 1982.

Meyers, M. H., and McKeever, F. M.: Fracture of the intercondylar eminence of the tibia. J. Bone Joint Surg., 41-A:209, 1959.

Meyers, M. H., and McKeever, F. M.: Fracture of the intercondylar eminence of the tibia. J. Bone Joint Surg., 52-A:1677, 1970.

Zaricznyj, B.: Avulsion fracture of the tibial eminence: Treatment by open reduction and pinning. J. Bone Joint Surg., 50-A:111, 1977.

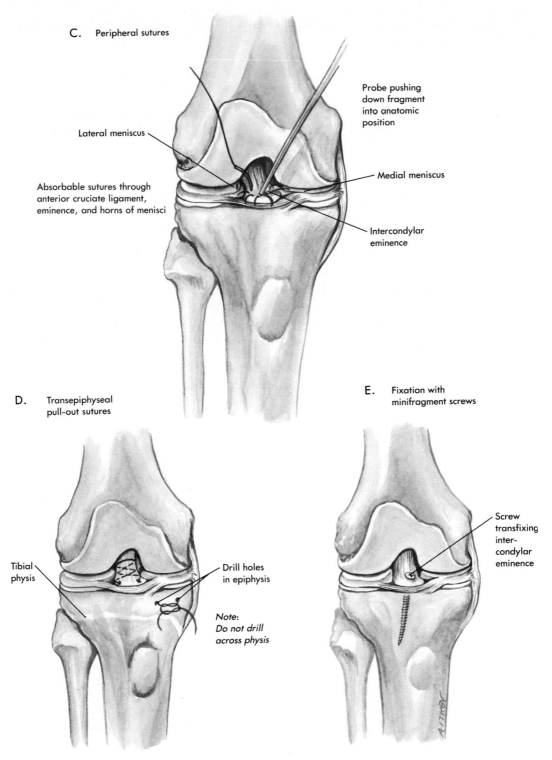

C.   Peripheral sutures

Probe pushing
down fragment
into anatomic
position

Lateral meniscus

Absorbable sutures through
anterior cruciate ligament,
eminence, and horns of menisci

Medial meniscus

Intercondylar
eminence

D.   Transepiphyseal
pull-out sutures

Tibial
physis

Drill holes
in epiphysis

Note:
Do not drill
across physis

E.   Fixation with
minifragment screws

Screw
transfixing
inter-
condylar
eminence

Plate 140. (Continued)

PLATE 141

Soft-Tissue Release to Correct Hyperextension Contracture of the Knee

Indications. Fixed hyperextension deformity of the knee not responding to conservative measures of stretching casts, traction, or physical therapy.

Patient Position. The patient is placed in the supine position with a pneumatic tourniquet placed high on the thigh. In an infant the procedure is performed with a sterile tourniquet.

Operative Technique

A. An anterolateral approach is used to expose the knee joint and the distal one third of the quadriceps. A longitudinal incision is made on the anterolateral aspect of the thigh because a midline incision is not cosmetically pleasing. The incision begins about 5 to 10 cm. superior to the proximal pole of the patella (depending on the size of the patient) and extends distally to the upper border of the patella. If it is necessary to perform a capsulotomy of the knee, the incision can be further extended distally to the medial joint line. Subcutaneous tissue and superficial fascia are divided in line with the skin incision.

B. The rectus femoris muscle and tendon are identified. The junction between the rectus femoris tendon and the anterior margin of the vastus medialis and vastus lateralis muscles is delineated. Divide the deep fascia along each side of the rectus femoris tendon and muscle. Make a long inverted "V" incision in the rectus femoris, leaving its distal attachment to the superior pole of the patella intact.

C. If the knee does not flex adequately (more than 90 degrees), the incision is extended over the anteromedial aspect of the knee. The wound flaps are undermined and retracted, and an anterior capsulotomy of the knee is performed. Any fibrous adhesions between the undersurface of the rectus femoris and patella are released. If there are intra-articular adhesions, they are sectioned and the knee is flexed to 110 to 120 degrees.

D. With the knee in 90 degrees of flexion, the proximally recessed vastus medialis and vastus lateralis are sutured together and distally to the displaced rectus femoris tendon.

The wound is closed in the usual fashion. An above-knee cast is applied with the knee in 90 degrees of flexion.

Postoperative Care. The cast is removed three weeks after surgery. Active assisted and gentle passive range of motion exercises are performed to develop motor strength of the quadriceps muscle and to maintain the full degree of flexion and extension of the knee.

REFERENCE

Curtis, B. H., and Fisher, R. L.: Congenital hyperextension with anterior subluxation of the knee. Surgical treatment and long-term observations. J. Bone Joint Surg., 51-A:255, 1969.

A.

B.

Rectus femoris
m.

Vastus medialis
m.

Vastus
lateralis
m.

Inverted V incision
in rectus tendon

C.

D.

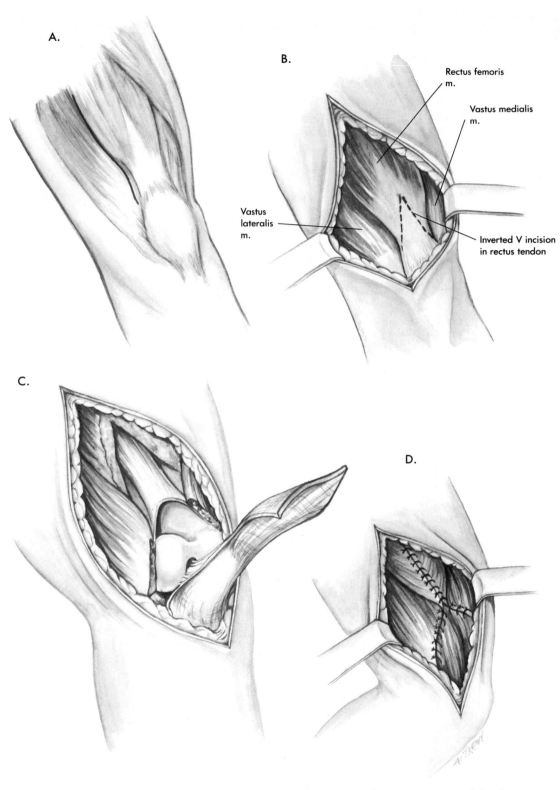

Plate 141. A.–D., Soft-tissue release to correct hyperextension contracture of the knee.

PLATE   142   ## Open Reduction of Congenital Dislocation of the Knee

Indications. When reduction is not achieved by closed methods.

Precautions. In grade III, in which there is total displacement of the upper tibial epiphysis in front of the femoral condyles (no contact between the articular surface of the two bones), the dislocation is rigid.

Caution! Closed methods usually fail, and physeal fracture-separation or tibial or femoral fractures do occur while traction is in use and during passive manipulation. Be gentle.

Perform MRI to detect fibrosis of the quadriceps femoris with obliteration of the quadriceps pouch. In such an instance, perform primary open reduction.

Blood for Transfusion. Yes.

Radiographic Control. Image intensifier.

Patient Position. The patient is placed in the supine position. In the infant, the pneumatic tourniquet may be too large for the small, short thigh; therefore, this author recommends the use of a narrow Esmarch or Martin bandage for tourniquet ischemia. The tourniquet ischemia period should not exceed 30 to 45 minutes. If more time is needed, take the tourniquet down and reapply after 10 minutes. To minimize blood loss, it is best to operate under tourniquet ischemia.

Operative Technique

A.–C. The knee joint is exposed through an anteromedial approach. Cosmetically, an anteromedial scar is more pleasing than a midline longitudinal scar. The skin incision begins over the medial aspect of the rectus femoris tendon about 4 to 5 cm. above the patella. It extends inferiorly to the medial border of the patella; at the inferior pole of the patella, the incision curves gently laterally and distally to end 1 cm. distal to the proximal tibial tubercle. The subcutaneous tissue is divided in line with the skin incision. The skin margins are mobilized, and the wound flaps are undermined. Keep close to the surface of the capsule to avoid inadvertent injury to the sensory nerves, which are located in the subcutaneous fat. Necrosis of wound flaps is ordinarily not a problem because the skin has adequate blood supply.

First, the pathologic anatomy is studied. The surgical procedure employed depends on the pathologic findings.

1. The patellar ligament is shortened and the anterior joint capsule is contracted.

2. The patella is underdeveloped and located more proximally than normal.

3. The rectus femoris and vastus intermedius muscles with the adjoining quadriceps mechanism are adherent to the femur by a mass of fibrous tissue, obliterating the suprapatellar pouch and fixing the patella to the femur.

4. The collateral ligaments and the medial hamstring and biceps femoris tendons are displaced anteriorly.

5. The iliotibial band and the lateral intermuscular septum may be contracted, causing valgus deformity and lateral subluxation of the knee.

Following assessment of the pathologic anatomy, make medial and lateral parapatellar longitudinal incisions, dividing parapatellar retinaculum, capsule, and synovium.

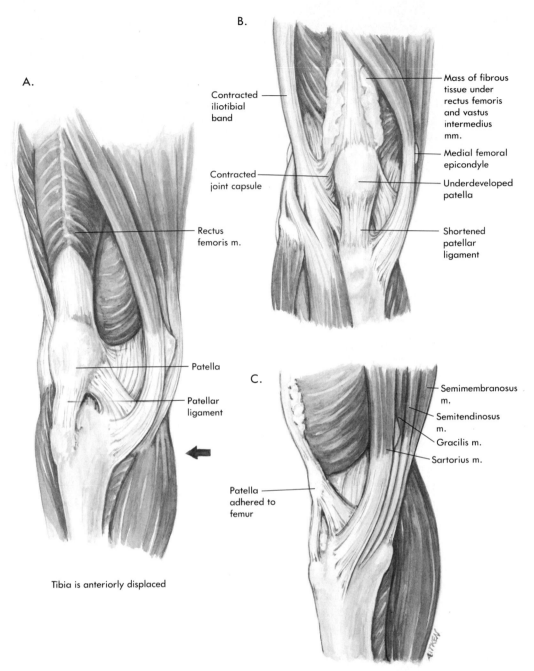

A.

B.

Contracted
iliotibial
band

Contracted
joint capsule

Rectus
femoris m.

Patella

Patellar
ligament

Tibia is anteriorly displaced

Mass of fibrous
tissue under
rectus femoris
and vastus
intermedius
mm.

Medial femoral
epicondyle

Underdeveloped
patella

Shortened
patellar
ligament

C.

Semimembranosus
m.

Semitendinosus
m.

Gracilis m.

Sartorius m.

Patella
adhered to
femur

Plate 142. **A.–H.,** Open reduction of congenital dislocation of the knee.

D. Dissect free the patellar tendon from the underlying capsule, and transversely divide the anterior joint capsule.

E. and **F.** Lengthen the iliotibial band by Z-plasty, and release the lateral intermuscular septum.

The vastus intermedius, rectus femoris, and adjoining vastus muscles are then freed from underlying bone. The rectus femoris tendon and quadriceps femoris are elongated by an inverted "V" lengthening. When the patella is very high-riding, with marked shortening of the quadriceps femoris, perform Z-plasty of the rectus femoris tendon and musculotendinous fractional lengthening of vastus medialis and lateralis. Occasionally excision of the hypoplastic patella is indicated to provide greater length of the quadriceps tendon.

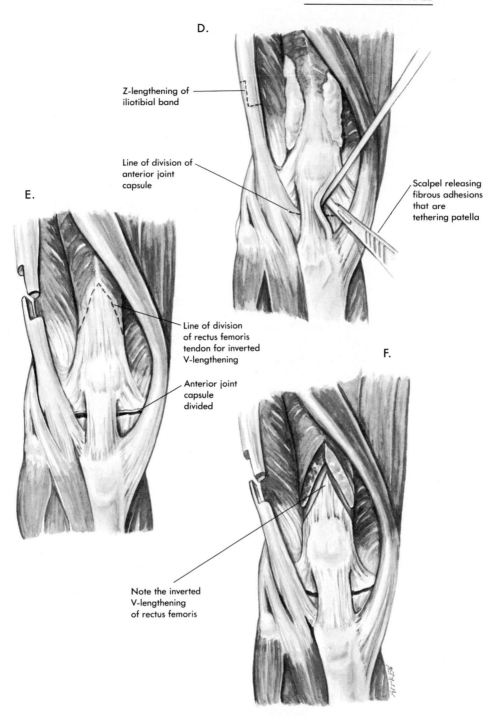

D.

Z-lengthening of iliotibial band

Line of division of anterior joint capsule

Scalpel releasing fibrous adhesions that are tethering patella

E.

Line of division of rectus femoris tendon for inverted V-lengthening

Anterior joint capsule divided

F.

Note the inverted V-lengthening of rectus femoris

Plate 142. (Continued)

G. and **H.** The cruciate ligaments are inspected next. If the anterior cruciate ligament is absent, stability to the knee joint is provided by using the semitendinosus tendon to reconstruct the anterior cruciate ligament.

An alternative method is to use the central one half of the patellar tendon to reconstruct the anterior cruciate ligament. This author recommends the use of semitendinosus tendon because the patellar ligament is contracted and not long enough.

If the anterior cruciate is present but elongated, its tibial attachment is transferred distally on the tibia to tauten it.

The knee is flexed and the anterior displacement of the tibia on the femur is reduced. This will bring the anteriorly displaced hamstring tendons and collateral ligaments into their anatomic relationship to the joint. The tourniquet is released and complete hemostasis is achieved.

The capsule and quadriceps mechanism are sutured in their lengthened position. Anteroposterior and lateral radiograms of the knee are made to confirm anatomic reduction of the knee.

The wound is closed in the usual manner. A hip spica cast is applied with the hips in neutral extension and rotation and the knees in 45 to 60 degrees of flexion.

Postoperative Care. The hip spica cast is removed in six weeks. A knee-ankle-foot orthosis (KAFO) with a stop to prevent hyperextension of the knee joint is used for ambulation. At night a posterior KAFO with the knee in 30 to 45 degrees of flexion is used. Gentle passive exercises are performed several times a day to maintain and increase range of knee motion. Active and progressive resistive exercises are performed to increase motor strength of the knee.

REFERENCES

Austwick, D. H., and Dandy, D. J.: Early operation for congenital subluxation of the knee. J. Pediatr. Orthop., 3:85, 1983.

Curtis, B. H., and Fisher, R. L.: Congenital hyperextension with anterior subluxation of the knee. Surgical treatment and long-term observations. J. Bone Joint Surg., 51-A:255, 1969.

Jacobsen, K., and Vopalecky, F.: Congenital dislocation of the knee. Acta Orthop. Scand., 56:1, 1985.

Katz, M. P., Grogono, B. J. S., and Soper, K. C.: The etiology and treatment of congenital dislocation of the knee. J. Bone Joint Surg., 49-B:112, 1967.

Niebauer, J. J., and King, D. E.: Congenital dislocation of the knee. J. Bone Joint Surg., 47-A207, 1960.

G.

MEDIAL VIEW

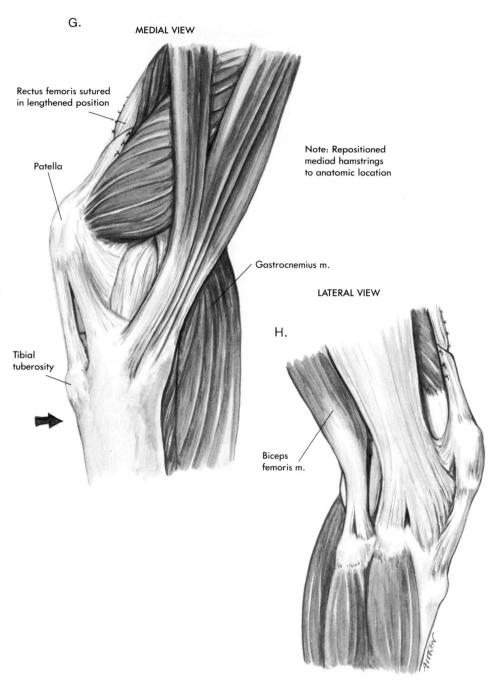

Rectus femoris sutured
in lengthened position

Patella

Note: Repositioned
mediad hamstrings
to anatomic location

Gastrocnemius m.

LATERAL VIEW

H.

Tibial
tuberosity

Biceps
femoris m.

Plate 142. (Continued)

PLATE 143

Quadriceps-Plasty for Recurrent Dislocation of the Patella (Green Technique)

Indications. Recurrent lateral subluxation for dislocation of the patella in which conservative nonoperative measures and partial proximal realignment by lateral patellar retinacular release have failed.

Patient Position. Supine with a pneumatic tourniquet placed high in the proximal thigh.

Operative Technique

A. The surgical approach is by two longitudinal skin incisions. The first incision is medial, beginning 3 cm. medial and 4 cm. proximal to the superior pole of the patella and extending distally to terminate at a point 2 cm. distal and 1 cm. medial to the proximal tibial tubercle. The lateral longitudinal skin incision begins at the joint line 2 cm. lateral to the lateral margin of the patellar tendon and extends proximally for a distance of 1 to 10 cm. The subcutaneous tissue and superficial fascia are divided, and the skin flaps are developed medially and laterally to expose the quadriceps muscle, patella, patellar tendon, patellar retinaculum, joint capsule, and iliotibial band.

B. and **C.** Starting at a level 3 cm. proximal to the lateral femoral condyle, a 7.5 cm. segment of the fascia lata and the lateral intermuscular septum are excised. Next, abnormal attachments of the iliotibial band are divided, and the vastus lateralis muscle is widely mobilized from the deep surface of the fascia lata and its origin from the femur to allow free medial displacement of the patella. During this procedure, several muscular branches of the perforating arteries may be encountered, requiring coagulation or ligation.

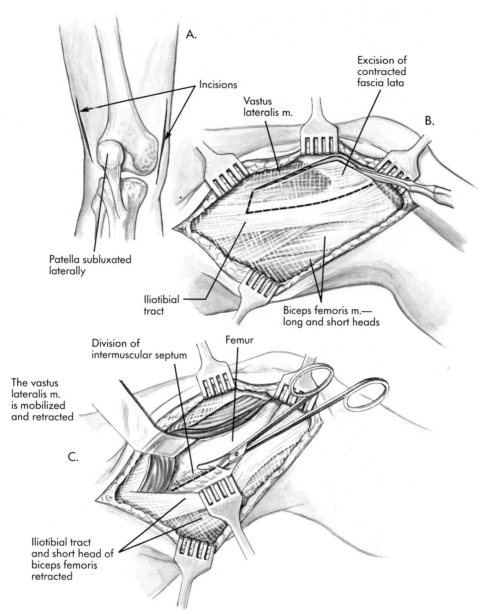

Plate 143. A.–F., Quadriceps-plasty for recurrent dislocation of the patella (Green technique).

D. and **E.** The contracted iliotibial tract, patellar retinaculum, and lateral joint capsule are then longitudinally divided in their posterolateral portion to allow medial displacement of the patella. The lax medial joint capsule and patellar retinaculum are longitudinally incised, and they are reefed later. The insertion of the vastus medialis, with its tendinous fibers and the periosteum of the patella, is detached from the medial and superior border of the patella by U-shaped incisions in the superoranterior and posteroinferior margins of the muscle. The synovial membrane is not incised unless visualization of the interior of the joint for loose bodies or chondromalacia of the patella is indicated. Next, the patella is displaced medially and the medial joint capsule is imbricated and tightly closed by reefing sutures. With the knee in complete extension, the medial patellar retinaculum is also imbricated by reefing sutures.

F. The superficial surface of the anterolateral third of the inferior half of the patella is then roughened with curved osteotomes and curet. The vastus medialis tendon is transferred laterally and distally deep to the patellar bursa and sutured to the lateral border of the patellar tendon. The wounds are closed in layers and a well-molded above-knee cylinder cast is applied with the knee in neutral position or flexed 5 degrees.

Postoperative Care. Immobilization in the solid cast is continued for three or four weeks. During this time the patient is permitted to walk with crutches with a three-point partial weight-bearing gait. Quadriceps muscle strength is maintained by isometric exercises in the solid cast. The cast is then removed, and knee motion and muscle strength are gradually developed by flexion-extension exercises. A knee orthosis holding the patella in reduced anatomic position and the knee in neutral extension is worn during the day for four weeks. Protection with crutches is continued until there is fair strength of the quadriceps muscle and 90 degrees of knee flexion.

REFERENCE

Green, W. T.: Recurrent dislocation of the patella. Its surgical correction in the growing child. J. Bone Joint Surg., 47-A:1670, 1965.

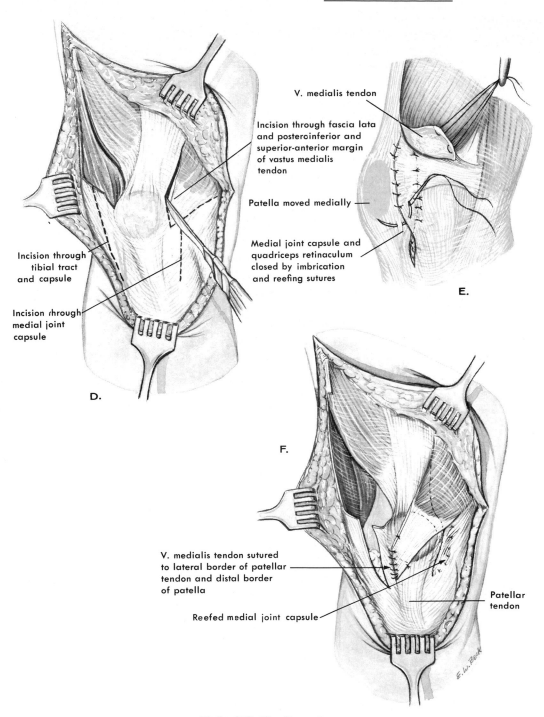

V. medialis tendon

Incision through fascia lata
and posteroinferior and
superior-anterior margin
of vastus medialis
tendon

Patella moved medially

Medial joint capsule and
quadriceps retinaculum
closed by imbrication
and reefing sutures

E.

Incision through
tibial tract
and capsule

Incision through
medial joint
capsule

D.

F.

V. medialis tendon sutured
to lateral border of patellar
tendon and distal border
of patella

Reefed medial joint capsule

Patellar
tendon

Plate 143. (Continued)

PLATE 144 **Medial and Distal Transfer of the Proximal Tibial Tubercle (Goldthwait-Hauser Procedure) for Recurrent Lateral Dislocation of the Patella**

Indications. Recurrent subluxation and dislocation of the patella in patients with patella alta and excessive increase in Q angle.

Precautions

1. Do not transfer the proximal tibial tubercle in children and adolescents with open physes and epiphyses because it will arrest growth from the anterior portion of the proximal tibial epiphysis and result in anterior tilting of the tibial plateau and genu recurvatum.

2. The procedure may cause distal migration of the patella and patellofemoral joint incongruity and early degenerative arthritis.

3. The transplanted tubercle may be pulled out like a traction apophysis and present as a large mass of bone at its new site.

4. Excessive lateral rotation of the tibia may result from medial transfer of the proximal tibial tubercle.

5. Anterior compartment syndrome may result from inadvertent division of or bleeding from the anterior tibial recurrent vessels.

6. Patellar compression may result from distal transfer of the patellar tendon.

This author does not recommend distal and medial transfer of the proximal tibial tubercle. It is best to treat the high-riding patella by lowering the patella to its anatomic position and stabilizing it there by tenodesis of the semitendinosus to the patella; the lax patellar tendon is shortened. The increased Q angle is treated by splitting the patellar tendon, detaching the lateral half and transferring it medially beneath the medial half, and anchoring it to the medial metaphysis of the tibia through drill holes (Roux-Goldthwait procedure).

Patient Position. Supine.

Operative Technique

A. An anteromedial incision is made, starting 2 cm. medial to the superior pole of the patella and extending distally to 3 cm. distal and 1 cm. medial to the proximal tibial tubercle. In this drawing, a U-shaped incision is illustrated over the anterior aspect of the knee; cosmetically the scar is ugly; therefore, this author does not recommend its use. The subcutaneous tissue and fascia are divided in line with the skin incision and the wound edges are retracted. Avoid injury to the infrapatellar branch of the saphenous nerve.

B. A longitudinal incision is made on each side of the patellar tendon, which is dissected free from its underlying fat pad. The patellar tendon should be left intact and attached at its insertion to the proximal tibial tubercle.

C. A rectangular block of bone (1 by 2 cm.) is resected from the tibial tuberosity at the site of insertion of the patellar tendon. The distal part is undercut as a wedge, following the method of McKeever. The joint capsule is incised on the medial and lateral side of the patella. The synovial membrane is left intact. The joint is not opened unless there are indications for inspection of the deep surfaces of the patella, menisci, and cruciate ligaments (such as patellar crepitation and locking of the knee). Next, a site for transplantation of the bone block is selected; it is 2 cm. medial and 1.5 to 2 cm. distal from its original location. The patella should lie betwen the femoral condyles in its normal position. A solid strut of bone should be present between the two blocks, in order to prevent fracture. It is best to use sharp drill points to control the extent of osteotomy. Too distal a position should be avoided, unless the patella was riding high. The periosteum is incised longitudinally and a similar-sized rectangular block of bone is removed.

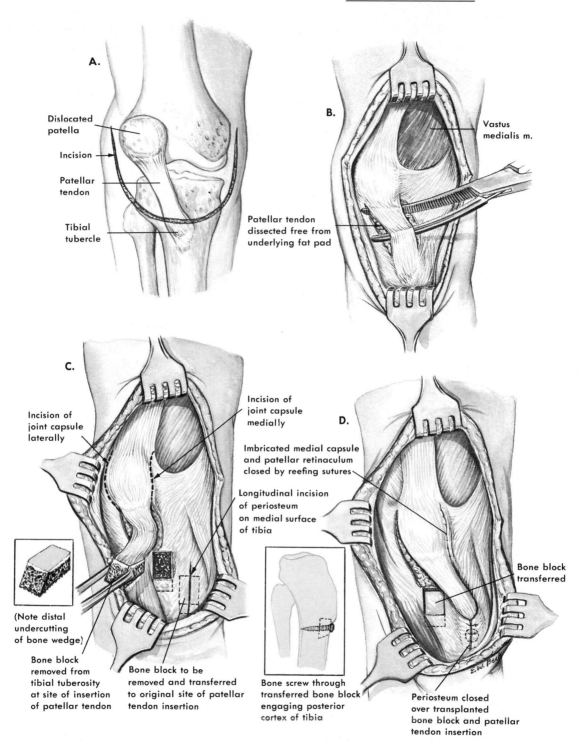

A.

Dislocated patella

Incision

Patellar tendon

Tibial tubercle

B.

Vastus medialis m.

Patellar tendon dissected free from underlying fat pad

C.

Incision of joint capsule laterally

Incision of joint capsule medially

Longitudinal incision of periosteum on medial surface of tibia

(Note distal undercutting of bone wedge)

Bone block removed from tibial tuberosity at site of insertion of patellar tendon

Bone block to be removed and transferred to original site of patellar tendon insertion

D.

Imbricated medial capsule and patellar retinaculum closed by reefing sutures

Bone block transferred

Bone screw through transferred bone block engaging posterior cortex of tibia

Periosteum closed over transplanted bone block and patellar tendon insertion

Plate 144. A.–D., Medial and distal transfer of the proximal tibial tubercle (Goldthwait-Hauser procedure) for recurrent lateral dislocation of the patella.

D. The first block of bone with the patellar tendon attached to it is firmly inserted and countersunk into the space created by removal of the second block. The bone block is transfixed internally with a screw, which should engage the posterior cortex of the tibia. The periosteum is closed with interrupted sutures, which should pass through the patellar tendon. The medial capsule is imbricated and reefed with interrupted sutures. The lateral capsule is left open. The second block of bone is inserted into the space created at the original site of patellar tendon insertion. The subcutaneous tissues and skin are closed in the routine manner, and the limb is immobilized in an above-knee cylinder cast with the foot and ankle free.

Postoperative Care. The patient is allowed to be ambulatory with crutches with a three-point partial weight-bearing gait when comfortable. Quadriceps isometric exercises are begun the day of operation. At four weeks, the cast is removed and radiograms are taken to determine the healing of the transplanted bone block. At this time, bony union is usually solid enough to allow side-lying knee flexion and extension exercises. A knee immobilizer holding the knee in extension is used for two or three weeks during walking. Then full weight-bearing is allowed. Quadriceps exercises are continued until full motor strength is regained. Full knee flexion may be difficult for some patients; hence, it is imperative to emphasize knee flexion as well as extension in the rehabilitation program.

REFERENCES

Goldthwait, J. E.: Dislocation of the patella. Trans. Am. Orthop. Assoc., 8:237, 1895.

Goldthwait, J. E.: Permanent dislocation of the patella. The report of a case of twenty years' duration, successfully treated by transplantation of the patellar tendon, with the tubercle of the tibia. Ann. Surg., 29:62, 1899.

Goldthwait, J. E.: Slipping or recurrent dislocation of the patella. With the report of eleven cases. Boston Med. Surg. J., 150:169, 1904.

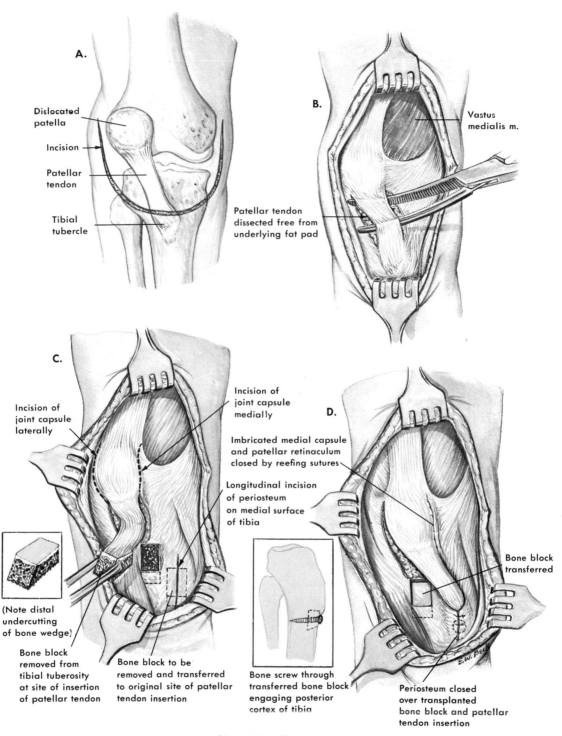

A.

Dislocated patella

Incision

Patellar tendon

Tibial tubercle

B.

Vastus medialis m.

Patellar tendon dissected free from underlying fat pad

C.

Incision of joint capsule laterally

Incision of joint capsule medially

Imbricated medial capsule and patellar retinaculum closed by reefing sutures

Longitudinal incision of periosteum on medial surface of tibia

(Note distal undercutting of bone wedge)

Bone block removed from tibial tuberosity at site of insertion of patellar tendon

Bone block to be removed and transferred to original site of patellar tendon insertion

Bone screw through transferred bone block engaging posterior cortex of tibia

D.

Bone block transferred

Periosteum closed over transplanted bone block and patellar tendon insertion

E.W. Beck

Plate 144. (Continued)

PLATE 145 **Semitendinosus Tenodesis to the Patella for Recurrent Lateral Subluxation of the Patellofemoral Joint**

Indications. Recurrent lateral subluxation or dislocation of the patellofemoral joint associated with high-riding patella (patella alta) and when there is marked generalized ligamentous hyperlaxity (familial or in syndromes such as Down, Marfan, or Ehlers-Danlos).

Patient Position. Supine.

Operative Technique

A. First, make a 4- to 5-cm. longitudinal incision over the proximal aspect of the lower third of the thigh, centered over the course of the semitendinosus tendon. The fusiform muscle of the semitendinosus ends a little below in the middle of the thigh in a long, rounded tendon that lies on the external surface of the semimembranosus. Identify the semitendinosus tendon by palpation and flexion-extension of the knee. Subcutaneous tissue and fascia are divided in line with the skin incision.

Caution! Do not injure the posterior femoral cutaneous nerve—in the back of the thigh it descends usually more laterally, medial to the biceps tendon.

B. and **C.** The semitendinosus tendon is sectioned at its musculotendinous junction; its muscle belly is sutured to the semimembranosus.

D. Next identify and follow the distal stump of the semitendinosus tendon to its insertion. It curves around the medial condyle of the tibia superficial to the medial collateral ligament of the knee, from which it is separated by a bursa. Pull on the semitendinosus tendon and palpate its tendon at its insertion. Make a 3 to 4 cm. oblique skin incision along the course of the tendon below the knee joint over the anteromedial aspect of the upper leg.

Caution! Do not injure the infrapatellar branch of the saphenous nerve.

E. The semitendinosus tendon is attached to the upper part of the medial surface of the tibia, posterior to the attachment of the sartorius and inferior to that of the gracilis. It is surprising how often the novice orthopedic resident has trouble identifying the semitendinosus tendon at its insertion. The semitendinosus tendon is delivered into the distal wound and left attached distally. If indicated, the synovium is incised and the interior of the knee joint is inspected. Determine the degree of chondromalacia—if marked or severe, shave the degenerated retro-patellar articular cartilage. Inspect for possible loose bodies in the knee joint; if any are present, remove them.

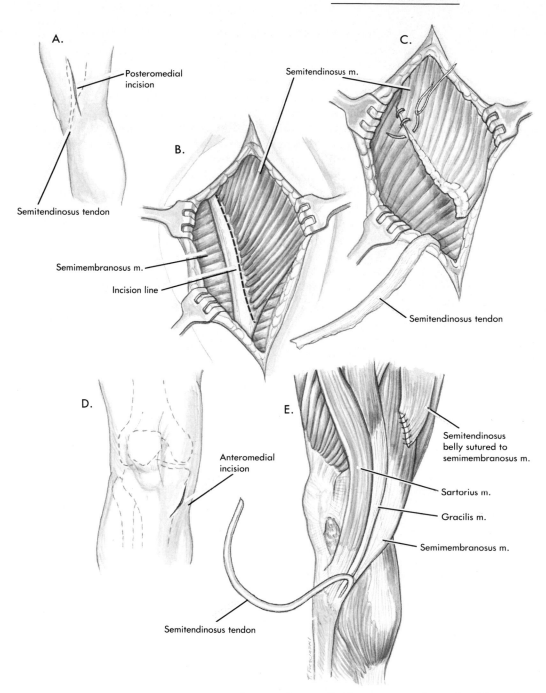

A.

Posteromedial incision

Semitendinosus tendon

B.

Semitendinosus m.

Semimembranosus m.

Incision line

C.

Semitendinosus m.

Semitendinosus tendon

D.

Anteromedial incision

Semitendinosus tendon

E.

Semitendinosus belly sutured to semimembranosus m.

Sartorius m.

Gracilis m.

Semimembranosus m.

Plate 145. A.–K., Semitendinosus tenodesis to the patella for recurrent lateral subluxation of the patellofemoral joint.

F. Next, make a medial parapatellar incision beginning 4 to 5 cm. proximal and 3 cm. medial to the superior pole of the patella. Extend it distally to terminate 2 cm. distal to the knee joint line and 2 cm. medial to the patellar tendon. The subcutaneous tissue and superficial fascia are divided in line with the skin incision. Avoid injury to the infrapatellar branch of the saphenous nerve.

G. The lateral and medial skin flaps are dissected and mobilized, exposing the anterior surface of the patella, patellar tendon, medial and lateral patellar retinaculi, vastus medialis, rectus femoris, vastus lateralis, and joint capsule. The lateral patellar retinaculum is divided to mobilize the patella medially; if the lateral joint capsule is contracted, it is also sectioned.

H. Next, an oblique hole is drilled across the patella in the line of tenodesis. Do not damage the articular cartilage on the deep surface of the patella!

I. The semitendinosus tendon is passed through the hole in the patella from its medial to its lateral side.

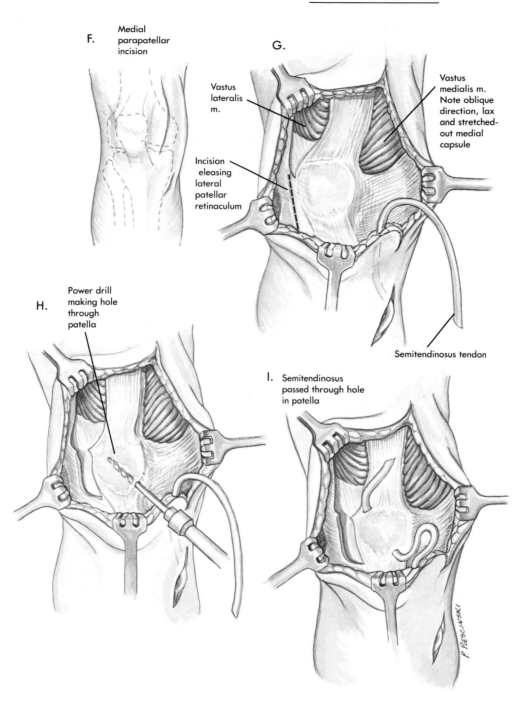

F. Medial parapatellar incision

G.

Vastus lateralis m.

Vastus medialis m. Note oblique direction, lax and stretched-out medial capsule

Incision eleasing lateral patellar retinaculum

Semitendinosus tendon

H. Power drill making hole through patella

I. Semitendinosus passed through hole in patella

P. PIECUINSKI

Plate 145. (Continued)

J. The patella is pulled down medially and distally and, while held there, the semitendinosus tendon is sewn back to itself; thereby the pull of the quadriceps is directed in line with the intercondylar notch of the femur. The patellar insertion is converted to a yoke of an inverted U.

K. The semitendinosus patellar tenodesis is combined with plication of the medial capsule and medial patellar retinaculum and realignment of the quadriceps mechanism. The vastus lateralis is released, and the vastus medialis is advanced distally and laterally. The oblique course of vastus medialis is corrected to a transverse course. If the patellar tendon is slack, it is tautened by distal-medial transfer of its lateral half; the medial half of the patellar tendon is shortened by plication.

Postoperative Care. The knee is immobilized in an above-knee cylinder cast for four to six weeks. The patient is allowed to be ambulatory with crutches with a three-point partial weight-bearing gait. Isometric exercises of the quadriceps femoris and hamstrings are begun the day of surgery. After four to six weeks, the cast is removed. This author prefers to admit the patient to the hospital for intensive physical therapy; active exercises (gravity eliminated and then against gravity) are performed to increase motor strength of the quadriceps femoris, hamstrings, and triceps surae. Side-lying active assisted knee flexion-extension exercises are performed to increase range of knee flexion. An above-knee orthosis is applied, holding the knee in extension and the patella in its relocated anatomic position. Initially the orthosis is worn day and night, except for exercise periods, and then its use is gradually decreased. When quadriceps femoris motor strength is normal and the knee has full range of motion, the use of the orthosis is discontinued. Running, jumping, and contact sports are not allowed for six months. The two failures that this author had were due to falls and injury in the immediate postoperative period. The importance of a meticulous physical therapy program to restore normal knee function cannot be overemphasized. Trauma to the knee should be avoided.

REFERENCES

Baker, R. H., Carroll, N., Dewar, F. P., and Hall, J. E.: The semitendinosus tenodesis for recurrent dislocation of the patella. J. Bone Joint Surg., 54-B:103, 1972.

Dewar, F. P., and Hall, J. E.: Recurrent dislocation of the patella. J. Bone Joint Surg., 39-B:798, 1957.

Galeazzi, R.: Nouve applicazioni del trapianto muscolare e tendineo. Arch. Orthop., 38:1922, 1921.

Hall, J. E., Micheli, L. J., and McNamara, G. B., Jr.: Semitendinosus tenodesis for recurrent subluxation or dislocation of the patella. Clin. Orthop., 144:31, 1979.

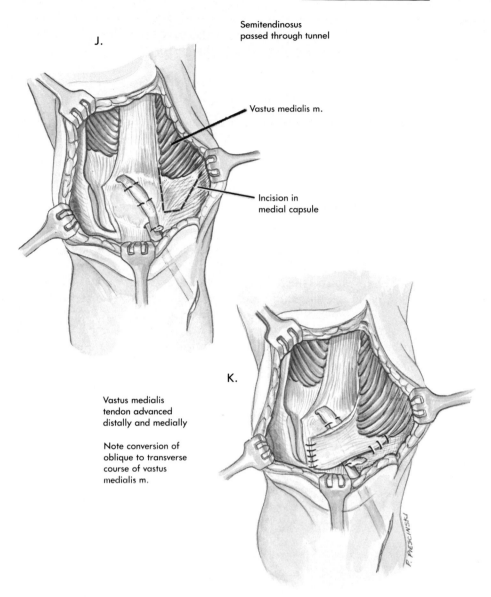

J.

Semitendinosus
passed through tunnel

Vastus medialis m.

Incision in
medial capsule

K.

Vastus medialis
tendon advanced
distally and medially

Note conversion of
oblique to transverse
course of vastus
medialis m.

Plate 145. (Continued)

PLATE 146   ## Patellar Advancement by Plication of the Patellar Tendon and Division of the Patellar Retinacula

Indications. High-riding patella due to elongation of patellar tendon with loss of full active extension of the knee (quadriceps lag).

Requisites. Complete correction of hamstring contracture and knee flexion deformity.

Patient Position. Supine.

Radiographic Control. Image intensifier.

Operative Technique

A. A transverse skin incision is made, centering over the knee joint and extending from the medial to the lateral condyle of the femur. Subcutaneous tissue and fascia are divided in line with the skin incision.

B. The wound flaps are retracted proximally and distally, exposing the high-riding patella, elongated patellar tendon, and patellar retinacula.

C. The wound flaps are approximated, and through separate stab wounds in the skin, a large threaded Steinmann pin is inserted transversely through the center of the patella and a similar pin is placed in the proximal tibia distal to the physis. Do not disturb growth. Use image intensifier. The distal pin should be drilled from the lateral side and should be directed somewhat anteroposteriorly to prevent pressure irritation of the common peroneal nerve.

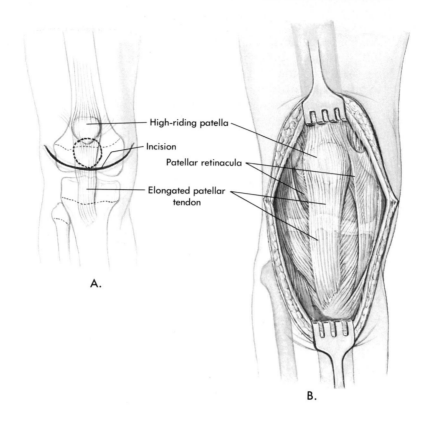

High-riding patella

Incision

Patellar retinacula

Elongated patellar tendon

A.

B.

C.

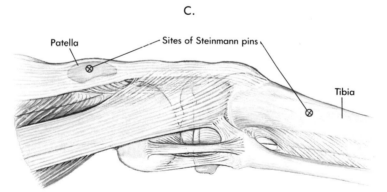

Patella

Sites of Steinmann pins

Tibia

Plate 146. A.–F., Patellar advancement by plication of the patellar tendon and division of the patellar retinacula.

D. The medial and lateral margins of the patellar tendon are identified. Longitudinal incisions are made on each side of the tendon, which is isolated and mobilized from subjacent and surrounding structures. Care should be taken not to open the capsule of the knee joint. Next, the patellar retinacula are divided medially and laterally.

E. The patella is pulled distally to its normal position in the intercondylar notch by traction on the proximal pin and manual pressure. The two pins are securely held together by a plate or external fixation apparatus. The patellar tendon is thoroughly freed from the underlying fat pad.

F. The patellar tendon is plicated, shortening it to the desired length. Its plicated ends are sutured together with 00 or 0 Tycron. Any bulky segment of the tendon is excised, if necessary. The wound is closed in layers and an above-knee cast is applied, which holds the knee in neutral position or 5 degrees of hyperextension. The pins are covered with petrolatum gauze to prevent skin slough from being incorporated in the cast. Adequate padding should be applied to prevent pressure sores.

Postoperative Care. About four to six weeks after surgery, the cast and pins are removed. Active and passive exercises are performed to regain muscle strength and range of motion. Weight-bearing is gradual and is protected with crutches. Full weight-bearing is allowed when the quadriceps is fair in motor strength.

REFERENCES

Chandler, F. A.: Re-establishment of normal leverage of patella in knee flexion deformity in spastic paralysis. Surg. Gynecol. Obstet., 57:523, 1933.

Chandler, F. A.: Patellar advancement operation. Revised technique. J. Int. Coll. Surg., 3:433, 1940.

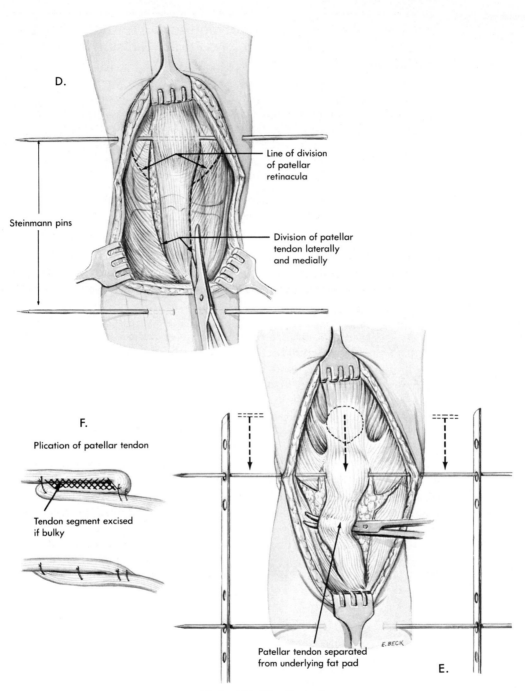

D.

Steinmann pins

Line of division
of patellar
retinacula

Division of patellar
tendon laterally
and medially

F.

Plication of patellar tendon

Tendon segment excised
if bulky

E. BECK

Patellar tendon separated
from underlying fat pad

E.

Plate 146. (Continued)

PLATE 147 | **Excision of the Discoid Lateral Meniscus—Total Excision by the Direct Lateral Approach and Partial Excision Through the Anterolateral Approach**

Indications. Frequent locking of the knees with pain and functional disability. First delineate the pathologic change by diagnostic arthroscopy. The entire meniscus is excised when the discoid meniscus is of the Wrisberg type (hypermobile) or when it is torn and when there is marked degeneration.

Partial resection of the discoid meniscus is indicated when it is of the complete or incomplete type and the following conditions exist:

1. There is minimal tearing or slight degeneration.
2. Capsular attachments are intact.
3. The discoid meniscus is not hypermobile (Wrisberg type).

Patient Position. With the tourniquet on the proximal thigh, the patient is placed in the supine position and the lower limb is prepared and draped so that full motion of the knee is permitted without contamination of the operative area.

Operative Technique

A. Diagrammatic representation of gross anatomy of discoid lateral meniscus.

B. The surgical approach is described by Bruser.

The affected knee is acutely (fully) flexed so that the heel almost touches the buttocks. This position also flexes the hip 80 degrees, relaxing the taut fibers of the iliotibial band. The skin incision is made over the lateral joint line, beginning at the patellar ligament anteriorly and ending at a point midway between the fibular head and the lateral femoral condyle. The subcutaneous tissue is divided and the wound edges are retracted with sharp rakes.

C. The shiny fibers of the iliotibial band are exposed; they lie almost parallel to the skin incision and the joint line. The fascial fibers are split or, if necessary, divided. The lateral (or fibular) collateral ligament traverses longitudinally in the posterior end of the fascial incision. Caution should be exercised so that the ligament is not divided inadvertently.

D. With a blunt right-angled knee retractor the lateral ligament and popliteus tendon are retracted posteriorly. The capsule and synovium are divided at the joint line along the superior margin of the discoid lateral meniscus.

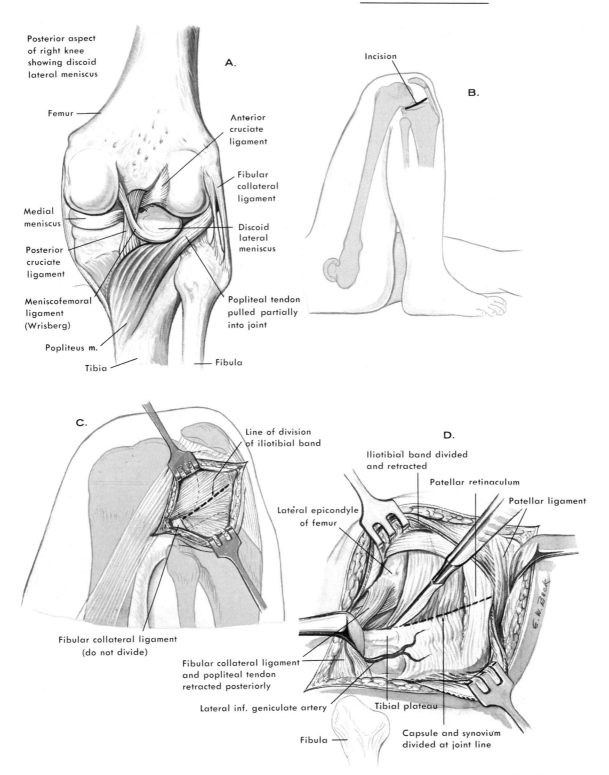

A. Posterior aspect of right knee showing discoid lateral meniscus

Femur

Anterior cruciate ligament

Fibular collateral ligament

Medial meniscus

Discoid lateral meniscus

Posterior cruciate ligament

Meniscofemoral ligament (Wrisberg)

Popliteal tendon pulled partially into joint

Popliteus m.

Tibia

Fibula

B. Incision

C. Line of division of iliotibial band

Fibular collateral ligament (do not divide)

D. Iliotibial band divided and retracted

Patellar retinaculum

Patellar ligament

Lateral epicondyle of femur

Fibular collateral ligament and popliteal tendon retracted posteriorly

Lateral inf. geniculate artery

Tibial plateau

Fibula

Capsule and synovium divided at joint line

Plate 147. A.–M., Excision of the discoid lateral meniscus—total excision by the direct lateral approach and partial excision through the anterolateral approach.

E.–H. Certain anatomic details should be considered next. The normal lateral meniscus is attached on the superior articular surface of the tibia at two sites, on the anterior and posterior aspects of the lateral intercondylar tubercle. Also, the ligament of Wrisberg or the meniscofemoral ligament connects the posterior horn of the lateral meniscus to the lateral surface of the medial femoral condyle, traversing obliquely behind the posterior cruciate ligament. (Humphry's ligament is the anterior branch of Wrisberg's ligament, and it runs in front of the anterior surface of the posterior cruciate ligament.)

When the knee is flexed, Wrisberg's ligament is relaxed, whereas the posterior cruciate ligament is relaxed during flexion and extension and runs almost vertically along the posterior midline. According to Kaplan, the discoid lateral meniscus does not have a posterior tibial attachment and is connected to the medial femoral condyle by the meniscofemoral ligament. When the knee is in extension, the discoid lateral meniscus is displaced posteromedially in the intercondylar area; in flexion it returns to its usual position. The popliteus tendon is attached anterior to the origin of the lateral ligament.

It is also important to remember that the popliteal artery is located 1 cm. posterior to the ligament of Wrisberg and that the lateral inferior genicular artery passes outside the synovium between the fibular collateral ligament and the posterolateral aspect of the meniscus. Injury to these vessels must be avoided. If the genicular vessels are divided inadvertently, they must be ligated to prevent hemarthrosis.

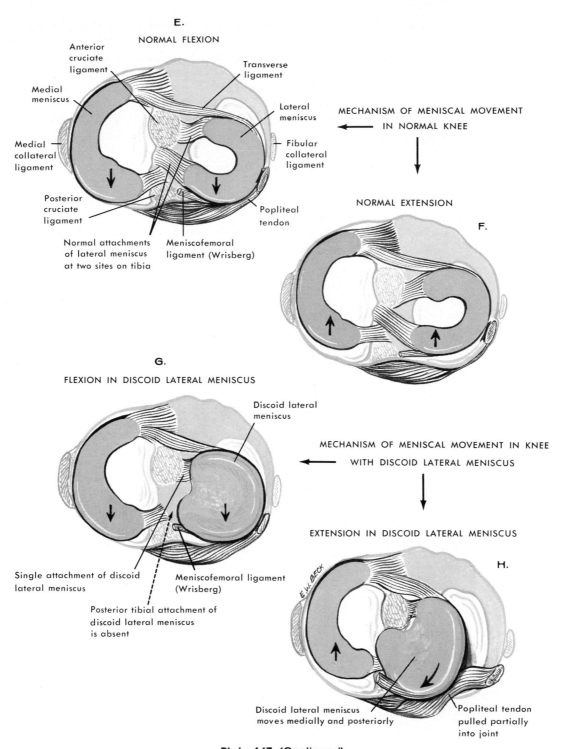

E.

NORMAL FLEXION

Anterior cruciate ligament

Transverse ligament

Medial meniscus

Lateral meniscus

Medial collateral ligament

Fibular collateral ligament

Posterior cruciate ligament

Popliteal tendon

Normal attachments of lateral meniscus at two sites on tibia

Meniscofemoral ligament (Wrisberg)

MECHANISM OF MENISCAL MOVEMENT IN NORMAL KNEE

NORMAL EXTENSION

F.

G.

FLEXION IN DISCOID LATERAL MENISCUS

Discoid lateral meniscus

MECHANISM OF MENISCAL MOVEMENT IN KNEE WITH DISCOID LATERAL MENISCUS

EXTENSION IN DISCOID LATERAL MENISCUS

H.

Single attachment of discoid lateral meniscus

Meniscofemoral ligament (Wrisberg)

Posterior tibial attachment of discoid lateral meniscus is absent

Discoid lateral meniscus moves medially and posteriorly

Popliteal tendon pulled partially into joint

E. W. BECK

Plate 147. (Continued)

I. and **J.** By sharp dissection the lateral meniscus is freed from its anterior, medial, and peripheral attachments. Forcibly bending the knee inward aids in visualization of the central portion of the joint. Posteriorly, the meniscus is freed by division of Wrisberg's ligament. After removal of the cartilage the lateral compartment of the joint is thoroughly inspected with the knee in flexion and extension; namely, the anterior and posterior cruciate ligaments, the popliteus tendon, the lateral femoral and tibial condyles, the lateral collateral ligament, and the lateral half of the articular surface of the patella. The tourniquet is released and complete hemostasis is obtained.

With the knee in 90 degrees of flexion the synovial membrane is closed with continuous plain catgut suture.

K. The knee is then extended, and the fascia is closed with interrupted sutures. The subcutaneous tissue and skin are closed in the usual manner. A compression dressing is applied. Protection of the joint with a posterior plaster of Paris cast or a light cylinder cast is not necessary, as the lateral collateral ligament is not divided.

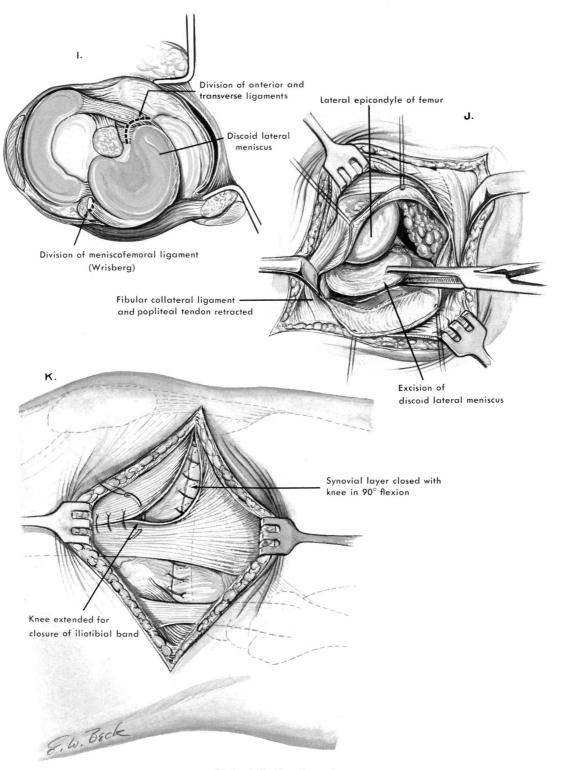

I.

Division of anterior and transverse ligaments

Discoid lateral meniscus

Division of meniscofemoral ligament (Wrisberg)

Fibular collateral ligament and popliteal tendon retracted

Lateral epicondyle of femur

J.

Excision of discoid lateral meniscus

K.

Synovial layer closed with knee in 90° flexion

Knee extended for closure of iliotibial band

Plate 147. (Continued)

Partial Excision. An open arthrotomy of the knee is performed through an antero-lateral approach with the knee flexed. The procedure can also be carried out through an arthroscope.

L. The femoral surface of the discoid meniscus is inspected. Determine the sagittal line of irregularity by fingertip palpation from the periphery toward the center. With a sharp scalpel excise the central-medial irregular part of the meniscus, leaving its anterior and posterior attachments intact.

M. Pull the anterior incised part toward the intercondylar fossa and with the help of a knife and scissors, the central and posterior parts of the meniscus are excised.

The incised part of the discoid meniscus is circular in outline. The meniscus is converted from discoid to a semilunar shape.

Next, carefully inspect the remaining lateral meniscus that is left behind. The meniscus left behind should not be loose, torn, or degenerated and its posterior horn should be intact.

The wound is closed in the usual fashion.

Postoperative Care. A compression dressing is applied. Protection of the joint with a posterior plaster of Paris or a light cylinder cast is not necessary, as the lateral collateral ligament is not divided.

On the day of surgery, isometric quadriceps and hamstring exercises and straight leg raising are performed. For several days after surgery the patient is allowed partial weight-bearing with crutches, and activities are gradually increased as they are tolerated.

Within seven to ten days (as soon as the soft tissues have healed) the knee is gently mobilized by side-lying flexion and extension exercises to redevelop muscle strength in the quadriceps, hamstrings, and triceps surae. These exercises are continued until normal motor power and full range of knee motion are obtained.

REFERENCE

Bruser, D. M.: A direct lateral approach to the lateral compartment of the knee joint. J. Bone Joint Surg., 42-B:348, 1960.

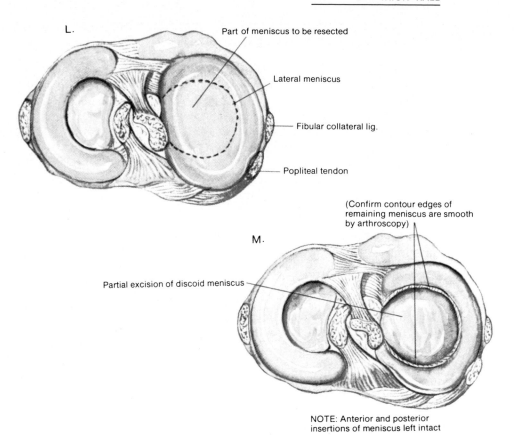

L.

Part of meniscus to be resected

Lateral meniscus

Fibular collateral lig.

Popliteal tendon

(Confirm contour edges of
remaining meniscus are smooth
by arthroscopy)

M.

Partial excision of discoid meniscus

NOTE: Anterior and posterior
insertions of meniscus left intact

Plate 147. (Continued)

PLATE 148 **Excision of a Popliteal Cyst**

Indications. Initially, popliteal cysts in children should be observed because most of them will regress and spontaneously disappear during a period of one-and-one-half to two years.

Surgical excision is indicated if, after a period of two to three years of observation, the cyst does not regress but instead remains large or increases in size and causes disabling symptoms.

Caution! Assess the popliteal mass by ultrasonography. The fluid-filled popliteal cyst depicts as an echo-free space. Magnetic resonance imaging is occasionally performed when definitive diagnosis is doubtful or when associated intra-articular pathology is suspected.

Patient Positioning. The patient should preferably be in prone position with a pneumatic tourniquet placed on the proximal thigh.

Operative Technique

A. The skin incision is oblique and centered directly over the swelling; it should *not* cross the popliteal crease.

The anatomic relationship of vessels and nerves in the popliteal areas is shown in this cross section of the knee.

B. Subcutaneous tissue and deep fascia are divided and the protruding mass is exposed. Every effort should be made not to rupture the cyst, as this will make it difficult to determine its outline and to dissect it to its pedicle or its point of contact with the joint. Excision of the sac should be complete to prevent recurrence. The knee is flexed, relaxing the hamstrings and both heads of the gastrocnemius.

The proper plane of dissection depends upon the site of the cyst. If it is located between the semimembranosus and the medial head of the gastrocnemius, the interval between the muscles is exposed by appropriate retraction. In this plane, neuromuscular structures should be avoided.

C. and **D.** With scissors and sharp knife dissection, the cyst is separated and traced to its base, which may be attached to the capsule synovium. The entire cyst is removed by division of the pedicle at its base.

E. Tight closure of any opening in the capsule is unnecessary, although, if possible, it is carried out. The wound is closed in layers.

Postoperative Care. A compression dressing is applied and the child is allowed to be ambulatory as soon as possible.

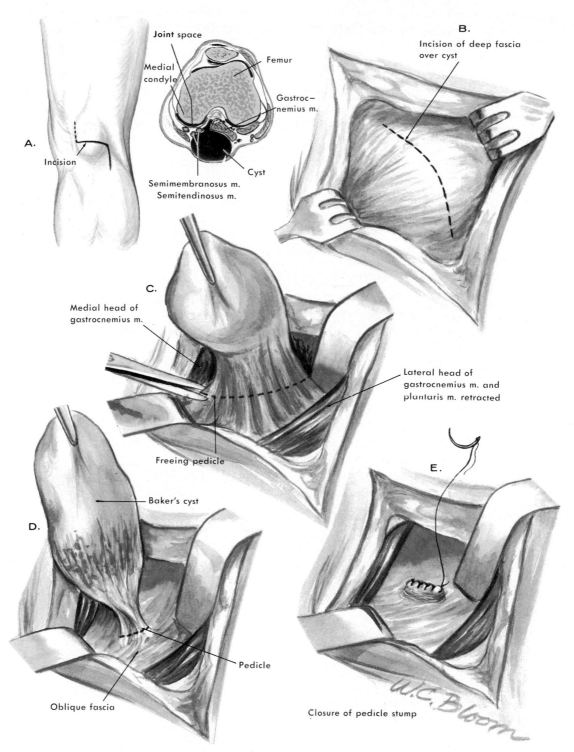

A.

Incision

Joint space

Medial condyle

Femur

Gastroc–nemius m.

Cyst

Semimembranosus m.
Semitendinosus m.

B.

Incision of deep fascia over cyst

C.

Medial head of gastrocnemius m.

Lateral head of gastrocnemius m. and plantaris m. retracted

Freeing pedicle

D.

Baker's cyst

Pedicle

Oblique fascia

E.

Closure of pedicle stump

W.C.Bloom

Plate 148. **A.–E.,** Excision of a popliteal cyst.

PLATE 149   Transphyseal Osteotomy for Elevation of the Medial Tibial Plateau

Indications. Neglected cases of tibia vara in the adolescent with marked ligamentous laxity of the knee and depression of the anteromedial part of the tibial plateau and hypermobility of the medial meniscus.

Note: Document pathologic condition by arthroscopy of the knee and magnetic resonance imaging.

Objective. To provide joint congruity and ligamentous stability of the knee and to prevent degenerative arthritis later in life.

Radiographic Control. Image intensifier.

Blood for Transfusion. Yes.

Patient Position. Supine with a pneumatic tourniquet on the proximal thigh.

Operative Technique

A. Make a 6- to 7-cm. incision on the anteromedial aspect of the upper tibia beginning 2 cm. above the joint line immediately medial to the patellar tendon and extending distally and somewhat posteriorly toward the medial cortex of the tibia.

B. The incision is carried through the subcutaneous tissue and deep fascia; avoid injury to the infrapatellar branch of the saphenous nerve. Incise the periosteum.

C. The medial collateral ligament and pes anserinus are elevated subperiosteally and reflected posteriorly, exposing the medial condyle and metaphyseal region of the anteromedial upper tibia. Next, the capsule is incised and the joint cavity is exposed and inspected.

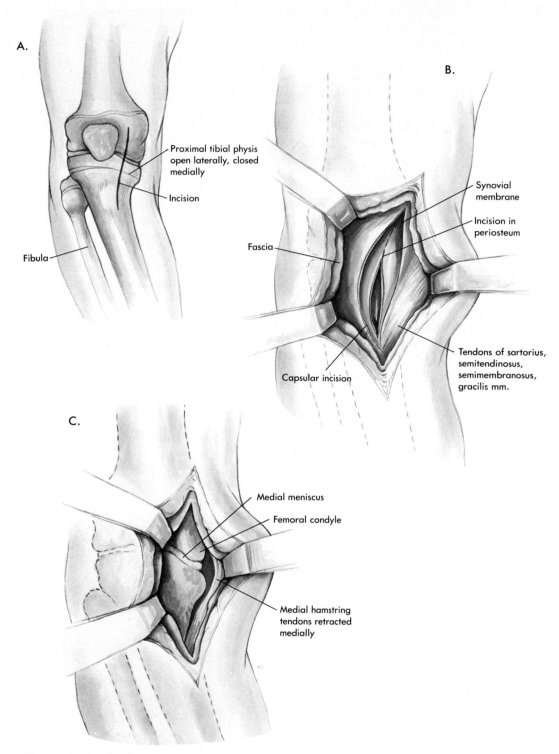

A.

Proximal tibial physis
open laterally, closed
medially

Incision

Fibula

B.

Synovial
membrane

Incision in
periosteum

Fascia

Tendons of sartorius,
semitendinosus,
semimembranosus,
gracilis mm.

Capsular incision

C.

Medial meniscus

Femoral condyle

Medial hamstring
tendons retracted
medially

Plate 149. A.–G., Transphyseal osteotomy for elevation of the medial tibial plateau.

D. With a straight-blade power saw, the anteromedial part of the medial condyle of the tibia is divided under direct vision. The osteotomy extends from immediately distal to the beak of the metaphysis, across the closed tibial physis, stopping just short of the subarticular bony plate of the intercondylar eminence.

E. Then, with wide osteotomes and periosteal elevators, the depressed medial tibial plateau is gently elevated. Observe the joint surface, and do not cause an intra-articular fracture.

F. Next, three or four triangular wedges of autogenous double-cortical iliac bone grafts taken from the innominate bone in the usual fashion, are firmly inserted into the resulting gap.

G. The elevated medial condyle of the tibia is secured in place by internal fixation with two cancellous screws or threaded Steinmann pins.

Anteroposterior, oblique, and lateral radiograms of the upper tibia, including the knee joint, are made to determine adequacy of correction. The medial collateral ligament and pes anserinus are sutured in place. It is vital that the medial collateral ligament be reattached very tautly.

The periosteum and wound are closed in the usual fashion, and an above-knee cast is applied with the knee in complete extension and the foot and ankle in neutral position.

Postoperative Care. The patient is allowed to ambulate with three-point crutch gait and partial weight-bearing. If threaded Steinmann pins are used for internal fixation, they are removed after four weeks; however, if cancellous screws are used, they are not removed until three or four months after surgery.

REFERENCES

Langenskiöld, A: Tibia vara. Osteochondrosis deformans tibiae. A survey of 23 cases. Acta Chir. Scand., 103:1, 1952.

Langenskiöld, A.: Tibia vara: Osteochondrosis deformans tibiae. Blount's disease. Clin. Orthop., 158:77, 1981.

Langenskiöld, A., and Riska, E. B.: Tibia vara (osteochondrosis deformans tibiae). J. Bone Joint Surg., 46-A:1405, 1964.

Sasaki, T., Yagi, T., Monji, J., Yasuda, K., and Kanno, Y.: Transepiphyseal plate osteotomy for severe tibia vara in children: Follow-up study of four cases. J. Pediatr. Orthop., 6:61, 1986.

Siffert, R. S.: Intraepiphyseal osteotomy for progressive tibia vara: Case report and rationale of management. J. Pediatr. Orthop., 2:81, 1982.

Støren, H.: Operative elevation of the medial tibial joint surface in Blount's disease. One case observed for 18 years after operation. Acta Orthop. Scand., 40:788, 1970.

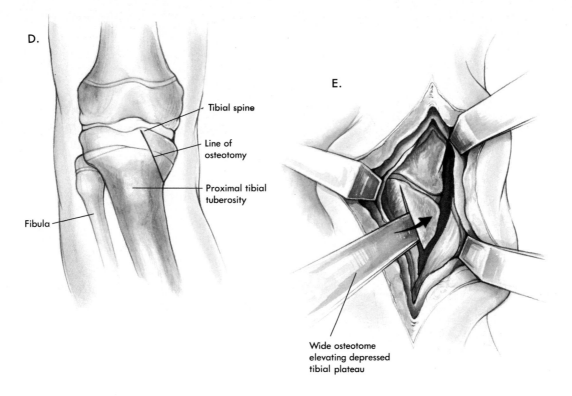

D.

Tibial spine

Line of
osteotomy

Proximal tibial
tuberosity

Fibula

E.

Wide osteotome
elevating depressed
tibial plateau

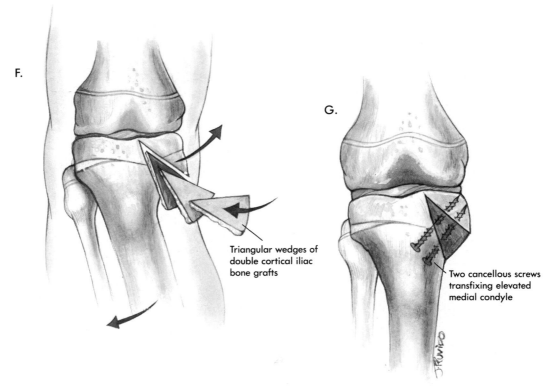

F.

Triangular wedges of
double cortical iliac
bone grafts

G.

Two cancellous screws
transfixing elevated
medial condyle

Plate 149. (Continued)

Index

Note: Page numbers in *italics* refer to illustrations; page numbers in **boldface** refer to surgical plates. Roman numerals refer to the principles of practice preceding Chapter 1.

I

ISBN 0-7216-5448-7

9 780721 654485

90038